ATLAS OF
Spine
Imaging

Donald L. Renfrew, MD
Center for Diagnostic Imaging

ATLAS OF
Spine
Imaging

SAUNDERS
An Imprint of Elsevier Science
Philadelphia   London   New York   St. Louis   Sydney   Toronto

SAUNDERS
An Imprint of Elsevier Science

The Curtis Center
Independence Square West
Philadelphia, Pennsylvania 19106

ATLAS OF SPINE IMAGING   ISBN 0–7216–9071–8

Notice

Medicine is an ever-changing field. Standard safety precautions must be followed, but as new research and
clinical experience broaden our knowledge, changes in treatment and drug therapy may become necessary
or appropriate. Readers are advised to check the most current product information provided by the
manufacturer of each drug to be administered to verify the recommended dose, the method and duration
of administration, and the contraindications. It is the responsibility of the treating physician, relying on
experience and knowledge of the patient, to determine the dosage and the best treatment for each
individual patient. Neither the publisher nor the editor assumes any liability for any injury and/or damage
to persons or property arising from this publication.

The Publisher

Library of Congress Cataloging-in-Publication Data

Renfrew, Donald L.
Atlas of spine imaging/Donald L. Renfrew.
    p.; cm.
        ISBN 0–7216–9071–8
    1. Spine–Imaging–Atlases. 2. Diagnostic imaging – Atlases. I. Title.
        [DNLM: 1. Spinal Diseases – diagnosis–Atlases. 2. Diagnostic Imaging – Atlases.
    WE 17 R411a 2003]
    RD768.R43 2003
617.5′60754–dc21   2002021192

Editor-in-Chief: Richard Lampert
Acquisitions Editor: Stephanie Donley
Project Manager: Mary Anne Folcher
Book Designer: Karen O'Keefe Owens

EH/MVY

Printed in the United States of America

Last digit is the print number: 9 8 7 6 5 4 3 2 1

To my wife, Susan

Contents

Contributors

Peter Bove, MD
Center for Diagnostic Imaging
Winter Park, Florida
> *Miscellaneous Diseases of the Spine*

Michael W. Hayt, MD
Center for Diagnostic Imaging
Winter Park, Florida
> *Congenital and Developmental Anomalies*
> *Imaging of Spine Tumors*

Kenneth B. Heithoff, MD
Medical Director and Chairman
Center for Diagnostic Imaging
St. Louis Park, Minnesota
> *Degenerative Disease*
> *Imaging of the Postoperative Spine*

Michael MacMillan, MD
Jewett Orthopedic Center
Winter Park, Florida
> *Imaging of the Postoperative Spine*

Donald L. Renfrew, MD
Center for Diagnostic Imaging
Winter Park, Florida
> *Anatomy*
> *Degenerative Disease*
> *Imaging of the Postoperative Spine*
> *Imaging of Spine Tumors*
> *Imaging of Trauma*
> *Infectious Spondylitis*
> *Congenital and Developmental Anomalies*
> *Spondylolysis*
> *Miscellaneous Diseases of the Spine*

Sanjay Saluja, MD
Assistant Professor, Radiology
Yale University School of Medicine
New Haven, Connecticut
Staff Radiologist
Veterans Administration Healthcare Systems
West Haven, Connecticut
> *Imaging of Spine Tumors*
> *Imaging of Trauma*
> *Congenital and Developmental Anomalies*

Preface

I have had a career-long interest in the spine and back pain. For the past few years, I've had the good fortune to be able to dedicate almost all of my professional time to imaging and to diagnostic and therapeutic injection of the spine. When I first began to perform predominantly spine radiology, I reviewed the available texts. For me, these texts lacked the appropriate focus. Although most imaging studies of the spine are obtained for evaluation of degenerative or postoperative conditions, the existing books seemed lacking in the treatment of these conditions. Furthermore, I found no single book that provided copious images obtained with current technology, concise descriptions of disease processes, and pragmatic approaches to interpretation. I decided to create such a textbook, and *Atlas of Spine Imaging* is the result of that effort.

I have included what I believe to be the most important points regarding the clinical aspects of spine imaging, based on multiple conferences and conversations with orthopedic spine surgeons and neurosurgeons and on review of journals such as *Spine* and *The Spine Journal*. In many cases, this approach results in categorizing patients into a particular "clinical scenario." The imaging workup, diagnostic possibilities, and importance of imaging findings may vary considerably from one clinical scenario to the next. In many cases, I have provided algorithms for clinical scenarios. Algorithms help make explicit a decision process, which may otherwise be difficult to understand or use.

A disease may manifest as one or several imaging findings. Imaging findings are often nonspecific, however, and may be the result of any one of several diseases. I have attempted to provide not only illustrations and descriptions of the imaging findings of several diseases, but also lists of diseases that may cause each finding. I also provide methods (clinical and imaging) to help sort out which disease is responsible for a particular imaging finding.

In addition to my interest in the spine and back pain, I also have an interest in reporting. For many imaging studies, the radiologist's main input into the clinical care of the patient takes the form of a radiology report. Agreed upon terminology facilitates construction of these reports. A combined task force of the North American Spine Society and the American Society of Neuroradiology has now developed a *Nomenclature and Classification of Disc Pathology*, which establishes a uniform lexicon for disc disease. I have incorporated this lexicon into Chapter 2, along with several examples. I advise what to include in radiology reports concerning other disease processes, based on my experience with referring clinicians and radiologists.

The process of collecting appropriate cases, reviewing the literature, formulating algorithms, and describing an approach to the various diseases that may be encountered in spine imaging took far more effort and time than I anticipated. The process was more illuminating and enjoyable than expected, and I hope that readers of *Atlas of Spine Imaging* share that experience when they read the book.

Donald L. Renfrew, MD

Acknowledgements

Many individuals contributed to the completion of this textbook. I would like to thank my mentor and friend Dr. Georges El-Khoury at the University of Iowa for his tireless commitment to superior radiology, patient care, and academic tradition. His enthusiasm for musculoskeletal radiology and his thoughtfulness have always served as a model that I strive to emulate.

I also thank Drs. William Mullin and Thomas Gilbert, who provided valuable training and insight into the imaging of the spine. I further wish to thank my co-authors, Drs. Kenneth Heithoff, Michael Hayt, Peter Bove, Sanjay Saluja, and Michael MacMillan. Their contributions to the text were numerous and valued.

In addition, I would like to thank the Center for Diagnostic Imaging (CDI). CDI is, on one hand, a corporation that owns and manages the facilities that allow me a unique radiology practice, and, on the other hand, a collection of exceptional and talented individuals. Technologists who were particularly helpful in the completion of this project included Shannon Risdon, Pamela Wagner, Merle Baylor, Gina Talantis, Teri Yost, and Charmaine Barclay.

My understanding of spine imaging would not be the same without the input of orthopedic spine surgeons. Drs. Mark Beckner, Reginald Tall, Michael MacMillan, and Gregory Munson from the Jewett Orthopedic Center; Drs. Joseph Flynn, Jr., and Geoffrey Stewart from The Spine and Scoliosis Center; Dr. Richard Smith from the Florida Center for Orthopedics; Dr. Stephane Lavoie from Florida Orthopedic Associates; and Drs. Stephen Goll, Grady McBride, and Steven Weber of Orlando Orthopedics Center have all been kind enough to share their knowledge and insight regarding care of spine patients.

Administrative assistants Laura Quist and Deena Foust did valuable work collating references, checking figures, and proofing text.

Stephanie Donley and Mary Anne Folcher at Elsevier Science provided encouragement and guidance at crucial times throughout the publication process.

Finally, I would like to thank my wife Susan for all her support during the work I did on *Atlas of Spine Imaging*.

Donald L. Renfrew, MD

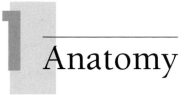

Anatomy

DONALD L. RENFREW

The spine is a complex, multisegmental structure consisting of 33 bones with dozens of joints and hundreds of ligamentous and muscular attachments. The cervical spine articulates superiorly with the skull, the thoracic spine articulates with the 12 ribs, and the sacral spine articulates inferiorly with the pelvis. The cervical spine demonstrates a lordotic (concave posterior) curve, the thoracic spine a kyphotic (concave anterior) curve, the lumbar spine a second lordotic curve, and the inferior sacrum and coccyx a second kyphotic curve. Vertebrae are numbered from superior to inferior, with C1 through C7 composing the cervical spine, T1 through T12 the thoracic spine, L1 through L5 the lumbar spine, S1 through S5 the sacral spine, and Co1 through Co4 the coccyx. From C3 through L5, each level consists of an anterior vertebral body and a posterior neural arch that, together, surround the spinal canal. The posterior neural arch is composed of paired pedicles, superior and inferior articular processes connected by pars interarticularia, transverse processes, laminae, and spinous processes. The spinal canal has a layered construction, with the spinal cord and nerve roots located centrally and covered in a thin layer of pia mater surrounded by cerebrospinal fluid (CSF) and housed in a lining of arachnoid mater and adjacent dura mater. A peridural membrane, external to the dura mater, forms the inner surface of the spinal canal. The subarachnoid space lies between the arachnoid and pia mater, the subdural space lies between the dura and arachnoid, and the epidural space lies between the peridural membrane and the dura. The vertebral bodies are separated by intervertebral discs, which are concentric structures with a central, gelatinous nucleus pulposus surrounded by the concentric lamellae of the annulus fibrosus. The superior and inferior articular processes meet at the facet or zygapophyseal joints. Major ligamentous structures include the anterior longitudinal ligament running along the anterior aspect of the vertebral bodies, the posterior longitudinal ligament running along the posterior aspect of the vertebral bodies, the ligamentum flavum (or yellow ligament) that runs between adjacent laminae, the interspinous ligament that runs between adjacent spinous processes, and the supraspinous ligament that connects the tips of the spinous processes.

The following images offer a concise review of anatomy pertinent to interpretation of spine imaging. The emphasis is on those structures likely to be involved by disease processes or to present a potentially confusing appearance. Nomenclature has been adopted from thelexicon developed by the North American Spine Society and the American Society of Spine Radiology (www.asnr.org/spine_nomenclature).

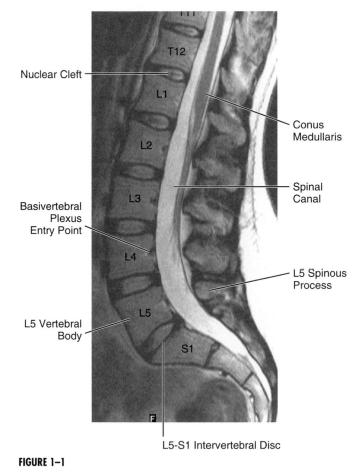

FIGURE 1–1
Lumbar spine. Sagittal T2WI.

Lumbar Spine [ED2]
SAGITTAL IMAGES

Sagittal T2-Weighted Image (T2WI) (Fig. 1–1)

1. The intervertebral disc height is usually greatest at L4–5. The L5–S1 disc height may be equal to or slightly less than the L4–5 disc height, and disc height usually gradually decreases from L3–4 through the thoracolumbar junction.
2. Intervertebral disc signal intensity is greater at its central aspect, which includes the nucleus pulposus and the inner portion of the annulus fibrosus.
3. A "nuclear cleft" may be seen within the intervertebral disc as a normal structure.
4. The conus (inferior terminus of the spinal cord) is mildly bulbous and ends at or above L2 is almost all normal people.
5. The entrance points of the basivertebral plexus veins along the dorsal aspect of the vertebral bodies are seen as foci of decreased signal intensity.

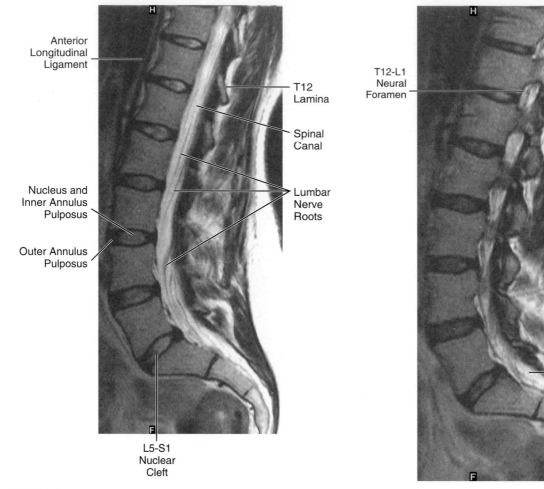

FIGURE 1–2
Lumbar spine. Right parasagittal T2WI, just to the right of Figure 1–1.

FIGURE 1–3
Lumbar spine. Right parasagittal T2WI, just to the right of Figure 1–2.

Right Parasagittal T2WI (Fig. 1–2)

1. On this image, which is slightly to the right of Figure 1–1, the laminae of the upper vertebrae are visible.
2. The anterior longitudinal ligament is seen as a stripe of decreased signal intensity along the anterior aspect of the vertebral bodies.
3. The lumbar nerve roots course obliquely through the lumbar thecal sac and are evenly distributed.
4. The "nuclear cleft" at L5–S1 is better seen on this image than on the midline study.
5. The basivertebral plexus entrance points are not seen on this parasagittal study.
6. The posterior margin of the intervertebral disc is usually at or only slightly posterior to a line connecting the posterior aspects of the vertebral bodies superior and inferior to the level of the disc. The posterior disc margins of the lower lumbar spine may normally extend slightly beyond the vertebral body margins.

Right Parasagittal T2WI (Fig. 1–3)

1. On this parasagittal image, just to the right of Figure 1–2, the pedicles of the upper lumbar spine and the laminae of the lower lumbar spine are in the plane. This is secondary to the increase of interpedicular distance from the superior to the inferior lumbar spine.
2. On parasagittal images, the more peripheral (lateral) aspect of the intervertebral discs is visualized, with lower signal intensity more typical of annulus fibrosus.
3. The spinal canal tapers laterally, with diminished anteroposterior dimension (compare the lower spinal canal in this image with the lower spinal canal in Fig. 1–1).

Right Parasagittal T2WI (Fig. 1–4)

1. On this parasagittal image, just to the right of Figure 1–3, the lower lumbar spine pedicles are in the plane of section, whereas the transverse processes are in plane in the upper lumbar and thoracic spine.
2. At each level, the nerve root ganglion resides in the superior aspect of the neural foramen (or intervertebral nerve root canal), exiting below the pedicle of the same

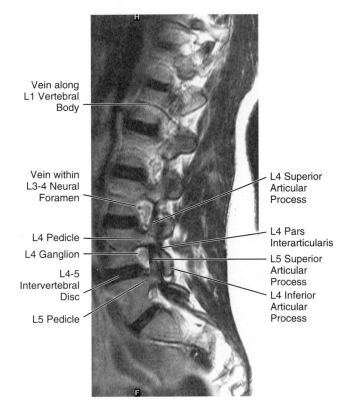

FIGURE 1–4
Lumbar spine. Right parasagittal T2WI, just to the right of Figure 1–3.

number (e.g., the L4 ganglion exits beneath the L4 pedicle). The inferior margin of the L4 pedicle defines the superior border of the L4–5 neural foramen, whereas the superior margin of the L5 pedicle defines the inferior border of this neural foramen. The posterior intervertebral disc margin forms the anterior border of the lower neural foramen, whereas the posterior aspect of the vertebral body forms the more superior border. The disc margin is thus normally below the exiting ganglion at the level of the foramen. The superior articular process of the subjacent vertebra forms the posterior margin of the neural foramen.
3. Small vessels also occupy the neural foramina.
4. The pars interarticularis connects the superior and inferior articular processes and should demonstrate intact marrow on at least one image.
5. A rich plexus of veins runs along the mid-vertebral bodies at their lateral margins.

AXIAL IMAGES

Axial T2WI Through the S1 Pedicles (Fig. 1–5)

1. The ventral rami of the L5 nerves lie on the ventral aspect of the sacrum.
2. The S1 nerve root sheaths are posterior to the S1 pedicles.
3. Epidural fat surrounds the S2 and S3 nerve root sheaths.

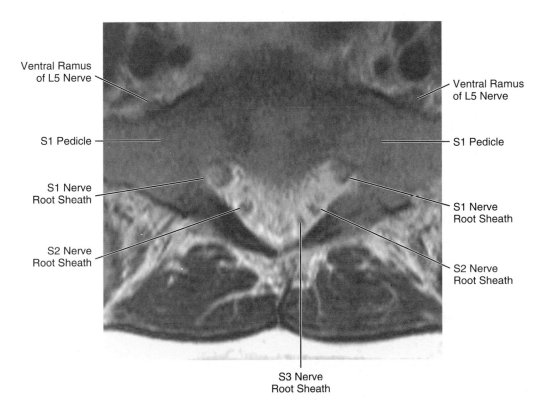

FIGURE 1–5
Lumbar spine. Axial T2WI through the S1 pedicles.

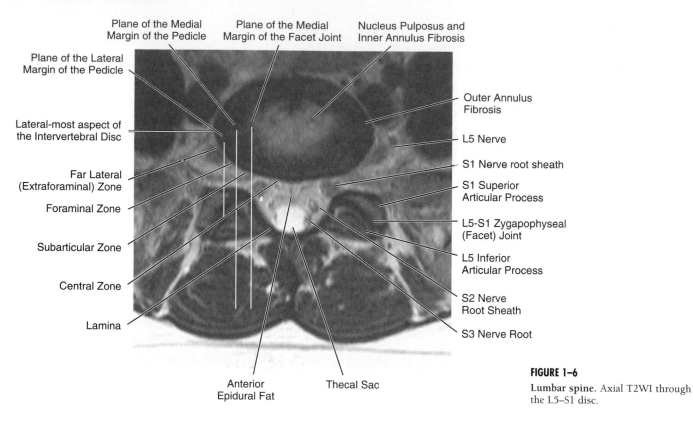

FIGURE 1–6

Lumbar spine. Axial T2WI through the L5–S1 disc.

Axial T2WI Through the L5-S1 Disc (Fig. 1–6)

1. The nucleus fibrosus and inner annulus fibrosis demonstrate T2 prolongation relative to the outer annulus and muscular tissue.

2. The disc margin is divided into several zones. The (single) *central zone* is that portion of the dorsal disc margin between two parasagittal planes along the medial margins of the facet joints. The (paired left and right) *subarticular zone* is that portion of the dorsal disc margin

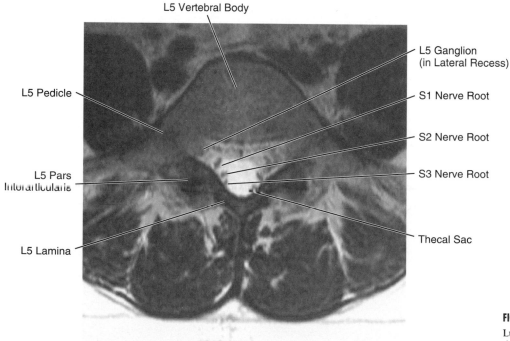

FIGURE 1–7

Lumbar spine. Axial T2WI through the L5 transverse process.

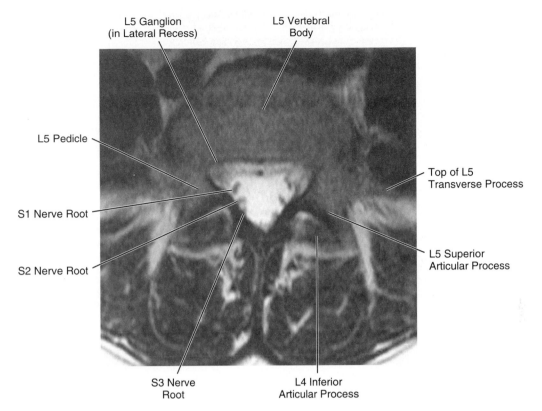

L5 Ganglion
(in Lateral Recess)

L5 Vertebral
Body

L5 Pedicle

Top of L5
Transverse Process

S1 Nerve Root

S2 Nerve Root

L5 Superior
Articular Process

S3 Nerve
Root

L4 Inferior
Articular Process

FIGURE 1–8

Lumbar spine. Axial T2WI through the L5 pedicles.

between the plane along the medial facet joint margin and a parasagittal plane through the medial aspect of the pedicle. The (paired left and right) *foraminal zone* is that portion of the dorsal disc margin between the parasagittal plane through the medial margin of the pedicle and the lateral margin of the pedicle. The (paired left and right) *extraforaminal zone* is that portion of the disc margin between the lateral aspect of the pedicle and the lateral-most portion of the disc margin. The anterior zone is along the anterior 180 degrees of the disc margin, anterior to the lateral-most aspects of the disc. The parasagittal planes through the pedicles need to be projected to the level of the disc from adjacent axial cuts or on sagittal examinations, since the pedicles are not in the same axial plane as the disc.

3. At the level of the disc, the foraminal zone of the disc constitutes the anterior border of the neural foramen. Above the level of the disc, the posterolateral aspect of the vertebral body constitutes the anterior border of the neural foramen. The posterior border is formed by the superior articular process of the vertebra below the disc.

4. The superior articular process lies anterior to the inferior articular process and articulates with the inferior articular process at the zygapophyseal or facet joint. These joints are normally symmetric and oblique. The facet joint capsule may extend well into the foramen along the anterior aspect of the superior articular process.

5. At this level on this individual, there is abundant epidural fat separating the dorsal disc margin from the ventral aspect of the thecal sac.

Axial T2WI Through the L5 Transverse Process (Fig. 1–7)

1. The inferior aspect of the pedicle, the transverse process, and the pars interarticularis lie in the same axial plane. The pars interarticularis may blend into the superior aspect of the facet joint below and the inferior aspect of the facet joint above (as at this level on the right side).

2. The L5 nerve root and proximal ganglion lie along the medial aspect of the L5 pedicle in the lateral recess.

3. The S1, S2, and S3 nerve roots are typically evenly and symmetrically located within the thecal sac.

Axial T2WI Through the L5 Pedicles (Fig. 1–8)

1. At the mid-pedicle level, the lateral recess is better defined than it is through the lower pedicle (Fig. 1–7). The L5 nerve roots are seen branching off the thecal sac in the nerve root sleeves (extensions of the dura that extend along the nerve roots and surround the ganglia).

2. The inferior articular processes from the L4 level project behind the superior articular processes from the L5 level.

3. The sacral nerve roots are evenly and symmetrically distributed within the thecal sac.

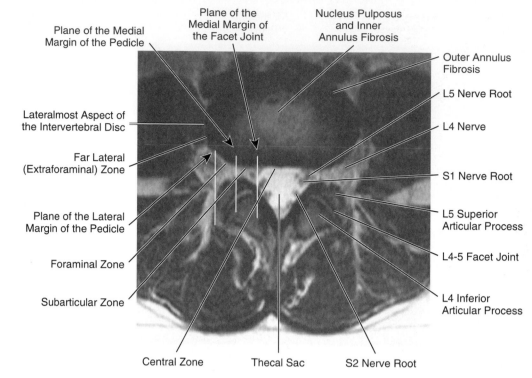

FIGURE 1–9

Lumbar spine. Axial T2WI through the L4–5 disc.

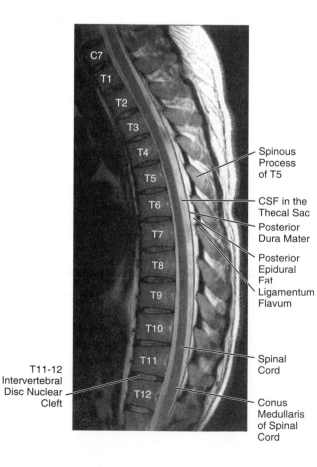

FIGURE 1–10

Thoracic spine. Sagittal T2WI.

Axial T2WI Through the L4-5 Disc (Fig. 1–9)

1. Features are similar to the L5–S1 intervertebral disc, with the following pertinent differences:
   a. There is no anterior epidural fat separating the ventral thecal sac from the dorsal disc margin.
   b. The dorsal disc margin is straight to slightly concave, whereas the dorsal disc margin at L5–S1 is convex.
   c. The facet joints are in a slightly more oblique plane at this level.

Thoracic Spine

Sagittal T2WI (Fig. 1–10)

1. Definite numbering in the thoracic spine relies on obtaining a scout view that includes the cervical region (not shown here).
2. The thoracic spine has a natural kyphotic (concave anterior) curve.
3. The thoracic spinal cord demonstrates slight fusiform expansion distally at the level of the conus medullaris.

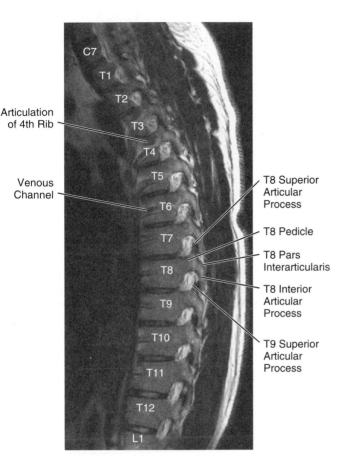

Articulation of 4th Rib

Venous Channel

C7
T1
T2
T3
T4
T5
T6
T7
T8
T9
T10
T11
T12
L1

T8 Superior Articular Process

T8 Pedicle

T8 Pars Interarticularis

T8 Interior Articular Process

T9 Superior Articular Process

FIGURE 1–11
Thoracic spine. Parasagittal T2WI.

Cervical Spine

Sagittal T2WI (Fig. 1–12)

1. On this somewhat oblique image, the upper cervical cord is imaged, but the more lateral aspect of the lower cervical spinal canal is seen with the neural foramina visible at T3–4 and T4–5.
2. A number of brain structures are visible at the superior margin of the examination. The cerebellar tonsils should end above the level of the foramen magnum.
3. The C1 and C2 vertebrae have unique features. The C1 vertebra has no body, but rather an anterior and posterior arch connecting two lateral masses. The C2 vertebral body extends upward at the dens, posterior to the anterior arch of C1. There may be (as in this case) a vestigial disc at the base of the dens.

4. The thoracic cord is typically directly applied to the posterior vertebral body and disc margin through the upper thoracic spine but is separated from these structures by CSF more inferiorly.
5. The intervertebral discs may show a greater proportion of T2 prolongation centrally than in the lumbar spine.
6. As in the lumbar spine, the central portion of the intervertebral discs may demonstrate a nuclear cleft.
7. The spinous processes through the lower thoracic spine demonstrate a relatively pronounced downward course.
8. CSF surrounds the spinal cord.
9. Fat separates the posterior aspect of the dura mater and the ligamentum flavum.

Parasagittal T2WI (Fig. 1–11)

1. The nerve root and ganglion occupy a much lesser percentage of the neural foramen within the thoracic spine than in the lumbar spine, and the disc margin forms a much smaller proportion of the anterior margin of the neural foramen.
2. A rich venous plexus with interconnecting channels runs along the lateral aspect of the vertebral bodies.
3. As in the lumbar spine, the superior articular process forms the posterior margin of the neural foramen and lies anterior the inferior articular process from the level above.
4. The ribs articulate with the transverse processes and also with the thoracic vertebra at the same level and at one level superior.

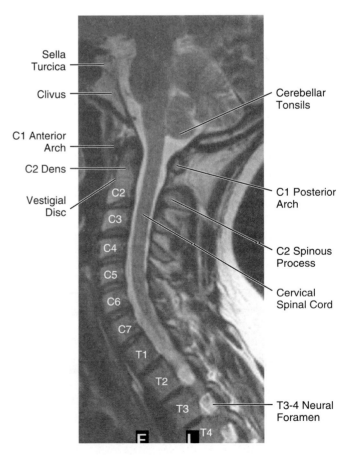

Sella Turcica

Clivus

C1 Anterior Arch

C2 Dens

Vestigial Disc

C2
C3
C4
C5
C6
C7
T1
T2
T3
T4

Cerebellar Tonsils

C1 Posterior Arch

C2 Spinous Process

Cervical Spinal Cord

T3-4 Neural Foramen

FIGURE 1–12
Cervical spine. Sagittal T2WI.

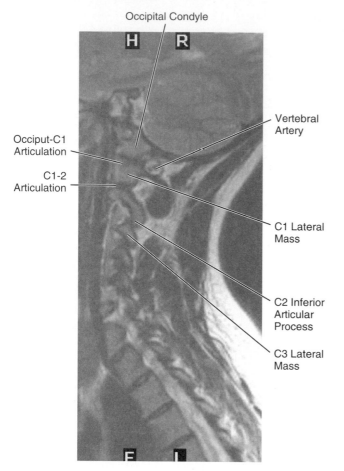

Occipital Condyle

Occiput-C1
Articulation

C1-2
Articulation

Vertebral
Artery

C1 Lateral
Mass

C2 Inferior
Articular
Process

C3 Lateral
Mass

FIGURE 1–13
Cervical spine. Parasagittal T2WI.

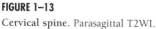

Parasagittal T2WI (Fig. 1–13)

1. The occipital condyle articulates with the superior margin of the lateral mass of C1.
2. The vertebral artery lies between the occiput and the posterior arch of C1 at the skull base.
3. The inferior aspect of the lateral mass at C1 articulates with C2.
4. C2–3 through C7–T1 have more typical spinal articulations, with the anterior aspect of the inferior articular process above articulating with the posterior aspect of the superior articular process from the level below.

Parasagittal T2WI (Fig. 1–14)

1. The C1 nerve exits the spinal canal above the C1 posterior arch. The spinal nerves at other levels in the cervical spine also exit over the pedicle of the same number (unlike in the thoracic and lumbar spine, where the nerves exit *under* the pedicle of the same number). The C7 nerve exits over the C7 pedicle, and the T1 nerve exits under the T1 pedicle; the nerve exiting over the T1 pedicle is called C8.
2. The lateral masses of the cervical spine articulate along superior and inferior margins and form the posterior

aspect of the neural foramina. The neural foramina in the cervical spine are at an oblique angle and not well visualized on sagittal images, unlike the foramina of the thoracic spine, which lie in a parasagittal plane and are relatively easily seen.

Axial T2WI (Fig. 1–15A) and Axial Gradient-Echo Image (Fig. 1–15B) at C4–5

1. The spinal cord occupies a relatively larger percentage of the overall cross-sectional area of the spinal canal than in the thoracic spine.
2. The T2WI and gradient-echo images are complementary for the following reasons:
   a. "Flow void" artifacts within the cerebrospinal fluid of the thecal sac on the T2WI may cause difficulty.
   b. "Bloom" artifacts on the gradient-echo images may cause the neural foramina to appear falsely narrowed.
   c. Soft tissue disc extrusions may appear to demonstrate T2 shortening on the T2WI but demonstrate T2 prolongation on gradient-echo images.

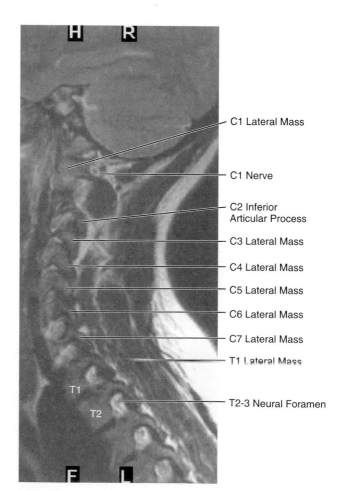

C1 Lateral Mass

C1 Nerve

C2 Inferior
Articular Process

C3 Lateral Mass

C4 Lateral Mass

C5 Lateral Mass

C6 Lateral Mass

C7 Lateral Mass

T1 Lateral Mass

T2-3 Neural Foramen

FIGURE 1–14
Cervical spine. Parasagittal T2WI.

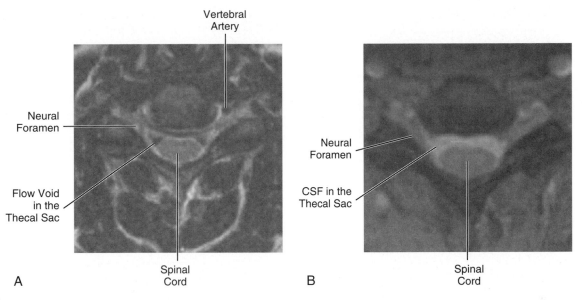

Vertebral
Artery

Neural
Foramen

Flow Void
in the
Thecal Sac

Spinal
Cord

A

Neural
Foramen

CSF in the
Thecal Sac

Spinal
Cord

B

FIGURE 1–15

Cervical spine. Axial T2WI (*A*) and axial gradient-echo image (*B*) at C4–5. CSF, cerebrospinal fluid.

3. Since the facet joints are more laterally located relative to the central spinal canal and pedicles than in the lumbar spine, there is no "subarticular zone." The disc may be divided into a central zone (between parasagittal planes along the medial aspect of the pedicles) and a foraminal zone (between parasagittal planes through the medial and lateral aspects of the pedicle. The interface between these two regions along the lateral aspect of the spinal canal may be called the *entrance zone of the neural foramen*.

4. The vertebral artery lies along the anterior aspect of the neural foramen.

2 Degenerative Disease

DONALD L. RENFREW • KENNETH B. HEITHOFF

Diagnosis and classification of degenerative disease forms the single most frequently performed task of the spine imager. This task often goes without the requisite attention to detail that enables the radiologist to be of maximum benefit to the referring clinician and patient. Many neuroradiologists regard degenerative processes of the spine as a nuisance. Musculoskeletal imagers may better understand degenerative processes of the bones and joints and interface more frequently with orthopedic surgeons (who probably order more spine magnetic resonance imaging [MRI] than any other single specialty). However, many musculoskeletal imagers do not read spine studies. Physicians who perform diagnostic and therapeutic spine injections often have an excellent grasp of degenerative processes of the spine, but most of these individuals are not radiologists and are not responsible for image interpretation.

This lack of focus on imaging of degenerative changes of the spine needs to be rectified. Between 70% and 80% of adults suffer from backache at some point in life (Andersson 1997, Waddell 1998). The number of back surgeries, the complexity of surgeries, and the number of repeat surgeries increase every year. Patients undergo more and more MRI studies. The overwhelming majority of these patients have one or more degenerative changes. The task of the imager of the spine is twofold: to provide a complete description of the abnormalities depicted on the examination, and to attempt to provide some sense of how the abnormalities detected relate to the patient's symptom(s). This chapter reviews our approach to these two tasks.

Pain and the Pain Diagram

Our patient information sheet, which is available to the radiologist at the time of imaging interpretation (Fig. 2–1), solicits not only demographic information but also requests information regarding any injury (if applicable), any prior surgery, and any prior imaging. In addition, there are three different locations soliciting information about patient symptoms. First, the patient is asked for a brief written description of his or her symptoms; second, a checkbox matrix asks for specific locations of symptoms; third, the patient is asked to generate a pain diagram on the cartoon figure of a body. Information provided by these three methods overlaps, and in some cases even conflicts, but the informa-

tion allows the radiologist to better assess the relative likelihood that a given imaging finding represents the cause of the patient's symptoms. As in any imaging study, correlation with the clinical history will help sort the clinically relevant from the clinically irrelevant abnormalities. Studies of subjects who have never experienced backache, or who have never lost work or sought medical care for backache, may demonstrate some features that overlap with patients having symptoms associated with similar-appearing abnormalities (Boden 1990a, Boden 1990b, Jarvik 2001, Jensen 1994, Matsumoto 1998, Stadnik 1998, Teresi 1987, Weinreb 1989, Weishaupt 1998, Wiesel 1984).

An abnormality on the side opposite radicular pain is unlikely to explain the present symptoms (although it may have been a cause of pain in the past), and the imager should be aware of the location of the symptoms. In some cases, the link between symptoms and a particular imaging finding is obvious: no one would doubt the association between the sudden-onset, severe pain shooting back down the back of the left leg associated with numbness and weakness in a 23-year-old man and the 12-mm disc extrusion smashing his left S1 left nerve root on his MRI scan.[*] Other instances may be considered more dubious: is the chronic central low back pain experienced by a 45-year-old woman secondary to a moderately dehydrated L4–5 disc or mild facet arthropathy at this level?

All imagers may not be familiar with one element of the information-gathering process just described: the pain diagram. Pain diagrams have been used for many years to help assess patient pain, and evaluation of such pain diagrams has been studied and found to be useful in analysis of radicular pain and associated disc herniations (Ljunggren 1988, Mann 1992, Uden 1987, Vucetic 1995) and to place patients in broadly defined diagnostic categories (Mann 1992) (Figs. 2–2 to 2–4). Pain diagrams have both a psychological and an anatomic component (Ohnmeiss 1995), and interevaluator repeatability and consistency within a single patient have been found high (Beattie 2000, Ohnmeiss 2000). Some investigators have used the pain diagram to test whether further psychological testing prior to surgery is necessary when the patient incorporates certain features in

---

[*]Although it may be less well known that the compression of the nerve root is generally not the cause of the patient's radicular pain (see later).

**PATIENT
INFORMATION
SHEET**

Center for Diagnostic Imaging

PLEASE PRINT

For Office Use Only
Date _____
FL Location _____
Account # _____
F/U Appt w/Ref MD _____

NAME _____   SOCIAL SECURITY # _____
        Last, First, Middle

AGE _____ BIRTHDATE _____ HEIGHT _____ WEIGHT _____   SEX: o M   o F

EMERGENCY CONTACT: NAME _____ NUMBER _____

FEMALES: Are you pregnant? o YES o NO When was your last menstrual period? _____ Are you breastfeeding? _____

REFERRING PHYSICIAN _____ DR. PHONE # _____

Briefly describe your problem/pain and how long you have had these symptoms? _____

_____

DATE OF INJURY (IF APPLICABLE) _____

DO YOU HAVE ANY ALLERGIES? o YES   o NO IF SO, WHAT ARE THEY? _____

HAVE YOU HAD SURGERY IN THE AREA TO BE SCANNED? ? o YES   o NO

IF YES, DESCRIBE WHAT WAS DONE AND WHEN THE SURGERY WAS PERFORMED _____

_____

IF SURGERY, ARE YOUR SYMPTOMS : BETTER   WORSE   SAME DIFFERENT (CIRCLE AND DESCRIBE)

_____

Please circle any **MEDICAL PROBLEMS** you have:

ASTHMA   BRONCHITIS   DIABETES   PANCREAS   GALLBLADDER   LIVER   KIDNEY   FEMALE ORGAN
Comment or **other medical problems:** _____

HAVE YOU HAD ANY OF THE FOLLOWING? IF SO, INDICATE WHEN, WHERE, AND RESULTS.

TEST	WHEN	WHERE	RESULTS
X-rays			
CT Scan			
MRI Scan			
Ultrasound			
Nuclear Medicine			
Therapeutic Injection			
Arthrogram			

INDICATE SYMPTOMS:

Please check:	RIGHT	LEFT	BOTH
Arm Pain			
Neck Pain			
Back Pain			
Leg Pain			
Tingling			
Weakness			
Numbness			

Scan Type_____

Pre-Scan_____

Scan Time_____

Bolus Rad Approved_____

Study #_____

Total # of images_____

C2/3 =
C3/4 =
C4/5 =
C5/6 =
C6/7 =
C7/T1 =
L1/2 =
L2/3 =
I 3/4 =
L4/5 =   Right
L5/S1 =

FRONT

**LOCATION
OF PAIN**
Please shade in
painful areas.

Left   Left

Lowest Full Body =
Lowest Disc Space =

BACK

Right

T1/2 =
T2/3 =
T3/4 =
T4/5 =
T5/6 =
T6/7 =
T7/8 =
T8/9 =
T9/10 =
T10/11 =
T11/12 =
T12/L1 =

FIGURE 2–1

MRI Information Sheet. The sheet requests symptom information in three locations: a prompt for a brief written description of pain, a matrix check-box, and a cartoon for provision of a pain diagram.

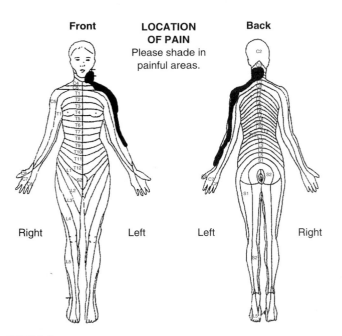

FIGURE 2–2

Pain diagram in a patient with C5 radicular pain. This pain diagram was drawn by a 33-year-old woman with neck and arm pain; MRI examination revealed a C4–5 disc herniation and accompanying C5 nerve root compression. A pain diagram that is unilateral and drawn as a thin strip suggests radicular pain.

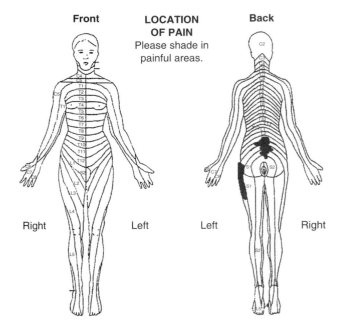

FIGURE 2–3

Pain diagram in a patient with spinal stenosis. A 77-year-old woman with severe spinal canal and subarticular recess stenosis at L4–5 drew this pain diagram. The patient also indicated bilateral leg weakness and numbness.

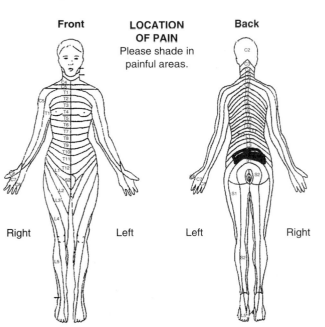

FIGURE 2–4

Pain diagram in a patient with degenerative disc disease. A 40-year-old woman with single-level degenerative disc disease at L4–5, with loss of disc height and hydration and subchondral marrow changes, drew this pain diagram.

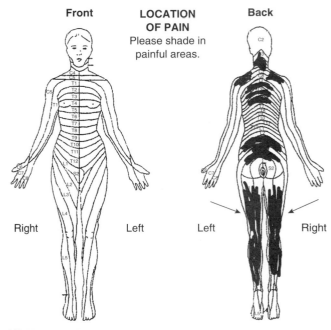

FIGURE 2–5

Pain diagram having characteristics of an "unreal" drawing. This 36-year-old woman had mild loss of L5/S1 disc height and moderate disc dehydration with a 2.1-mm disc protrusion. There are several features of the pain diagram (including a nonanatomic distribution of the pain and "I hurt here" markers), suggesting that further psychological testing might be in order before surgery is contemplated.

the drawing (e.g., "unreal drawings" not consistent with any anatomic structure and "I particularly hurt here" indicators such as added arrows or lengthy printed explanations) (Fig. 2–5) (Ransford 1976).

Our pain diagram has lines, letters, and numbers on it that follow the dermatome chart first published by Keegan and Garret in 1948 (Fig. 2–1). They based this dermatome

chart on their own work (including nerve root compression and traction of an exposed root at operation, section of nerve roots, and nerve root blocks on medical student volunteers) as well as multiple prior studies and previous charts, including those of Foerster (1933). Keegan and

Garret's dermatome chart was *a map of hyposensitivity to cutaneous sensation following nerve root lesioning or anesthetization*, and the first sentence of their discussion states that "the exact anatomical significance of these dermatome areas of primary hyposensitivity from single nerve root loss is somewhat uncertain." Given their uncertainty, it is ironic that the chart they published is now ubiquitous, appearing in innumerable medical textbooks, wall charts, and patient handouts. This dermatome chart is a simplification and may be helpful but is also potentially misleading. Review of the literature used by Keegan (Foerster 1933), other literature contemporaneous with Keegan (Kellgren 1939, Kellgren 1941), and more recent work (Bogduk 1997, van Akkerveeken 1993) demonstrate that there is a great deal of diversity in the location and shape of particular dermatomes. Exclusive use of Keegan and Garret's chart may result in the misperception that pain radiating straight down the back of the leg *must* be from S1, and cannot originate from L5, but this is simply not the case. A narrow band of pain radiating straight down the back of the leg to the heel is *usually* from S1, but it may originate from L5 or S2 in many individuals. Similarly, pain in the lateral thigh is usually from L5 (but may be from L4 or S1), and pain in the groin is usually from L4 (or higher) (Vucetic 1995). In the upper extremity, pain radiating to the long finger is more likely from C7 (than from C6 or C8), and in the thumb more likely from C6 (than from C5 or C7). The side and character of pain, however, are more important than the exact physical location, unless there is a two- or three-level variance between the location and the imaged abnormality.

The pain diagram does not fully communicate the character of the pain. *Radicular pain* is described as sharp, shooting, and confined to a narrow band (Bogduk 1997). Radicular pain originates in irritation of the spinal nerve or its roots. Compression of the nerve root alone may produce *radiculopathy* (conduction block associated with numbness or weakness in the nerve root's distribution) but not radicular pain (with the exception of compression of the dorsal root ganglion). To produce radicular pain, compression must be accompanied by inflammation of the spinal nerve or nerve root (Bogduk 1997, Garfin 1991, Howe 1977, Kelly 1956, Kuslich 1991). *Referred pain* is perceived to be deeper and broader than radicular pain, is more difficult to localize, and has an aching quality. Referred pain occurs because sensory neurons from different peripheral sites link to common neurons in the spine and brain. Many structures in the cervical spine may cause referred pain in the shoulders and arms, and many structures in the lumbar spine may cause referred pain in the buttocks and legs. Pain drawn on the pain diagram as a narrow band running from the neck down the entire arm into a single digit (Fig. 2–2), or drawn as a narrow band down the length of the leg, is more likely radicular pain. Pain drawn in as a broad area covering most of one shoulder or buttock is much more likely referred pain.

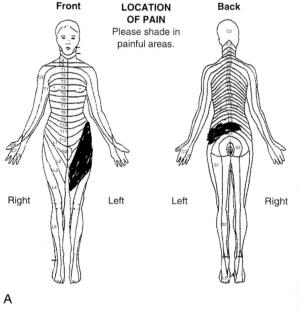

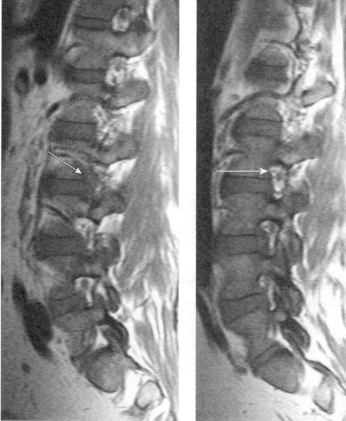

FIGURE 2–6

Pain diagram that called attention to a subtle foraminal disc herniation. A 42-year-old woman with low back and left anterior thigh pain. A, Pain diagram. B, Parasagittal T1WI through the foramina with an L2–3 foraminal disc extrusion (arrow) causing compression of the exiting L2 nerve. C, Parasagittal T1WI through the foramina on the contralateral (normal) side. Note widely patent foramina at the L2–3 level (arrow). The lesion within the left foramen could have gone undetected without scrutiny of the images directed at finding a cause of high lumbar radicular pain.

Although the pain diagram, as well as the other information about symptoms solicited on the intake sheet, helps the spine imager correlate the imaging findings with the patient's symptoms, no single piece of information can indicate the "cause" of the patient's pain, or, more important, the likelihood of success of specific therapeutic measures. The probability of success in treatment of back pain depends on multiple variables. These variables include the lesions discovered at imaging and the patient's pain diagram and written report of pain. Additional variables include, but are not limited to, the chronicity of pain, the patient's psychological makeup and response to pain, and possible secondary gain (from both the litigation and workers' compensation systems) (Boos 1995, Ohnmeiss 1995, Spengler 1979, Taylor 1984). Certainly, patients may fabricate a radiculopathy on pain diagrams and thus mislead the spine imager; patients may also claim to feel pain that is not really there in their written descriptions. Although reliance on the pain diagram is susceptible to failure secondary to such misrepresentation, we think that the benefits outweigh the detriments: we have encountered several patients wherein the pain diagram caused us to further scrutinize the imaging study and thus to detect a subtle lesion that would have been undiagnosed without reference to the pain diagram (Fig. 2–6; see also Figs. 2–37, 2–42, and 2–43 in the section, "Disc Herniation").

We noted that the notion that any specific lesion is the cause of a given patient's pain might be subject to attack by critics. Patients and asymptomatic volunteers may demonstrate similar imaging findings (Boden 1990a, Boden 1990b, Jensen 1994, Matsumoto 1998, Stadnik 1998, Teresi 1987, Weinreb 1989, Weishaupt 1998, Wiesel 1984). Diagnostic injection whereby a patient's typical pain is stimulated by needle placement with injection of a small amount of contrast material, and then relieved by injection of local anesthetic, is subject to the placebo effect. Van Akkerveeken (1993) demanded not only imaging and surgical observation of disc abnormalities to accept these as the cause of the patient's pain, but also relief of pain following surgical

removal of the offending lesion. However, even these stringent criteria do not avoid the placebo effect of surgery. In addition, back pain and radicular pain may wax and wane with time, and ascribing improvement to a particular therapeutic maneuver may be incorrect. Indeed, the basic model widely employed in most of the literature regarding spine pain diagnosis and treatment, namely, the existence of stimulated nociceptors, which result in brain activity perceived as pain, has been challenged as not accounting for all observed phenomena. For example, Kibler and Nathan (1960) have documented that pain "from" lesions of peripheral nerves, nerve roots, the posterior columns, and the spinothalamic tract can be blocked (often for a duration outlasting the pharmacologic effect) by anesthetizing the peripheral nerve distal to the lesions. Patients with amputations commonly experience phantom limb pain, and sectioning of nerves in ever more proximal locations is infamously unsuccessful at eradicating such pain (Foerster 1933). Melzack and Wall (1965) proposed a new theory of pain to account for these observations. Although their theory has generated considerable interest, it cannot be said to have become a clinical mainstay at this time: most of the attention of the surgical and imaging community continues to focus (for better or worse) on the discovery and categorization of "pain generators" in the spinal column, and the remainder of this chapter is devoted to the display and explanation of degenerative changes that may be held responsible for pain.

Imaging of Degenerative Disease

PLAIN FILMS

Patients with neck and back pain usually have plain films taken at some point in their evaluation. Plain films allow assessment of alignment and position and such findings as degenerative narrowing of intervertebral discs as well as subchondral sclerosis and osteophyte formation (Fig. 2–7).

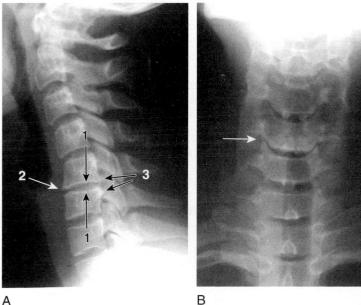

A   B

FIGURE 2–7

Plain films of degenerative disc disease in the cervical spine. A 30-year-old patient with neck and shoulder pain. A, Lateral plain film examination of the cervical spine demonstrates C5–6 intervertebral disc space narrowing (arrows 1), anterior (arrow 2) and posterior (arrow 3) osteophyte formation, and reversal of normal cervical lordosis centered at the C5–6 level. B, Anteroposterior examination demonstrates C5–6 uncinate spurring, particularly on the right (arrow).

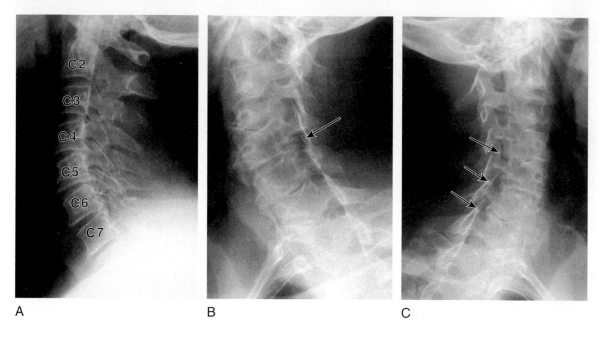

FIGURE 2–8

Oblique plain films demonstrating foraminal stenosis. A 60-year-old man with neck pain and hand numbness. A, Lateral examination shows disc narrowing and osteophytic spurring at C4–5, C5–6, and C6–7. The foramina cannot be evaluated on this view. B, Left oblique view demonstrates severe left C5–6 foraminal stenosis from osteophytic spurring (arrow), with lesser degrees of stenosis elsewhere in the cervical spine. C, Right oblique view shows C4–5, C5–6, and C6–7 foraminal stenosis (arrows) from osteophytic spurring. Oblique plain films are quite helpful in delineating bony stenosis in cervical neural foramina.

Oblique cervical radiographs allow evaluation of bony foraminal stenosis (Fig. 2–8). Central spinal canal stenosis is difficult to evaluate, and soft tissues cannot be directly visualized on plain films, limiting the usefulness of plain film evaluation of degenerative changes of the spine.

MYELOGRAPHY

Myelography may be helpful in evaluation of spinal canal stenosis. For many years, diagnosis of disc herniations was based on features such as indentation of the contrast column, distortion of nerve roots, or asymmetric filling of nerve root sleeves. Many of these findings can be subtle, and myelography today is usually performed in conjunction with computed tomography (CT). One beneficial feature of plain film myelography that is difficult or impossible to recreate with most MRI scanners is the dynamic evaluation of spinal canal stenosis with lateral flexion/extension views.

COMPUTED TOMOGRAPHY

CT revolutionized evaluation of degenerative disc disease by allowing the diagnosis of disc herniation and degenerative stenosis without use of contrast material. Although CT has largely been supplanted by MRI, it is often still used in three situations: (1) when implants (e.g., aneurysm clips, pacemakers) preclude MRI; (2) as an adjunct to myelography, particularly in the evaluation of spinal stenosis; and (3) to evaluate the relative contributions of calcification/ bone versus soft tissue in a lesion discovered on MRI (Fig. 2–9).

When CT is done, axial slices should not be limited to the intervertebral discs but rather be performed in a stack that includes all levels: migrated disc fragments, spondy-

lolysis, and synovial cysts all may occur at positions significantly cephalad or caudad from the disc.

NUCLEAR MEDICINE

Bone scans often demonstrate increased radiotracer localization at areas of degeneration, either at the level of the disc or the facet joints. Single photon-emission computed tomography images better localize the degenerative change. However, bone scans are limited in their ability to evaluate soft tissue abnormalities.

MAGNETIC RESONANCE IMAGING

MRI is currently the imaging technique of choice for evaluation of degenerative changes of the spine. Image sequences usually consist of axial and sagittal T1-weighted images (T1WI) and/or proton density and T2-weighted images (T2WI). Imaging parameters vary greatly from institution to institution and from machine to machine. We offer the following generalizations:

1. In most instances, open configuration scanners lack sufficient field strength to obtain excellent images in a reasonable time. Either the matrix size, number of signal averages, slice thickness, or number of sequences is usually attenuated relative to what would be obtained in the same time for a high-field system, resulting in lesser image quality.
2. Contrast injection is not routinely necessary for evaluation of degenerative changes.
3. Contiguous axial slices should be obtained in the lumbar spine from S1 through L3 and in the cervical

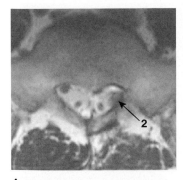

A

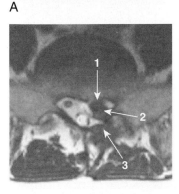

B

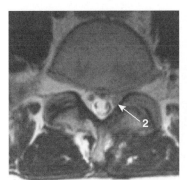

C

D

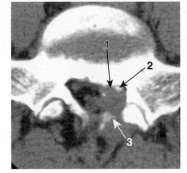

F

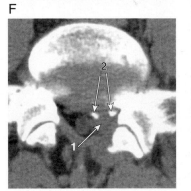

G

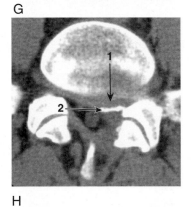

H

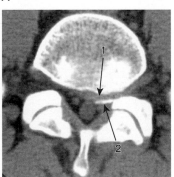

I

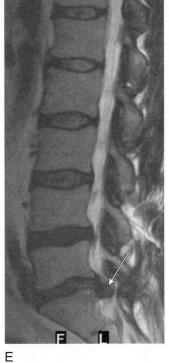

E

J

FIGURE 2–9

Additional information added by CT scan in disc herniation. A 40-year-old man with persistent low back and left buttock pain s/p discectomy. A–D, Sequential, inferior to superior axial T2WIs through the L5–S1 intervertebral disc show a left caudally dissecting disc extrusion (arrow 1) with posterior displacement of the left S1 nerve root (arrow 2). Note the posterior laminectomy defect (arrow 3). E, Right parasagittal T2WI confirms a caudally dissecting disc extrusion (arrow). F–I, Sequential, inferior to superior axial CT studies demonstrate the disc extrusion (arrows 1) with extensive calcification along the margin (arrows 2). Again noted is a posterior laminectomy defect (arrows 3). J, Sagittal reconstruction view also demonstrates calcification along the disc margin (arrow). In some cases, CT may be requested as an adjunct to MRI to define and differentiate calcified or ossified material, since this may alter any surgical approach.

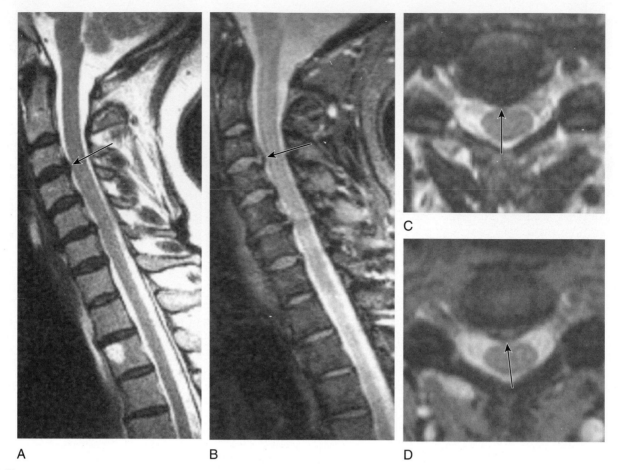

A   B   C   D

FIGURE 2–10

Additional information added by gradient-echo images of the cervical spine. A 48-year-old woman with right neck, shoulder, and arm pain. A, Sagittal fast spin-echo T2WI shows multilevel degenerative disc disease. Note that the lesion at C3–4 (arrow) has uniformly decreased signal intensity, making differentiation of disc extrusion and osteophytic spurring difficult. B, Sagittal gradient-recalled echo T2WI shows increased signal intensity within the cranially dissecting component of the lesion (arrow), consistent with disc herniation (and not with osteophyte). C, Axial fast spin-echo T2WI at the level of the C3–4 lesion again demonstrates uniform decreased signal intensity. D, Axial gradient-recalled echo T2WI, as on the sagittal view, shows a more complex appearance with a central focus of increased signal intensity consistent with disc extrusion.

spine from T1 through C2. As noted earlier, significant pathology including migrated disc fragments, synovial cysts, and pars defects will be seen only if imaging includes the area between the discs, as well as the discs themselves. In the thoracic spine, axial slices are usually confined to the intervertebral discs.

4. In the cervical spine, the combination of a gradient-echo and a fast spin-echo T2WI sequence usually allows the best differentiation from osteophytic spurring, disc protrusion, and fat (Fig. 2–10). Comparison of the two sequences is particularly helpful in the neural foramina.

Disc Degeneration and Internal Disc Disruption

The term *disc degeneration* has been used to indicate various histopathologic processes and radiographic findings, including disc narrowing, dehydration, annular fissures, and subchondral marrow changes (Modic 1988a, Resnick 1985). Some of these findings are held to be a manifestation of aging alone, whereas others are thought to be pathologic.

Controversy continues over the relationship between degenerative changes and patient symptoms. In this section we describe the MRI and CT findings of disc degeneration. We also review the entity of "internal disc disruption" and briefly discuss the topic of spine "instability."

DISC DEHYDRATION

On T2WI, the intervertebral discs demonstrate increased signal intensity relative to bone marrow, with signal intensity approaching that of cerebrospinal fluid in younger patients. Water content and signal intensity decreases with age (Luoma 2001, Sether 1990), but the signal intensity of the central portion of the disc should be uniform from level to level and should be appreciably greater than bone marrow. Recognizing that disc signal intensity (reflecting hydration) exists as a continuous variable and may assume an infinite number of values, it is nonetheless reasonable to categorize individual discs as having normal hydration, or having mild, moderate, or severe dehydration (Fig. 2–11) (Buirski 1992, Ito 1998). At the opposite end of the spectrum from normal disc hydration is the severely degenerat-

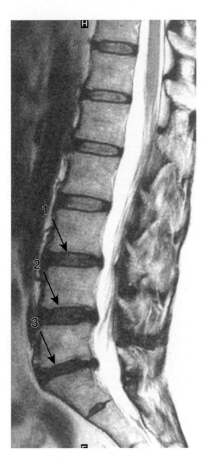

FIGURE 2–11

Disc dehydration. A 50-year-old woman with central low back pain for 10 years. Sagittal T2WI. There is normal hydration for age at the T11–12 through L2–3 levels, with mild dehydration at L3–4 (arrow 1), moderate dehydration at L4–5 (arrow 2), and severe loss of disc height and dehydration at L5–S1 (arrow 3). There is also degenerative disc bulging at L3–4, L4–5, and L5–S1.

ed disc containing a vacuum phenomenon, with absence of signal on all imaging sequences in a narrow linear channel usually located in the mid-portion of the disc (Fig. 2–12). Because of the contrast characteristics of gas, the vacuum phenomenon is often easier to recognize on plain films and CT scans than on MRI studies (Grenier 1987).

Disc dehydration, or at least decreased signal intensity on T1WI and T2WI, may not always accompany disc degeneration. Calcification of the disc may lead to increased signal intensity on T1WI (Bangert 1995) (Fig. 2–13). Occasionally, even markedly narrowed discs with osteophytes and predominantly decreased signal intensity on all other imaging sequences demonstrate areas of increased signal intensity on T2WI (Stabler 1996) (Fig. 2–14). These areas do not represent a normal nucleus pulposus surviving the apparent degeneration of the annulus but rather granulation tissue within the degenerated disc.

Fused discs may undergo a transformation from calcification to ossification and eventual conversion to marrow. The end result of this process of autofusion may be fat signal from the intervertebral disc, similar to marrow with the vertebral bodies (Fig. 2–15).

DISC NARROWING

Intervertebral disc narrowing, as disc dehydration, exists as a continuous variable and ranges from normal, preserved height to complete loss of disc height. Height determination requires comparison with other levels in the same patient or (explicit or implicit) comparison with other patients. As with dehydration, one may categorize individual discs as demonstrating normal height, or mild, moderate, or severe loss of disc height (Ito 1998) (Figs. 2–11, 2–12, and 2–16). Although it is not necessary to measure each and every disc to use this categorization scheme, we use the cutoffs shown in Table 2–1 for use of the corresponding terms.

Usually dehydration accompanies narrowing. As noted earlier, however, if *apparently* normally hydration is present in a moderately or severely narrowed disc, an abnormality resulting in abnormal disc signal intensity (e.g., granulation tissue from motion at the level) should be suspected (Fig. 2–14). Conversely, severe or even moderate disc dehydration in a full-height disc indicates an annular fissure (Yu 1989) and may be the clue to the presence of a disc herniation (Fig. 2–17).

SUBCHONDRAL MARROW DEGENERATIVE CHANGES

De Roos (1987) and Modic (1988a, 1988b) and their colleagues first described subchondral marrow changes adjacent to degenerated discs (Table 2–2). Three types have been described: Type I changes demonstrate T1 and T2 prolongation (Fig. 2–18), Type II changes demonstrate T1 shortening and T2 prolongation (Fig. 2–19), and Type III changes demonstrate T1 prolongation and T2 shortening (Fig. 2–20). Modic and coworkers (1988b) found that Type I changes converted to Type II changes in five of six patients studied over a 3-year period. Type I changes probably represent an earlier stage of the same process, in which disruption of the cartilaginous end plate separating the nucleus from the subchondral marrow is followed by subsequent subchondral marrow histologic (and accompanying imaging) changes and disc degeneration. Stabler and associates (1996) have noted contrast enhancement of subchondral marrow degenerative changes, with bands of increased signal intensity paralleling the intervertebral disc on postcontrast T1WI (Fig. 2–21).

ANNULAR FISSURE

An annular fissure is an abnormal discontinuity of the concentrically arranged collagen fibers forming the annulus fibrosus. The term *fissure* is generally preferred to "tear" (Fardon 1997). MRI depicts annular fissures either as foci of T2 prolongation (Yu 1989) or as areas of contrast enhancement on postinjection T1WI (Ross 1990). Aprill and Bogduk (1992) defined a high-intensity zone (HIZ) as a focus of increased signal intensity (relative to the nucleus at the same level) in the posterior annulus of the disc on T2WI obtained with thin sections (Fig. 2–22). They found a strong correlation of HIZs and concordant pain on discography and believed that these lesions represented symptomatic annular fissures. Subsequent articles have both supported (Milette 1999, Saifuddin 1998, Schellhas 1996) and

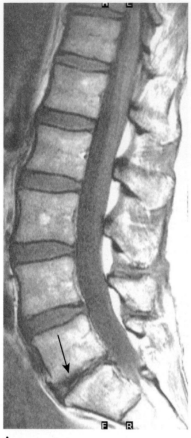
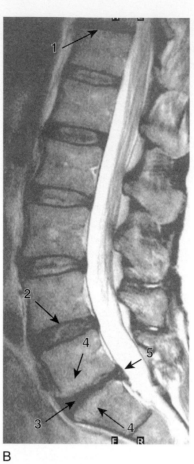

A

B

FIGURE 2–12

Vacuum disc. A 62-year-old patient with chronic low back pain. A, Sagittal T1WI shows severe narrowing at L5–S1 along with complete absence of signal from the mid-anterior L5–S1 intervertebral disc (arrow). B, Sagittal T2WI shows normal height and hydration of T12–L1 through L3–4. T11–12 demonstrates moderate loss of disc height and hydration (arrow 1). L4–5 shows mild dehydration and degenerative disc bulging (arrow 2). L5–S1 demonstrates severe loss of disc height and disc hydration (arrow 3), Modic Type II subchondral marrow degenerative changes (arrows 4), and degenerative bulging (arrow 5). Because of the lack of signal intensity from the disc on T2WI, the vacuum phenomenon is easier to appreciate on T1WI.

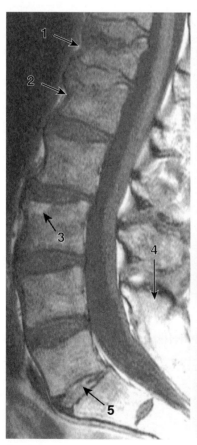
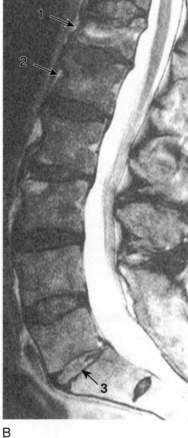

A

B

FIGURE 2–13

Calcified disc demonstrating T1 shortening and T2 prolongation. A 78-year-old man with chronic L5–S1 fusion and acute low back pain. A, Sagittal T1WI shows loss of height at T12 (arrow 1) and L1 (arrow 2), anterior Modic Type II subchondral marrow degenerative changes at L3–4 (arrow 3), and posterior fusion at L5–S1 (arrow 4) with anterior T1 shortening at the level of the disc (arrow 5). B, Sagittal T2WI confirms loss of height with T2 prolongation at T12 (arrow 1) (indicating an acute or subacute fracture [see Chapter 5]); loss of height with isointensity at L1 (arrow 2) (indicating a chronic fracture); moderate disc dehydration at L1–2, L2–3, and L3–4; and mild disc dehydration at L4–5. At L5–S1, there is T2 prolongation (arrow 3). The findings at L5–S1 are secondary to chronic fusion at this level; immobilized discs may undergo calcification and/or ossification with eventual marrow formation (with fat signal) at the level of the disc.

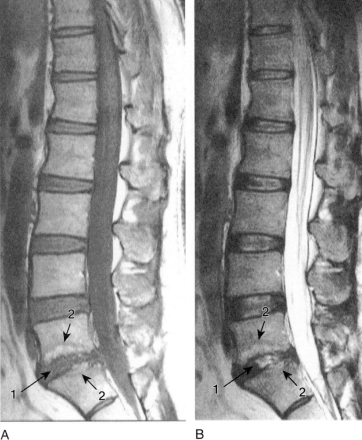

A

B

FIGURE 2–14

T2 prolongation within a narrowed disc indicating disc degeneration. A 51-year-old patient with left low back and leg pain and tingling. A, Sagittal T1WI shows mild loss of L5–S1 disc height (arrow 1) and subchondral Modic Type II marrow degenerative changes (arrows 2). B, Sagittal T2WI shows T2 prolongation relative to other (normal) discs of the lumbar spine (arrow 1). Such T2 prolongation, in this case, is not a sign of normal hydration but rather a marker of degenerative disc disease, similar to the high-intensity zone of the posterior annulus. Also noted are Modic Type II degenerative changes (arrows 2).

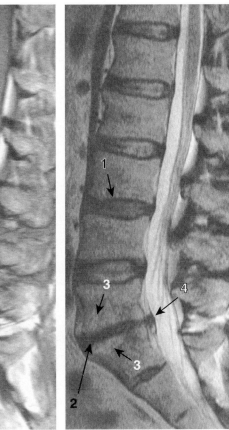

A

B

FIGURE 2–16

Disc narrowing. A 51-year-old man with chronic right paraspinal low back pain. A, Sagittal T1WI shows mild loss of height at L3–4 (arrow 1), severe loss of disc height at L5–S1 and a vacuum phenomenon with a linear focus of absent signal (arrow 2), and subchondral Modic Type II degenerative changes (arrows 3). B, Sagittal T2WI shows mild loss of disc height and hydration at L3–4 (arrow 1), severe loss of disc height and hydration at L5–S1 (arrow 2), along with subchondral Modic Type II degenerative changes (arrows 3). There is also L5–S1 degenerative disc bulging with a superimposed disc protrusion (arrow 4).

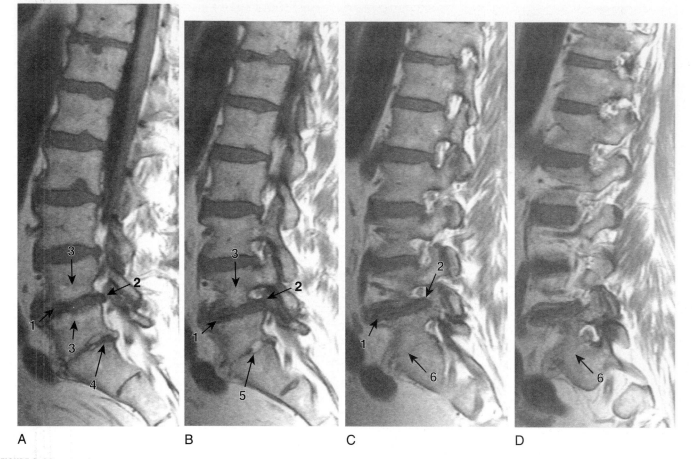

A B C D

FIGURE 2–15

Autofusion with fatty conversion of disc. A 76-year-old man with chronic central low back pain. A–D, Sequential right parasagittal T1WIs show L4–5 degenerative disc narrowing (arrow 1), bulging (arrow 2), and Modic Type II degenerative changes (arrow 3). At L5–S1, there is marked narrowing of the disc, with severe disc dehydration (arrow 4); laterally, there is a focus of fat crossing the disc (arrow 5) and, more laterally yet, complete fusion of the disc (arrow 6).

TABLE 2–1. Definition of Descriptors for Disc Height

Term	Percentage (%) of Height Compared to Normal Level
Mild	75–99
Moderate	50–74
Severe	<50

TABLE 2–2. Subchondral Marrow Changes

Modic Type	MRI Findings	Histologic Correlate
I	T1 prolongation T2 prolongation	Vascularized fibrous tissue
II	T1 shortening T2 prolongation	Red marrow replacement with yellow marrow
III	T1 prolongation T2 shortening	Bone

challenged (Carragee 2000, Rankine 1998, Ricketson 1996, Smith 1998) the value of the HIZ as an imaging finding. Stadnik and coworkers (1998) found HIZs in 56% of asymptomatic volunteers, demonstrating that the finding is not always associated with symptoms (Fig. 2–23).

INTERNAL DISC DISRUPTION

What is the clinical significance of the degenerative changes mentioned earlier? We know that many asymptomatic individuals manifest imaging findings of degenerative disc disease, including disc narrowing, dehydration, subchondral marrow degenerative changes, and HIZs. Certainly, disc narrowing may lead to foraminal stenosis and ganglionic compression and thus have associated clinical symptoms. Absent neural compression, can degenerative change cause back pain?

Bogduk (1997) has defined internal disc disruption as a painful condition that is diagnosed by provocation of typical pain by discography, and demonstration of an annular fissure extending to the outer third of the annulus on a CT performed after discography (Fig. 2–22). He supports the notion that internal disc disruption (along with zygapophyseal and sacroiliac joint pain) may account for a large proportion of the back pain that approximately 70% to 80% of the population will suffer at some point in life. In an analysis of data from a study by Ito and colleagues (1998) on MR signs of internal disc derangement, Bogduk noted that severe disc narrowing, severe loss of nuclear signal, the HIZ, and subchondral bone changes all carried a likelihood ratio of 4.2 or greater for indicating internal disc disruption.

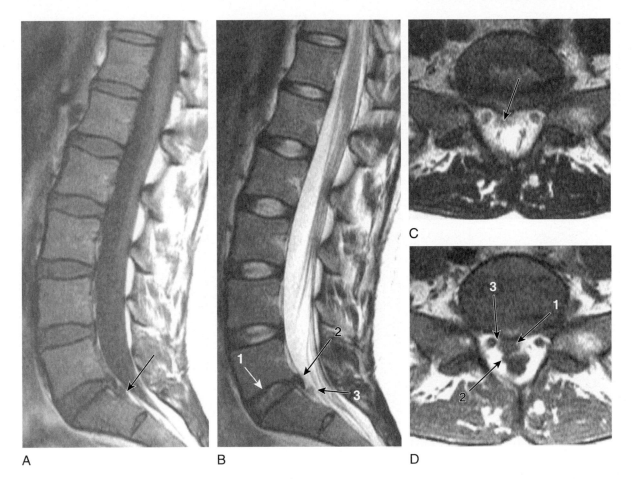

FIGURE 2–17

Disc dehydration in a normal-height disc as a clue to disc herniation. A 30-year-old woman with low back and right posterior thigh and calf pain. A, Sagittal T1WI shows a subtle soft tissue density inferior to the disc margin that displaces normal anterior epidural fat seen in this location (arrow). B, Sagittal T2WI shows preserved disc height and hydration at all levels except for L5–S1, where there is mild dehydration (arrow 1) and an apparent small disc protrusion (arrow 2). There is also abnormal soft tissue posterior to the upper margin of the sacrum that is quite subtle on the T2WIs (arrow 3). C, Axial T2WI shows a subtle soft tissue abnormality in the anterior epidural fat on the right side (arrow). D, Axial T1WI shows a caudally dissecting disc extrusion (arrow 1) posteriorly displacing the right S2 nerve root (arrow 2) and contacting the medial aspect of the right S1 nerve root sleeve (arrow 3). Because of the location of the lesion in the anterior epidural fat, it is much easier to appreciate on T1WI.

Moderate disc space narrowing had a likelihood ratio of only 2.0, whereas moderate loss of disc signal had a likelihood ratio of 0.6, indicating that moderate loss of disc signal actually made internal disc disruption less likely in a given patient. Subchondral bone marrow enhancement on contrast examinations was not specifically evaluated in this study.

In subsequent studies, Milette and associates (1999) found that loss of disc height and signal intensity predicted symptomatic tears shown at discography, and Weishaupt and colleagues (2001) found that moderate and severe endplate changes had a high specificity and positive predictive value for internal disc disruption using discography as a reference standard. Sandhu and coworkers (2000), however, found no correlation between end-plate changes and discography results.

If one accepts internal disc disruption as a cause of back pain, then the imaging findings of degenerative disc disease mentioned earlier are important markers of internal disc disruption. The reference standard for the diagnosis of

internal disc disruption remains discography,† which is not universally accepted as a diagnostic tool (Carragee 1999, Jackson 1997). The literature is replete with articles noting that MR findings are imperfect predictors of response to discography (Brightbill 1994, Buirski 1992, Horton 1992, Milette 1999, Moneta 1994, Osti 1992, Sandhu 2000, Weishaupt 2001). In general, patients who have a normal disc on MRI and an abnormal discogram fare more poorly at surgery: Gill and Blumenthal (1992) found a 50% rate of functional success in such patients, versus a 75% rate of success in those with both an abnormal MRI and an abnormal discogram. Thus, MRI findings of degeneration of the disc may increase or decrease the likelihood of a given patient having internal disc disruption, and for some clinicians they may even obviate discography. The report of MRI

---

†However, as noted in Chapter 3, some authorities advocate a trial of external fixation in patients suspected of internal disc derangement as a predictor of surgery, and this may be a better "reference standard."

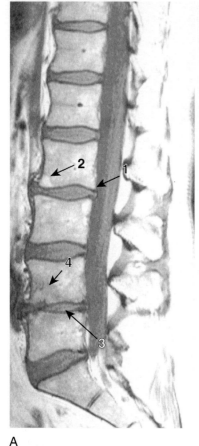

A

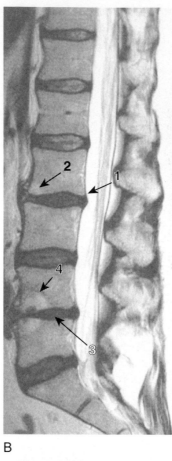

B

FIGURE 2–18

Subchondral Modic Types I and II degenerative changes. A 53-year-old woman with chronic central and right-sided low back pain. A, Sagittal T1WI shows slight retrolisthesis of L2 on L3 (arrow 1) with T1 shortening in the anterior subchondral marrow (arrow 2) along with L4–5 severe disc space narrowing (arrow 3) and extensive subchondral T1 prolongation (arrow 4). B, Sagittal T2WI again demonstrates retrolisthesis at L2–3 (arrow 1). There is also T2 prolongation at L2–3 (arrow 2) indicating Modic Type II changes. At the L4–5 level, there is disc narrowing (arrow 3) and T2 prolongation (arrow 4). Given the T1 prolongation on A, the findings at L4–5 are those of Modic Type I degenerative change. There is also moderate loss of disc height and hydration at L2–3 with degenerative disc bulging, mild dehydration at L3–4, and severe loss of disc height and hydration with degenerative disc bulging and anterior herniation at L4–5. Finally, there is mild dehydration at L5–S1.

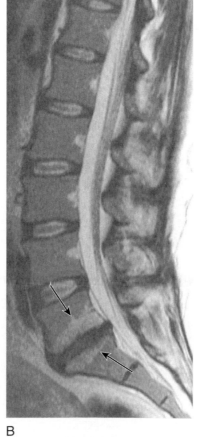

A

B

FIGURE 2–19

Subchondral Modic Type II degenerative change. A 33-year-old woman with chronic central low back pain. A, Sagittal T1WI shows moderate loss of L5–S1 disc height and extensive subchondral T1 prolongation adjacent to the disc (arrows). B, Sagittal T2WI shows moderate disc dehydration and extensive subchondral T2 prolongation matching the abnormality on the T1WI (arrows), or Modic Type II subchondral degenerative change.

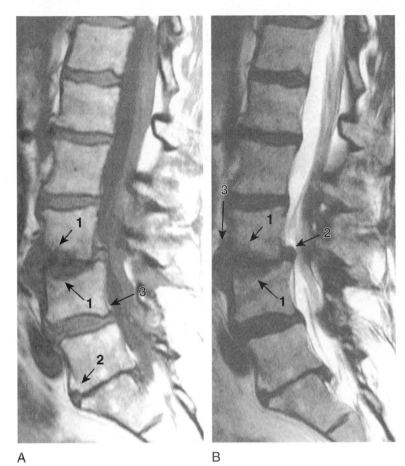

A   B

FIGURE 2–20

Subchondral Modic Type III degenerative change. A 71-year-old woman with left low back and left leg pain. A, Sagittal T1WI shows severe loss of disc height at L3–4 along with 15% degenerative spondylolisthesis and extensive subchondral T1 prolongation (arrows 1). L5–S1 is severely narrowed and demonstrates minimal Modic Type II degenerative change (arrow 2), and L4–5 demonstrates 5% degenerative spondylolisthesis (arrow 3). B, Sagittal T2WI shows moderate dehydration at T12–L1 and L4–5 and severe dehydration elsewhere. Matching the T1 prolongation at L3–4 is extensive T2 shortening (arrows 1). There is also a disc extrusion posteriorly (arrow 2). Anteriorly, there is extensive excess tissue (arrow 3). The marrow abnormalities (which correspond to erosions and sclerosis on plain films) have been termed "hemispheric sclerosis" and "discovertebral trauma" and are one manifestation of severe degenerative disc disease.

studies must therefore include a complete description of all degenerative findings. Attribution of symptoms to these findings is far less straightforward than in other disease processes (e.g., unilateral radiculopathy and radicular pain with a corresponding large disc extrusion in the appropriate location), and is often done by excluding other processes. Internal disc disruption has no specific historical or physical examination features allowing differentiation from other sources of back pain (Schwarzer 1995). Therefore, the radiology report regarding the MRI study should refrain from any strong conclusions about the causative role of commonly seen degenerative changes on MRI and a given patient's back pain.

Controversy surrounding treatment of internal disc disruption probably exceeds the controversy surrounding the diagnosis. Waddell (1998) advises against fusion surgery for internal disc disruption and advocates conservative management. Intradiscal steroids have been studied with mixed results (Feffer 1956, Feffer 1969, Graham 1985, Leao 1960, Simmons 1992, Wilkinson 1980). Fusion surgery has produced favorable results in some reports (Gill 1992, Kuslich 1998, Ray 1997), but others claim that fundamental questions regarding the scientific foundation of fusion surgery remain unanswered (Muggleton 2000). Saal and Saal (2000) have developed a device that allows percutaneous delivery of thermal energy to the disc and reported improved functional outcome in treated patients. If one does not accept such thermal therapy or fusion surgery as a valid treatment of internal disc disruption, it is difficult to justify the pain, expense, and risks of discography for other than research purposes. We encourage radiologists to keep abreast not only of the local surgeons' viewpoints but forthcoming scientific literature in this controversial area.

DISC AND FACET DEGENERATION AND "INSTABILITY"

Kirkaldy-Willis and Farfan (1982, Yong-Hing 1983) developed the notion of a "degenerative cascade" in the spine, with facet degeneration accompanying disc degeneration. Disc degeneration generally precedes facet degeneration (Butler 1990). Some authors have claimed a relationship between facet joint tropism (asymmetric alignment of facet joints) and disc degeneration (Farfan 1967, Noren 1991), whereas others deny such a relationship (Boden 1996). When disc degeneration and facet arthropathy coexist at a level, particularly when there is malalignment at the level, the patient may have spinal "instability." Different authors use the term *instability* in different ways (Bogduk 1997), and some authors propose multiple subtypes (Frymoyer 1985, Sato 1993). Use of the term *instability* in a report of a static study (the overwhelming majority of spine imaging) should probably be limited. Some specialized MRI units may allow dynamic studies of seated patients (Schmid 1999, Weishaupt 2000), and some devices may allow dynamic imaging of the cervical spine (Muhle 1998) and lumbar spine (Willen 2001). In these circumstances, reports of exaggerated motion and other findings on motion and loading at a given level may benefit the surgeon.

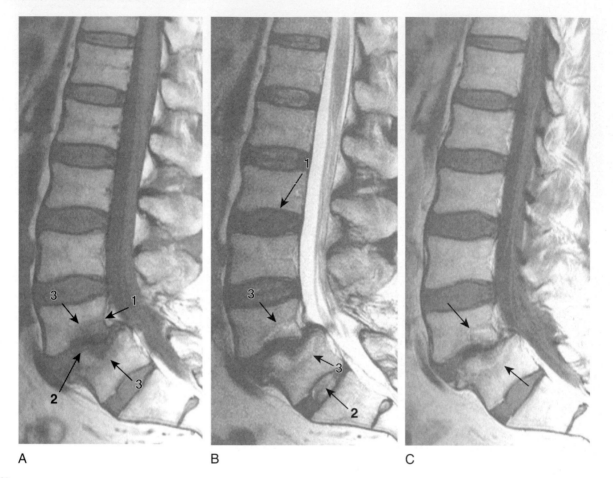

A   B   C

FIGURE 2–21

Contrast enhancement of subchondral Modic Type I degenerative change. A 71-year-old man with right back pain and bilateral leg tingling. A, Sagittal T1WI shows 20% lytic spondylolisthesis at L4–L5 (arrow 1) with severe loss of disc height (arrow 2). Note subchondral T1 prolongation (arrows 3). B, Sagittal T2WI shows mild L2–3 dehydration (arrow 1) and mixed signal intensity of the L5–S1 intervertebral disc (arrow 2) consistent with degenerative disc disease. At the L4–5 level, there is severe narrowing and dehydration with subchondral T2 prolongation (arrows 3) that, combined with the findings on the T1WI, indicate Modic Type I subchondral degenerative changes. C, Postcontrast T1WI shows contrast enhancement of the abnormal subchondral marrow (arrows) (compare to A).

Disc Herniation

MECHANISM OF SYMPTOM PRODUCTION

At present, two camps offer opposing theories regarding the mechanism of symptom production in disc herniation. Mixter and Barr (1934) first proposed mechanical neural compression as the source of symptom production. Studies have established that larger disc herniations are more likely to be symptomatic (and to benefit from surgery) (Hurme 1987, Spangfort 1972), that (generally larger) extrusions are more likely to be associated with symptoms and are rarely seen in asymptomatic individuals whereas (generally smaller) protrusions can often be seen in asymptomatic individuals (Boden 1990a, Boden 1990b, Jensen 1994, Matsumoto 1998, Stadnik 1998, Weishaupt 1998), and that neural compression from disc herniation is associated with symptoms (Beattie 2000, Boos 1998, Debois 1999). Although mechanical compression cannot immediately cause radicular pain with the exception of pressure on the dorsal root ganglion, continued pressure may impair axonal transport, resulting in a damaged nerve root that may then be painful (Garfin 1991, Heithoff 1987). In comparison, members of the chem-

ical irritation camp propose that a substance (phospholipase A$_2$ [Franson 1992, Lee 1998, Ozaktkay 1998, Saal 1990], matrix metalloproteinases [Kang 1996, Roberts 2000], nitrous oxide [Furusawa 2001, Kang 1996], cytokines [Kang 1996], tumor necrosis factor alpha [Igarashi 2000, Olmarker 1998], and free glutamate [Harrington 2000] all have been proposed) incites a biochemical cascade that results in excessive macrophages in the vicinity of the nerve (Gronblad 1994, Habtemariam 1998), with subsequent abnormal nerve conduction and resultant pain.[†] Studies have demonstrated the inflammatory nature of autologous nuclear material placed in the epidural space (Kayama 1998, McCarron 1987, Olmarker 1993), and an animal model of sciatica has shown both the existence of inflammatory changes in the epidural space and a beneficial effect from corticosteroids (Lee 1998). Saal (1995) has gone so far as to

---

[†]Note, however, that Gronblad and colleagues (2000) could demonstrate no relationship between the amount of inflammatory cells within resected transligamentous disc herniations and motor weakness or a positive straight leg–raising sign in patients having resection of symptomatic disc herniations.

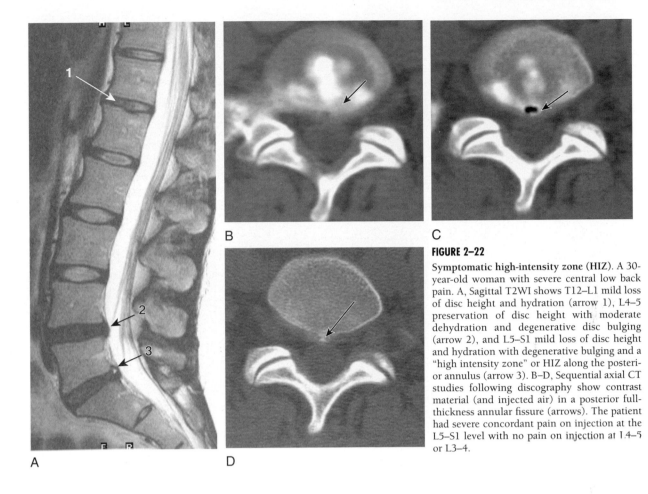

FIGURE 2–22

Symptomatic high-intensity zone (HIZ). A 30-year-old woman with severe central low back pain. A, Sagittal T2WI shows T12–L1 mild loss of disc height and hydration (arrow 1), L4–5 preservation of disc height with moderate dehydration and degenerative disc bulging (arrow 2), and L5–S1 mild loss of disc height and hydration with degenerative bulging and a "high intensity zone" or HIZ along the posterior annulus (arrow 3). B–D, Sequential axial CT studies following discography show contrast material (and injected air) in a posterior full-thickness annular fissure (arrows). The patient had severe concordant pain on injection at the L5–S1 level with no pain on injection at L4–5 or L3–4.

propose that most pain from disc herniation is chemical and that excision of the disc may actually exacerbate the pain; in his opinion, the pain should be controlled by oral or locally applied corticosteroids.

These theories may be regarded as forming complements of a larger whole rather than being mutually antagonistic. In some individuals, mechanical compression may predominate as the cause of radicular symptoms (Fig. 2–24), whereas in other patients chemical irritation predominates. Yet other patients may suffer from a combination of compression and irritation. Approaches to treatment may vary depending on which factor predominates: anti-inflammatory medication (oral or local) makes sense for chemical irritation, whereas surgery may be required for relief of mechanical compression. Later studies have evaluated schemes for grading compression and correlating compression with clinical symptoms (Beattie 2000, Boos 1998). Imaging is capable of indirectly showing the cause of chemical irritation, but the link between the imaging findings of chemical irritation and symptoms in a given patient is often tenuous.

NOMENCLATURE AND DESCRIPTION OF DISC HERNIATIONS

In 1999, Milette and coworkers noted:

The clinical usefulness of [MRI] is still being hindered by the lack of a standardized nomenclature for disc abnormalities. This lack of uniform terminology is probably partly responsible for the persistent controversy regarding prevention of back pain and sciatica.

As these authors note, traditional medical dictionary definitions are of little benefit. As noted by Fardon and colleagues (1993), confusing use of terminology runs rampant, and the situation is in many ways analogous to the status of mammography reporting in the 1980s, prior to the unifying force of the American College of Radiology's (ACR) lexicon. The advent of the ACR's lexicon did much to improve communications between mammography readers and clinicians. Recently, efforts at The North American Spine Society (NASS) led by David F. Fardon, and at the American Society of Neuroradiology (ASNR) and the associated American Society of Spine Radiology (ASSR) led by Pierre C. Milette, have resulted in a lexicon for lumbar disc pathology (Fardon 2001). This lexicon has received widespread support not only from NASS, ASNR, and ASSR but also from the Joint Section on Disorders of the Spine and Peripheral Nerves of the American Association of Neurological Surgeons (AANS), the Congress of Neurological Surgeons (CNS), and the CPT and ICD Coding Committee of the American Academy of Orthopaedic Surgeons (AAOS). This lexicon may do for spine imaging what the ACR lexicon did for mammography. The terminology outlined in the following sections is based on the NASS/ASNR/ASSR lexicon.

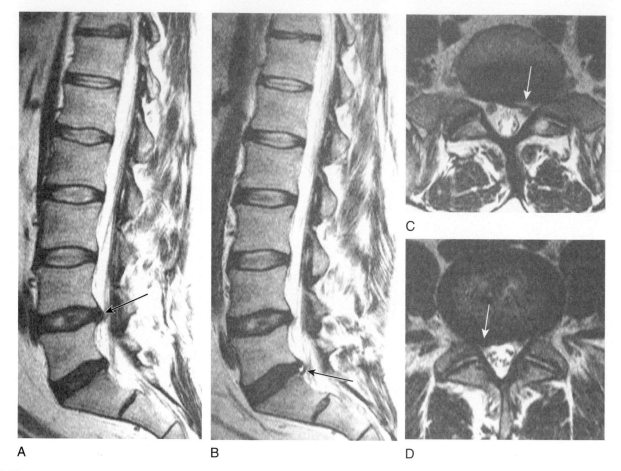

A B C D

FIGURE 2-23

Asymptomatic high-intensity zone (HIZ). A 44-year-old patient with exclusively right low back pain and right "hip" and lateral thigh pain. The patient had a remote history (17 years ago) of severe left low back, buttock, and posterior thigh pain that remitted after hospitalization and epidural steroid injections. A, Right parasagittal T2WI shows mild L4–5 disc dehydration and moderate L5–S1 disc dehydration. In addition, there is a disc protrusion at the L4–5 level (arrow). B, Left parasagittal T2WI shows similar findings, with, in addition, an HIZ (and small associated disc protrusion) (arrow). C, Axial T2WI at the L5–S1 disc level shows a small right central disc protrusion and HIZ directly adjacent to the left S1 nerve root (arrow). The patient's imaging findings at this level presumably represent the sequelae of remote injury and are not presently symptomatic. D, Axial T2WI at the L4–5 disc level shows a right central, subarticular, and foraminal disc protrusion with associated subarticular recess narrowing and compression of the traversing L5 nerve root (arrow). The patient obtained dramatic relief from a right L5 transforaminal epidural steroid injection, consistent with right L5 nerve root irritation as the cause of symptoms.

Disc Contour

Description of the disc margin contour uses several terms (Table 2–3). A *normal* disc contour is one in which the disc does not extend beyond the margin of the vertebral body by more than 1 to 2 mm. "Normal" includes the rare disc that actually demonstrates an indentation in the sagittal imaging plane (Fig. 2–25). Abnormalities of disc contour may be *generalized*, arbitrarily defined as involving more than 180 degrees or 50% of the disc circumference, and *localized*, defined as involving less than 180 degrees of the disc circumference. Generalized disc contour abnormalities, also known as *bulges*, extend beyond the vertebral body margin. This extension is generally limited to approximately 3 mm, although some bulges may be quite large (Fig. 2–26). Contour abnormalities involving less than 180 degrees (50%) of the disc circumference are called *localized displacements* or *disc herniations*. Disc herniations may be further divided into two categories: protrusions and extrusions. A *protrusion* is a localized abnormality of disc contour wherein the base of the abnormality measured along the circumference

of the disc is *greater than* the extension beyond the circumference, measured perpendicular to the base (Fig. 2–27). One may subclassify protrusions into focal protrusions, which involve less than 25% of the disc circumference, and broad-based protrusions, which involve between 25% and 50% of the disc circumference. An *extrusion* is a focal abnormality of disc contour wherein the base of the abnormality measured along the circumference is *less than* the extension beyond the circumference, measured perpendicular to the base (Fig. 2–28). Note that in most cases, the differentiation between protrusion and extrusion is made by reference to the axial images. In cases where disc material migrates cranially or caudally, however, it is necessary to measure from the vertebral end plate cranial or caudad on the sagittal images to see if the criteria of extrusion have been met by a disc contour abnormality (Figs. 2–29 and 2–30). What seems to be a relatively "flat" disc protrusion on axial scans may meet criteria for extrusion when sagittal images are reviewed, because the base of the disc herniation in the craniocaudad direction can be at most the height of the intervertebral disc. This implies that virtually all disc her-

TABLE 2–3. Disc Contour Abnormalities

Term	Definition
Normal	The disc contour does not extend beyond the margin of the vertebral body by more than 1–2 mm
Bulge	A *generalized* extension of the disc beyond the vertebral body margin, usually limited to approximately 3 mm. The contour abnormality involves at least 180 degrees (50%) of the disc circumference
Herniation	
Protrusion	A *localized* abnormality of disc contour wherein the base of the abnormality measured along the circumference of the disc is *greater than* the extension beyond the circumference, measured perpendicular to the base. *Focal protrusions* involve <25% of the disc circumference, whereas *broad-based protrusions* involve between 25% and 50% of the disc contour
Extrusion	A *localized* abnormality of disc contour wherein the base of the abnormality measured along the circumference of the disc is *greater than* the extension beyond the circumference, measured perpendicular to the base
Sequestration	Disc material that is no longer attached to the parent disc and is thus free in either the epidural (commonly) or subarachnoid (rarely) space

niations demonstrating cranial or caudal dissection are extrusions.

Although not a disc contour abnormality, a sequestration is another type of herniated disc: a *sequestration (or sequestered disc)* is a fragment of disc material that has broken free from the parent disc and is free in either the epidural space (the usual situation) or in the subarachnoid space (rarely) (Fig. 2–31).

Although the terms *bulge, protrusion,* and *extrusion* were once maintained to convey not only imaging characteristics but also to imply pathoanatomic significance (regarding the status of the annulus and so forth) (Masaryk 1988, Modic 1994), these terms are best regarded as strictly morphologic descriptors of imaging studies. For example, although a "bulge" was once thought to imply intact annular fibers, Yu and associates (1989) found full-thickness annular fissures in 84% of disc bulges. Similarly, disc contour abnormalities classified as "protrusions" do not necessarily have intact outer annular fibers covering nuclear material, and extrusions may consist of a combination of nuclear and annular material or exclusively annular material (Yasuma 1990). In addition, the terms do not specifically convey whether a given disc contour abnormality is a symptom-producing lesion or not. Although disc extrusions are rarely seen in asymptomatic patients (Boden 1990a, Boden 1990b, Jensen 1994, Matsumoto 1998, Stadnik 1998, Weishaupt 1998) and are more likely to be symptomatic than disc protrusions, a disc extrusion is not guaranteed to be the patient's problem (Boos 1998), and disc protrusions may be large (particularly if broad), and thus to be symptomatic, particularly if superimposed on a small spinal canal or neural

FIGURE 2–24

Disc herniation without accompanying radicular pain, but with conduction block (radiculopathy). A 42-year-old woman with left posterior thigh, calf, and heel numbness and decreased ankle jerk reflex. The patient had no back or leg pain. A, Sagittal T2WI shows moderate loss of disc height and hydration at the L5–S1 level and a large disc extrusion (arrow). B, Axial T2WI shows a left central disc extrusion (arrow 1) with posterior displacement and moderate compression of the traversing left S1 nerve root (arrow 2). Usually, such significant neural compression is associated with radicular pain, but in this patient the symptoms were limited to those of conduction block. Physical examination showed a decreased heel jerk on the left along with decreased sensation over the posterior left thigh and calf.

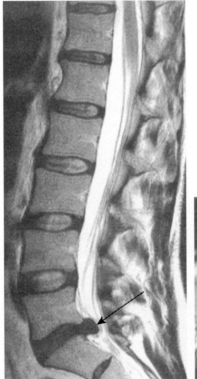

A

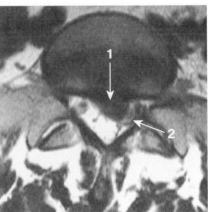

B

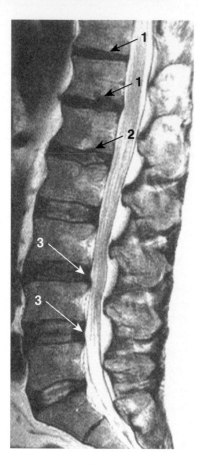

FIGURE 2–25

Normal variant of the intervertebral disc with an indentation of the disc margin. A 52-year-old patient with central low back pain. Sagittal T2WI shows multilevel degenerative disc disease with mild loss of disc height and moderate dehydration at T11–12 and T12–L1 (arrows 1). At L1–2, there is mild dehydration and a Schmorl's node (arrow 2), and there is similar mild dehydration at L3–4 and L4–5. Note that the posterior margins of L3–4 and L4–5 demonstrate a concavity (arrows 3), which is an infrequently seen but normal variation.

foramen (Fig. 2–32). Therefore, not only the type of disc contour abnormality but its size and associated neural compression must be noted.

Disc Herniation Size

Terms to describe the size of an abnormal disc contour are necessarily arbitrary, because disc herniations can range in size from 1 to more than 20 mm in greatest dimension. Our use of the terms *small, medium,* and *large* employs different cutoffs in the lumbar and cervical spine in recognition of the space available before neural compression ensues (Table 2–4). The abnormal contour is measured (in millimeters) from a line connecting the posteroinferior corner of the vertebra at the level above and the posterosuperior corner of the vertebra below the disc. Use of such terminology is optional, and the degree of neural compression is more important than the size of the disc herniation.

Disc Herniation and Neural Compression

As noted earlier, careful studies of the description of neural compression have appeared since 1998 (Beattie 2000, Boos

TABLE 2–4. Disc Herniation Size

Term	Lumbar (mm)	Cervical (mm)
Small	<5	<2.5
Moderate	6–10	2.6–5.0
Large	>10	>5.0

1998). Within our group, we have employed terms denoting neural compression for more than 15 years, with a system of internal training and peer review to ensure consistency of reporting. This system uses terms in a different manner than described by Beattie and associates (2000) but makes use of mild, moderate, and severe in a consistent, reproducible manner that conveys to the referring physician the degree of neural compression (Table 2–5) (Figs. 2–33 and 2–34). Compression causes a change in the configuration of the spinal cord, nerve root, ganglion, or nerve. In almost all instances, these structures are round or nearly round (oval) in cross section. Compression is indicated by loss of this circular configuration, with the structure first deformed into an oblong oval, and eventually flattening into a thin ribbon of tissue. In some cases, particularly in the subauricular recesses and cervical neural foramina, the degree of neural compression may be difficult to determine. In this case, if there is undoubtedly neural compression, then this should be noted without qualification of mild, moderate, or severe (Fig. 2–35).

Imaging is nearly always performed in a supine, non-weight-bearing position, and this may underestimate the degree of neural compression (Schmid 1999, Weishaupt 2000, Willen 2001). Note that although studies have demonstrated that the degree of neural compression is predictive in a general way with respect to symptom production and relief with surgery, there is a large amount of variation in the degree of symptom production for the same amount of neural compression in different patients (Wada 1999). Elucidation of the source of this variation remains uncertain, but possible reasons include the presence of additional compression elsewhere along the course of the same nerve (Olmarker 1992, Porter 1992) and the rapidity of onset of compression. Thus, acute disc herniations producing moderate or even mild degrees of neural compression may cause pronounced symptoms, whereas the same degree of compression caused by a gradually developing process (e.g., foraminal stenosis secondary to osteophytic spurring and loss of disc height) may produce no symptoms.

TABLE 2–5. Neural Compression Definitions

Term	Definition
Mild	75–99% of normal diameter of the structure maintained
Moderate	50–74% of the diameter of the structure maintained
Severe	<50% of the diameter of the structure maintained

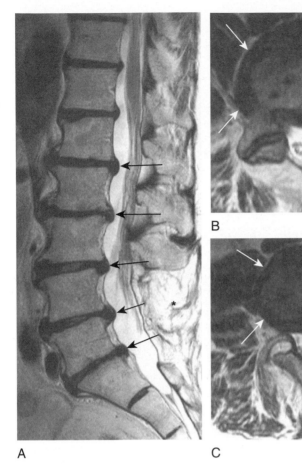

A

B

C

FIGURE 2–26

Large disc bulges. A 71-year-old man with chronic central low back pain. A, Sagittal T2WI showing universal severe loss of disc height and hydration and disc bulging. Anteroposterior dimension of the bulges exceeds 5 mm at all levels in the lumbar spine (arrows). There is also posterior decompression from L3–4 through L5–S1 (*). B, Axial T2WI at L4–5 showing circumferential nature of the disc contour abnormality (arrows) and posterior decompression (*). C, Axial T2WI at L3–4 showing similar circumferential disc contour abnormality (arrows).

Disc Herniation Position

The position of disc herniations determines the route of administered drugs in epidural steroid injections and the surgical approach if an operation is required. The position of focal disc contour abnormalities needs to be reported in terms of the circumference of the parent disc (Table 2–6) (Figs. 2–27 to 2–29, 2–33). Note that many disc contour abnormalities involve more than one location, and hence a disc protrusion may be, for example, "left central, subarticular, and foraminal" (Figs. 2–32 and 2–34). Note that the term *lateral recess* is not used in the description of the position of disc contour abnormalities at the level of the disc, because the lateral recess is the portion of the spinal canal along the medial aspect of the pedicle, and as such is not *at* the level of the disc. Cranially and caudally dissecting discs might *reach* the lateral recess, in which case this term may be used (Fig. 2–30).

Disc Herniation Dissection

Dissection is described as "cranial" or "caudal" and is measured in millimeters from the posteroinferior corner of the vertebral body above in cranial dissection, and the postero-superior corner of the vertebral body below in caudal dissection (Figs. 2–28 to 2–30).

Disc Herniation Signal Intensity

The signal intensity of the abnormal disc contour may demonstrate variable degrees of T1 and T2 shortening

TABLE 2–6. Location of Disc Contour Abnormalities

Term	Definition
Central	In the mid-posterior disc. Left or right central may be used if the disc contour abnormalities favor one side or the other
Subarticular	Lateral to a parasagittal plane through the medial edge of the articular facet but medial to a parasagittal plane through the medial aspect of the ipsilateral pedicle
Foraminal	Along the foraminal portion of the disc; that is, between the parasagittal planes defined by the medial and lateral aspects of the pedicle
Extraforaminal (or "far lateral")	Lateral to the foramen; that is, lateral to the parasagittal plane defined by the lateral border of the pedicle

and prolongation (Fig. 2–36). Although most disc contour abnormalities are easily detected on T2WI, occasional lesions may be seen much more easily (or exclusively) on T1WI. Foraminal lesions and those dissecting caudally from the L5/S1 level are most likely to exhibit these characteristics (Figs. 2–17 and 2–37). Occasionally, disc contour abnormalities may demonstrate T2 prolongation (relative to the parent disc) (Glickstein 1989, Masaryk 1988). Inhomogeneity of disc signal should be specifically noted,

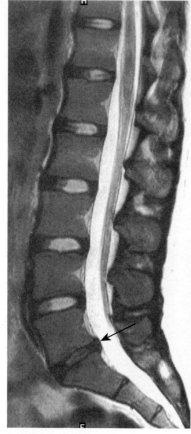

A

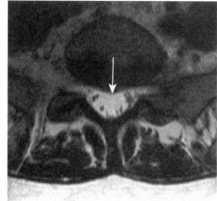

B

FIGURE 2–27

Disc protrusion. A 19-year-old patient with central low back and bilateral leg pain. A, Sagittal T2WI demonstrates moderate loss of disc height and dehydration at L5–S1. In addition, there is a central 3.3-mm disc protrusion (arrow). B, Axial T2WI demonstrates minimal thecal sac indentation from the disc protrusion (arrow).

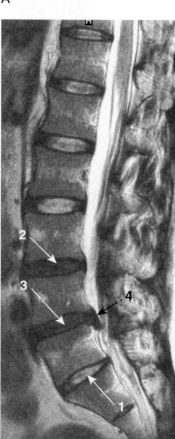

A

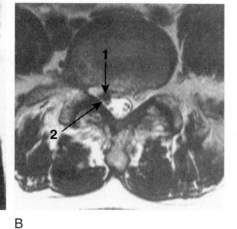

B

FIGURE 2–28

Disc extrusion. A 40-year-old man with a 5-month history of posterior right thigh and leg pain. A, Right parasagittal T2WI. The patient has transitional anatomy, with the lowest most well-developed disc termed 31–2 (arrow 1). There is mild loss of disc height and moderate disc dehydration at the L4–5 (arrow 2) and L5–S1 (arrow 3) levels. There is also a small, caudally dissecting right subarticular disc extrusion at the L5–S1 level (arrow 4). B, Axial T2WI slightly inferior to the level of the L5–S1 disc. The caudally dissecting portion of the disc (arrow 1) lies directly in front of and compresses the traversing right S1 nerve root (arrow 2).

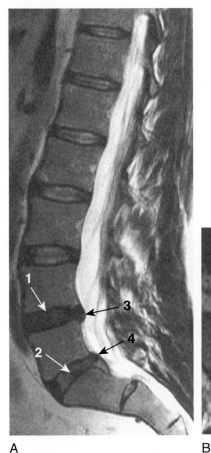

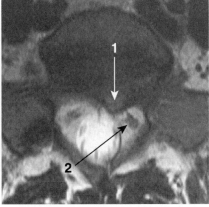

A

B

FIGURE 2–29

Disc extrusion. A 49-year-old man with left low back and buttock pain. A, Sagittal T2WI shows moderate L4–5 disc dehydration (arrow 1) and mild L5–S1 disc dehydration at L5–S1 (arrow 2). There is an L4–5 disc protrusion (arrow 3) and an L5–S1 caudally dissecting disc extrusion (arrow 4). B, Axial T2WI below the level of the disc shows the left central, caudally dissecting component of the disc extrusion (arrow 1) with intermediate signal intensity and slight displacement of the S1 nerve root (arrow 2). Note that on axial images, the disc contour abnormality does not meet the criteria of extrusion (with the dimension of the extension beyond the base exceeding the dimension of the base), whereas on sagittal images it clearly does meet the criteria (since the base can be no wider than the disc at the level of the abnormality).

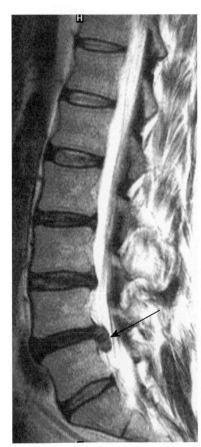

A

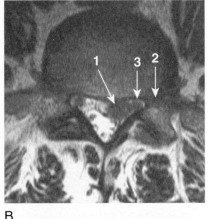

B

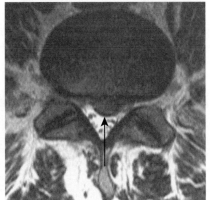

C

FIGURE 2–30

Disc extrusion. A 46-year-old man with low back and left "hip," lateral thigh, and calf pain. A, Left parasagittal T2WI shows L2–3 and L3–4 mild and L4–5 moderate disc dehydration. In addition, there is a caudally dissecting disc extrusion at the L4–5 level (arrow). B, Axial T2WI at the level of the L5 pedicles. The disc extrusion (arrow 1) has reached the "lateral recess" adjacent to the medial aspect of the L5 pedicle (arrow 2), where there is mild compression of the preganglionic L5 nerve root (arrow 3). C, Axial T2WI at the level of the disc shows a central disc contour abnormality (arrow). Although the base of this abnormality is of greater dimension than its anteroposterior measurement on axial images, the lesion is classified as an "extrusion" based on the appearance on sagittal images.

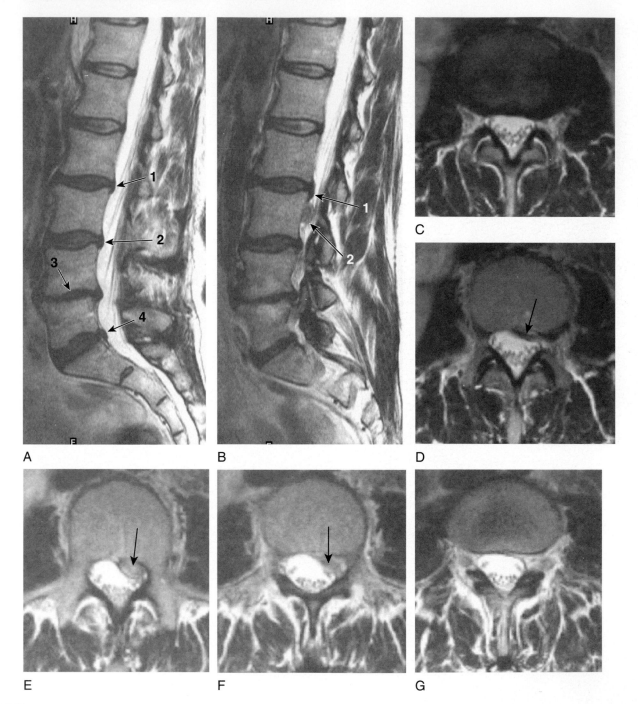

FIGURE 2–31

Sequestered disc. A 52-year-old woman with low back and left anterior thigh pain. A, Sagittal T2WI shows multilevel degenerative change including L2–3 mild loss of disc height and moderate disc dehydration with degenerative disc bulging (arrow 1), L3–4 mild disc dehydration with minimally abnormal disc contour (arrow 2), L4–5 severe loss of disc height and hydration (arrow 3) with degenerative disc bulging and Modic Type I subchondral degenerative changes, and L5–S1 moderate disc dehydration and disc bulging (arrow 4). B, Left parasagittal T2WI shows a small L2–3 disc extrusion with caudal and cranial dissection (arrow 1). In addition, there is a 7 × 12 mm apparently sequestered fragment posterior to the upper half of the L2 vertebral body (arrow 2). C–G, Sequential axial T2WIs from the L3 to the L2–3 disc level demonstrate the caudally dissecting sequestered fragment (arrow) in the left lateral recess medial to the L3 pedicle. No connection exists between the free fragment and parent disc (more likely L2–3 than L3–4, given the appearance on D).

because this may be an indication of a combination of displaced nuclear and annular material or associated hemorrhage (Gundry 1993) (Fig. 2–38) (see following discussions).

Disc Herniation Imaging Findings

Disc herniations may have a variety of imaging findings, and each finding has a differential diagnosis (Table 2–7). Other disc contour abnormalities are discussed in previous sections. Synovial cysts are discussed later in this chapter in

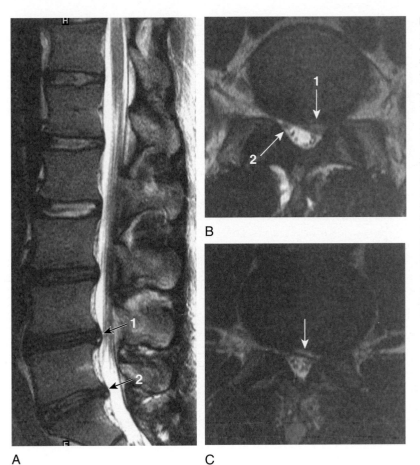

A   **C**

FIGURE 2–32

Symptomatic disc protrusion. A 22-year-old man with sudden-onset low back and left leg pain. A, Sagittal T2WI shows multilevel disease with L5–S1 mild loss of disc height and hydration, L4–5 moderate loss of disc height and hydration, and mild dehydration at T12–L1, L1–2, and L3–4. The patient has an inherently small spinal canal with superimposed disc protrusions at L4–5 (arrow 1) and L5–S1 (arrow 2). B, Axial T2WI at the level of the L5–S1 disc. There is a left central and subarticular disc protrusion (arrow 1) with severe subarticular recess narrowing. Although the right S1 nerve root may be slightly posteriorly displaced (arrow 2), the left S1 nerve root is not seen as a distinct entity and is thus severely compressed in the subarticular recess. C, Axial T2WI at the L4–5 disc level. There is a left central and subarticular disc protrusion (arrow) with severe left subarticular narrowing and compression of the traversing left L5 nerve root. This case shows several interesting features, including (1) the coexistence of multilevel Schmorl's nodes and degenerative disc disease in the lower lumbar spine (juvenile discogenic disease); (2) symptomatic disc protrusions secondary to superimposition of small lesions on an inherently small spinal canal; and (3) limited soft tissue contrast secondary to a general lack of fat in this young, muscular man.

the section, "Facet Arthropathy," and tumors are discussed in Chapter 4.

Disc Herniation, Hematomas, and Fluid Collections

Hematomas and fluid collections may accompany disc herniations or other degenerative changes and be associated with radicular symptoms and/or back pain with a presentation similar to disc herniations (Chiba 2001, Gundry 1993, Watanabe 1997). Anatomically, such collections lie anterior to the peridural membrane as described by Wiltse and associates (1993). The imaging characteritics of such hematomas and fluid collections may bear a striking resemblance to disc extrusions (Chiba 2001, Gundry 1993, Watanabe 1997) (Figs. 2–38 and 2–39). Clues to differentiation of hematomas and fluid collections from extruded disc herniations are the often small disc contour abnormalities at the level of the disc; the variation in signal intensity between the lesion away from the disc and the disc contour abnormality; an obtuse margin along the posterior aspect of the vertebral body; and maximum dimension at or near the mid-vertebral body (Fig. 2–39). Such lesions may be constrained by the central septum, a sagittal structure that tacks the posterior longitudinal ligament to the posterior vertebral body away from the disc margin (Schellinger 1990) (Fig. 2–39). The hematomas and fluid collections may explain the rapid resolution of imaging abnormalites documented in some individuals (Mochica 1998) and the

TABLE 2–7. Disc Herniation Imaging Findings

Finding	Differential Diagnosis
Generalized (>180 degrees or 50%) extension beyond adjacent vertebral body on sequential axial images	Disc bulge "Pseudodisc" caused by spondylolisthesis Remodeling with osteoporosis
Focal soft tissue lesion apparently extending from the intervertebral disc	Disc protrusion Disc extrusion Disc sequestration still adjacent to the parent disc Hematoma or fluid collection Gas collection (Tamburrelli 2000) Tumor adjacent to the disc (see Chapter 4)
Epidural soft tissue lesion	Extruded disc Sequestered disc Epidural hematoma Synovial cyst Tumor (see Chapter 4)

lack of surgical findings in some (first noted, interestingly, by Mixter and Barr [1934]). Such hematomas and fluid collections may resolve spontaneously or persist until relieved by surgical decompression. Even if specifically sought at surgery, they may not be identified since puncture of the margin of the lesion may be followed by aspiration of a small

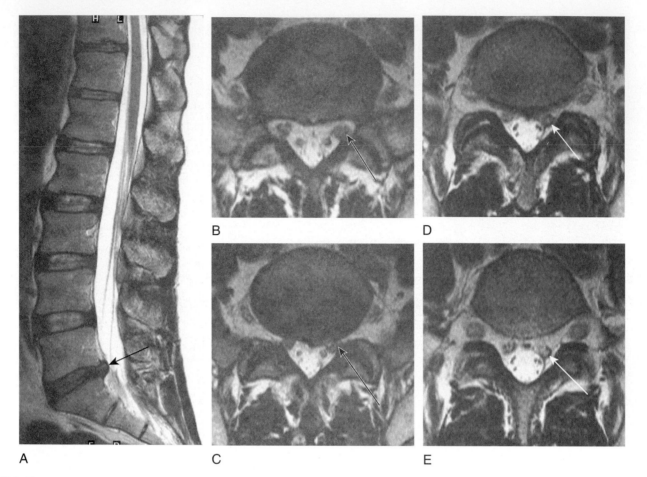

FIGURE 2–33

Mild neural compression. A 54-year-old man with left buttock, posterior thigh, and calf pain. A, Sagittal T2WI shows mild loss of disc height and hydration at L5–S1 along with a small disc protrusion (arrow). B–E, Sequential axial T2WIs from the top of the S1 pedicles through the mid-neural foramen level show posterior displacement and mild compression of the left S1 nerve root (arrow) by the left central disc protrusion. The nerve root sleeve is flattened by less than 25%.

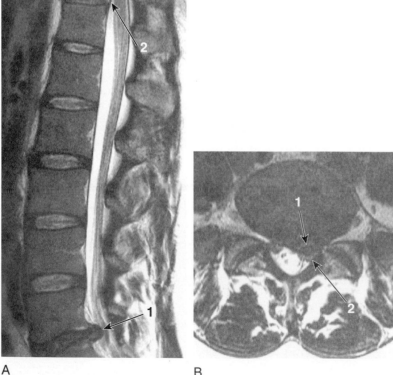

FIGURE 2–34

Severe neural compression. A 34-year-old man with posterior right thigh and calf pain. A, Sagittal T2WI shows L5–S1 moderate loss of disc height and hydration and a large disc contour abnormality (arrow 1). There is also T11–12 mild disc dehydration and an additional disc protrusion (arrow 2). B, Axial T2WI at the level of the L4–S1 disc demonstrates the large left central and subarticular disc protrusion (arrow) that causes posterior displacement and more than 50% (severe) compression of the S1 nerve root (arrow 2).

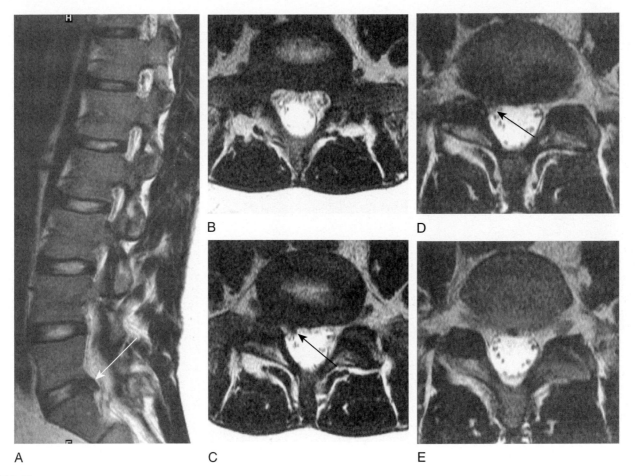

FIGURE 2–35

Neural compression in the subarticular recess and thus difficult to quantify. A 23-year-old patient with right buttock and posterior thigh pain for 5 weeks. A, Right parasagittal T2WI shows a small, caudally dissecting disc extrusion at the L5–S1 level (arrow). B–E, Sequential axial T2WIs from the S1 pedicle through the level of the L5–S1 disc confirm a small lesion in the subarticular zone of the disc margin (arrow), but quantification of S1 neural compression is not possible since the degree of deformity of the traversing S1 nerve root cannot be confidently estimated; in these instances the neural compression should be noted but not quantified as "mild," "medium," or "moderate."

amount of bloody fluid taken to be a consequence of surgical dissection. The main clinical significance of such collections is that related symptoms may resolve relatively, rapidly without specific treatment. This may explain the lack of impressive surgical findings at a level with what appears to be a large disc extrusion on MR imaging.

Unusual Findings of Disc Herniations

Disc extrusions and sequestrations may have a number of unusual findings, particularly when the connection with the parent disc is tenuous and the extruded or sequestered material has a linear or filamentous rather than a rounded appearance (Figs. 2–40 and 2–41). Careful correlation with the patient's pain diagram and symptoms of radiculopathy and radicular pain may help focus attention on particular "trouble spots" where material may be somewhat difficult to see (see "Pain Diagram" section and Fig. 2–6). This includes alongside the S1 nerve roots in the anterior epidural fat at the L5/S1 level (Figs. 2–17 and 2–42), within the lateral recess or paralleling the dorsal root ganglion (Fig. 2–41), in the neural foramen (Figs. 2–37, 2–40, and 2–43), or lateral to the neural foramen. Cervical foraminal

disc protrusions may be difficult to diagnose because of the crowded nature of structures in this region (see later). Similarly, herniations in muscular individuals where soft tissue contrast is decreased may result in difficulty in diagnosis (Fig. 2–32). On occasion, bubbles of gas along the disc margin, presumably emanating from a degenerated disc with a vacuum phenomenon and sometimes assumed to represent a type of disc herniation, cause radiculopathy (Tamburrelli 2000). Such gas collections may be difficult to recognize on MRI, since the uniform decreased signal intensity on all imaging sequences may mimic displaced annular material.

Cauda Equina Syndrome

Cauda equina syndrome is bilateral lower extremity symptoms (pain and/or weakness), saddle anesthesia, and urinary incontinence or retention (Ahn 2000, Shapiro 2000). These symptoms may be caused by large disc herniations within the lumbar spine compressing traversing nerve roots, or even moderate-sized disc herniations superimposed on an inherently small spinal canal. Whereas most disc herniations are not medical emergencies and treatment may be post-

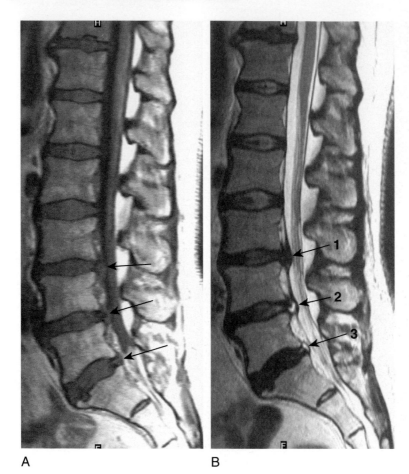

A   B

FIGURE 2–36

Variable signal intensity within disc herniations. A 54-year-old woman with low back pain radiating into the left leg. A, Sagittal T1WI. The disc contour abnormalities at L3–4, L4–5, and L5–S1 (arrows) are isointense with the parent discs. B, Sagittal T2WI. L3–4, L4–5, and L5–S1 all demonstrate mild loss of disc height with associated mild disc dehydration at L3–4 and L4–5 and moderate disc dehydration at L5–S1. The disc herniation at L3–4 (arrow 1) is isointense with the parent disc, whereas the lesions at L4–5 (arrow 2) and L5–S1 (arrow 3) demonstrate T2 prolongation and are hyperintense relative to the parent discs.

poned without adverse consequences, delay in operation on patients with the cauda equina syndrome may result in persistent loss of bladder control, permanent severe motor deficit, and permanent sexual dysfunction (Ahn 2000, Shapiro 2000). Any patient suspected to have cauda equina syndrome should undergo imaging immediately. Any clinician referring a patient who has severe spinal canal narrowing from a disc herniation should be called with the results of the study.

Disc Herniation and Anomalous Nerve Roots

Nerve roots may arise at anomalous locations from the thecal sac, either too high (cranial origin, seen in less than 1% of subjects), too low (caudal origin, seen in approximately 1% to 2% of subjects), or two sets of nerve roots may occupy a single nerve root sleeve (conjoined nerve roots, seen in <1% of subjects) (Haijiao 2001). These anomalies are not necessarily intrinsically painful, but they complicate the presentation and treatment of disc herniation. If two sets of nerve roots exit via the same neural foramen, the clinical presentation of a disc herniation may be confusing since two adjacent dermatomes may be involved with radicular pain. In addition, any space-occupying lesion within the foramen is liable to produce symptoms that are both earlier in onset and more severe than if only one root occupied the neural foramen (Bogduk 1997). Furthermore, White and colleagues (1982) have noted that discectomy

for a herniated disc at the level of a conjoined nerve root will have poor results unless it is accompanied by a pediculectomy. Therefore, the coexistence of these two conditions needs to be explicitly mentioned in the report. Cranial-origin nerve roots are infrequently accompanied by clinical manifestations, but caudal origin of nerve roots brings the nerve roots and ganglion into a lower position relative to the neural foramen of the lumbar spine, where small foraminal disc protrusions and disc bulges that would otherwise not compress the ganglion may be more likely to present with symptoms (Fig. 2–44).

Disc Herniation and Contrast Enhancement

Evaluation of degenerative disc disease certainly does not require contrast medium; occasionally, however, contrast medium is given to evaluate other findings in patients with simultaneous degenerative disease or to help elucidate a puzzling finding. In general, disc herniations do not demonstrate contrast enhancement, but exceptions to this rule occur. A single nerve root occasionally enhances in a linear fashion, and this enhancement has been associated with breakdown of the blood-brain barrier, radiculopathy, and radicular pain (Crisi 1993, Georgy 1996, Kobayashi 1993). The finding is not uniformly found in cases of herniated discs and associated radiculopathy and has little clinical value in routine evaluation of degenerative disease of the spine.

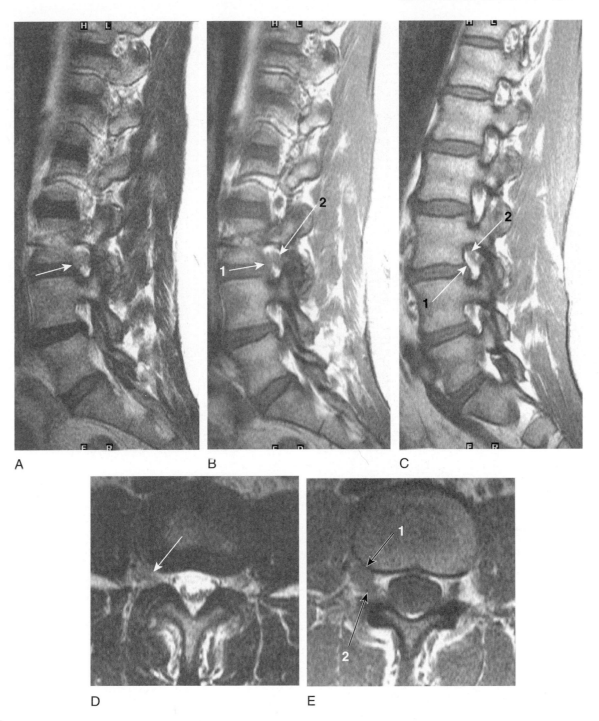

FIGURE 2–37

Disc herniation more conspicuous on T1WI. A 50-year-old woman with right anterior thigh and groin pain. *A,* Parasagittal T2WI at the level of the right neural foramina demonstrates subtle excess soft tissue at the L3–4 foraminal level (arrow), which could easily be attributed to a prominent ganglion. *B,* Parasagittal T1WI at the same level as A, more clearly showing the anterior disc extrusion (arrow 1) with posterior displacement of the exiting L3 ganglion (arrow 2). *C,* Parasagittal T1WI of the contralateral side, showing a small disc protrusion inferior to the disc at the L3–4 level (arrow 1) but clear fat anterior to the L3 ganglion (arrow 2). *D,* Axial T2WI at the level of the lesion shows subtle asymmetry of the foramen (arrow), with more soft tissue within the right neural foramen. *E,* Axial T1WI at the level of the lesion shows the disc extrusion (arrow 1) more clearly, with posterior displacement of the exiting ganglion (arrow 2). As seen on this study, foraminal lesions frequently demonstrate greater conspicuity on T1WI.

Disc Herniation: Special Considerations in the Cervical Spine

As pediatricians repeatedly admonish medical students, children are not miniature adults. Similarly, the cervical spine is no scale model of the lumbar spine. Major differ-

ences between the cervical and lumbar spine include the following:

1. A thinner posterolateral disc annulus (Mercer 1999). This anatomic difference predisposes toward posterolateral herniation of disc material (Fig. 2–45).

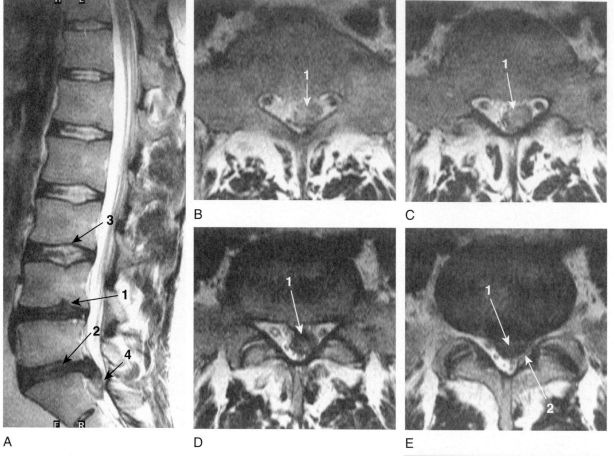

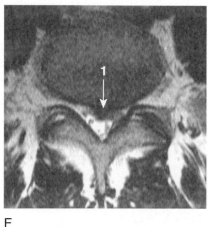

FIGURE 2–38

Disc herniation with accompanying hematoma fluid. This 29-year-old patient had sudden onset of severe low back and left buttock and leg pain after lifting weights. A, Sagittal T2WI demonstrates mild loss of disc height and moderate disc dehydration at L4–5 (arrow 1) and L5–S1 (arrow 2) as well as mild disc dehydration at L3–4 (arrow 3) and multilevel Schmorl's node formation. There is a large, caudally dissecting disc extrusion at the L5–S1 level with signal intensity inhomogeneity (arrow 4). B–F, Sequential axial T2WIs from the S1 pedicle to the level of the L5–S1 disc show that the spinal canal is nearly filled with herniated disc material (arrow 1), with the thecal sac compressed along the posterolateral, right side of the spinal canal. The lesion causes severe compression of the traversing S1 nerve root (arrow 2). There is inhomogeneity of signal intensity of the extruded material. At surgery, the amount of extruded disc material was much smaller than that demonstrated on the MRI, with the more caudally located tissue (demonstrating different signal intensity than the parent disc) felt to represent hematoma fluid.

2. Differences in composition of the nucleus (Mercer 1999). The amount of nuclear material and its fluidity, particularly in any spine past juvenile development, is greatly decreased relative to the lumbar spine.
3. The upturning lateral margins known as the *uncinate processes*, which may have associated joints of Luschka. Whether these are true joints or a manifestation of (nearly universal) degenerative change is a matter of controversy. Osteophytic spurring along these joints narrows the intervertebral nerve root canals, contributing to neural compression. This makes small disc protrusions more likely to be symptomatic because of decreased capacity within the intervertebral nerve root canals and at the

same time more difficult to diagnose because of the smaller size of the foramen.
4. The spinal cord is immediately adjacent to the disc margin (Fig. 2–46). Compression of the spinal cord may produce symptoms of myelopathy, particularly if this compression is acute or severe. Patients may present with lower extremity weakness or even bowel and bladder problems secondary to cord compression. Grading of spinal cord compression is the same as grading compression of other neural structures (see Table 2–5).
5. The more lateral location of the facet joints relative to the central spinal canal. The facet joints basically form the posterior wall of the intervertebral nerve root canals

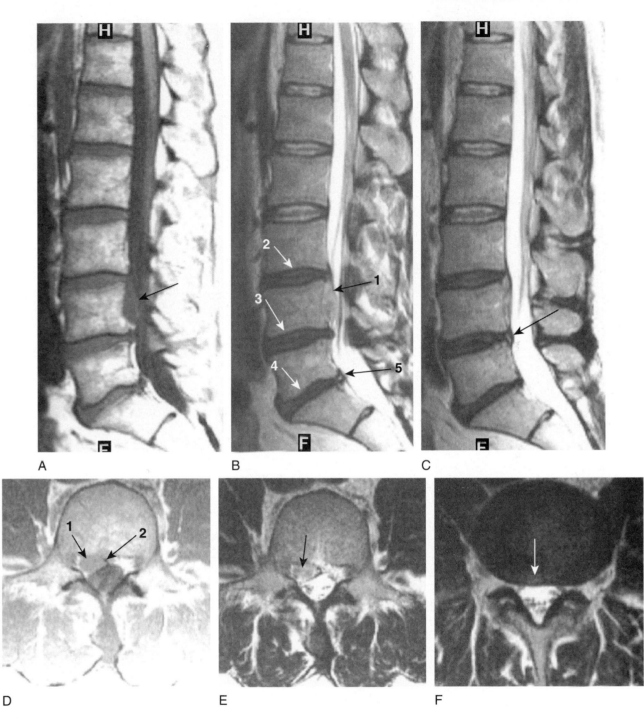

FIGURE 2–39

Disc herniation with accompanying hematoma. A 45-year-old man with right foot drop and severe right leg pain. A, Right parasagittal T1WI shows a relatively subtle lens-shaped hematoma posterior to the L4 level (arrow). B, Right parasagittal T2WI shows the same hematoma, now much more conspicuous, with intermediate and mixed signal intensity (arrow 1). Also noted are mild loss of disc height and moderate disc dehydration at L3–4 (arrow 2) and L4–5 (arrow 3) and severe loss of disc height at L5–S1 (arrow 4). At the L5–S1 level, there is degenerative disc bulging and a posterior high-intensity zone (arrow 5). C, Right parasagittal T2WI closer to midline (than B). The cranially dissecting component of the hematoma is much less conspicuous, whereas the disc margin at L4–5 demonstrates a small disc protrusion with a focus of T2 prolongation (arrow). D, Axial T1WI at the level of the L4 pedicles shows the hematoma (arrow 1) displacing the thecal sac posteriorly. Note that, medially, the hematoma is constrained by the central septum (Schellinger 1990) (arrow 2). E, Axial T2WI at the level of the L4 pedicles again shows inhomogeneity and intermediate signal intensity of the hematoma (arrow). F, Axial T2WI through the level of the L4–5 disc shows the small focus of T2 prolongation (arrow). Characteristics of hematoma demonstrated in this case include minimal mass at the level of the disc, the lens shape of the lesion, the mixed signal intensity within the lesion, and the fact that the anteroposterior dimension of the lesion is maximum well away from the disc, at about the mid-L4 vertebral body.

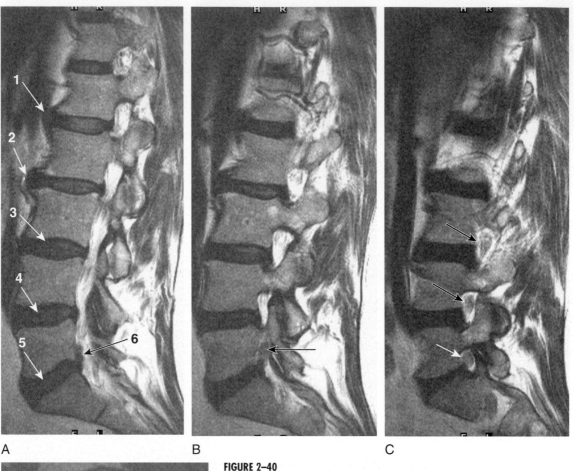

A

B

C

D

FIGURE 2–40

Unusual appearance of disc herniation with a linear appearance of extruded material. A 58-year-old woman with low back pain, right "hip" pain, and lateral thigh pain. A, Right parasagittal T2WI shows multilevel degenerative changes, including L1–2 anterior osteophytic spurring and subchondral marrow changes (arrow 1), L2–3 mild loss of disc height, anterior osteophytic spurring (arrow 2), L3–4 mild disc dehydration (arrow 3), L4–5 moderate disc dehydration (arrow 4), and L5–S1 mild loss of disc height and moderate disc dehydration (arrow 5). Posterior to the lower aspect of the L5 vertebra is a linear lesion measuring 4.4 mm in anteroposterior dimension and showing 11 mm of cranial dissection (arrow 6). B, Right parasagittal T2WI (slightly more lateral than A) shows intermediate signal intensity filling the right L4–5 neural foramen (arrow), with an appearance suggestive of a ganglion. C, Right parasagittal T2WI (more lateral yet) shows the dorsal root ganglia at the L3–4, L4–5, and L5–S1 levels (arrows). D, Axial T2WI just above the level of the L5–S1 disc shows the L5 ganglia (arrow 1) to have intermediate signal intensity bilaterally. The disc extrusion mimicking a ganglion on image B lies medial to the ganglion and is of lesser signal intensity (arrow 2).

(neural foramina). Thus, there is no "subarticular recess" in the cervical spine (as there is in the lumbar spine). The descriptors of the disc margin are thus *central* (or *left central* or *right central*), *foraminal*, and *far lateral* (Fig. 2–47).

6. Numbering of the nerves. Whereas lumbar nerves exit under the same numbered pedicle (e.g., L3 exits the spinal canal under the L3 pedicle), the cervical nerves exit over the same numbered pedicle (e.g., the C6 nerve leaves the spinal canal via the C5–6 intervertebral nerve root canal, above the C6 pedicle). C8 exits at the C7–T1

level, and T1 exits under the T1 pedicle at the T1–2 level (so the thoracic spine is numbered as the lumbar spine).

Disc Herniation: Special Considerations in the Thoracic Spine

As in the cervical spine, thoracic disc herniations may cause cord compression and result in myelopathy. Disc herniations of the thoracic spine are less frequent than those of the cervical and lumbar spine and are often accompanied by Scheuermann's disease (see the section "Scheuermann's

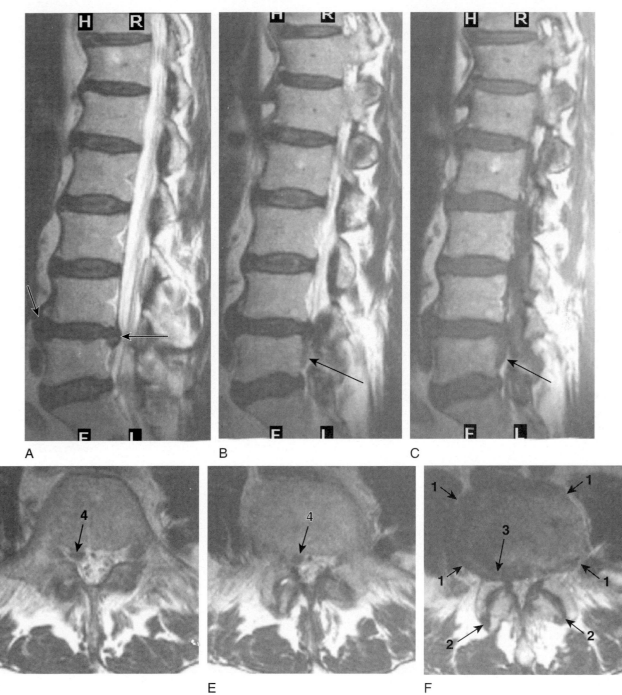

FIGURE 2–41

Unusual appearance of disc herniation with a linear appearance of extruded material. A 78-year-old man with low back and right "hip" and lateral thigh pain. A, Right parasagittal T2WI shows multilevel degenerative disc disease with T12–L1 mild loss of disc height and hydration and L1–2, L2–3, L3–4, and L5–S1 mild disc dehydration. L4–5 demonstrates mild loss of disc height and moderate disc dehydration as well as degenerative disc bulging (arrows). There are anterior osteophytes at all levels. B, Right parasagittal T2WI (lateral to A) shows a linear focus of T2 shortening along the dorsal surface of the L5 vertebral body (arrow). C, Right parasagittal T1WI (matching B) shows the lesion to have the same signal characteristics as the intervertebral disc (arrow). D–F, Sequential axial T2WIs from inferior to superior ending at the level of the L4–5 intervertebral disc. At the level of the disc, there is degenerative disc bulging (arrows 1) and moderate facet arthropathy (arrows 2), with a superimposed right central, subarticular, and foraminal disc contour abnormality (arrow 3). Inferior to the disc, there is caudally dissecting disc extrusion medial to the L5 ganglion (arrow 4).

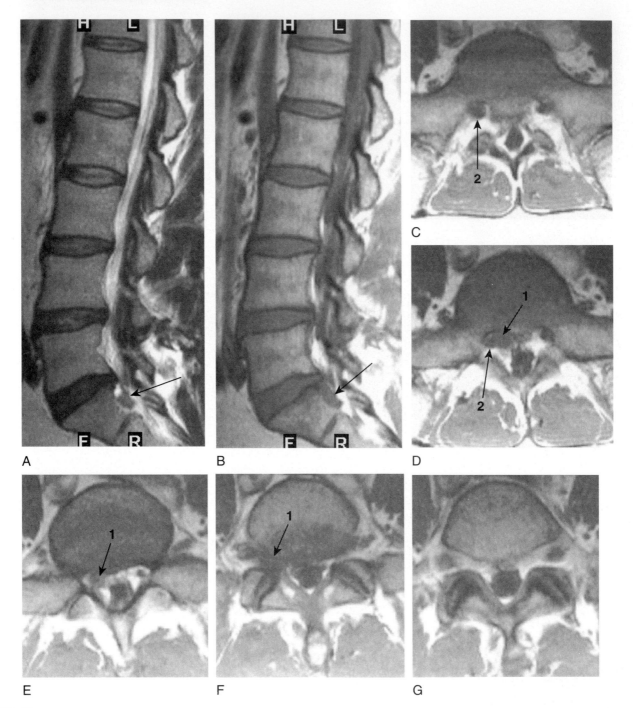

FIGURE 2–42

Unusual appearance of disc herniation with a linear appearance of extruded material along the S1 nerve root sleeve. A 53-year-old man with pain in right buttock, posterior thigh, and calf and right foot numbness. A, Parasagittal T2WI shows abnormal intermediate signal intensity soft tissue along the dorsum of the proximal S1 segment (arrow) that could be mistaken for the S1 nerve root. B, Parasagittal T1WI at a similar location to A confirms abnormal soft tissue (arrow). C–G, Sequential axial T1WIs from the S1 pedicle to just above the L5–S1 disc show a right subarticular and foraminal disc herniation at the level of the disc (D) (arrow 1), with a caudally dissecting extrusion paralleling the medial aspect of the S1 nerve root (F).

Disease, Thoracolumbar Osteochondrosis, and Juvenile Discogenic Disease").

TREATMENT

Treatment of disc herniation varies greatly. Surgical removal clearly offers great benefit to correctly chosen patients, but

the choice depends on a great deal more than whether the lesion meets the criteria of "protrusion" or "extrusion." As noted earlier, studies have found multiple variables related to outcome from surgery. Spengler and Freeman (1979) achieved good results by basing the decision to operate on a combination of four findings: neurologic signs, sciatic tension signs, personality factors (Minnesota Multiphasic

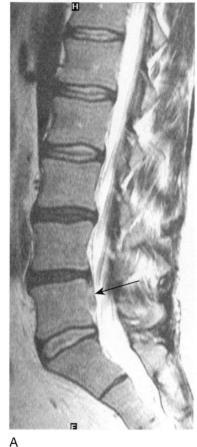

A

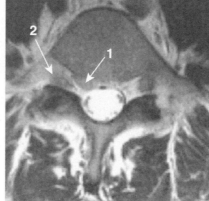

B

FIGURE 2–43

Unusual appearance of disc herniation with a linear appearance of extruded material. A 37-year-old man with low back and right "hip" and lateral thigh pain, along with right leg tingling, weakness, and numbness. A, Sagittal T2WI shows mild loss of disc height and moderate disc dehydration at L3–4 and L4–5, as well as prominence of soft tissue behind the posterior, superior aspect of the L5 vertebral body resembling a nerve root (arrow). B, Axial image just below the L5 pedicle shows a disc extrusion (arrow 1) causing lateral displacement and compression of the exiting L5 ganglion (arrow 2).

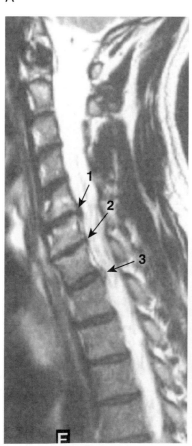

A

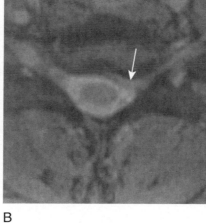

B

FIGURE 2–45

Paracentral cervical disc extrusion. A 44-year-old man with severe left neck, shoulder, and arm pain. A, Left parasagittal T2WI shows disc narrowing and osteophytic spurring at both the C5–6 (arrow 1) and C6–7 (arrow 2) levels. At C7–T1, there is a 3.0-mm anteroposterior dimension disc extrusion demonstrating minimal cranial and caudal dissection (arrow 3). B, Axial gradient-recalled echo T2WI at the level of the disc shows the disc extrusion (arrow) filling the entrance zone of the neural foramen with right C8 nerve root compression.

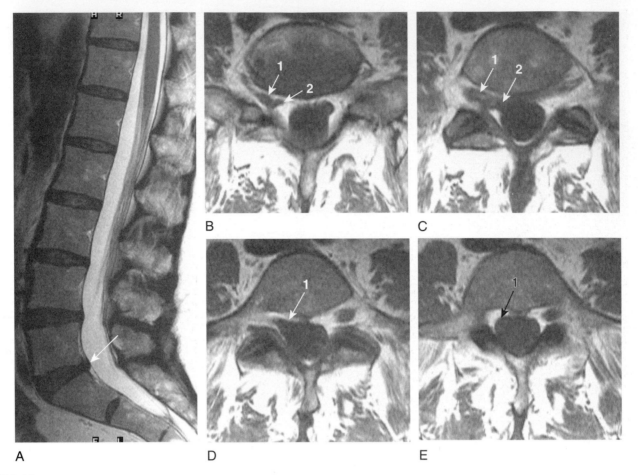

FIGURE 2–44

Conjoined nerve roots at L5 and S1. A 61-year-old woman with central low back pain and right hip and lateral thigh pain. A, Sagittal T2WI shows multilevel degenerative disc disease with mild disc dehydration at T12–L1 and L2–3 and moderate dehydration at L3–4, L4–5, and L5–S1. In addition, there is degenerative disc bulging at L5–S1 (arrow). B–E, Sequential axial T2WIs from below to above the L5–S1 disc level show asymmetry of the nerve roots at the L5 and S1 levels with a lower than normal location of the right L5 nerve root sleeve (arrow 1) and a higher than normal appearance of the right S1 nerve root sleeve (arrow 2) secondary to conjoined nerve roots. The low position of the L5 nerve root puts it in contact with the disc margin within the foramen, at a lower position than the L5 ganglion would normally occupy.

Personality Inventory scores) and lumbar myelography (the imaging modality of that era). Similarly, Boos and associates (1998) found not only the type of disc contour abnormality but also nerve root compromise, related to symptomatic disc herniation; they also found that work perception and psychosocial factors were helpful in discriminating between symptomatic and asymptomatic disc herniations. As noted in "Mechanism of Symptom Production," at least two distinct theories exist regarding the cause of symptoms in patients with disc herniation. If the patient's symptoms are predominantly those of conduction block (numbness and weakness), then mechanical compression would seem more likely to be the cause of symptoms and efforts at relieving mechanical compression (i.e., surgery) make the most sense. If the patient's symptoms are predominantly those of radicular pain, then chemical irritation would seem likely to be the cause of the symptoms and oral or locally applied anti-inflammatory medications make the most sense (Saal 1995). Many patients undergo both treatments, sometimes simultaneously (McNeill 1995). Regardless of the mechanism of symptom production, the natural history of herniated disc is, in general, a benign one: multiple studies have

shown that herniated material tends to regress with time (Bozzao 1992, Mochicha 1998, Teplick 1985)[§] (Fig. 2–48), and in one of the few controlled trials evaluating disc surgery, Weber (1983) found most of the differences between the control and operated group decreased or vanished with time. (However, for a discussion of methodology issues in Weber, see Bessette 1996.) Atlas and colleagues (2001) similarly reported diminishing differences between operated and nonoperated patients through time, although in their noncontrolled study there were still significant differences favoring the operated group at 5 years.

All this leads to the conclusion that disc herniation surgery is not an emergency and in many patients may not even be necessary. The exception, as noted earlier, is the patient presenting with cauda equina syndrome: emergency work-up and surgery needs to be performed for this condition (Ahn 2000, Shapiro 2000). Clinicians treat most other

---

[§]Note, however, that some of the apparent "regression of disc herniations" may be secondary to accompanying hematomas or fluid collections.

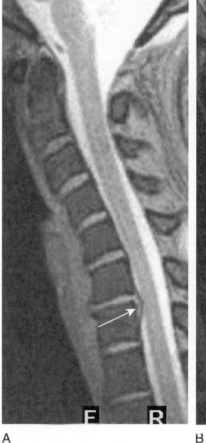

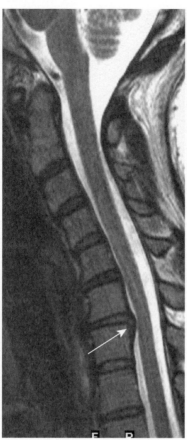

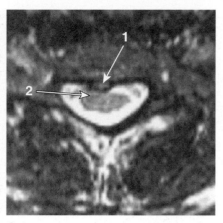

FIGURE 2–46

Disc extrusion with contact of the immediately adjacent spinal cord. A 31-year-old woman with neck and right arm pain, right shoulder tingling, and numbness in the right arm and hand. A, Sagittal gradient-recalled echo (GRE) T2WI shows reversal of normal cervical lordosis centered at the C6–7 level and a 3.5-mm, caudally dissecting disc extrusion (arrow) with contact of the ventral aspect of the spinal cord. B, Sagittal fast spin-echo (FSE) T2WI shows the disc herniation (arrow). Note the decreased signal intensity within the extruded material compared to the GRE T2WI (A). C, Axial FSE T2WI at the C6–7 disc level shows the right central disc extrusion (arrow 1) with contact of the ventral aspect of the spinal cord (arrow 2).

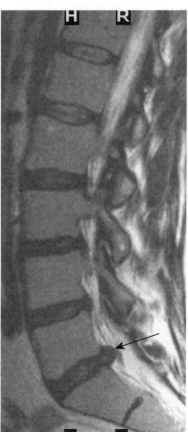

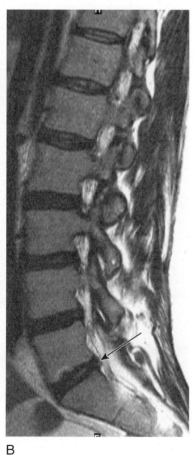

FIGURE 2–48

Spontaneous regression of disc herniation. A 43-year-old woman with right low back and buttock pain. A, Parasagittal right T2WI just medial to the pedicle at L5 shows a moderate-sized disc protrusion (arrow). B, Parasagittal right T2WI at the same level 6 months later shows resolution of almost all the disc protrusion at this level (arrow).

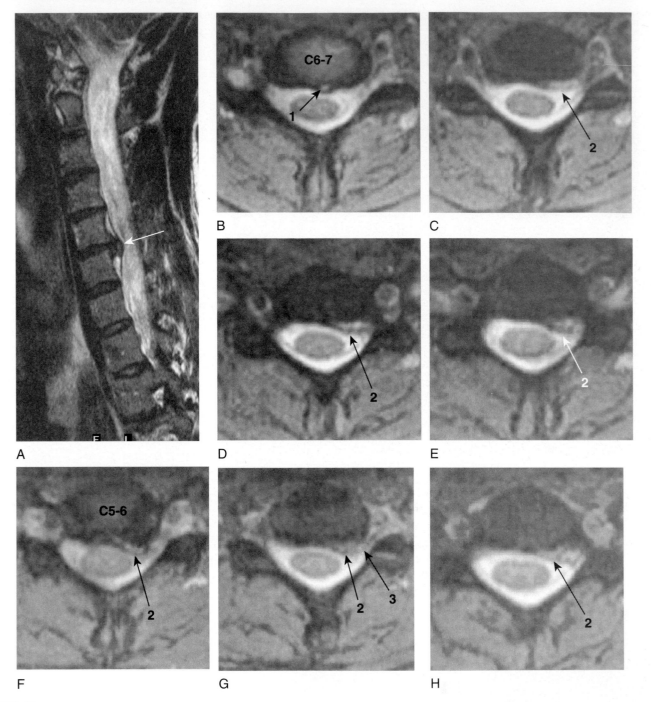

FIGURE 2–47

Cervical disc contour abnormalities illustrating descriptors of the disc margin. A 37-year-old man with neck and left arm pain, weakness, and numbness. A, Left parasagittal T2WI shows a 5-mm left paracentral disc extrusion with cranial and caudal dissection (arrow). B–H, Sequential axial gradient-recalled echo T2WIs from the C6–7 disc through the C4–5 neural foramen. There is a 2- to 3-mm disc protrusion along the left central aspect of C6–7 with contact and slight displacement of the spinal cord (arrow 1). A much larger left central and foraminal disc extrusion (arrow 2) arises from the C5–6 level with both cranial and caudal dissection and narrowing of the left C5–6 neural foramen, with contact of the exiting left C6 nerve root (arrow 3).

patients with disc herniations conservatively (with a variety of methods) unless progressive neurologic deficit becomes apparent. Those who fail conservative treatment and have intractable radicular pain and/or findings of conduction block then undergo surgery for their disease, and 80% to 95% of these patients do well. We address imaging evaluation of the other 10% to 15% in Chapter 3.

Spinal Stenosis

MECHANISM OF SYMPTOM PRODUCTION

One of the main symptoms ascribed to spinal stenosis is *neurogenic claudication*, or exercise-induced back and leg pain that worsens with continued effort and requires a vari-

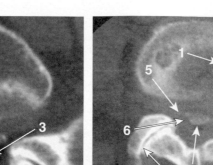

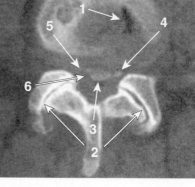

A

B

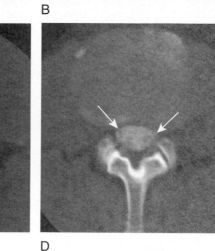

C

D

FIGURE 2–49

Spinal canal and subarticular recess stenosis demonstrated on a CT-myelogram. A 45-year-old man with low back and bilateral leg pain. A, L5–S1 level. There is moderate facet arthropathy (arrows 1), but no spinal canal or subarticular recess stenosis is present. There is no distortion of the S1 nerve root sleeves (arrows 2) or thecal sac (arrow 3). B, L4–5 level. There is degenerative disc bulging with a vacuum phenomenon (arrow 1). There is bilateral severe facet arthropathy (arrows 2). These result in severe (>50% anteroposterior diameter reduction) spinal canal stenosis (arrow 3) and moderate left (arrow 4) and severe right (arrow 5) subarticular recess stenosis. On the right side, a focal abnormality of the facet joint capsule (arrow 6) further narrows the subarticular recess; this may represent a small synovial cyst. C, L3–4 level. Findings are similar to the L4–5 level, with degenerative disc bulging and facet arthropathy combining to cause severe spinal canal and subarticular recess stenosis (arrow). D, L2–3 level. The spinal canal and subarticular recesses (arrows) have normal caliber at this level.

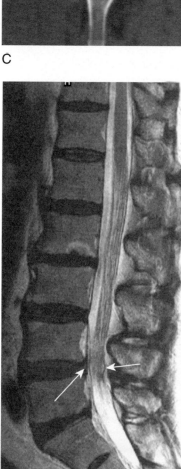

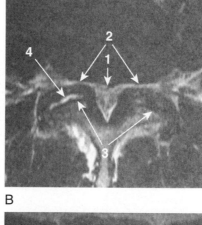

B

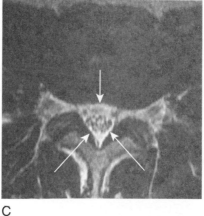

A

C

FIGURE 2–51

Trefoil central spinal canal with mild stenosis. A 76-year-old man with low back and left leg pain. A, Sagittal T2WI shows multilevel disc dehydration, mild at T12–L1 and L1–2, moderate at L2–3, L3–4, and L4–5, and severe at L5–S1. Note subchondral marrow degenerative changes at L2–3 and anteriorly at L3–4, as well as mild loss of disc height at T12–L1 and L2–3, with severe loss of disc height at L5–S1. The sagittal image does little to indicate that there is spinal canal stenosis at L4–5 (arrows). B, Axial T2WI at the L4–5 disc level shows a trefoil configuration of the spinal canal with mild spinal canal (arrow 1) and subarticular recess (arrows 2) stenosis. The facet joints are somewhat coronally oriented (arrows 3), and there is moderate facet arthropathy with a right joint effusion (arrow 4). C, Axial T2WI at the L3–4 disc level shows a normal-dimension (and normal-configuration) spinal canal (arrows).

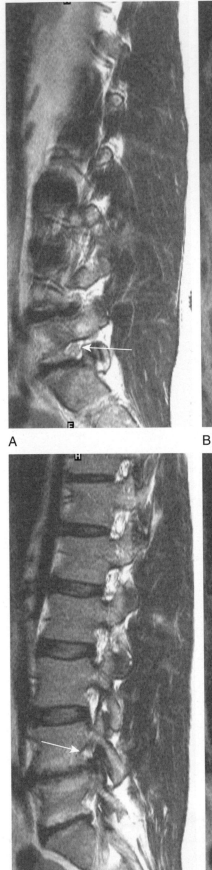

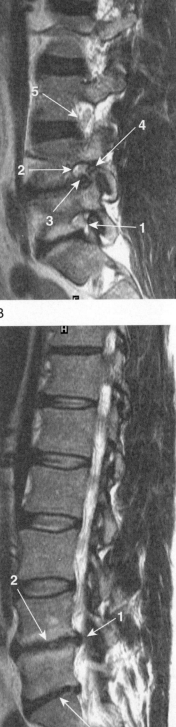

FIGURE 2–50

Foraminal stenosis demonstrated on MRI. A 42-year-old man with lower back pain, "pinching" in right hip, and numbness in left foot for 1 month. Sequential right parasagittal T2WIs from the lateral aspect of the L5 pedicle past the medial aspect of the pedicle to the right side of the spinal canal. A, There is greater than 50% reduction in the up-down dimension of the L5–S1 foramen (arrow), but no associated ganglionic deformity is present, so the stenosis is graded as "moderate, without associated ganglionic deformity." B, Moderate stenosis is again seen at L5–S1 (arrow 1). At L4–5, there is severe combined up-down and front-back foraminal stenosis (arrow 2) from a combination of degenerative disc narrowing, degenerative disc bulging (arrow 3), and facet arthropathy (arrow 4); there is associated mild compression of the L4 ganglion. No L3–4 narrowing is identified (arrow 5). C, At the level of the medial aspect of the neural foramina, no L5–S1 narrowing is seen, but there continues to be severe L4–5 narrowing (arrow). D, At the lateral aspect of the spinal canal, subarticular recess stenosis is seen at the L4–5 level (arrow 1). There is severe loss of disc height and disc dehydration at L4–5 (arrow 2) and L5–S1 (arrow 3) and subchondral Modic Type II degenerative changes at L4–5.

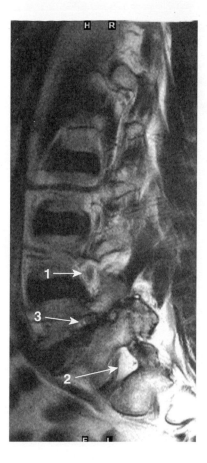

FIGURE 2–52

Severe up-down foraminal stenosis. A 71-year-old man with right back pain and leg tingling. This patient had 20% lytic spondylolisthesis and severe loss of disc height and hydration at L5–S1 (not shown here). Right parasagittal T2WI at the level of the neural foramina shows normal up-down dimension of the L3–4 (arrow 1) and L5–S1 (arrow 2) foramina with severe up-down narrowing of the L4–5 (arrow 3) foramen with associated moderate compression of the exiting L4 ganglion.

able period for recovery (Porter 1996, St. Amour 1994). Patients often suffer from central low back pain, which may precede the symptoms of neurogenic claudication by years. Occasionally, radicular pain accompanies the other symptoms, and findings of conduction block (numbness and weakness) may be present. Patients may also complain that they feel that their lower extremities are clumsy or ill-coordinated. Extension typically exacerbates symptoms, probably because of increased pressure within the spinal canal (Takahashi 1995). As with disc herniation, authorities offer different theories regarding the mechanism of symptom production in spinal stenosis. Postacchini (1989) summarized the three main contenders as mechanical compression, ischemia from arterial insufficiency, and venous congestion. The mechanical compression of nerve tissue can impair axonal transport and nutrition, leading to damage and swelling of the nerve, further impairing axonal transport and resulting in a vicious cycle (Garfin 1991, Heithoff 1987). Ischemia results from arterial insufficiency when stenosis impairs flow from the spinal artery branches and recurrent radicular branches. Stenosis impairs venous outflow at lower pressures than arterial inflow, and venous congestion may be the largest factor in producing neuro-

genic claudication from spinal stenosis (Olmarker 1992, Porter 1996, Porter 1992).

NOMENCLATURE AND DESCRIPTION OF SPINAL STENOSIS

In an article on conservative treatment of spinal stenosis published in 2000, Simotas and coworkers stated that "no validated system for radiographic rating of stenosis exists." The same problems that plague nomenclature with disc herniation (see earlier) also hinder the evaluation, study, and reporting of spinal stenosis. In studies of stenosis, authors use various terms or scales that are usually unique to that particular study. Measurements of intraobserver and interobserver variability are rarely reported; when measured, there seems to be poor agreement between different observers (Drew 2000, Yousem 1991). We present here a simplified version of the terminology used within our organization for more than 15 years.

We use the term *stenosis* to denote relatively fixed narrowing of the spinal canal, subarticular recesses, or neural foramina.‖ Most clinical cases of spinal stenosis follow from degenerative changes of the intervertebral discs and facet joints. Although osteophytes along the disc and facet joints contribute to narrowing, soft tissue abnormalities usually account for more of the narrowing than do bony abnormalities (Schonstrom 1985). Soft tissue abnormalities include thickening of the ligamentum flavum (Yoshida 1992), bulging of the disc, and capsular swelling of the facet joints. Such changes more frequently cause symptoms when superimposed on an inherently small bony canal (Heithoff 1987). Although an inherently small canal may be seen in any of a number of rare specific systemic conditions (e.g., achondroplasia), such inherent narrowing is usually idiopathic (St. Amour 1994). This narrowing may merely represent one end of a spectrum in canal size, or be secondary to as-yet-unrecognized defects or variations of the molecular biology.

Some authors (Arnoldi 1976, Schonstrom 1985, St. Amour 1994) use the term *stenosis* to denote *any* narrowing of the canal, whether from the relatively fixed bony and soft tissue structures (mentioned earlier) or from acute disc herniation, tumor, or epidural abscess. Others (Verbiest 1973, Verbiest 1980) reserve use of the term *stenosis* for fixed bony reductions in canal size. We use the term *stenosis* for fixed bony or relatively fixed soft tissue reductions in canal size and use the term *narrowing* for more evanescent reductions in canal size.

Attempts to find a specific fixed numerical value for a given measurement (either anteroposterior [AP] diameter or cross-sectional area) predictive of symptom production or surgical outcome have not been particularly successful (Amundsen 1995, Bolender 1985, Schonstrom 1985, Verbiest 1980, Weisz 1983). Use of only bony measurements makes little sense in light of the contributions of soft tissue to spinal canal narrowing (Bolender 1985, Schonstrom 1985). Use of dural sac dimensions makes more sense but is still only roughly predictive of symptoms or surgical results. In fact, some studies have shown poorer outcomes when operating on more severe degrees of

---

‖Note that the anatomic descriptors for stenosis are the same as those for disc herniation.

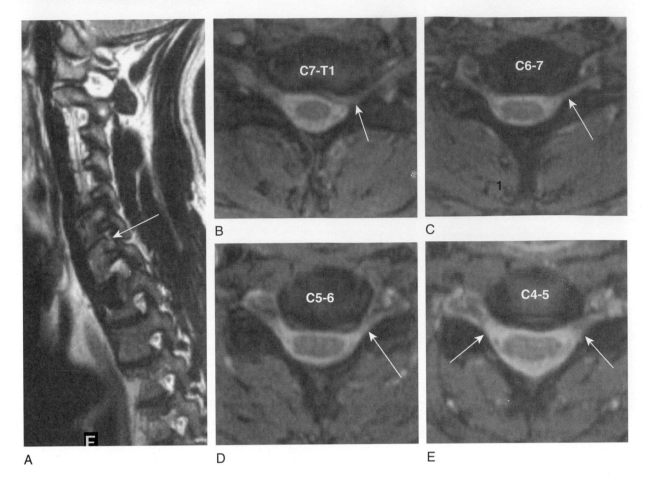

FIGURE 2–53

Cervical spine foraminal stenosis. A 44-year-old man with neck and left arm pain radiating into the small finger. A, Left parasagittal T2WI shows osteo-phytic spurring with narrowing of the left C6–7 neural foramen (arrow). Note that it is difficult to judge foraminal stenosis on the parasagittal spine images because of the obliquity of the foramen with respect to the sagittal plane. B, Axial gradient-recalled echo (GRE) T2WI at C7–T1 demonstrates a disc extru-sion filling the entrance zone of the neural foramen (arrow). This lesion was also well seen on sagittal images (not shown). C, Axial GRE T2WI at C6–7 demonstrates moderate left foraminal stenosis (arrow). D, Axial GRE T2WI at C5–6 demonstrates mild left foraminal steno-sis (arrow). E, Axial GRE T2WI at C4–5 demonstrates normal size neural foramina (arrows).

narrowing, perhaps because of the permanent damage of the nerve roots prior to operation. Thus, although absolute measurements of a linear dimension or (with markedly greater difficulty) cross-sectional area of the spinal canal, subarticular recess, or neural foramen may be reported, their significance in a given case is questionable. Factors contributing to the lack of correlation between measure-ments of narrowing and symptoms or surgical outcomes include the necessity of a second location of stenosis for symptom production (Olmarker 1992, Porter 1992), the rapidity of onset of stenosis (slowly progressive stenosis is better tolerated than rapidly progressive stenosis), super-imposed minor trauma (Heithoff 1987), and psychosocial factors.

We grade spinal canal, subarticular, and foraminal steno-sis not only relative to other levels in the same patient (and, when necessary because of an inherently small canal, an ide-alized norm from other patients) but also taking into account the degree of neural compression (Tables 2–8 to 2–10) (Figs. 2–49 and 2–50). Reliance solely on percentages of narrowing will over-rate the severity of stenosis in pa-tients with inherently large canals while under-rating the

severity of stenosis in patients with small canals. In addition to grading the degree of stenosis, note may be made in appropriate cases that the spinal canal has a "trefoil" config-uration, a characteristic of congenital/developmental ("short pedicle") spinal stenosis (Fig. 2–51).

Spinal canal stenosis and lumbar foraminal stenosis and neural compression may almost always be graded relatively easily. However, because of scan quality for technical or patient-related reasons, crowding of neural structures, or other factors, grading of subarticular recess stenosis tends to be more difficult. As an alternative to grading subarticu-lar stenosis in these cases, it may be preferable to note that subarticular recess narrowing is present and whether com-pression of the traversing nerve root is likely or not, rather than attempting to specifically grade the degree of stenosis and compression.

With lumbar foraminal stenosis, in addition to grading the degree of stenosis, the predominant *direction* of narrow-ing may be noted. The overwhelming majority (>90%) of cases of lumbar foraminal stenosis are secondary to loss of disc height and/or disc margin osteophytic spurring and degenerative bulging (Heithoff 1987). This produces loss of the cephalocaudad dimension or "craniocaudal" or "up-down" stenosis (Figs. 2–50 and 2–52). If facet arthropathy is the cause of AP narrowing, the stenosis may be "AP" or "front-back." A combination of both is called, logically enough, *combined stenosis.* Foraminal stenosis in the cervical spine is considerably more difficult to grade because the foramen is not as large to begin with and because it is oblique with respect to the usual sagittal imaging plane (Fig. 2–53)

In a few patients, bony stenosis may occur between the transverse process of L5 and the sacral ala (Wiltse 1984). Occasionally, a pseudarthrosis between a transitional transverse process/sacral ala and the vertebral body of the next higher segment may cause compression of the ventral ramus of the spinal nerve, producing radicular pain. Similar stenosis may be produced by lateral osteophytic spurring off of the L5–S1 disc with narrowing of the space between the disc margin and the ipsilateral sacral ala (Fig. 2–54).

Stenosis and Neural Compression

The same grading scheme of neural compression applies to spinal stenosis as to disc herniation (see Table 2–5), and the prior discussion is germane to compression caused by

stenosis as well. Note, however, that much larger degrees of compression may be tolerated with few accompanying symptoms. This follows from the gradual onset of the lesion in stenosis compared to disc herniation.

Special Considerations in Stenosis No. 1: Degenerative Spondylolisthesis

Spondylolisthesis, or forward displacement of one vertebra on the next lower segment, has multiple causes (see Chapter 8). One of these causes is degeneration of the facet joints and intervertebral disc that occurs most frequently at the L4–5 level in middle-aged to elderly women (Macnab 1950, Matsunaga 1990, Moller 2000, Nagaosa 1998, Newman 1955, Rosenberg 1975, Vogt 1998). Degenerative spondylolisthesis probably occurs because of alignment of the facet joints in either a more nearly sagittal (Grobler 1993) or axial (Macnab 1950, Nagaosa 1998) plane at the afflicted level than at other spinal segments. Degenerative spondylolisthesis, invariably associated with moderate or severe facet arthropathy, produces associated stenosis, particularly of the subarticular recesses and spinal canal and usually somewhat less dramatically of the neural foramina (Figs. 2–55 to 2–57). Differentiation of degenerative and

TABLE 2–8. Spinal Canal Stenosis Grading Scheme

Term	Description
Mild	The spinal canal has 75–99% of the AP dimension of a normal level.
	Lumbar spine: There is no crowding of the nerve roots within the spinal canal.
	Cervical and thoracic spine: There is partial effacement of CSF around the spinal cord but no distortion of the cord is present.
Moderate	The spinal canal has 50–74% of the AP dimension of a normal level.
	Lumbar spine: If the patient has an inherently small canal and this degree of narrowing produces a crowded appearance of the nerve roots with scant CSF around the nerve roots, the degree of stenosis should be upgraded to "severe." If the patient has an inherently very generous spinal canal and there is abundant CSF around the nerve roots, the stenosis may be graded as "mild" or it may be explicitly noted that "although there is moderate narrowing of the spinal canal, the patient has an inherently large canal and this produces no crowding of nerve roots or neural compression."
	Cervical spine: If the patient has an inherently small canal and this degree of narrowing produces flattening of the spinal cord and moderate cord compression (with >25% reduction in AP diameter), then the stenosis should be upgraded to "severe." If the patient has a very large spinal canal and there remains abundant CSF around the cord despite moderate canal narrowing, the stenosis may be downgraded to "mild," or it may be explicitly noted that "although there is moderate narrowing of the spinal canal, the patient has an inherently large canal and no contact or compression of the spinal cord is identified."
Severe	Severe spinal canal stenosis. The spinal canal has <50% of the AP dimension of a normal level.
	Lumbar spine: Typically, there is no visible CSF around the nerve roots at the level of severe stenosis. If the patient has an inherently generous spinal canal so that there is still abundant CSF around the nerve roots with little crowding of these structures, the stenosis may be graded as "moderate," or it may be explicitly noted that "although there is >50% loss in the AP dimension of the spinal canal, the patient has an inherently large canal and this stenosis produces no crowding of nerve roots or neural compression."
	Cervical spine: Typically, there is at least moderate (25–50%) narrowing of the cervical spinal cord. If the patient has an inherently large spinal canal so that there is mild or no cord compression, the stenosis may be graded as "moderate," or it may be explicitly noted that "although there is >50% loss in the AP dimension of the spinal canal, the patient has an inherently large canal and this produces no (or minimal) cord flattening."

AP, anteroposterior; CSF, cerebrospinal fluid.

TABLE 2–9. Subarticular Recess Stenosis Grading Scheme

Term	Description
Mild	The subarticular recess has 75–99% of the AP dimension of a normal level, and the traversing nerve root has ample surrounding CSF, without displacement or compression of the nerve root.
Moderate	The subarticular recess has 50–74% of the AP dimension of a normal level. If the patient has an inherently narrow subarticular recess and this degree of narrowing produces compression of the traversing of the nerve root, the degree of stenosis should be upgraded to "severe." If the patient has an inherently generous subarticular recess and there is abundant CSF around the nerve root, the stenosis may be graded as "mild" or it may be explicitly noted that "although there is moderate narrowing of the subarticular recess, the patient has an inherently large subarticular recess and this produces no compression of the traversing nerve root."
Severe	The subarticular recess has <50% of the AP dimension of a normal level. There is no visible CSF around the nerve root at the level of severe stenosis. If the patient has an inherently generous subarticular recess so that there is still abundant CSF around the nerve root, the stenosis may be graded as "moderate," or it may be explicitly noted that "although there is >50% loss in the AP dimension of the subarticular recess, the patient has an inherently large subarticular recess and this produces no compression of the traversing nerve root."

AP, anteroposterior; CSF, cerebrospinal Fluid.

TABLE 2–10. Foraminal Stenosis Grading Scheme

Term	Description
Mild	The neural foramen has 75–99% of the AP *and* cephalocaudad dimension of a normal level, and the traversing nerve root has ample surrounding CSF or perineural fat, without displacement or compression of the nerve root.
Moderate	The neural foramen has 50–74% of the AP *and* cephalocaudad dimension of a normal level. If the patient has an inherently small neural foramen and this degree of narrowing produces at least moderate compression of the exiting nerve root or ganglion, the degree of stenosis should be upgraded to "severe." If the patient has an inherently generous neural foramen and there is abundant perineural fat around the nerve root and ganglion, the stenosis may be graded as "mild," or this may be explicitly noted by stating that "there is moderate narrowing of the neural foramen but no associated neural compression."
Severe	The neural foramen has <50% of the AP dimension of a normal level. There is no visible perineural fat around the nerve root at the level of maximal stenosis.* If the patient has an inherently large neural foramen so that there is still abundant fat around the nerve root and ganglion and there is no neural compression, the stenosis may be graded as "moderate," or it may be explicitly noted that "although there is >50% loss in the ["front-back," "up-down," or "combined," as appropriate] dimension of the neural foramen, the patient has inherently large foramina and this produces no compression of the exiting nerve root."

*Note that there may be abundant fat in the *posterior* aspect of the neural foramen, but this is not around the nerve root and ganglion.

AP, anteroposterior; CSF, cerebrospinal fluid.

lytic/dysplastic spondylolisthesis relies on the location of the spondylolisthesis (more frequently L4/5 in degenerative spondylolisthesis and L5/S1 in spondylolysis), associated facet arthropathy (moderate or severe in degenerative spondylolisthesis and usually absent in spondylolysis), spinal canal diameter (decreased in degenerative spondylolisthesis and increased in spondylolysis), and appearance of the pars interarticularis (intact in degenerative spondylolisthesis and interrupted in spondylolysis). In some patients, the two entities coexist (Fig. 2–58).

The development of synovial cysts sprouting off degenerated facet joints in patients with degenerative spondylolisthesis frequently contributes to symptoms (Heithoff 1987), and this complication should be suspected when a patient develops superimposed radicular pain on long-standing low back pain (see section, "Facet Joint Disease."). Of course, an acute disc herniation may be seen in the same clinical scenario, and imaging will be required to make this differentiation (Fig. 2–59).

Special Considerations in Stenosis No. 2: The Cervical Spine and Spondylotic Myelopathy

As in the case of disc herniation, special considerations apply to cervical spinal stenosis. Severe narrowing of the neural foramina is more likely to be accompanied by nerve root symptoms, probably secondary to the lower location of the ganglion and nerve root in relation to the neural foramina compared with the lumbar spine (Kaiser 1998). For another, compression of the spinal cord may produce *spondylotic myelopathy*, or abnormality of the spinal cord secondary to degenerative narrowing of the spinal canal (Krauss 2000, Nurick 1972). Such myelopathy may manifest clinically as upper extremity weakness and muscle atrophy (with sometimes little corresponding sensory deficit), lower extremity weakness and hyperreflexia, and disturbances of bladder function (Kameyama 1998, Ono 1987, Takahashi 1989, Wada 1995). This myelopathy may be accompanied by areas of T2 prolongation within the spinal cord (Kaiser

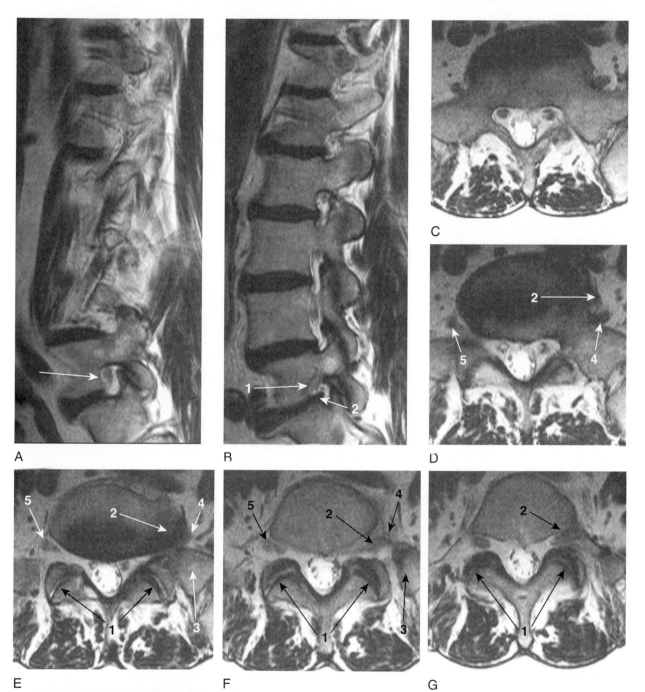

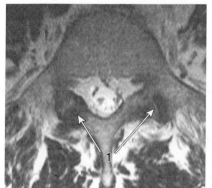

FIGURE 2–54

Stenosis between far-lateral osteophytic spurring and the sacral ala producing radicular pain. A 67-year-old man with low back and left leg pain in the hip, lateral thigh, and lateral calf. A, Right parasagittal T2WI shows a widely patent neural foramen (arrow) without L5 ganglionic compression. B, Left T2WI shows severe up-down foraminal stenosis (arrow 1) secondary to loss of disc height and osteophyte formation (arrow 2), with associated compression of the exiting right L5 ganglion. C–H, Sequential axial T2WIs from the S1 pedicle through the L5 pedicle show moderate facet arthropathy (arrows 1) and degenerative disc bulging. Furthermore, there is extensive left-sided osteophytic spurring (arrow 2) that projects along the left lateral aspect of the L5 vertebral body and narrows the space between the vertebral body and the left sacral ala (arrow 3), with displacement and compression of the L5 ventral ramus (arrow 4) (compare to the position of the left L5 ventral ramus [arrow 5]).

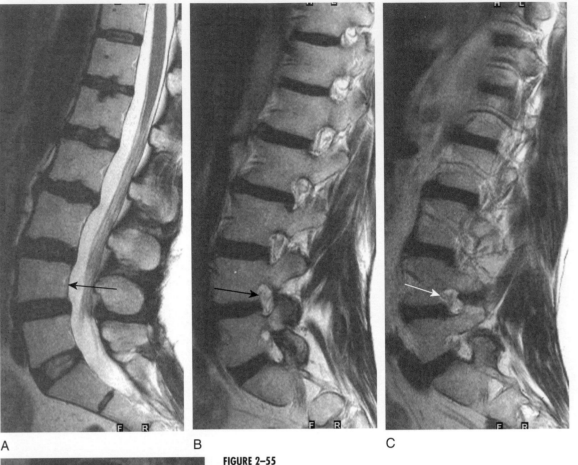

A   B   C

FIGURE 2–55

Mild degenerative spondylolisthesis. A 59-year-old woman with central low back pain radiating into both legs. A, Sagittal T2WI shows multilevel degenerative disc disease, with T12–L1 and L1–2 mild loss of disc height with extensive Schmorl's node formation, L2–3 moderate disc dehydration, disc bulging, and Schmorl's node formation, L3–4 moderate disc dehydration, and L4–5 mild disc dehydration. In addition, at the L4–5 level, there is minimal (<5%) degenerative spondylolisthesis: note the forward shift of L4 on L5 (arrow). B, Right parasagittal T2WI through the level of the foramina shows mild (<25%) front-back foraminal stenosis (arrow). C, Left parasagittal T2WI shows no front-back L4–5 narrowing (arrow). D, Axial T2WI at the level of the L4–5 disc shows moderate facet arthropathy (arrows 1), a trefoil appearance of the spinal canal, and mild spinal canal (arrow 2) and subarticular recess (arrows 3) stenosis. No neural compression is present.

D

1998, Kameyama 1998, Krauss 2000, Takahashi 1989, Wada 1995, Wada 1999) (Fig. 2–60). Histologically, such abnormal signal intensity may correspond to (reversible) edema, particularly if there is no corresponding T1 prolongation. If there *are* corresponding areas of T1 prolongation, increased signal intensity on T2WI more likely represents (irreversible) cavitations or cystic necrosis (Wada 1999). The prognostic significance of abnormal signal intensity in the cord is still being studied, with some authors maintaining a relationship between these abnormal signal intensities and prognosis and surgical outcome (Okada 1994, Takahashi 1989, Wada 1999), whereas others deny that such a relationship exists (Wada 1995). Wada and associ-

ates (1999) found that the cross-sectional area of the spinal cord correlated better to prognosis than increased signal intensity within the spinal cord.[¶] Morio and coworkers (2001) reported that prognosis was better predicted by T1 prolongation than T2 prolongation. Extensive flattening of the spinal cord and multiple abnormal foci of T2 prolongation may be accompanied by a surprisingly benign clinical course (Krauss 2000).

[¶]However, the correlation coefficient was .584 and review of a plot of recovery rate percent as a function of transverse area of the cord fails to reveal any obvious cut-point to use as a decision criterion.

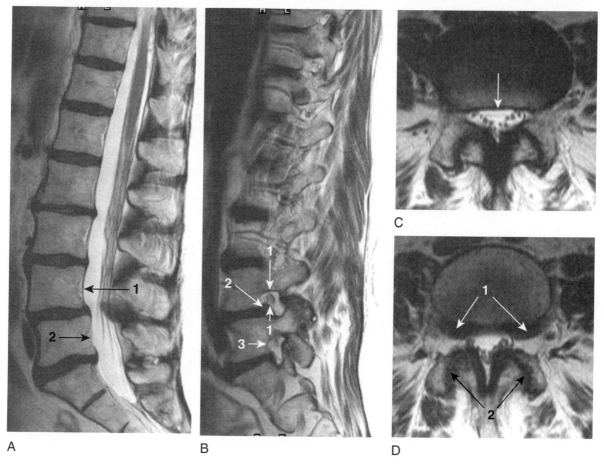

FIGURE 2–56

Moderate degenerative spondylolisthesis. A 74-year-old patient with constant backache radiating into both hips and legs, with superimposed sharp pain with walking. A, Sagittal T2WI shows multilevel degenerative disc disease with moderate disc dehydration at T12–L1, mild dehydration at L1–2, mild loss of disc height, moderate dehydration, degenerative disc bulging and anterior osteophyte formation at L2–3, mild loss of disc height with moderate disc dehydration and disc bulging at L3–4, and mild loss of disc height and moderate disc dehydration at L4–5 and L5–S1. At L4–5, there is 15% degenerative spondylolisthesis (arrow 1), and at L5–S1 there is 3 mm of retrolisthesis (arrow 2). B, Parasagittal right T2WI shows mild L4–5 up-down narrowing (arrows 1) from a foraminal disc protrusion (arrow 2) and mild front-back L5–S1 foraminal stenosis (arrow 3) from retrolisthesis of L5 on S1. C, Axial T2WI just below the L4–5 disc shows a trefoil configuration of the spinal canal from facet arthropathy and again demonstrates mild spinal canal stenosis (arrow). D, Axial T2WI at the superior margin of the L4–5 disc shows a "pseudodisc" appearance because of spondylolisthesis (arrows 1), moderate facet arthropathy (arrows 2), and mild spinal canal and subarticular recess stenosis.

Special Considerations in Stenosis No. 3: Scoliosis and Stenosis

Scoliosis of the lumbar spine may be associated with extensive degenerative disc and facet disease, particularly on the concave side of the scoliotic curve. This may lead to multilevel foraminal, lateral recess, and occasionally even spinal canal stenosis (Figs. 2–61 and 2–62).

TREATMENT

As is the case with disc herniation, treatment of spinal stenosis varies greatly. Many publications have supported conservative treatment (Johnsson 1993, Simotas 2000), with a combination of exercise, nonsteroidal anti-inflammatory medication, or epidural steroid injection (Ferrante 1989, Jenis 2000, Simotas 2000, St. Amour 1994). Since symptom production follows from not only single level narrowing but also any additional areas of narrowing (Olmarker 1992, Porter 1992), the rapidity of onset of the narrowing, such

superimposed soft tissue abnormalities as disc herniations and synovial cysts, and minimal trauma (Heithoff 1987), as well as additional, as yet unidentified factors, addressing only the stenosis at a single level will not invariably lead to a favorable outcome. However, in a meta-analysis of 74 articles on spinal stenosis, Turner and coworkers (1992) found favorable outcomes reported in an average of 64% of cases. In a more recent publication, Atlas and associates (2000) compared 4-year outcomes in a matched, prospective, observational study and found that surgical treatment was associated with a greater improvement in patient-reported outcomes than nonsurgical treatment. The decision to perform surgery usually hinges more on clinical symptoms (particularly on neurogenic claudication interfering with activities of daily living or progressive neurologic dysfunction [Herkowitz 1989]) than it does on imaging appearance. Controversy continues regarding whether fusion should accompany decompression (Grob 1995, Mc Cullough 1998).

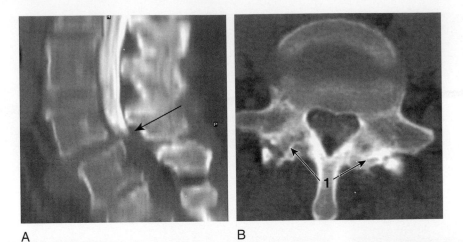

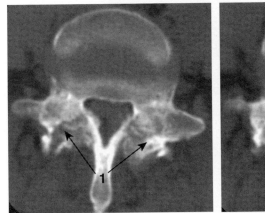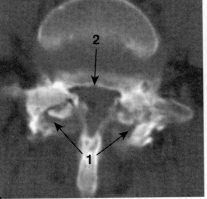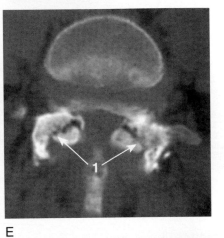

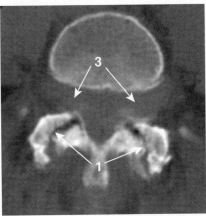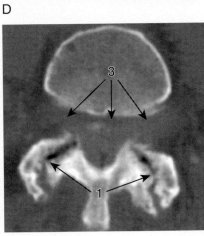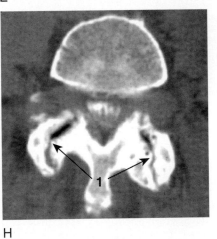

FIGURE 2–57

Severe degenerative spondylolisthesis. A 62-year-old patient with low back and bilateral leg pain and right leg weakness. A, Sagittal reconstruction CT examination shows moderate L4–5 and severe L5–S1 disc narrowing. There is 20% degenerative spondylolisthesis of L4 on L5 and complete block to flow of myelographic contrast material at the L4–5 level (arrow). B–H, Sequential 3-mm CT-myelogram slices from the L5 pedicle through the L4–5 disc demonstrate severe degenerative changes of the facet joints (arrows 1) with vacuum phenomenon bilaterally. There is a trefoil appearance of the spinal canal at the level of the L4–5 disc, along with severe spinal canal stenosis (arrow 2). Note the pseudodisc appearance on the cut immediately above the L4–L5 level (arrows 3) secondary to volume averaging through the spondylolisthesis.

In the special case of degenerative spondylolisthesis, Vogt and colleagues (1998) in a population study found no relationship between anterolisthesis and back pain. Kauppila and colleagues (1998) found it problematic to ascribe back pain to degenerative spondylolisthesis, and Matsunaga and

coworkers (1990) thought that autostabilization prevented progression of disease and that the natural history of the disease was thus benign. Iguchi and associates (2000) found most patients did well even without surgery. On the other hand, Moller and colleagues (2000) found that surgery

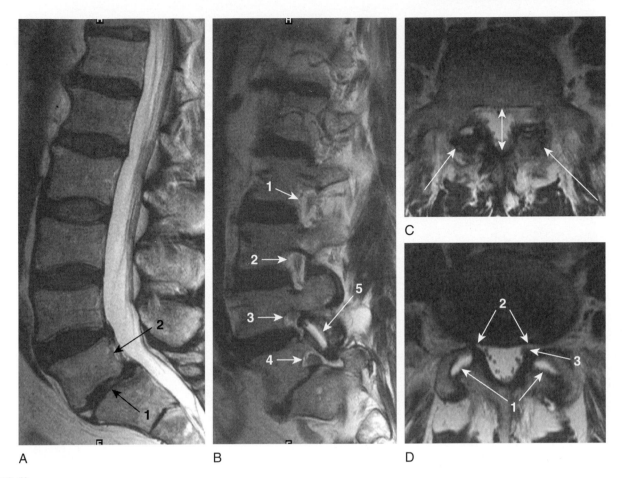

A   B   C   D

FIGURE 2–58

Coexistent lytic and degenerative spondylolisthesis. A 77-year-old man with low back and bilateral leg pain. A, Sagittal T2WI shows multilevel degenerative changes with moderate disc dehydration at T12–L1, L1–2, L3–4, and L4–5, with mild disc dehydration at L2–3. At L5–S1, there is severe loss of disc height and disc dehydration (arrow 1) with 25% lytic spondylolisthesis (arrow 2). L4–5 shows minimal (<5%) degenerative spondylolisthesis. B, Right parasagittal T2WI at the level of the right foramen shows normal-appearing foramina at L2–3 (arrow 1) and L3–4 (arrow 2) with moderate combined up-down and front-back stenosis at L4–5 (arrow 3) and moderate up-down stenosis at L5–S1 (arrow 4) with associated flattening of the L5 ganglia. Note the joint effusion within the right L4–5 facet joint (arrow 5). C, Axial T2WI at the level of the L5 pars shows bilateral pars defects with proliferative changes along the pars defects (arrows) and anteroposterior elongation of the spinal canal (double-headed arrow). D, Axial T2WI at the level of the L4–5 disc shows degenerative disc bulging and bilateral severe facet arthropathy with large joint effusions (arrows 1). There is minimal spinal canal narrowing, but there is moderate subarticular recess narrowing (arrows 2) with compression of the traversing left L5 nerve root (arrow 3).

provided better pain relief and functional outcome than an exercise program.

In the special case of spondylotic myelopathy, surgical treatment consists of decompression of the compressed segment of the spinal cord, often with accompanying fusion (Krauss 2000). Sampath and colleagues (2000) compared groups of surgically and nonsurgically treated patients and found that those undergoing surgery had better results despite having more symptoms and disability prior to surgery.

As in the case of disc herniation, most patients undergoing surgery have a favorable outcome. Chapter 3 deals with the evaluation of those who return for further imaging.

Facet Joint Disease

A three-joint complex (the intervertebral disc anteriorly and the facet joints posteriorly) composes each motion segment within the spine. However, the facet joint generally receives much less attention both in terms of published literature and clinical focus than does the intervertebral disc. Disc and facet joints tend to degenerate together (Kirkaldy-Willis 1982, Yong-Hing 1983), with disc degeneration preceding facet degeneration (Butler 1990). Although disc degeneration and herniation is a widely recognized source of back pain, many authorities minimize the role of the facet joints in back and neck pain. Studies on both conscious patients undergoing discectomy (Kuslich 1991) and volunteers (Dwyer 1990, Kaplan 1998, Kellgren 1939) support the notion that the facet joint may represent a source of pain in at least some patients. The large numbers of patients with back pain implies that even if facet joint abnormalities are the cause of pain in a relatively low percentage, there will still be many patients with pain arising from the facet joints.

No specific clinical syndrome accompanies facet joint pain, and no set of symptoms is predictive of the pain relief accompanying joint anesthetization (Jackson 1988, Revel 1998, Schwarzer 1994). The correlation between imaging

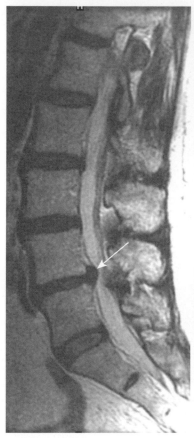

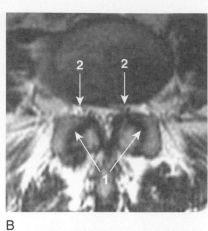

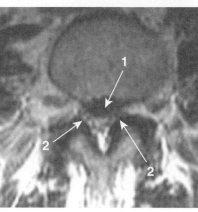

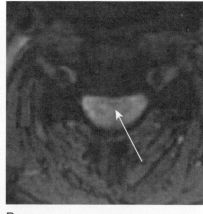

A

B

C

FIGURE 2–59

Degenerative spondylolisthesis with superimposed disc herniation. A 66-year-old woman with chronic low back pain and new-onset left leg pain. A, Sagittal T2WI demonstrates multilevel degenerative disc disease with mild disc dehydration at L1–2, L2–3, and L5–S1 with degenerative disc bulging at L2–3. L3–4 and L4–5 show moderate disc dehydration, and L4–5 shows mild loss of disc height with a cranially dissecting 6.3-mm disc extrusion (arrow). Also present is approximately 5% degenerative spondylolisthesis. B, Axial T2WI at the level of the L4–5 disc demonstrates severe facet arthropathy (arrows 1) and moderate spinal canal and subarticular recess stenosis (arrows 2) with a trefoil appearance of the spinal canal. C, Axial T2WI just above the level of the L4–5 disc demonstrates the cranially dissecting disc extrusion (arrow 1) with severe spinal canal and bilateral subarticular recess narrowing (arrows 2) with compression of the traversing L5 nerve roots (left > right).

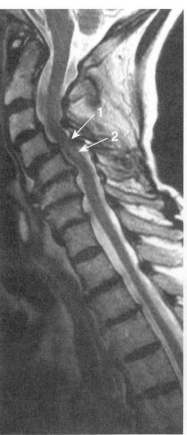

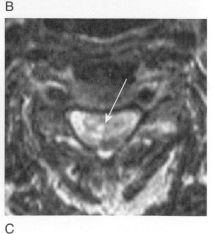

A

B

C

FIGURE 2–60

Spondylotic myelopathy. A 79-year-old patient with bilateral leg pain and weakness, bilateral arm pain, and neck pain. A, Sagittal T2WI demonstrates extensive multilevel degenerative change with reversal of normal cervical lordosis and spinal canal stenosis at C4–5 (arrow 1) from a combination of degenerative disc narrowing and spondylolisthesis and also at C5–6 and C6–7 from degenerative disc bulging, osteophyte formation, and facet arthropathy. Between the C4–5 and C5–6 levels there is T2 prolongation within the central aspect of the spinal cord (arrow 2) consistent with spondylotic myelopathy. B, Axial gradient-recalled echo T2WI just below the C4–5 disc level demonstrates T2 prolongation within the cord (arrow) (the window and level of the image have been adjusted to emphasize cord signal). C, Axial fast spin-echo T2WI at the same level also shows T2 prolongation within the spinal cord (arrow).

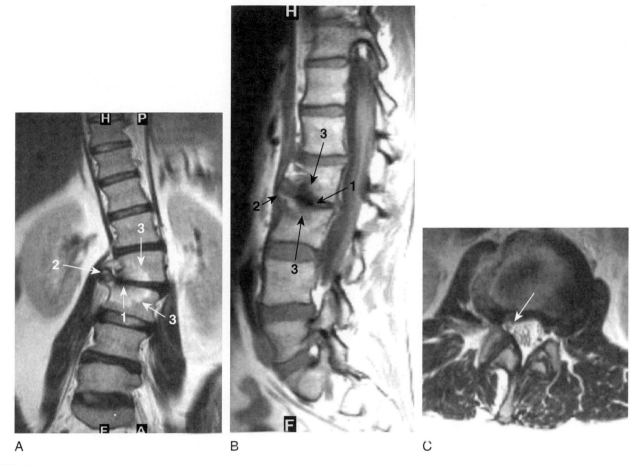

A   B   C

FIGURE 2–61

Scoliosis with accompanying degenerative disc disease and mild subarticular recess stenosis. A 42-year-old woman with right-sided low back pain. A, Coronal T2WI demonstrates marked scoliosis apex to the left at the L2–3 level. On the concave (right) side of the curve, there is marked disc narrowing (arrow 1), osteophytic spurring, and lateral disc extrusion (arrow 2) with accompanying Modic Type I subchondral degenerative changes (arrows 3). B, Sagittal T1WI through the lateral aspect of the L2–3 disc (but more medial at levels above and below because of scoliosis) again shows disc narrowing (arrow 1), osteophytic spurring (arrow 2), and Modic Type I subchondral degenerative changes (arrows 3). C, Axial T2WI at the L2–3 disc level demonstrates degenerative disc bulging and mild narrowing of the right subarticular recess (arrow).

morphology and symptoms is as imperfect in facet arthropathy as it is in disc degeneration, and patients with minimal morphologic abnormalities may have pronounced symptoms whereas those with severe degenerative changes report little or no pain (Schwarzer 1995). The facet joints should nonetheless be evaluated when reporting imaging studies of the spine. The presence of degeneration and other abnormalities within these structures may indicate that they are symptomatic and lead to appropriate treatment. At present, treatment options include conservative management with

TABLE 2–11. Facet Arthropathy Grading Scheme

Term	Description
Mild	There is mild undulation of the facet joint margins with small (1–3 mm) osteophytes and minimal subchondral sclerosis. The articular cartilage is minimally narrowed. There is a 0–25% increase in overall size of the facet joint transverse dimension.
Moderate	There is more pronounced undulation of the facet joint margins. There is definite loss of articular cartilage and there is subchondral sclerosis. There are medium-sized osteophytes (3–5 mm at most). There is a 25–50% increase in the overall size of the facet joint transverse dimension.
Severe	There is pronounced undulation along the facet joint margins. There is nearly complete or complete elimination of the joint space with or without a vacuum phenomenon, with large (>5 mm) osteophytes along the facet joint margins. There is increased size of the joints, which may be >50% of normal.

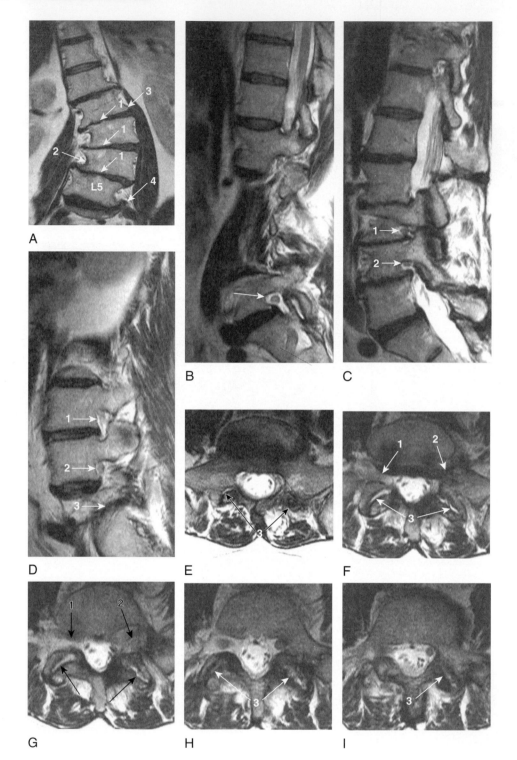

FIGURE 2–62

Scoliosis with accompanying degenerative disc disease and multilevel foraminal stenosis. A 66-year-old man with low back pain and left hip and lateral thigh pain and left leg weakness and numbness. A, Coronal T2WI demonstrates scoliosis apex to the left at the L3–4 level. L2–3, L3–4, and L4–5 (arrows 1) all demonstrate severe disc narrowing and dehydration, particularly along the concave, right side of the curve where there are accompanying osteophytes. There is also a right-sided shift of L4 on L5 (arrow 2) and a left-sided shift of L2 on L3 (arrow 3). Because of the L5 scoliotic tilt, the left side of the L5–S1 disc is narrowed with associated osteophytes (arrow 4). B, Right parasagittal T2WI through the plane of the right L5 pedicle shows mild up-down narrowing of the foramen and no right L5 ganglionic compression (arrow). Note that L2 through L4 are medial to the plane of the image. C, Right parasagittal T2WI through the plane of the L3 and L4 pedicles, approximately 1 cm medial to B. This image demonstrates severe up-down foraminal stenosis at the L3–4 (arrow 1) and L4–5 (arrow 2) levels with moderate compression of the exiting L3 and L4 ganglia. D, Left parasagittal T2WI through the plane of the left L4 and L5 pedicles. Note that on the convex side of the curve, the L3–4 (arrow 1) and L4–5 (arrow 2) neural foramina are not narrowed. However, the L5–S1 neural foramen is severely stenotic (arrow 3), with abutment of the L5 pedicle and sacral ala and resulting severe compression of the L5 ganglion. E–I, Sequential axial T2WIs from the S1 through the L5 pedicle level demonstrate no right foraminal or spinal canal stenosis (arrow 1), but there is severe left foraminal stenosis (arrow 2) with left L5 ganglionic compression. Also note severe bilateral facet arthropathy with effusions (arrows 3).

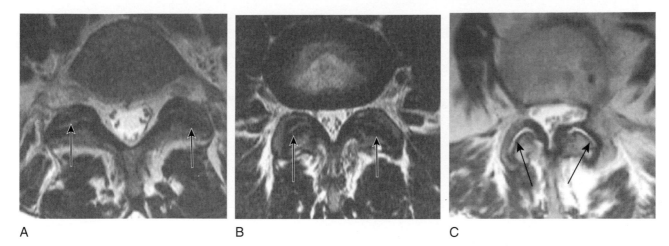

FIGURE 2–63

Facet joint grading scheme with MRI. A, Axial T2WI of mild facet arthropathy (arrows). Note that there is also mild facet joint tropism, with the left facet joint in a slightly more sagittal plane than the right joint. B, Axial T2WI of moderate facet arthropathy (arrows). C, Axial T2WI of severe facet arthropathy (arrows).

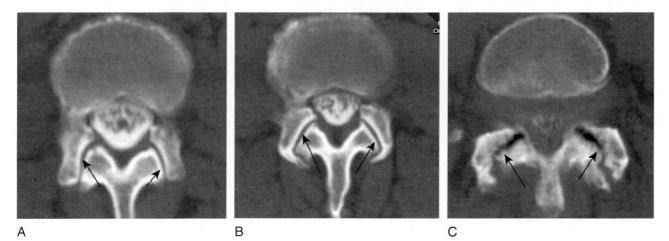

FIGURE 2–64

Facet joint grading scheme with CT. A, Axial postmyelogram CT of mild facet arthropathy (arrows). B, Axial postmyelogram CT of moderate facet arthropathy (arrows). C, Axial postmyelogram CT of severe facet arthropathy (arrows).

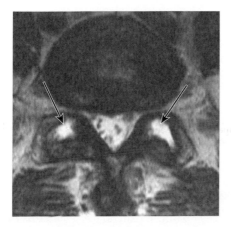

FIGURE 2–65

Facet joint effusions. Axial T2WI shows bilateral large joint effusions, with T2 prolongation within the facet joints bilaterally (arrows).

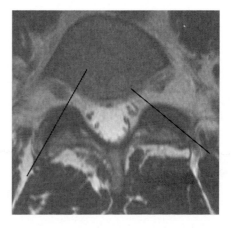

FIGURE 2–66

Facet joint tropism. Axial T2WI shows facet joint tropism, with a more sagitally oriented right joint and bilateral mild facet arthropathy (compare the lines drawn down the joint space on the right and left).

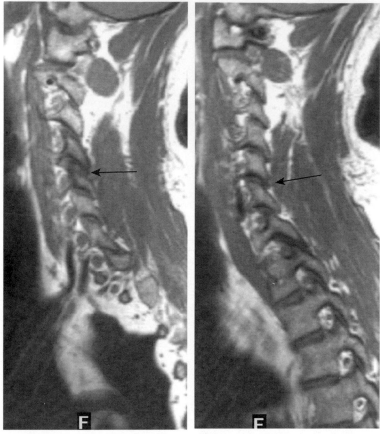

A   B

FIGURE 2–67

Asymmetric facet arthropathy of the cervical spine. A 51-year-old man with right-sided mid-neck pain. A, Right parasagittal T1WI shows joint space narrowing and subchondral marrow changes of the right C4–5 facet joint (arrow). B, Left parasagittal T1WI (for comparison) shows a normal-appearing C4–5 facet joint (arrow).

oral medication and physical therapy, intra-articular injection of steroids (Carette 1991,** El-Khoury 1991, Lippitt 1984), percutaneous rhizotomy (Dreyfuss 2000, van Kleef 1999), and fusion surgery (often accompanied by posterior decompression in cases of stenosis).

Grading facet arthropathy has received little attention in the literature (Fujiwara 2000a; Fujiwara 2000b, Grogan 1997). Our scheme for grading facet arthropathy is presented in Table 2–11 and illustrated in Figures 2–63 and 2–64. Facet arthropathy may lead to subarticular recess and foraminal stenosis, and this should be graded as noted earlier in the section on "Spinal Stenosis." Facet arthropathy may also lead to displacement or compression of neural structures, and this should also be graded as noted earlier. Facet joints may demonstrate effusions indicative of synovitis, with or without other manifestations of degenerative changes; the presence of such effusions should be noted (Fig. 2–65). The presence of tropism, or an asymmetry, of the facet joints should be noted: some authorities (Bogduk 1997, Farfan 1967, Noren 1991) believe that tropism contributes to degenerative disc disease, although others have denied such a relationship (Boden 1996, Grogan 1997) (Fig. 2–66).

Facet arthropathy disproportionate in comparison to the opposite side and other levels suggests a post-traumatic abnormality (Woodring 1982). Such unilateral abnormality is usually encountered in the cervical spine (see Chapter 5). Sometimes these patients have a specific history of trauma, but on occasion patients will not recall any specific event that may have resulted in significant damage to the facet joints (Fig. 2–67). Small intra-articular fractures with resultant intracapsular hemorrhage and/or incongruous joint surfaces, or cartilaginous fractures, may both lead to subsequent asymmetric facet arthropathy.

SYNOVIAL CYSTS

Fluid-filled pockets with a synovial lining, or *synovial cysts*, may sprout from the facet joints and produce symptoms through neural compression. *Ganglion cysts* may also contain fluid but are not lined by synovium and do not communicate with the facet joint. Ganglion cysts may be synovial cysts that have lost their communication with the parent facet joint and degenerated (Awwad 1990, Jackson 1989, St. Amour 1994, Yuh 1991) or arise directly from the ligamentum flavum (Abdullah 1984). A variety of chemicals may occupy the cyst including serous, gelatinous, or mucinous fluid as well as hemosiderin or blood; this gives rise to imaging inhomogeneity (Apostolaki 2000, Awwad 1990, St. Amour 1994), but in general synovial cysts demonstrate T1 and T2 prolongation (Fig. 2–68). Contrast enhancement varies, with early contrast enhancement of some portions of the cyst and delayed or absent enhancement of other por-

---

**Note that although the authors of this study claim no efficacy for intra-articular steroid injection, the results indicate a threefold difference in percentage of patients improved at 6-month follow-up, which was statistically significant.

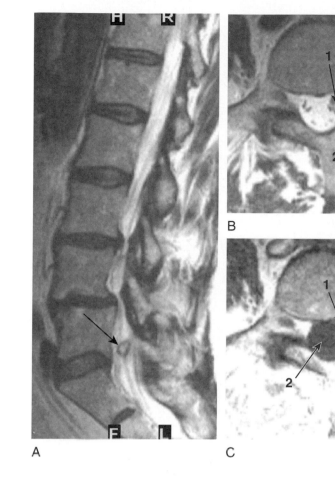

A

C

FIGURE 2–68

Synovial cyst. A 62-year-old woman with central low back pain. A, Sagittal T2WI shows a lesion projecting in the middle of the thecal sac behind the L5 vertebral body (arrow). Note multilevel degenerative disc disease, L3–4 degenerative disc bulging, L4–5 degenerative spondylolisthesis, and spinal canal stenosis. B, Axial T2WI shows that the apparently "floating" lesion seen on the sagittal represents a synovial cyst (arrow 1) projecting off the medial aspect of the left L5–S1 facet joint, which demonstrates severe degeneration (arrow 2). C, Axial T1WI demonstrates that it is difficult to visualize the cyst (arrow 1) against the background of cerebrospinal fluid. It is barely discernible, with only slightly more signal intensity than the adjacent cerebrospinal fluid (arrow 2).

tions; some lesions may demonstrate characteristic "rim" enhancement (Howling 1997, Silbergleit 1990, Yuh 1991). Although some articles refer to synovial cysts as "uncommon" (Kurz 1985, Liu 1990, Yuh 1991) or a "rare cause of radiculopathy" (Jackson 1989, Silbergleit 1990), we encounter symptomatic synovial cysts on a weekly and sometimes daily basis. A report on 25 patients undergoing imaging for acute radiculopathy (Modic 1995) supports the common occurrence of these lesions, with 2 of the 25 patients having symptomatic synovial cysts (vs. 18 patients with symptomatic herniated discs). Figures illustrating synovial cysts typically demonstrate lesions projecting off the medial aspect of the joint margin into the spinal canal, sometimes with associated spinal canal narrowing, or projecting off the anteromedial aspect of the joint into the subarticular recess with subarticular recess narrowing and traversing nerve root compression. We have encountered many lesions in a far more anterior and lateral location: in the neural foramen (Fig. 2–69). Such lesions may cause pain by compression of the dorsal root ganglion.

Kurz and associates (1985) reported surgical results of four cases of symptomatic synovial cysts in 1985 and noted that percutaneous aspiration and injection of synovial cysts with steroid should be considered. Subsequently, Bjorkengren and colleagues (1987) reported opacification of three synovial cysts via facet joint injection. They also reported relief of symptoms following injection of intra-articular steroids. Parlier-Cuau and coworkers (1999) reported the results of 30 such intra-articular injections and

reviewed the existing literature; they concluded that between one third and one half of patients would achieve good to excellent long-term (≥6 months) relief of pain from intra-articular injection. Such injection constitutes a viable first step in management of these patients (Fig. 2–69). The injection provides diagnostic information: if injection of the facet joint (and inflation of the cyst) provokes symptoms, then the cyst is likely the symptom-producing lesion. The injection in many patients also appears to offer long-term therapeutic benefit, although many patients will require surgery for pain relief (Jonsson 1999, Howington 1999, Hsu 1995, Kurz 1985, Lyons 2000, Onofrio 1988, Sabo 1996).

L4/5 is the most frequent level of synovial cysts, and such cysts frequently accompany degenerative spondylolisthesis (Howington 1999, Hsu 1995, Lyons 2000, Wang 1987). In fact, images of patients with degenerative spondylolisthesis and unilateral radiculopathy should be scrutinized with special care for the presence of such lesions (Fig. 2–70). Although most synovial cysts are of the lumbar spine, cervical (Chang 2000, Howington 1999, Onofrio 1988) and thoracic (Aksoy 2000, Howington 1999, Lynn 2000) synovial cysts have also been reported, frequently in association with myelopathy (Stoodley 2000). Because of the possibility of pressurizing the cyst (and exacerbating myelopathy), synovial cysts within the spinal canal at the thoracic and cervical regions are generally treated surgically rather than via percutaneous injection.

Although the imaging characteristics of synovial cysts generally allow confident diagnosis, identical findings may

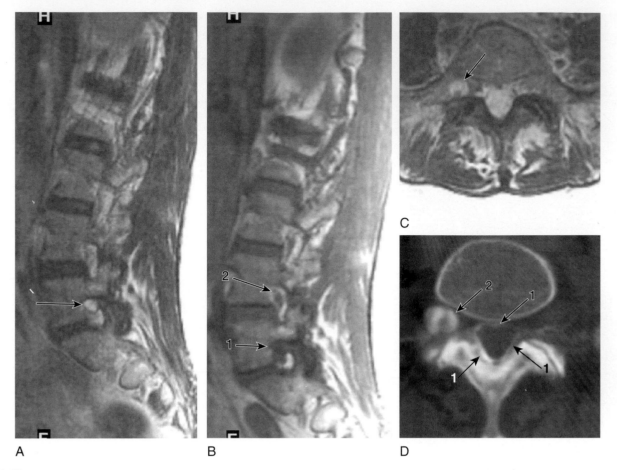

FIGURE 2–69

Foraminal synovial cyst. A 57-year-old woman with right low back pain radiating into the hip and lateral aspect of the thigh. A, Right parasagittal T2WI at the level of the right neural foramen demonstrates a focus of T2 prolongation with a well-delineated margin occupying the superior aspect of the neural foramen (arrow). B, Matching right parasagittal T1WI demonstrates a focus of T1 prolongation within the upper foramen (arrow 1), consistent with fluid (in this case, a synovial cyst). This area of the neural foramen should demonstrate a thin rim of fat above the ganglion, as at the L4–5 level (arrow 2). C, Axial T2WI at the level of the L5–S1 foramina demonstrates a focus of T2 prolongation in the mid-to-lateral aspect of the right L5–S1 foramen (arrow). There is volume averaging through the right S1 pedicle on this cut. D, Axial CT through the L5–S1 foramen performed after injection of the right L5–S1 facet joint. There is contrast medium in the epidural space (arrow 1) and also in the synovial cyst within the neural foramen (arrow 2). Although the cyst was not ruptured at the time of injection, local anesthetic and steroids resulted in prolonged pain relief.

be seen in pigmented villonodular synovitis (PVNS) of the facet joint (Khoury 1991). This is an extremely rare entity, however, compared to the common synovial cyst. Treatment of PVNS is complete joint excision; these lesions do not respond to percutaneous injection.

OTHER NONDISCAL DEGENERATIVE PROCESSES

Interspinous Degenerative Changes

Baastrup's disease, or "kissing spines," results from apposition of the spinous processes posteriorly, which leads to periostitis along the spinous processes and inflammation of the afflicted ligament (Bogduk 1997, Resnick 1995) (Fig. 2–71). Such changes may be a cause of central low back pain. MRI allows classification of interspinous ligament signal into several types (Fujiwara 2000). It would appear that medial branch blocks could assess whether this finding was symptomatic in a given patient, since enervation comes from this nerve. However, treatment with rhizotomy has not been evaluated, and treatment with surgery has met with limited success (Beks 1989).

Posterior Longitudinal and Ligamentum Flavum Calcification and Ossification

Ossification of the posterior longitudinal ligament (OPLL) is generally regarded as an idiopathic, rather than a degenerative, condition, but is included here as one manifestation of degenerative disease. OPLL has been associated with diabetes mellitus, abnormal calcium metabolism, ankylosing spondylitis, diffuse idiopathic skeletal hypertrophy, and fluoride overdose (St. Amour 1994). This condition is several times as frequent in Japanese people as compared to North Americans. Although usually asymptomatic, OPLL may result in symptoms of myelopathy if extensive or superimposed on an inherently small spinal canal. Patients with mild symptoms are usually treated conservatively, whereas those with severe or rapidly developing symptoms usually undergo surgery (St. Amour 1994) (Fig. 2–72).

Ossification of the yellow ligament causes shortening of both T1 and T2 with lack of signal, whereas CT demonstrates increased density (Fig. 2–73) (Hanakita 1990, Okada 1991, van Oostenbrugge 1999, Sugimura 1992). Although often an asymptomatic finding, in some cases extensive

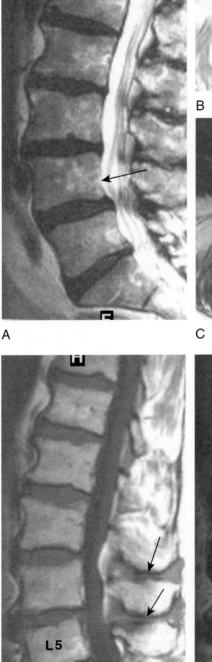

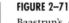

A

B

C

FIGURE 2–70

Degenerative spondylolisthesis with accompanying subarticular recess synovial cyst. An 82-year-old man with central low back pain and lower extremity weakness. A, Sagittal T2WI shows multilevel disc dehydration and L4–5 degenerative spondylolisthesis (arrow). B, Axial T1WI shows severe facet arthropathy (arrows 1) and a slightly trefoil configuration of the spinal canal. C, Axial T2WI confirms the findings seen on the T1WI. In addition, note the 5-mm lesion in the left subarticular recess demonstrating T2 prolongation (arrow). This cannot be fat: there is T1 prolongation apparent on the T1WI. This is a small synovial cyst projecting off the anterior aspect of the facet joint and further compromising the left subarticular recess and contributing to compression of the traversing left L5 nerve root.

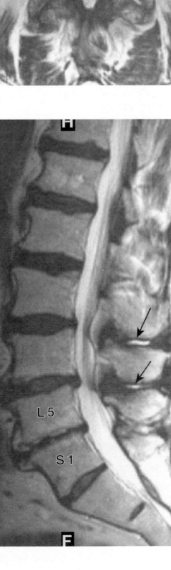

A

B

FIGURE 2–71

Baastrup's disease. A 74-year-old man with central low back pain. A, Sagittal T1WI demonstrates transitional anatomy with a well-developed S1–2 intervertebral disc and multilevel disc degeneration and degenerative disc bulging. The degenerative disc disease is worst at L5–S1, where there is severe loss of disc height and disc dehydration as well as subchondral Modic Type II degenerative changes. Note the areas of intermediate signal intensity between the L3–4 and L4–5 spinous processes, as well as the apparent cortical thickening manifested by absence of signal along the spinous process margins (arrows). B, Sagittal T2WI shows linear streaks of T2 prolongation between the L3–4 and L4–5 spinous processes (arrows), consistent with fluid or inflammatory tissue.

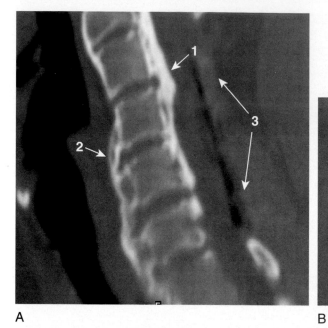

A

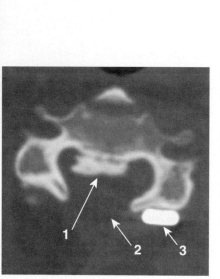

B

FIGURE 2–72

Ossification of the posterior longitudinal ligament. A 53-year-old woman with neck pain s/p multilevel fusion/decompression for extensive ossification of the posterior longitudinal ligament. A, Sagittal reconstruction demonstrates multilevel exuberant ossification of the posterior longitudinal ligament (arrow 1). There is also lesser anterior longitudinal ligament ossification (arrow 2), and there is multilevel posterior decompression (arrow 3). B. Axial CT study done at the C3 pedicle level demonstrates dense bone in the anterior cervical canal posterior to the vertebral body (arrow 1) and posterior decompression (arrow 2) with a metallic plate (arrow 3).

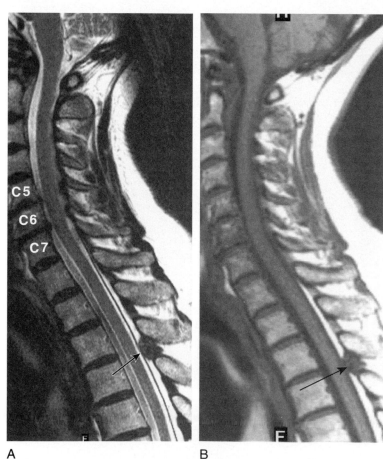

A   B

FIGURE 2–73

Ossification of the ligamentum flavum (also known as ossification of the yellow ligament). An 83-year-old woman with bilateral shoulder and arm pain. A, Sagittal T2WI demonstrates C5–6 and C6–7 degenerative disc narrowing and bulging with osteophyte formation. Posteriorly, between the anterior aspects of the T3 and T4, there is marked thickening of the ligamentum flavum with T2 shortening (arrow). B, Sagittal T1WI demonstrates that the abnormally thickened yellow ligament also demonstrates T1 prolongation. The imaging findings are typical of ossification of the yellow ligament.

ossification causes indentation of the posterior aspect of the spinal cord with associated radiculopathy and/or myelopathy (Hanakita 1990, Sugimura 1992, van Oostenbrugge 1999). Such ossification may occur secondary to degenerative change or from any one of several metabolic diseases. Laminectomy may be required to relieve pressure on the spinal cord (Okada 1991, van Oostenbrugge 1999).

Scheuermann's Disease, Thoracolumbar Osteochondrosis, and Juvenile Discogenic Disease

As the title of this section might suggest, controversy regarding terminology of this subject abounds. Authorities have debated the definition, characteristic lesion, and clini-

TABLE 2–12. Scheuermann's Disease Terminology

Term	Source	Definition
Scheuermann's disease	Lowe 1990	Irregularity of the vertebral body margins with wedging of at least 5 degrees in at least three adjacent vertebral bodies
	Dorland's Illustrated Medical Dictionary	A form of osteochondrosis. Synonyms include "juvenile kyphosis," "vertebral epiphysitis," and "kyphosis dorsalis juvenilis"
	Alexander 1977	A primary irregularity of ossification of one or more vertebral end plates. Neither symptoms nor wedging are appropriate criteria for the diagnosis.
Lumbar Scheuermann's disease	Lowe 1990	"Irregularity of the vertebral end-plates, the presence of Schmorl nodes, and narrowing of the intervertebral discs, without wedging of the vertebral bodies or kyphosis."
Juvenile vertebral osteochondrosis	Milsom 1961	The preferred synonym for Scheuermann's disease. The presence of Schmorl's nodes or the presence of at least two of four other criteria: deep and irregular notching of the anterior corners of the vertebral centra, anterior wedging, irregular sclerosis, and narrowing of the disc space
Lumbar and dorsolumbar forms of Scheuermann's disease	Greene 1985	Dorsolumbar vertebral changes without kyphosis and variable combinations of end-plate irregularity, Schmorl's node formation, and narrowing of the disc space
Classic Scheuermann's disease	Blumenthal 1987	Vertebral wedging of ≥5 degrees at (at least) three consecutive levels
Atypical Scheuermann's disease	Blumenthal 1987	Vertebral end-plate irregularities, anterior Schmorl's nodes, and disc space narrowing
	Paajanen 1989	Vertebral end-plate irregularities, Schmorl's nodes, and interspace narrowing
Thoracolumbar Scheuermann's disease	Heithoff 1994	Schmorl's node formation, end-plate irregularity, and/or wedging of the anterior vertebral body margins, often accompanied by disc space narrowing and dehydration

cal manifestations of these processes for more than 50 years. The term *Scheuermann's disease* is usually taken to mean irregularity of the vertebral body margins; a more stringent definition requires accompanying kyphosis of at least 5 degrees at three adjacent levels of the lumbar spine (Blumenthal 1987, Lowe 1990). Although Scheuermann initially offered this definition, he later wrote that one- to five-level involvement qualified as the disease (Resnick 1995). Table 2–12 provides some of the multiple definitions of the term *Scheuermann's disease* as well as related terms.

Schmorl's Nodes

Approximately 20% of asymptomatic subjects demonstrate lumbar Schmorl's nodes on MRI examination (Jensen 1994). Schmorl himself called these abnormalities *knorpelknotchen* and defined them as intraosseous herniations of the intervertebral disc (Soderberg 1955). Schmorl's nodes are generally held to be asymptomatic and are often regarded as a normal variant. However, intraosseous disc herniation is on occasion a painful process (Blumenthal 1987, Fahey 1998, McCall 1985, Stabler 1997, Walters 1991, Wood 1999) (Fig. 2–74), and the presence of multiple Schmorl's nodes is not normal variation, although the prognostic significance of having one, two, or several Schmorl's nodes and what term to use to describe a patient with multiple Schmorl's nodes remains a matter of ongoing controversy (see further discussion).

"CLASSIC," "ATYPICAL," "LUMBAR," AND "THORACOLUMBAR" SCHEUERMANN'S DISEASE

As is evident from perusal of Table 2–12, different authors use the term *Scheuermann's disease* to mean different things. Furthermore, some authors attach adjectives (e.g., "classic," "lumbar," "atypical") to indicate whether the earlier definition, requiring wedging of three adjacent vertebral bodies of at least 5 degrees, or some later variation is meant. Other authors (Alexander 1977) redefine the term entirely. Although some authors (Blumenthal 1987) maintain that classic Scheuermann's disease and atypical Scheuermann's disease are two distinct entities, it is more likely that there is only one underlying disease process that manifests as a spectrum of clinical and imaging findings. The characteristic lesion of Scheuermann's disease is irregularity of ossification of one or more vertebral end plates (Alexander 1977). This irregularity of ossification most frequently manifests itself as one or more Schmorl's nodes or vertebral marginal abnormalities (Fig. 2–75). Thoracic disc space narrowing and dehydration may develop as secondary phenomena. In many cases, the thoracic vertebral body and disc abnormalities of Scheuermann's disease are accompanied by lumbar disc degenerative changes and herniations, the combination of which has been termed *juvenile discogenic disease* (Heithoff 1994). There are mild cases wherein there are two or three thoracolumbar discs with Schmorl's nodes and minimal irregularity along the vertebral body

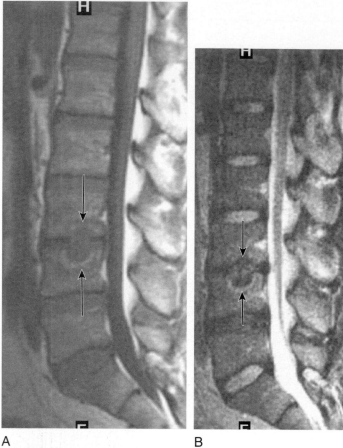

A

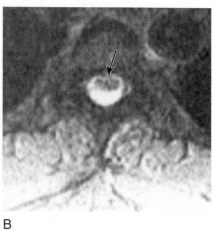

B

FIGURE 2-74

Symptomatic Schmorl's node. A 30-year-old man with severe central low back pain. A, Sagittal T1WI demonstrates L3–4 moderate loss of disc height as well as Schmorl's node formation both within the inferior aspect of L3 and the superior aspect of L4 (arrows). B, Sagittal T2WI again demonstrates Schmorl's node formation (arrows) with L3–4 disc dehydration and reactive changes in the bone marrow adjacent to the Schmorl's node with T2 prolongation.

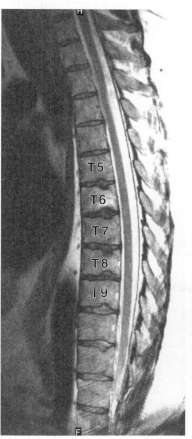

A

B

FIGURE 2-75

Scheuermann's disease with accompanying thoracic disc herniation. A 35-year-old man with upper mid-back pain. A, Sagittal T2WI shows multilevel extensive Schmorl's nodes and irregularity along the vertebral body margins. There is dehydration of T5–6 through T8–9 with narrowing of T6–7 and T8–9. B, Axial gradient-recalled echo T2WI at the T3–4 level shows a small disc protrusion (arrow) indenting the ventral aspect of the spinal cord.

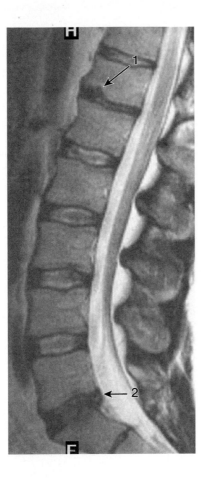

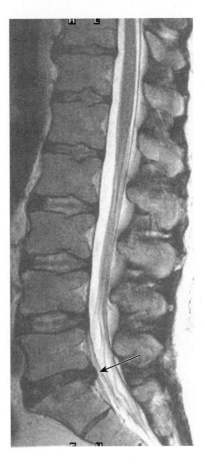

FIGURE 2–76

Mild juvenile discogenic disease. A 38-year-old man with low back pain and right leg pain and weakness. Sagittal T2WI demonstrates T11–12 mild loss of disc height and vertebral margin irregularity, T12–L1 moderate loss of disc height and hydration with Schmorl's node formation (arrow 1) and anterior vertebral marginal irregularity, L1–2 vertebral marginal irregularity, L3–4 Schmorl's node formation, and L5–S1 moderate disc dehydration with a 4-mm disc protrusion (arrow 2). There was no associated neural compression.

FIGURE 2–77

Moderate juvenile discogenic disease. A 46-year-old man with low back and bilateral leg pain and right leg numbness. Sagittal T2WI demonstrates T11–12 mild loss of disc height with moderate disc dehydration, minimal irregularity of the vertebral body margins, and degenerative disc bulging; T12–L1 and L1–2 mild loss of disc height and hydration with Schmorl's node formation; L2–3, L3–4, and L4–5 mild loss of disc hydration and Schmorl's node formation; and L5–S1 moderate loss of disc height and hydration with extensive (>3 mm) degenerative disc bulging (arrow).

margins (Fig. 2–76), moderate cases wherein there are multiple levels of Schmorl's nodes, thoracolumbar disc marginal irregularity (Fig. 2–77), disc space narrowing and dehydration, and severe cases wherein young individuals have severe multilevel thoracolumbar marginal abnormalities, and disc space narrowing with dehydration, frequently with accompanying disc herniations and IIIZs (Fig. 2–78). No sharp dividing line exists between those with mild, moderate, or severe disease; rather, there is a spectrum of abnormality where one grade of disease shades into the next. We use the term *Scheuermann's disease* in the same way that Alexander does, denoting Schmorl's nodes and vertebral marginal irregularity with or without wedging.

The underlying cause of Scheuermann's disease is unknown (Lowe 1990). Alexander (1977) maintains that trauma to the spine, particularly in patients with a somewhat weak spine undergoing rapid growth, causes end-plate fractures of the spine. Such fractures appear as either Schmorl's nodes or irregular vertebral end plates. These fractures lead to "disturbed cell vectoring and traumatic growth arrest," followed by narrowed intervertebral discs, wedging of the vertebral bodies, and kyphosis. Histologic

evidence from Aufdermaur (1981) and Scoles and associates (1991) supports this hypothesis. This theory most adequately accounts for the manifestations of the process as seen on MRI.

SCHEUERMANN'S DISEASE SYMPTOMS

There are at least four causes of pain in patients with Scheuermann's disease:

1. Scheuermann's disease occasionally produces symptoms in the thoracic spine, particularly if accompanied by considerable kyphosis (Aufdermaur 1991, Lowe 1990, Wassman 1946) (Fig. 2–79).
2. With or without pronounced kyphosis within the thoracic spine, posterior disc herniation within the thoracic spine (often at the level of Schmorl's nodes) may lead to thoracic pain and radiculopathy (Hafner 1952) (Fig. 2–80). As noted earlier in the section, "Disc Herniation," most thoracic disc herniations accompany Scheuermann's disease. Degenerated thoracic discs may demonstrate "nuclear tails" on CT examinations, with a

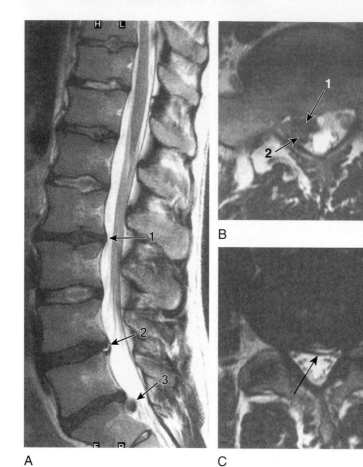

A   C

FIGURE 2–78

Severe juvenile discogenic disease. A 30-year-old man with a 3-week history of low back pain radiating down the posterior aspect of the right thigh and associated foot numbness. A, Sagittal T2WI shows extensive multilevel Schmorl's node formation from T10–11 through L2–3, mild loss of disc height and hydration at T10–11 and T12–L1, mild loss of disc height and moderate disc dehydration at L2–3 and L4–5, and severe loss of disc height and moderate dehydration at L5–S1. In addition, L2–3 shows degenerative disc bulging (arrow 1), L4–5 shows disc protrusion and associated T2 prolongation (high-intensity zone) along the annulus (arrow 2), and L5–S1 demonstrates a large disc extrusion (incompletely seen on this single sagittal image) (arrow 3). B, Axial T2WI at the level of the S1 pedicle shows a large, caudally dissecting disc extrusion (arrow 1) with posterolateral displacement and severe compression of the S1 nerve root sleeve (arrow 2). C, Axial T2WI at the L4–5 level shows degenerative disc bulging with a superimposed left central disc protrusion and accompanying linear focus of T2 prolongation (high-intensity zone) paralleling the disc margin (arrow).

tail of calcification leading from a degenerated nucleus to the disc margin (Fig. 2–81). Degenerative changes of discs in the thoracic spine may cause spinal stenosis with associated symptoms (Tallroth 1990).

3. As noted earlier, Scheuermann's disease may be accompanied by lumbar spine disc disease, remote from the location of the multilevel Schmorl's nodes (Cleveland 1981, Paajanen 1989, Salminen 1999, Soderberg 1955, Swischuk 1998), an association that has been called *juvenile discogenic disease* (Heithoff 1994). This degeneration usually occurs at the L4/5 and L5/S1 levels, although multilevel involvement is not uncommon (Figs. 2–76 to 2–78, 2–82).

4. Scheuermann's disease may be accompanied by spondylolysis of the lower lumbar spine, again remote from the Schmorl's nodes of the thoracic spine (Alexander 1977, Greene 1985, Milsom 1961, Ogilvie 1987, Stoddard 1979). The spondylolysis usually involves the L5 pars (Fig. 2–83).

The coexistence of degenerative changes and Scheuermann's disease exceeds what would be expected by chance: the disc abnormalities occur earlier in life, involve more levels, and are more severe in patients with Scheuermann's disease than in patients without Scheuermann's disease. Similarly, the incidence of spondylolysis appears to be higher in patients with Scheuermann's disease than in patients without. The association of Scheuermann's disease and spondylolysis has been attributed to accentuation of lumbar lordosis (Ogilvie 1987), but

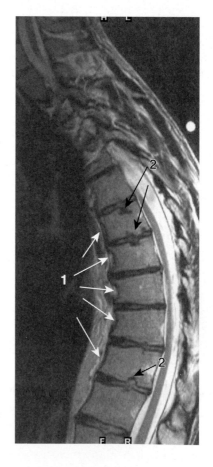

FIGURE 2–79

Scheuermann's disease with associated painful kyphosis. A 27-year-old man with upper back pain. Sagittal T2WI of the thoracic spine shows multilevel intervertebral disc narrowing, dehydration, and degenerative bulging. Note extensive multilevel wedging of vertebral bodies (arrows 1), Schmorl's node formation (arrows 2), and irregularity of vertebral end plates. There is accentuation of thoracic kyphosis.

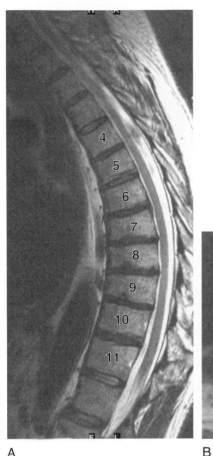

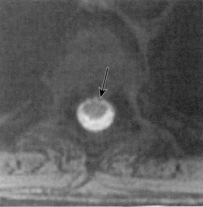

FIGURE 2–80

Scheuermann's disease with associated thoracic disc herniations. A 41-year-old patient with central upper back pain. A, Sagittal T2WI shows moderate intervertebral disc narrowing and dehydration from T6–7 through T10–11, as well as irregular vertebral body margins and Schmorl's nodes through these areas. In addition, there is wedging of T7 through T9. B, Axial gradient-recalled echo T2WI through the T6–7 disc shows a small left central disc protrusion (arrow) minimally indenting the ventral aspect of the spinal cord. Similar disc protrusions were seen at T7–8 through T9–10 (not shown).

A   B

this does not explain the high rate of disc disease. Alexander posited that Scheuermann's disease represented one end of a biologic spectrum and that patients with Scheuermann's disease had somewhat inherently weaker tissue. Whether such weakness results from one or several enzymatic or biochemical deficiencies is a subject of ongoing research (Paassilta 2001).

SCHEUERMANN'S DISEASE TREATMENT

Treatment of Scheuermann's disease aims at treating the cause of the patient's pain. For painful kyphosis, bracing has been recommended with surgery held in reserve for cases of severe kyphosis (Lowe 1990). For degenerative disc disease, conservative or surgical treatment as outlined in the section "Disc Herniation" may be employed. In general, it may be advisable to avoid fusion surgery in patients with coexistent Scheuermann's disease and lumbar disc degeneration, for such fusion appears to accelerate degenerative changes at the adjacent segment, necessitating further back surgery. Diagnosis and treatment of spondylolysis are discussed in Chapter 8; as with fusion for degenerative disc disease, fusion for spondylolysis in patients with Scheuermann's disease may be accompanied by a higher complication rate than in patients without Scheuermann's disease.

Reporting

Ideally, the report describing degenerative changes of the spine should concisely and accurately convey the status of the disc (height, hydration, and contour); the spinal canal, subarticular recess, and neural foramina (normal or mild, moderate, or severe stenosis); and the facet joints (normal, or showing mild, moderate, or severe facet arthropathy). In addition, the degree of nerve root compression (none, mild, moderate, or severe) and (in the cervical and thoracic spine) spinal cord compression should be evaluated. On a usual lumbar spine study (including at least T12/L1 through L5/S1), there are thus 6 levels × 1 disc/level × 3 evaluations (height, hydration, contour) plus 6 levels × three locations of possible stenosis (central, subarticular, and foraminal) plus 6 levels × 2 facet joints plus 6 levels × 4 (main) nerve roots to evaluate (left and right traversing and exiting) = 6 × 3 + 6 × 3 + 6 × 2 + 6 × 4 = 18 + 18 + 12 + 24 = 72 assessments. This is even before reporting such possible additional features as tumor, infection, fracture, and subchondral marrow degenerative changes. A given report has two parts: a body (cataloging these findings), and an impression, which may reiterate certain findings and which correlates the imaging findings with other available data (such as the history, the pain diagram, and additional imaging) to come to a conclusion. In some cases, the imager may definitely

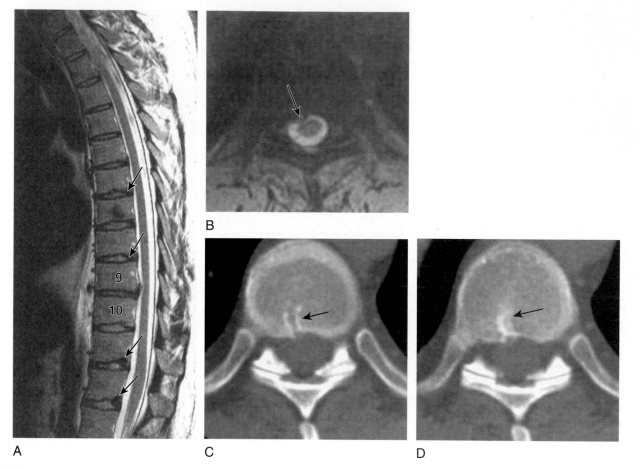

A   C   D

B

FIGURE 2–81

Scheuermann's disease with disc herniations and "nuclear tails." A 37-year-old man with mid-thoracic spine pain radiating to beneath the right scapula. A, Sagittal T2WI demonstrates multilevel degenerative disc disease with vertebral marginal irregularity and areas of T2 shortening along the posterior vertebral bodies adjacent to the intervertebral discs (arrows). There is a cranially dissecting disc extrusion at the T9–10 level. B, Axial gradient-recalled echo T2WI at the T9–10 disc level demonstrates a right central disc extrusion with associated cord indentation (arrow). C, Axial CT study done at the level of the T9–10 disc demonstrates calcification along the disc annulus (arrow) leading to the location of the disc protrusion (a nuclear tail). On this nonmyelographic CT study, the disc protrusion itself is difficult to appreciate. D, Axial CT scan just superior to C demonstrates calcification (the nuclear tail) along the undersurface of the T9 vertebral body (arrow).

ascribe symptoms to imaging findings; in other cases, the imager may suggest that the imaging findings are likely to be the source of symptoms; and in yet other cases, the imager may not be able to come to any definite conclusion based on the imaging findings and available clinical data.

The art of constructing a concise and accurate report requires time and experience. At least in the beginning, a systematic approach usually provides significant advantages. Remembering the status and measurement of the various structures to maintain consistency between the body and conclusion in a given report may be next to impossible. Relatively simple forms for the lumbar and cervical spine (Fig. 2–84A and B) with appropriate blanks can provide both a reminder to evaluate structures and also, once evaluated, a valuable memory aid in dictating cases (to ensure consistency between the body and conclusion of the report).

With regard to specific report formatting, we make the following recommendations, recognizing that the preferences of not only the dictating radiologist but the referring clinician will result in a wide range of practice.

1. Break up the report into a level-by-level format.
2. Report findings in a systematic fashion. This makes editing new and reviewing old reports easier. It is also possible to alter dictations in mid-stride (so to speak) when realizing that something has not been included.[††] One format is as follows:

[††] For example, for some reason it is easy to forget to report the height/hydration status of a disc when the level demonstrates spondylolisthesis. After providing a paragraph describing 15% degenerative spondylolisthesis of L4 on L5 secondary to severe facet arthropathy, and grading spinal canal, subarticular recess, and foraminal stenosis and neural compression along with description of a disc protrusion and synovial cyst, one may be starting the L3/4 level before one remembers that the moderate loss of disc height and hydration have not been mentioned. If one reports each level in a consistent manner, one may then state to the transcriptionist: "Time out. Go back to the L4/5 level and as the first sentence of that level say 'There is moderate loss of disc height and hydration.' End time out. Now go on with the L3/4 level as follows." Consistency in report formatting will allow placement of such statements without the annoying task of rewinding past a perfectly good description of the other findings at L4/5.

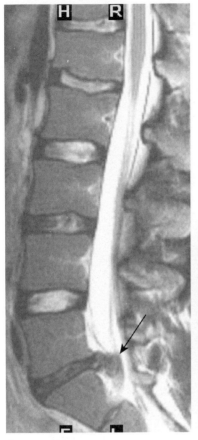

A

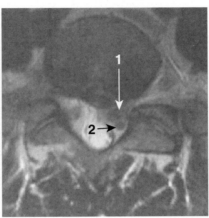

B

FIGURE 2–82

Juvenile discogenic disease with a large disc extrusion in a young man. A 23-year-old man with low back and left leg pain. A, Sagittal T2WI shows preservation of disc height and hydration but considerable irregularity along the vertebral body margins at T12–L1 and L1–2, a normal disc at L2–3, a mildly dehydrated disc with a Schmorl's node at L3–4, a normal disc at L4–5, and moderate loss of disc height and hydration at L5–S1. In addition, there is a large disc extrusion at L5–S1 (arrow). B, Axial T2WI at the L5–S1 level shows a complex, large, left central and subarticular disc extrusion (arrow 1) with posterior displacement and mild compression of the S1 nerve root sleeve (arrow 2).

a. Disc status
  i. Height
  ii. Hydration
  iii. Associated subchondral degenerative changes (if present)
b. Spondylolisthesis if present
  i. Percentage of spondylolisthesis
  ii. Cause of spondylolisthesis
    1. Degenerative from facet arthropathy
      a. Grade facet arthropathy
    2. Lytic
      a. State levels of pars abnormalities
  iii. Associated stenosis and neural compression
c. Disc contour abnormality
  i. Bulge
  ii. Protrusion or extrusion
    1. Size (small, medium, large)
    2. AP dimension (usually reported from sagittal)
    3. Neural compression (usually reported from axial)

d. Facet arthropathy
  i. Grade
  ii. Associated stenosis
  iii. Associated neural compression
e. Stenosis and compression not described as part of above processes
  i. Location
  ii. Degree
  iii. Cause
3. In the impression, convey a sense of the likelihood of the cause of the patient's symptoms and the relationship between the imaging findings and these symptoms.

We conclude this chapter by providing several imaging examples to flesh out these recommendations. We selected the included cases not because of their rarity or complexity but rather to illustrate what we believe are everyday disease processes with complete reports. The reports included with these studies are typical of our usual reporting process.

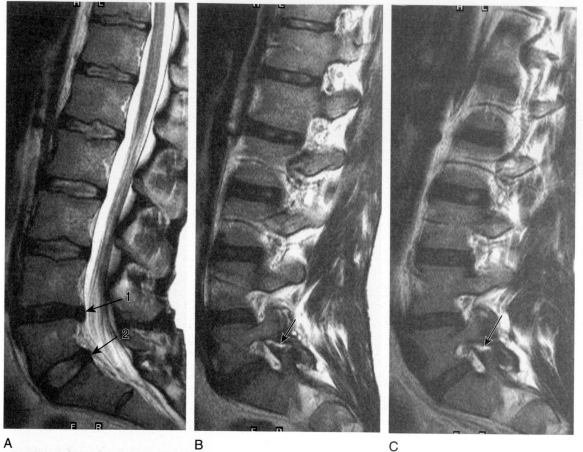

A   B   C

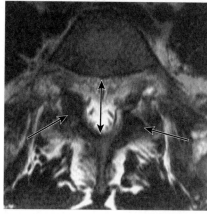

D

FIGURE 2–83

Scheuermann's disease with accompanying spondylolysis. A 35-year-old patient with chronic low back and left leg pain. A, Sagittal T2WI shows Schmorl's nodes at T12–L1, L1–2, and L3–4; L2–3 shows vertebral marginal irregularity. L4–5 shows mild loss of disc height and moderate disc dehydration as well as a disc protrusion (arrow 1). L5–S1 shows minimal loss of disc height and degenerative disc bulging (arrow 2). L4 is slightly posteriorly displaced relative to L5. B, Right parasagittal T2WI shows a right pars defect with T2 prolongation through the pars (arrow). C, Left parasagittal T2WI shows similar findings on the left side, with a left pars defect and a focus of T2 prolongation through the pars (arrow). D, Axial T2WI at the level of the L5 pars shows fibroproliferative changes along the pars (arrows) and anteroposterior elongation of the spinal canal (double-headed arrow).

LEVEL	RIGHT NEURAL FORAMEN	SPINAL CANAL	LEFT NEURAL FORAMEN
L5/S1			
L4/5			
L3/4			
L2/3			
L1/2			
T12/L1			

A

LEVEL	RIGHT NEURAL FORAMEN	SPINAL CANAL	LEFT NEURAL FORAMEN
C2/3			
C3/4			
C4/5			
C5/6			
C6/7			
C7/T1			
T1/2			
T2/3			

B

FIGURE 2–84

Paper form. A, Lumbar form. B, Cervical form. These forms serve as a reminder to evaluate each level, and they also provide a valuable memory aid when dictating the conclusion by ensuring that grading and measurements are consistent with the body.

FIGURES AND REPORT EXAMPLES

EXAMPLE 1 (FIG. 2–85)

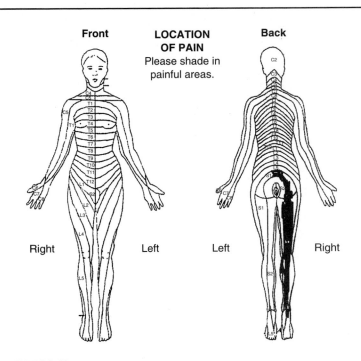

FIGURE 2–85

Example 1. A 34-year-old woman with right-sided low back pain radiating into the right leg, with right leg tingling, weakness, and numbness. See accompanying complete report and pain diagram. Axial images were obtained through the L3–4 level, but not displayed as these were normal.

(*continued on page 84*)

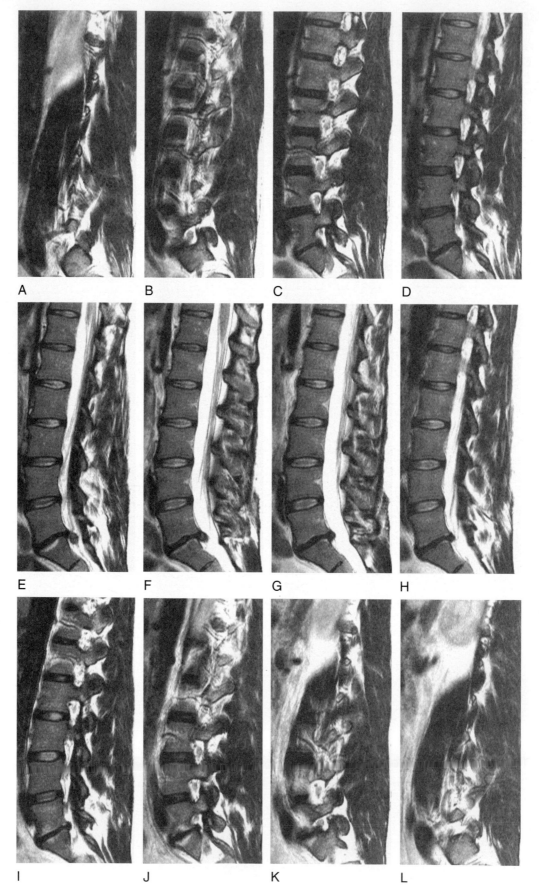

FIGURE 2–85 (*continued*)

Example 1. A–L, Sequential right-to-left sagittal T2WIs.

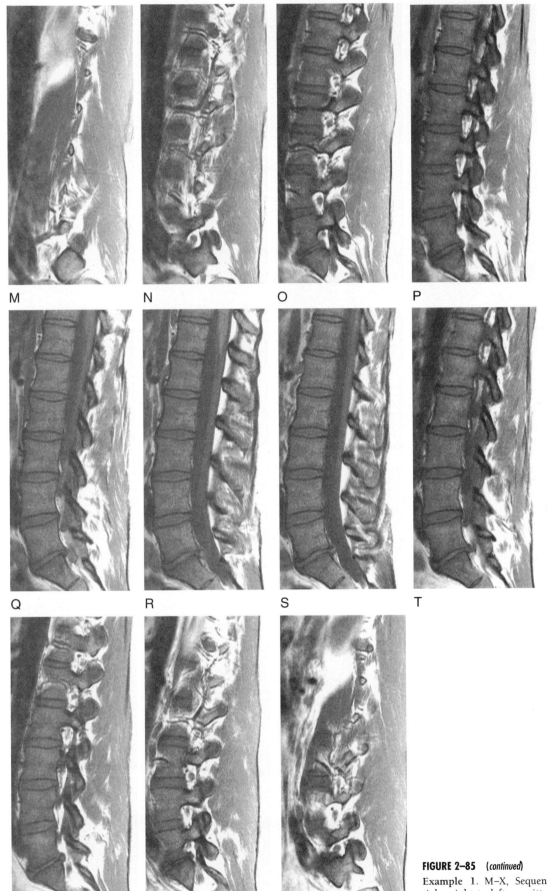

M   N   O   P

Q   R   S   T

U   W   X

FIGURE 2–85 (*continued*)
Example 1. M–X, Sequential right-to-left sagittal T1WIs.

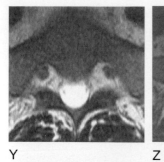
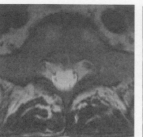
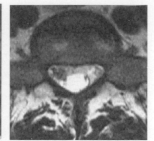

Y

Z

AA

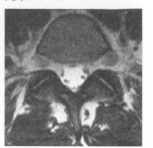

BB

CC

DD

FIGURE 2–85 *(continued)*

Example 1. Y–DD, Sequential inferior-to-superior axial T2WI from the S1 through the L5 pedicles.

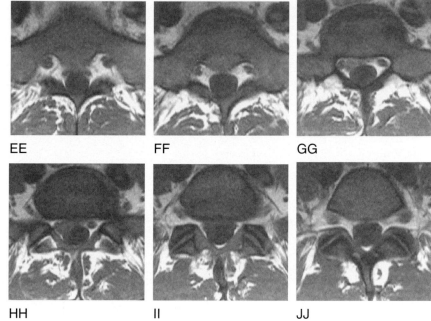

EE   FF   GG

HH   II   JJ

FIGURE 2–85 (*continued*)

Example 1. EE–JJ, Sequential inferior-to-superior T1WI from the S1 through the L5 pedicles.

Clinical Information: Evaluate for lumbar pain. Furthermore, the patient indicates that she has right low back pain and right leg pain and right leg tingling, weakness, and numbness.

Technical Information: The following imaging sequences were performed:

1. Sagittal fast spin-echo T1WIs.
2. Sagittal fast spin-echo T2WIs.
3. Axial fast spin echo T1WIs.
4. Axial fast spin echo T2WIs.

Interpretation: The conus is normal and ends at the T12 level.

L5–S1: There is moderate loss of disc height and severe disc dehydration as well as Modic Type I degenerative change on sagittal images 11 (Fig. 2–85*E*) and 24 (Fig. 2–85*R*). There is a right central and subarticular, caudally dissecting disc extrusion measuring 8.3 mm in AP dimension on sagittal image 11 (Fig. 2–85*E*), and showing 11 mm of caudal dissection on that image. Axial image 50 (Fig. 2–85*BB*) shows posterolateral displacement and severe compression of the right S1 nerve root. There is also flattening of the right side of the thecal sac. There is some heterogeneity of signal intensity within the disc extrusion as well as a globular appearance of the inferior aspect of the extrusion. Because of disc narrowing, there is bilateral mild up-down foraminal stenosis but no exiting L5 ganglionic compression is identified.

T11–12 through L4–5: Disc height and hydration is preserved. No focal disc contour abnormality, spinal canal stenosis, or foraminal stenosis is identified at any of these levels.

Conclusion

1. L5–S1 degenerative changes including moderate loss of disc height, severe disc dehydration, and subchondral Modic Type I marrow changes. In addition, there is a right central and subarticular, caudally dissecting disc extrusion with posterolateral displacement and compression of the right S1 nerve root. Signal inhomogeneity and a somewhat globular appearance of the inferior aspect of the lesion suggest the possibility of a sequestered fragment. Considering the patient's right lower extremity symptoms and lack of neural compressive pathology elsewhere, this disc extrusion in all likelihood represents the symptom-producing lesion.
2. Other levels are unremarkable.

Comments Regarding Report

1. In the "Clinical Information" section, information provided on the patient's prescription is usually listed first, preceded by the words "Evaluate for." Following this, and preceded by the word "Furthermore," information gleaned from the patient's completed "MRI Information Sheet" is provided.
2. In the "Technical Information" section, pulse sequences are enumerated. We have found that listing the sequences makes it easy to determine how many (and which) sequences were performed. Generally, this information is dictated and transcribed as "Standard technical macro for the lumbar spine No. 1" ("No. 2" is the same with the addition of "5. Sagittal gradient echo T2-weighted images" obtained when infection, tumor, or fracture is suspected).
3. In the "Interpretation" section:
   i. References to specific scans in the original reports have been supplemented to fit the format of figures within this chapter.
   ii. The section provides a description of the findings.
   iii. We usually provide the location of the conus and its appearance. Some may not feel that this is necessary, while others may wish to comment on paraspinal soft tissues, the overall appearance of the bone marrow, and so forth.
   iv. Specific figures are cited in description of the findings.
   v. To save space in the report and time dictating and transcribing, normal levels are combined.
4. In the "Conclusion" section:
   i. Some overlap of descriptive terminology with the "Interpretation" section is necessary.
   ii. An attempt is made to offer a specific diagnosis and also to provide an indication as to how the imaged abnormality (or abnormalities) relates to the patient's symptoms. In this case, the relationship is straightforward.

EXAMPLE 2 (FIG. 2–86)

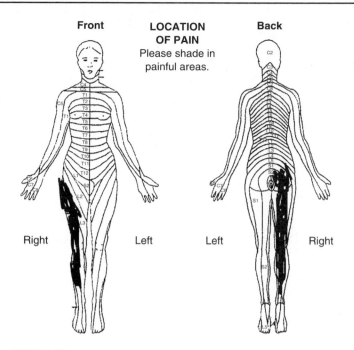

FIGURE 2–86

Example 2. A 42-year-old man with right low back, hip, and leg pain. See accompanying complete report and pain diagram.

(*continued on page 92*)

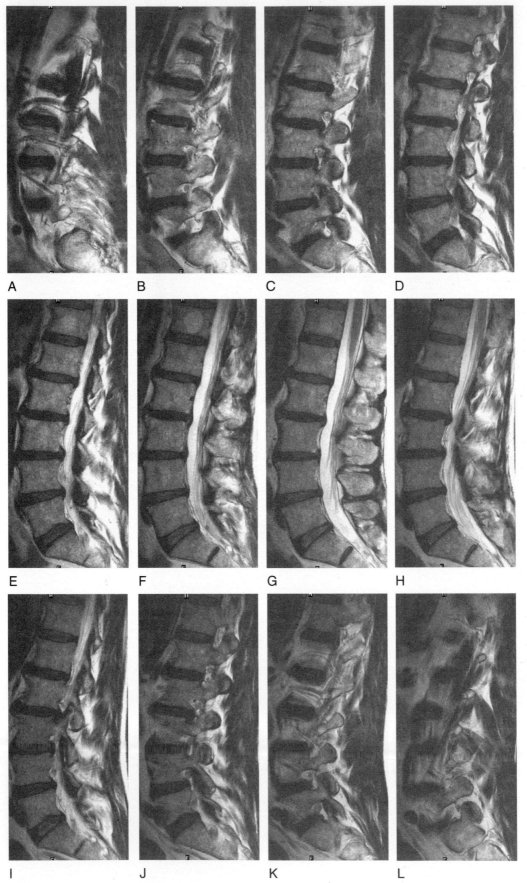

FIGURE 2–86 *(continued)*

Example 2. A–L, Sequential right-to-left sagittal T2WI.

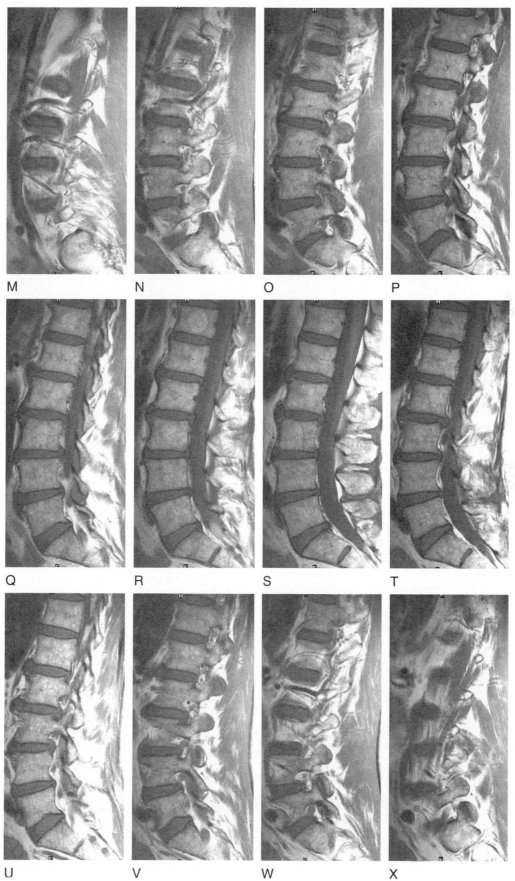

FIGURE 2–86 (*continued*)

Example 2. M–X, Sequential right-to-left sagittal T1WI.

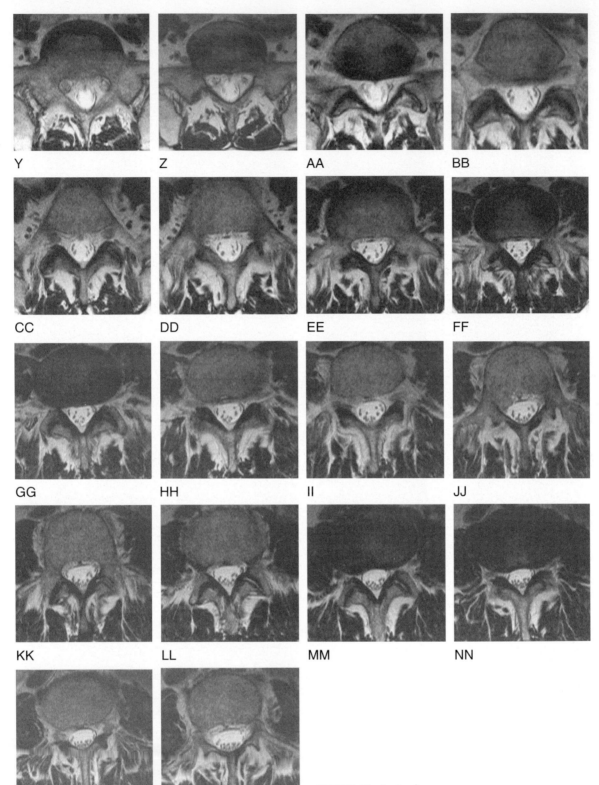

FIGURE 2–86 (*continued*)

Example 2. Y–PP, Sequential inferior-to-superior axial T2WI from the S1 through the inferior aspect of the L3 pedicle.

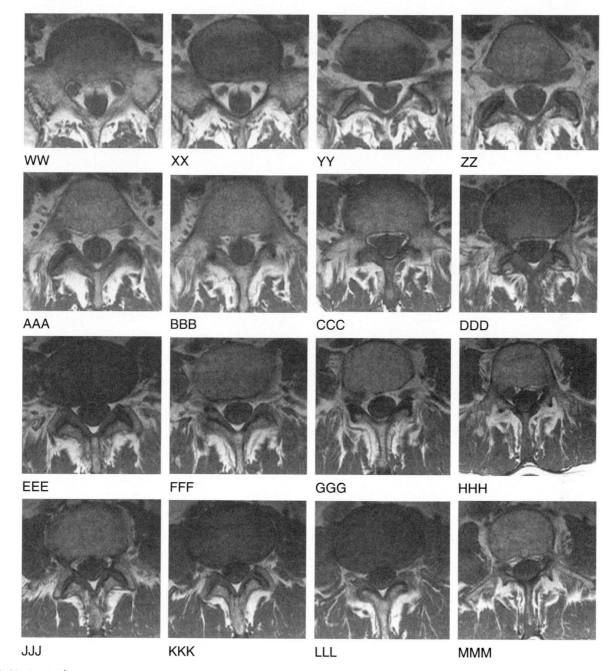

WW   XX   YY   ZZ

AAA   BBB   CCC   DDD

EEE   FFF   GGG   HHH

JJJ   KKK   LLL   MMM

FIGURE 2–86 (*continued*)
Example 2. WW–MMM, Sequential inferior-to-superior axial T1WI from the S1 through the inferior aspect of the L3 pedicle.

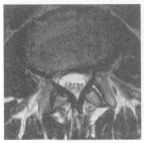
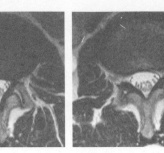

QQ   RR   SS

FIGURE 2–86   (*continued*)
Example 2. QQ–SS, Axial T2WI from inferior to superior, centered at the L2–3 disc.

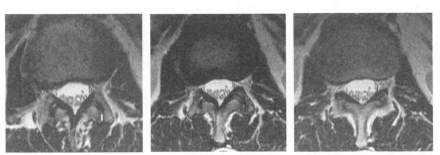

TT   UU   VV

FIGURE 2–86   (*continued*)
Example 2. TT–VV, Axial T2WI from inferior to superior, centered at the L1–2 disc.

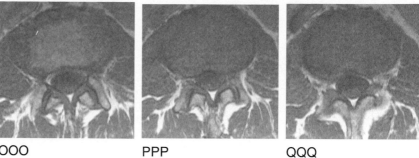

OOO   PPP   QQQ

FIGURE 2–86 (*continued*)

Example 2. OOO–QQQ, Axial T1WI from inferior to superior, centered at the L2–3 disc.   (*continued*)

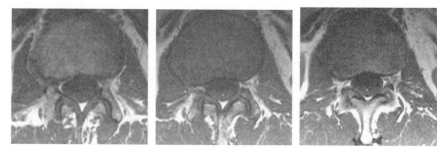

RRR   SSS   TTT

FIGURE 2–86 (*continued*)

Example 2. RRR–TTT, Axial T1WI from inferior to superior, centered at the L1–2 disc.

Clinical Information: Evaluate for right leg pain. Furthermore, the patient indicates that he has right hip and low back pain.

Interpretation: The conus is normal and ends at the L1 level.

L5–S1: There is preservation of disc height and hydration. There is mild facet arthropathy. No spinal canal stenosis or foraminal stenosis is identified.

L4–5: There is mild loss of disc height and hydration, and there is degenerative disc bulging. There is a right foraminal disc extrusion isointense to the parent disc measuring 5.0 mm in AP dimension at the level of the disc on sagittal image 10 (Fig. 2–86*D*). In addition, and superimposed on the other findings, there is a cranially dissecting extension of the foraminal disc extrusion. This is much better seen on the T1WIs than on the T2WIs, and is seen for example on sagittal image 22 (Fig. 2–86*P*) as an extra density along the posterior aspect of the L4 vertebral body, posteriorly displacing the right preganglionic L4 nerve root. On axial studies, the lesion is seen on axial image 43 (Fig. 2–86*JJ*) as an approximately 4 × 6 mm mass adjacent to the right L4 pedicle in the lateral recess. On the T1WIs, the lesion is seen on axial image 97 (Fig. 2–86*HHH*), where there is compression of the preganglionic L4 nerve root at its point of origin from the thecal sac.

L3–4: There is moderate loss of disc height and moderate disc dehydration. There is a right subarticular and foraminal disc protrusion measuring 7.0 mm in AP dimension on sagittal image 11 (Fig. 2–86*D*), narrowing the inferior aspect of the intervertebral nerve root canal. There is also left foraminal disc protrusion measuring 4.8 mm in AP dimension on sagittal image 15 (Fig. 2–86*I*) narrowing the inferior aspect of the intervertebral nerve root canal without exiting ganglionic compression. No traversing nerve root compression is identified.

L2–3: There is mild loss of disc height and moderate disc dehydration along with degenerative disc bulging. As at the next lower level there are bilateral foraminal disc protrusions measuring 5.2 mm in AP dimension on the left as measured on image 9 (Fig. 2–86*C*) and 5.5 mm in AP dimension on the right as measured on image 15 (Fig. 2–86*I*), causing bilateral moderate up-down foraminal stenosis without exiting ganglionic compression.

L1–2: There is mild loss of disc height and moderate disc dehydration. There is circumferential disc bulging and a superimposed right 5.2-mm disc protrusion seen on sagittal image 9 (Fig. 2–86*C*) and axial image 32 (Fig. 2–86*UU*) . There is bilateral moderate up-down foraminal narrowing without exiting L1 ganglionic compression.

T12–L1: There is preservation of disc height with mild disc dehydration. No posterior disc contour abnormality, spinal canal stenosis, or foraminal stenosis is seen.

Incidentally noted is a 2.0-cm hemangioma of the T12 vertebral body demonstrating T1 shortening and T2 prolongation relative to adjacent normal marrow.

Conclusion

1. L4–5 right subarticular, cranially dissecting disc extrusion with compression of the preganglionic right L4 nerve root. Considering the patient's right hip and leg symptoms, this is in all likelihood the symptom-producing lesion.
2. There are additional degenerative changes at other levels, including L3–4, where there is moderate loss of disc height and dehydration with bilateral foraminal disc protrusions without associated neural compression, L2–3 mild loss of disc height and moderate disc dehydration with bilateral foraminal disc protrusions with moderate foraminal stenosis but no exiting ganglionic compression, and L1–2 mild loss of disc height and moderate disc dehydration with a right foraminal disc protrusion without associated neural compression.

Comments Regarding Report

1. The "Technical Information" section identical to Example 1 has been omitted.
2. Sequential axial images were obtained through the mid L3 vertebral body, with images through the discs at the L2–3 and L1–2 levels. Limited image sets through upper lumbar or lower thoracic discs may be obtained, but imaging from L3–4 through L5–S1 should always include everything, and not skip the area between the discs. This lesion, for example, is most conspicuous at the mid-L4 level and could be missed if no axial views had been obtained through the mid-vertebral body.
3. This is a relatively subtle lesion. Both finding the lesion and ascribing significance to it require the patient's pain diagram and history.
4. Foraminal disc contour abnormalities are sometimes difficult to describe. In this case, the term *protrusion* was used, although technically the lesions dissect slightly from the level of the disc and thus meet criteria for *extrusion*. This term is not used for the small "mushroom cap"–appearing lesions seen in this case but is used for the dissecting component of the L4–5 abnormality. Small, bilateral foraminal protrusions (or even extrusions) that narrow the lower aspect of the neural foramina are a frequently seen degenerative phenomenon.
5. The hemangioma is included not so much for medical necessity but to avoid misunderstanding on the part of clinicians who might see the lesion and incorrectly ascribe significance to it.

EXAMPLE 3 (FIG. 2–87)

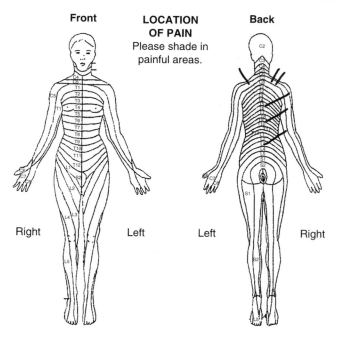

Front   **LOCATION OF PAIN**   **Back**

Please shade in painful areas.

Right   Left   Left   Right

FIGURE 2–87

Example 3. A 53-year-old woman with central mid and lower back pain. See accompanying complete report and pain diagram.

(*continued on page 98*)

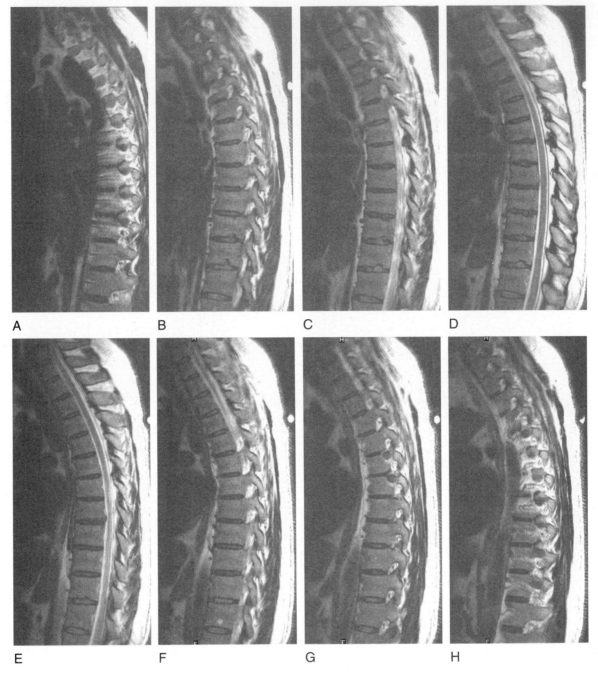

A   B   C   D

E   F   G   H

FIGURE 2–87 *(continued)*
Example 3. A–H, Sequential T2WI from the right to the left of the thoracic spine.

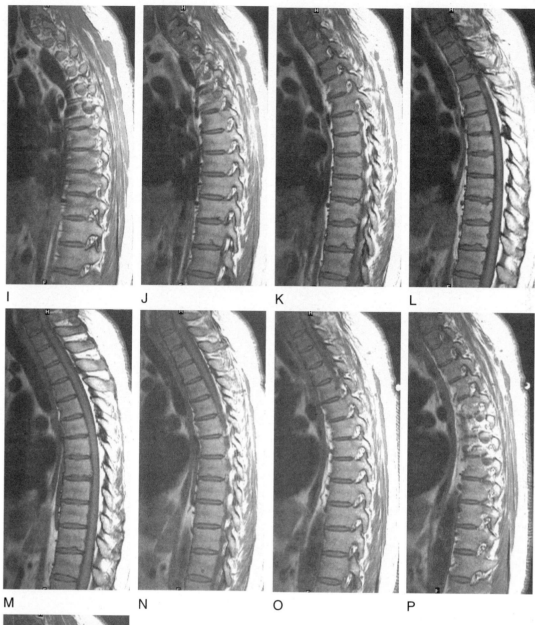

I

J

K

L

M

N

O

P

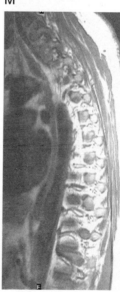

Q

FIGURE 2–87 (*continued*)

Example 3. I–K, Sequential T1WI from the right to the left of the thoracic spine.

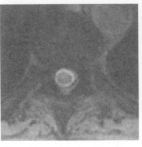
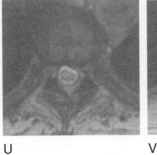
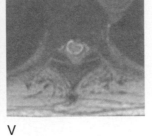

T   U   V

FIGURE 2–87 (*continued*)

Example 3. T–V, Sequential inferior-to-superior axial images centered at the T8–9 disc.

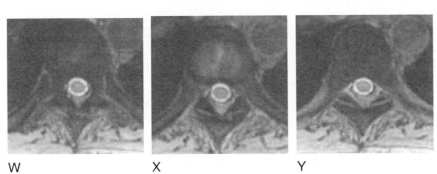

W   X   Y

FIGURE 2–87 (*continued*)

Example 3. W–Y, Sequential inferior-to-superior axial images centered at the T7–8 disc.

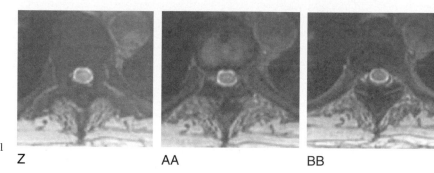

Z   AA   BB

FIGURE 2–87   (*continued*)

Example 3. Z–BB, Sequential inferior-to-superior axial images centered at the T6–7 disc.

Clinical Information: Evaluate for thoracalgia and lumbalgia. Rule out HNP. In addition the patient indicates she has central mid back pain and low back pain.

Technical Information: The following imaging sequences were performed:

1. Sagittal fast spin-echo T1WIs.
2. Sagittal fast spin-echo T2WIs.
3. Axial gradient-echo T2WIs at select levels.

The patient received 10 mg of liquid diazepam orally. The patient's O_2 saturation and heart rate were monitored throughout the procedure, and values remained within their normal range.

Interpretation: The thoracic spinal cord is of normal caliber and signal intensity. No syrinx or tumor is identified.

Sagittal images demonstrate multilevel degenerative changes of the intervertebral discs with disc narrowing, Schmorl's node formation, and irregularity of the vertebral body margins seen from the T6–7 through the T9–10 levels.

T8–9: There is a left central, cranially dissecting disc extrusion measuring 3.3 mm in AP dimension on axial image 47 (Fig. 2–87 V), with indentation of the left side of the spinal cord.

T7–8: Axial image 45 (Fig. 2–87 X) suggests a "nuclear tail" consistent with nuclear degeneration. No disc protrusion or cord compression is seen.

T6–7: Axial image 42 (Fig. 2–87 AA) shows a 1-mm central disc protrusion without contact or compression of the spinal cord.

Sagittal images 21 (Fig. 2–87 C) and 34 (Fig. 2–87 L) demonstrate abnormal thickening with T1 prolongation and T2 shortening of the ligamentum flavum between the T5–6 and T6–7 levels and to a lesser extent along the T3–4 level. The findings are consistent with ossification of the ligamentum flavum.

Conclusion

1. Multilevel degenerative change of the thoracic discs as described earlier, particularly at T6–7 through T9–10, with disc narrowing and dehydration, Schmorl's node formation, and irregularity of vertebral body margins consistent with Scheuermann's disease.
2. At T8–9, there is a 3.3-mm, cranially dissecting disc extrusion with indentation of the left ventral lateral spinal cord.
3. There is ossification of the ligamentum flavum. This is generally an asymptomatic finding unless sufficient ossification is present to produce neural compression (which it is not in this case).

Reference

van Oostenbrugge RJ, Herpers MJ, de Kruijk JR. Spinal cord compression caused by unusual location and extension of ossified ligamenta flava in a Caucasian male. Spine 1999; 24:486–488.

Comments Regarding Report

1. The thoracic technique is different than the lumbar technique: T1 axials are not routinely obtained, and the T2 axials are gradient echo rather than fast spin echo because of flow-related artifacts in thoracic imaging using axial fast spin-echo images. Axials are usually obtained through only selected levels at the discretion of the reviewing radiologists (or, if the technologist is well trained, the discretion of the technologist).
2. The patient was sedated with oral diazepam for claustrophobia. With short-bore high-field magnets, almost all claustrophobic patients can be scanned with oral or intravenous diazepam.
3. As noted earlier (see section, "Scheuermann's Disease, Thoracolumbar Osteochondrosis, and Juvenile Discogenic Disease") our criteria for the diagnosis of Scheuermann's disease do not include wedging of three adjacent levels by 5 degrees but rather relies on the presence of multiple levels of disc narrowing, dehydration, and marginal irregularity.
4. When describing an infrequently seen entity (such as ossification of the ligamentum flavum), it is often helpful to include a reference with the dictation.

EXAMPLE 4 (FIG. 2–88)

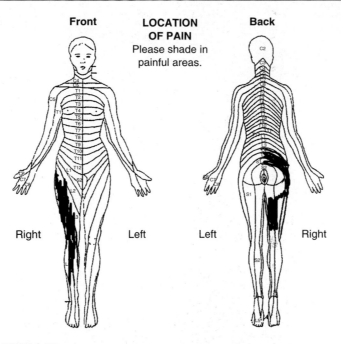

Front

LOCATION OF PAIN
Please shade in painful areas.

Back

Right   Left   Left   Right

FIGURE 2–88

Example 4. A 69-year-old man with low back and right hip and anterior thigh pain. See accompanying complete report and pain diagram.

(*continued on page 106*)

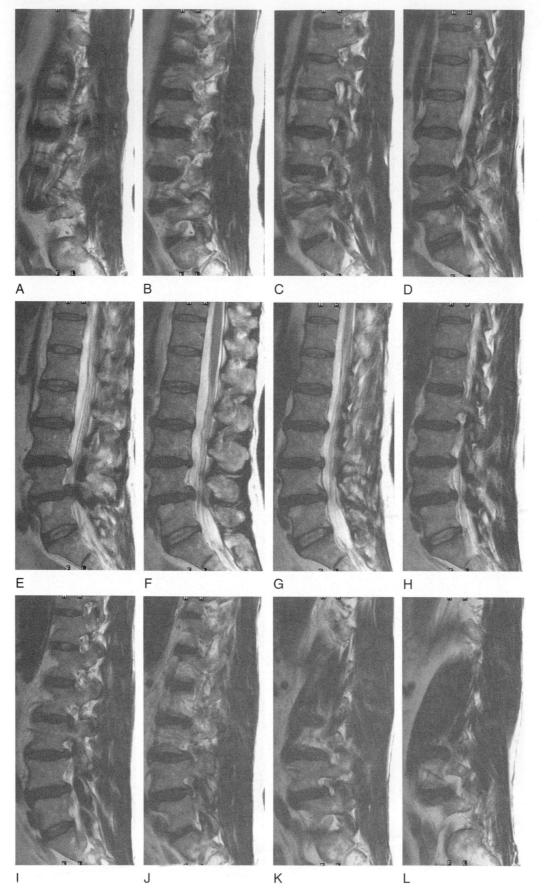

FIGURE 2–88 *(continued)*
Example 4. A–L, Sequential right-to-left sagittal T2WI.

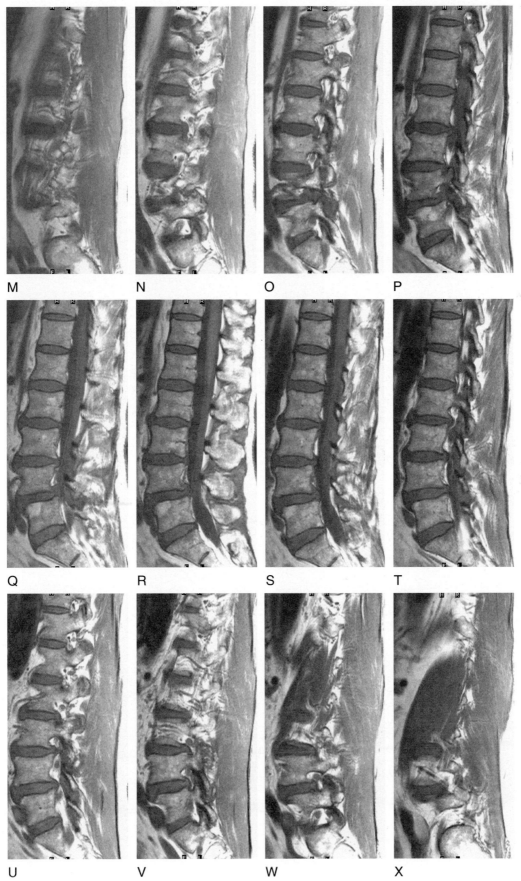

M N O P

Q R S T

U V W X

FIGURE 2–88 (*continued*)

Example 4. M–X, Sequential right-to-left sagittal T1WI.

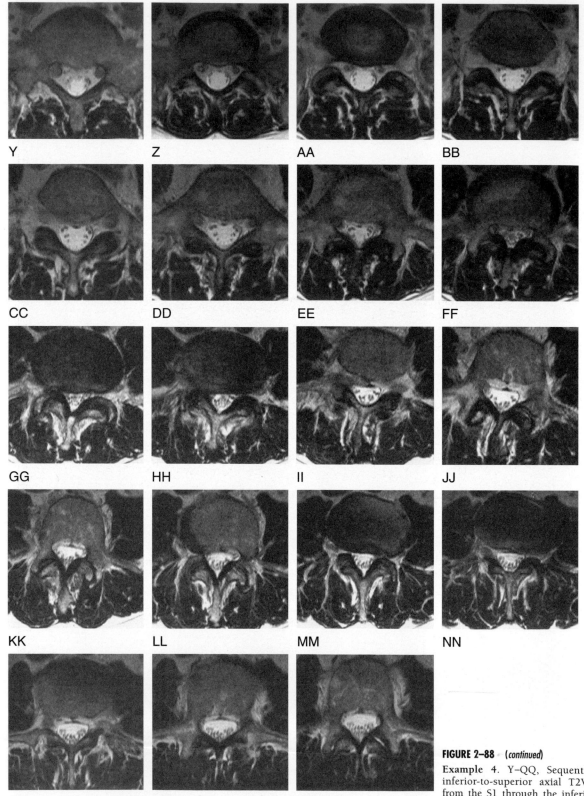

Y   Z   AA   BB

CC   DD   EE   FF

GG   HH   II   JJ

KK   LL   MM   NN

OO   PP   QQ

FIGURE 2–88 (*continued*)

Example 4. Y–QQ, Sequential inferior-to-superior axial T2WI from the S1 through the inferior aspect of the L3 pedicle.

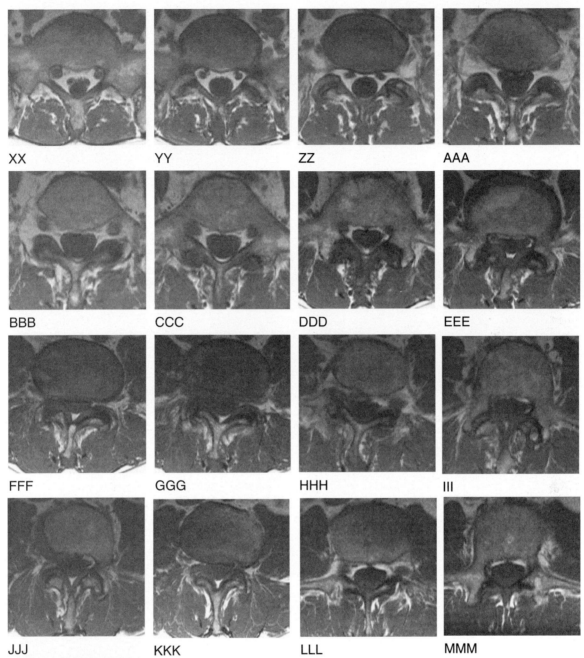

XX   YY   ZZ   AAA

BBB   CCC   DDD   EEE

FFF   GGG   HHH   III

JJJ   KKK   LLL   MMM

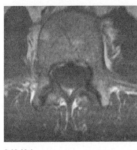

NNN

FIGURE 2–88 (*continued*)

Example 4. XX–NNN, Sequential inferior-to-superior axial T1WI from the S1 through the inferior aspect of the L3 pedicle.

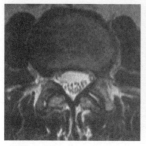
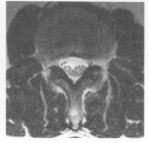

RR   SS   TT

FIGURE 2–88 *(continued)*

Example 4. RR–TT, Axial T2WI from inferior to superior, centered at the L2–3 disc.

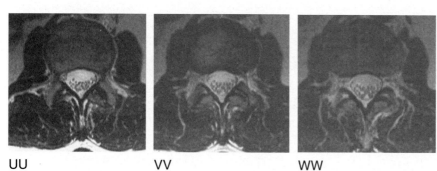

UU   VV   WW

FIGURE 2–88 *(continued)*

Example 4. UU–WW, Axial T2WI from inferior to superior, centered at the L1–2 disc.

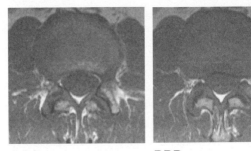
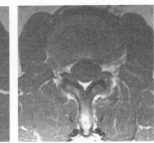

QQQ   RRR   SSS

FIGURE 2–88   (*continued*)

Example 4. QQQ–SSS, Axial T1WI from inferior to superior, centered at the L2–3 disc.

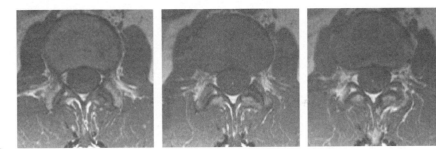

TTT   UUU   VVV

FIGURE 2–88   (*continued*)

Example 4. TTT–VVV, Axial T1WI from inferior to superior, centered at the L1–2 disc.

Clinical Information: Evaluate for HNP. Furthermore, the patient indicates that he has low back and right leg pain along the right hip and in front and back of the right leg.

Interpretation: The conus is normal and ends at the L1 level.

L5–S1: Disc height and hydration are preserved. No disc contour abnormality, spinal canal stenosis, or foraminal stenosis is identified. There is mild facet arthropathy.

L4–5: There is mild loss of disc height and moderate disc dehydration. There is anterior subchondral Modic Type II degenerative change along the superior margin of the L5 vertebral body seen on images 12 (Fig. 2–88*I*) and 24 (Fig. 2–88*R*). There is approximately 10% degenerative spondylolisthesis seen on sagittal image 12 (Fig. 2–88*F*), with bilateral severe facet arthropathy seen on axial image 47 (Fig. 2–88*GG*). This causes moderate spinal canal stenosis. Superimposed on this is a right subarticular and foraminal disc extrusion measuring approximately 7.6 mm in AP dimension on sagittal image 11 (Fig. 2–88*E*), with some associated cranial dissection. There is severe up-down right foraminal narrowing with moderate compression of the exiting right L4 ganglion seen on sagittal image 9 (Fig. 2–88*C*). The right subarticular recess is also narrowed with compression of the traversing right L5 nerve root on axial image 47 (Fig. 2–88*GG*). On the left side, there is moderate up-down foraminal stenosis without exiting left L4 ganglionic compression.

L3–4: There is preservation of disc height with mild disc dehydration. There is circumferential degenerative disc bulging. Image 42 (Fig. 2–88*LL*) demonstrates bilateral severe facet arthropathy. There is a superimposed left subarticular and foraminal disc protrusion measuring 4.2 mm in AP dimension on sagittal image 15 (Fig. 2–88*I*). Axial image 45 (Fig. 2–88*II*) demonstrates right subarticular recess narrowing and compression of the traversing right L4 nerve root. There is bilateral moderate up-down foraminal stenosis without exiting L3 ganglionic compression.

L2–3: There is preservation of disc height with mild disc dehydration. There are bilateral foraminal disc protrusions measuring 4 to 5 mm and narrowing the inferior aspect of the neural foramina exiting L2 ganglionic compression. There is mild facet arthropathy.

L1–2: Disc height and hydration are preserved. No disc contour abnormality, spinal canal stenosis, or foraminal stenosis is identified.

T12–L1: Disc height and hydration are preserved. No disc contour abnormality, spinal canal stenosis, or foraminal stenosis is identified.

T11–12: Disc height and hydration are preserved. No disc contour abnormality, spinal canal stenosis, or foraminal stenosis is identified.

Conclusion

1. L4–5 demonstrates mild loss of disc height and moderate disc dehydration along with 10% degenerative spondylolisthesis from severe facet arthropathy. There is a superimposed right subarticular and foraminal disc extrusion with compression of the preganglionic and ganglionic right-sided L4 nerve and also compression of the traversing L5 nerve root.
2. L3–4 demonstrates mild loss of disc hydration and severe facet arthropathy. There is degenerative disc bulging with a superimposed right subarticular and foraminal disc protrusion causing narrowing of the right subarticular recess and possible compression of the traversing right L4 nerve root, but this is on the side opposite the patient's clinical symptoms. Please correlate.
3. L5–S1 demonstrates mild facet arthropathy.

Comments Regarding Report

1. The patient has multilevel disease. The degree of L4–5 right-sided subarticular recess stenosis and L3–4 left-sided subarticular recess stenosis are similar, but as noted in the "Conclusion," the patient's symptoms were predominantly right-sided. The right-sided symptoms could be coming from either the traversing L5 or exiting L4 nerve root compression, or from inflammation associated with the cranially dissecting disc herniation.
2. As in Example 2, the patient has multilevel disease with focal abnormalities of disc contour at many different locations. Without the pain diagram and a full clinical history (and sometimes even with these items), it is difficult to ascribe causality to lesions.

EXAMPLE 5 (FIG. 2–89)

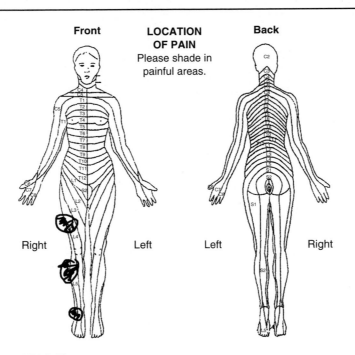

Front   **LOCATION OF PAIN**   **Back**
Please shade in painful areas.

Right   Left   Left   Right

FIGURE 2–89

Example 5. A 72-year-old woman with tingling in the right leg from the thigh to the foot. See accompanying complete report and pain diagram.

(*continued on page 113*)

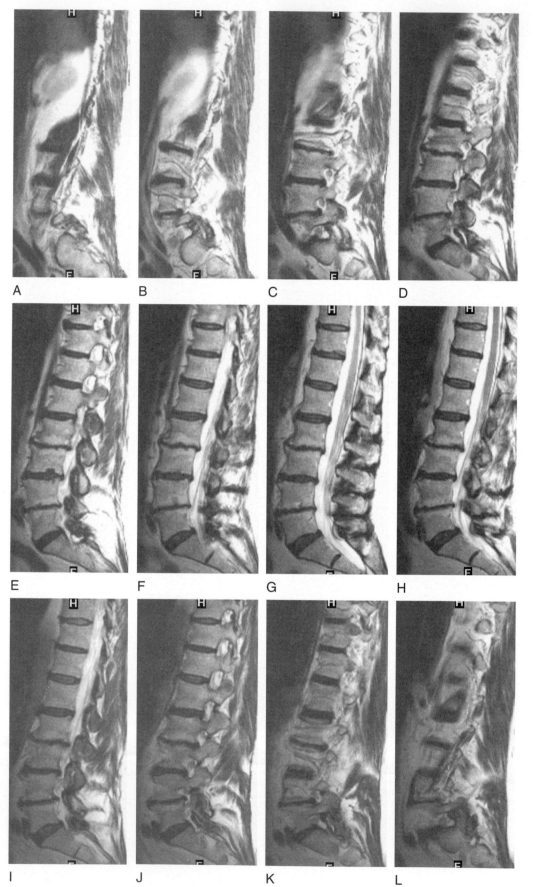

FIGURE 2–89 *(continued)*

Example 5. A–L, Sequential right-to-left sagittal T2WI.

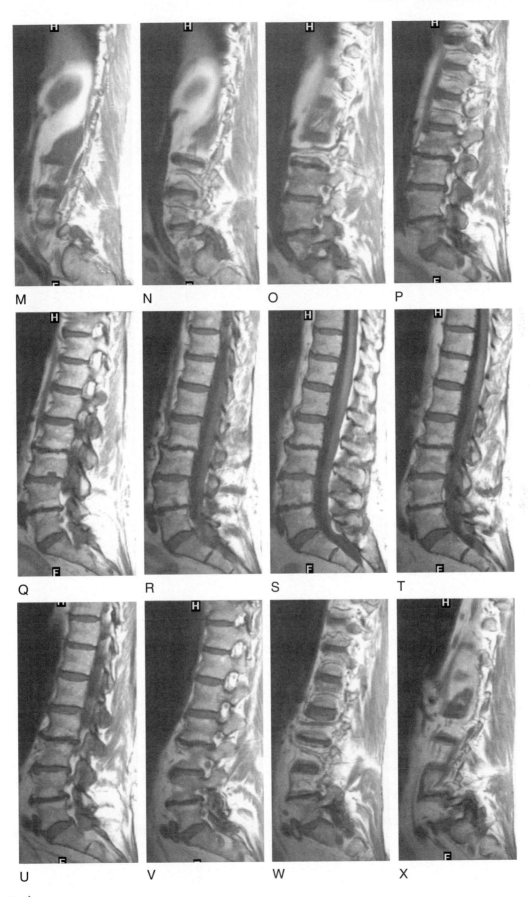

M N O P

Q R S T

U V W X

FIGURE 2–89 (*continued*)

Example 5. M–X, Sequential right-to-left sagittal T1WI.

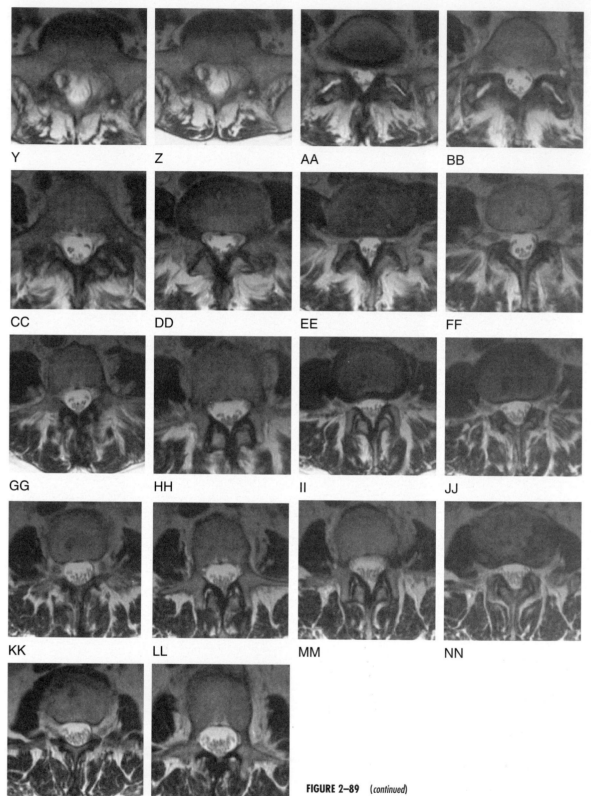

FIGURE 2–89 (*continued*)

Example 5. Y–PP, Sequential inferior-to-superior axial T2WI from the S1 through the inferior aspect of the L3 pedicle.

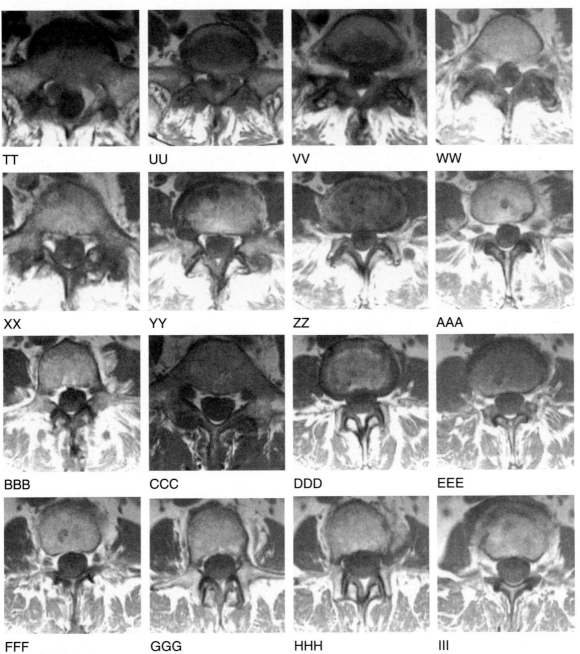

TT   UU   VV   WW

XX   YY   ZZ   AAA

BBB   CCC   DDD   EEE

FFF   GGG   HHH   III

JJJ

FIGURE 2–89 *(continued)*
Example 5. TT–JJJ, Sequential inferior-to-superior axial T1WI from the S1 through the inferior aspect of the L3 pedicle.

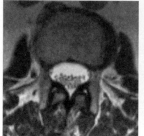
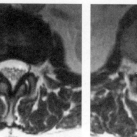
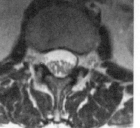

QQ   RR   SS

FIGURE 2–89   (continued)
Example 5. QQ–SS, Axial T2WI from inferior to superior, centered at the L2–3 disc.

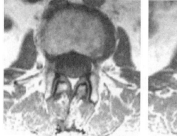
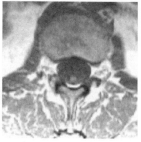

LLL   MMM

FIGURE 2–89   (continued)
Example 5. LLL–MMM, Axial T1WI from inferior to superior, centered at the L2–3 disc.

Clinical Information: Tingling in the right leg from thigh to foot for approximately 2 months.

Interpretation: The conus is normal and ends at the L1 level.

L5–S1: There is preservation of disc height with moderate disc dehydration. No focal disc contour abnormality is identified. The patient has severe bilateral facet arthropathy with joint effusions on both sides. There is a synovial cyst projecting off the medial, inferior aspect of the right facet joint as seen on sagittal image 11 (Fig. 2–89*E*) and axial image 74 (Fig. 2–89*Y*). This anteriorly displaces and compresses the right S1 nerve root. There is also bilateral subarticular recess narrowing, greater on the left than on the right, secondary to facet arthropathy. There is bilateral moderate combined up-down and front-back foraminal stenosis without, however, exiting L5 ganglionic compression.

L4–5: There is severe loss of disc height and severe disc dehydration along with Modic Type II subchondral marrow degenerative changes, osteophytic spurring along the disc margin, and degenerative disc bulging. There is moderate left up-down foraminal stenosis with mild exiting L4 ganglionic compression. There is mild right up-down foraminal stenosis without exiting right L4 ganglionic compression. There is bilateral moderate facet arthropathy. No severe spinal canal stenosis is identified.

L3–4: There is moderate loss of disc height and moderate disc dehydration. There is Schmorl's node formation seen on sagittal image 11 (Fig. 2–89*E*). There is osteophytic spurring along the disc margin and degenerative disc bulging. Sagittal image 13 (Fig. 2–89*G*) suggests 1- to 2-mm retrolisthesis of L3 on L4. No disc extrusion is identified. There is some mild up-down foraminal stenosis without exiting L3 ganglionic compression. There is mild facet arthropathy.

L2–3: There is severe loss of disc height and severe disc dehydration along with subchondral Modic Type II marrow degenerative changes. There is extensive left lateral osteophytic spurring. Sagittal image 13 (Fig. 2–89*G*) shows 3 to 4 mm of retrolisthesis of L2 on L3. There is mild facet arthropathy. No disc protrusion or severe spinal canal or foraminal stenosis is identified.

L1–2: There is preservation of disc height with mild disc dehydration. There is degenerative disc bulging without spinal canal or foraminal stenosis.

T12–L1: There is preservation of disc space height with mild disc dehydration. No focal disc contour abnormality, spinal canal stenosis, or foraminal stenosis is identified.

T11–12: There is moderate loss of disc height and dehydration with minimal irregularity along the vertebral body margin. No focal disc contour abnormality, spinal canal stenosis, or foraminal stenosis is identified.

T10–11: There is mild loss of disc height and dehydration with anterolateral right-sided osteophyte formation. No posterior disc contour abnormality, spinal canal stenosis, or foraminal stenosis is identified.

Sagittal images 13 (Fig. 2–89*G*) and 26 (Fig. 2–89*S*) demonstrate apposition of spinous processes posteriorly ("kissing spines").

Conclusion

1. L5–S1 severe facet arthropathy and subarticular recess stenosis. In addition, there is a right synovial cyst measuring 7 mm in transverse dimension on axial image 74 (Fig. 2–89*Y*), anteriorly displacing and compressing the right S1 nerve root. Considering the patient's right lower extremity tingling, this could be a cause of conduction block and right lower extremity symptoms. Please correlate. Occasionally, such patients obtain relief with injection of the associated facet joint, which may pressurize and rupture the synovial cyst.
2. The patient has multiple additional degenerative change, including severe loss of disc height and hydration at L2–3 and L4–5, and moderate loss of disc height and hydration at L3–4. There is also degenerative disc bulging and osteophytic spurring along the disc margin at these levels and moderate facet arthropathy at L4–5. However, no additional neural compression is identified.
3. I spoke with the physician's office regarding the results of the study.

Comments Regarding Report

1. Extensive multilevel disease requires a lengthy and detailed catalog of the degenerative changes.
2. In this case, there seems to be a particular lesion (the synovial cyst) that may be amenable to relatively simple therapy that would benefit the patient. This was noted in the report and communicated to the referring physician, as documented in the "Conclusion" section.

EXAMPLE 6 (FIG. 2–90)

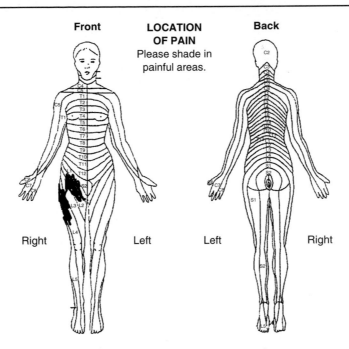

**LOCATION
OF PAIN**
Please shade in
painful areas.

Front

Back

Right

Left

Left

Right

FIGURE 2–90

Example 6. A 71-year-old woman with right leg pain, weakness, and tingling. See accompanying complete report and pain diagram.

(*continued on page 122*)

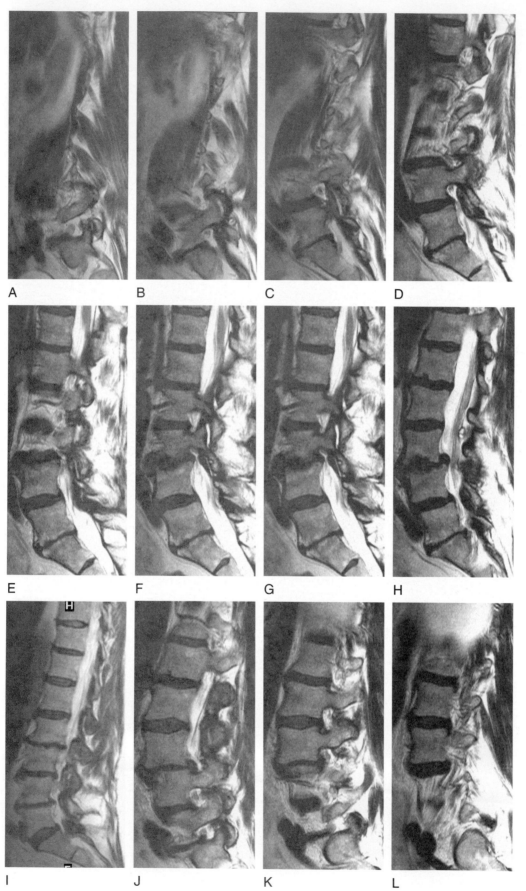

FIGURE 2–90 *(continued)*

Example 6. A–L, Sequential right-to-left sagittal T2WI.

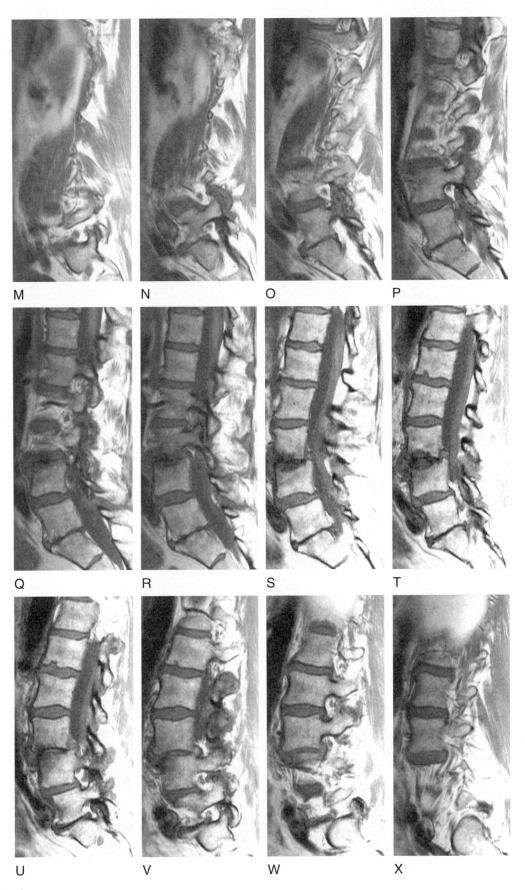

FIGURE 2–90 (*continued*)

Example 6. M–X, Sequential right-to-left sagittal T1WI.

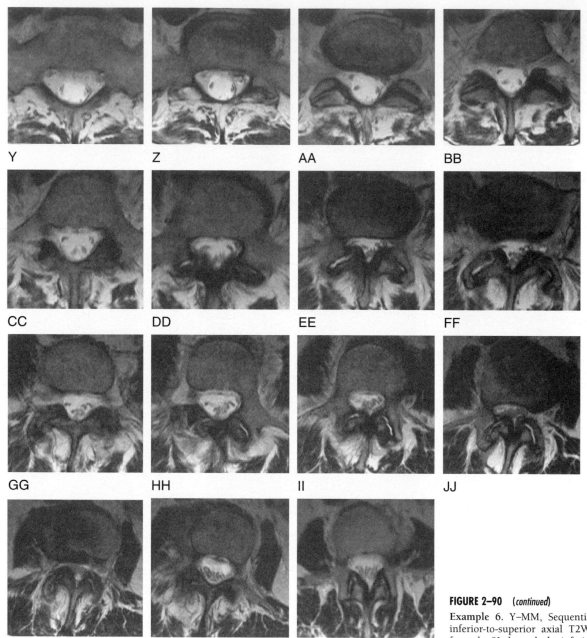

Y Z AA BB

CC DD EE FF

GG HH II JJ

KK LL MM

FIGURE 2–90 *(continued)*
Example 6. Y–MM, Sequential inferior-to-superior axial T2WI from the S1 through the inferior aspect of the L3 pedicle.

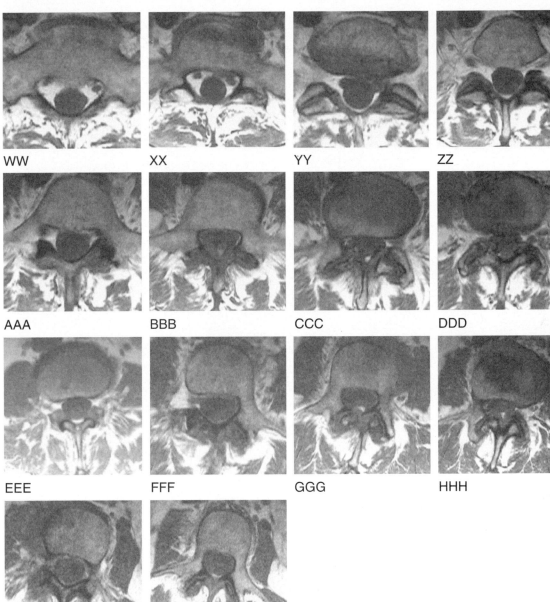

WW   XX   YY   ZZ

AAA   BBB   CCC   DDD

EEE   FFF   GGG   HHH

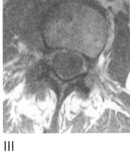   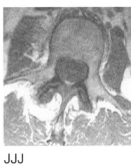

III   JJJ

FIGURE 2–90 (*continued*)

Example 6. WW–JJJ, Sequential inferior-to-superior axial T1WI from the S1 through the inferior aspect of the L3 pedicle.

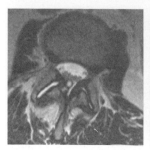
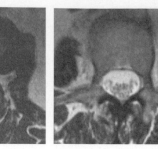

NN   OO   PP

FIGURE 2–90 (*continued*)
Example 6. NN–PP, Axial T2WI from inferior to superior, centered at the L2–3 disc.

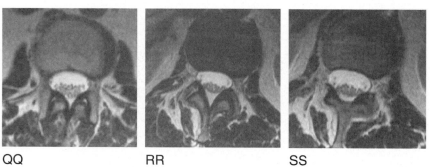

QQ   RR   SS

FIGURE 2–90 (*continued*)
Example 6. QQ–SS, Axial T2WI from inferior to superior, centered at the L1–2 disc.

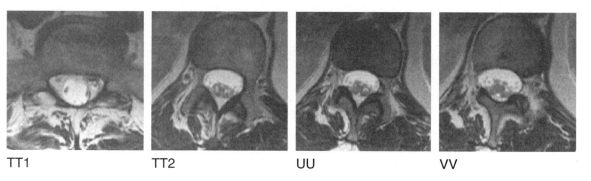

TT1   TT2   UU   VV

FIGURE 2–90 (*continued*)
Example 6. TT1–VV, Axial T2WI from inferior to superior, centered at the T12–L1 disc.

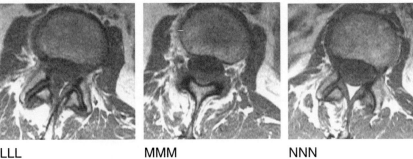

FIGURE 2–90 (*continued*)
Example 6. LLL–NNN, Axial T1WI from inferior to superior, centered at the L2–3 disc.

LLL   MMM   NNN

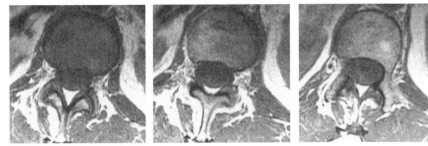

FIGURE 2–90 (*continued*)
Example 6. OOO–QQQ, Axial T1WI from inferior to superior, centered at the L1–2 disc.   (*continued*)

OOO   PPP   QQQ

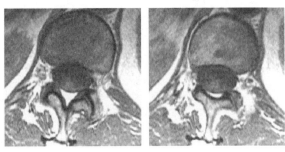

FIGURE 2–90 (*continued*)
Example 6. RRR–SSS, Axial T1WI from inferior to superior, centered at the T12–L1 disc.

RRR   SSS

Clinical Information: Right leg pain, tingling, and weakness.

Interpretation: The conus is normal and ends at the T12 level. There is scoliosis apex to the left at the L3–4 level.

L5–S1: There is severe loss of disc height and severe disc dehydration as well as Modic Type II subchondral marrow degenerative changes. There is a right subarticular, caudally dissecting disc extrusion measuring 5.5 mm in AP dimension on sagittal image 13 (Fig. 2–90*G*), with approximately 5 mm of caudal dissection on that image. Axial images 56 (Fig. 2–90*Z*) and 57 (Fig. 2–90*AA*) demonstrate posterior displacement of the left S1 nerve root. Axial image 55 (Fig. 2–90*BB*) demonstrates mild right and moderate left facet arthropathy. There is no right foraminal narrowing, but there is moderate front-back foraminal narrowing from facet arthropathy that is most severe medial to the exiting left L5 ganglion and that causes no neural compression.

L4–5: There is mild loss of disc height and moderate disc dehydration. There is approximately 5% degenerative spondylolisthesis seen on sagittal image 13 (Fig. 2–90*G*), with bilateral severe facet arthropathy seen on axial image 51 (Fig. 2–90*FF*). There is mild spinal canal stenosis at the level of spondylolisthesis. There is also bilateral mild combined up-down and front-back foraminal stenosis, without exiting ganglionic compression. On the left side, there is a foraminal synovial cyst measuring 5 × 4 mm as seen on axial image 51 (Fig. 2–90*FF*) and sagittal image 15 (Fig. 2–90*I*), without any associated neural compression.

L3–4: There is severe loss of disc height and hydration and there are combined Modic Type II and III subchondral degenerative changes particularly along the right side of the intervertebral disc. There is approximately 15% degenerative spondylolisthesis at this level with axial image 47 (Fig. 2–90*JJ*) showing severe facet arthropathy. There is rightward shift and rotation of L3 with respect to L4, contributing to moderate spinal canal stenosis as seen on axial image 46 (Fig. 2–90*KK*). Exacerbating the narrowing is a central and bilateral paracentral disc protrusion measuring approximately 6 mm in AP dimension on sagittal image 14 (Fig. 2–90*H*). There is right subarticular recess narrowing with compression of the traversing right L4 nerve root. There is severe right up-down foraminal stenosis with compression of the exiting right L3 ganglion, as well as mild front-back left foraminal stenosis without exiting left L3 ganglionic compression.

L2–3: There is preservation of disc height with mild disc dehydration. There is moderate facet arthropathy with bilateral joint effusions, and there is an accompanying dorsal synovial cyst seen on sagittal image 14 (Fig. 2–90*H*) and axial image 43 (Fig. 2–90*NN*). This measures 7 mm in AP dimension on axial image 43 (Fig. 2–90*NN*), but does not cause any neural compression or significant spinal canal narrowing. No significant foraminal narrowing or exiting nerve root compression is identified.

L1–2: There is mild loss of disc height and moderate disc dehydration. There is Schmorl's node formation. No disc contour abnormality, spinal canal stenosis, or foraminal stenosis is seen.

T12–L1: There is mild loss of disc height and moderate disc dehydration. There is Schmorl's node formation. No focal disc contour abnormality, spinal canal stenosis, or foraminal stenosis is seen.

Conclusion

Multilevel degenerative changes of the lumbar spine with specific findings as follows:

1. L3–4 shows severe loss of disc height and hydration with extensive subchondral marrow Modic Type II and Type III degenerative changes suggesting hemispheric sclerosis. There is also 15% degenerative spondylolisthesis from severe facet arthropathy. There is a superimposed disc protrusion, and there is moderate spinal canal stenosis as well as severe right subarticular stenosis with traversing right L4 nerve root compression and severe right up-down foraminal stenosis with compression of the exiting right L3 ganglion. The patient's right leg symptoms could be secondary to compression of L3 or L4. Please correlate.
2. L4–5 shows 5% degenerative spondylolisthesis from severe facet arthropathy, with some mild spinal canal stenosis and mild foraminal stenosis but no ganglionic compression.
3. L2–3 shows moderate facet arthropathy and a 7-mm posterior synovial cyst without associated neural compression.
4. L5–S1 shows severe loss of disc height and hydration and a small left paracentral disc protrusion with slight posterior displacement of the left S1 nerve root, apparently opposite of the side of the patient's clinical symptoms.

Comments Regarding Report

1. As with Example 5, extensive multilevel disease requires a lengthy and detailed catalog of degenerative changes.
2. Scoliosis and accentuation of lordosis or abnormal kyphosis (which involve several segments) may be addressed in a separate paragraph prior to the level-by-level description of degenerative changes.
3. The patient's leg pain could represent radicular pain secondary to compression of the right L3 ganglionic or L4 nerve root, but it could also represent somatic referred pain from any of several degenerated facet joints or discs.

References

Andersson GB. Low back pain. J Rehabil Res Dev 1997; 34:ix–x.

Waddell G. The Back Pain Revolution. New York, Churchill Livingstone, 1998.

Pain and the Pain Diagram

Beattie PF, Meyers SP, Stratford P, Millard RW, Hollenberg GM. Associations between patient report of symptoms and anatomic impairment visible on lumbar magnetic resonance imaging: associations between patient report of symptoms and anatomic impairment visible on lumbar magnetic resonance imaging. Spine 2000; 25:819–828.

Boden SD, Davis DO, Dina TS, Patronas NJ, Wiesel SW. Abnormal magnetic resonance scans of the lumbar spine in asymptomatic subjects. J Bone Joint Surg Am 1990a; 72:402–408.

Boden SD, McCowin PR, Davis DO, Dina TS, Mark AS, Wiesel S. Abnormal magnetic resonance scans of the cervical spine in asymptomatic subjects. J Bone Joint Surg Am 1990b; 72:1178–1184.

Bogduk N. Clinical Anatomy of the Lumbar Spine, 3rd ed. New York, Churchill Livingstone, 1997.

Boos N, Rieder R, Schade V. The diagnostic accuracy of magnetic resonance imaging, work perception, and psychosocial factors in identifying symptomatic disc herniations. Spine 1995; 20:2613–2625.

Foerster O. The dermatomes in man. Brain 1933; 56:1–39.

Garfin SR, Rydevik BL, Brown RA. Compressive neuropathy of spinal nerve roots: a mechanical or biological problem? Spine 1991; 16:162–166.

Howe JF, Loeser JD, Calvin WH. Mechanosensitivity of dorsal root ganglia and chronically injured axons: a physiological basis for the radicular pain of nerve root compression. Pain 1977; 3:25–41.

Jarvik JJ, Hollingworth W, Heagerty P, Haynor DR, Deyo RA. The longitudinal assessment of imaging and disability of the back (LAIDBack) study. Spine 2001; 26:1158–1166.

Jensen MC, Brant-Zawadski MN, Obuchowski N, Modic MT, Malkasian D, Ross J. Magnetic resonance imaging of the lumbar spine in people without back pain. N Engl J Med 1994; 331:69–73.

Keegan JJ, Garret FD. The segmental distribution of the cutaneous nerves in the limbs of man. Anat Rec 1948; 102:409–437.

Kellgren JH. On the distribution of pain arising from deep somatic structures with charts of segmental pain areas. Clin Sci 1939; 4L:35–46.

Kellgren JH. Sciatica. Lancet 1941; 1:561–564.

Kelly M. Is pain due to pressure on nerves? Neurology 1956; 6:32–36.

Kibler RF, Nathan PW. Relief of pain and paraesthesiae by nerve block distal to a lesion. J Neurol Neurosurg Psychiatry 1960; 23:91–98.

Kuslich SD, Ulstrom CL, Michael CJ. The tissue of origin of low back pain and sciatica: a report of pain response to tissue stimulation during operations on the lumbar spine using local anesthesia. Orthop Clin North Am 1991; 22:181–187.

Ljunggren AE, Jacobsen T, Osvik A. Pain descriptions and surgical findings in patients with herniated lumbar intervertebral discs. Pain 1988; 35:39–46.

Mann NH, Brown MD, Enger I. Expert performance in low back disorder recognition using patient pain drawings. J Spinal Disord 1992; 5:254–259.

Matsumoto M, Fujimura Y, Suzuki N, Nishi Y, Nakamura M, Yabe Y, Shiga H. MRI of the cervical intervertebral discs in asymptomatic patients. J Bone Joint Surg Br 1998; 80:19–24.

Melzack R, Wall PD. Pain mechanisms: a new theory. Science 1965; 150:971–979.

Ohnmeiss DD. Repeatability of pain drawings in a low back pain population. Spine 2000; 25:980–988.

Ohnmeiss DD, Vanharanta H, Guyer RD. The association between pain drawings and computed tomographic/discographic pain responses. Spine 1995; 20:729–733.

Ransford AO, Cairns D, Mooney V. The pain drawing as an aid to the psychologic evaluation of patients with low back pain. Spine 1976; 1:127–134.

Spengler DM, Freeman CW. Patient selection for lumbar discectomy: an objective approach. Spine 1979; 4:129–134.

Stadnik TW, Lee RR, Coen HL, Neirynck EC, Buisseret TS, Osteaux MJC. Annular tears and disk herniation: prevalence and contrast enhancement on MR images in the absence of low back pain or sciatica. Radiology 1998; 206:49–55.

Taylor WP, Stern WR, Kubiszyn TW. Predicting patients' perceptions of response to treatment for low back pain. Spine 1984; 9:313–316.

Teresi LM, Lufkin RB, Reicher MA, et al. Asymptomatic degenerative disk disease and spondylosis of the cervical spine: MR imaging. Radiology 1987; 164:83–88.

Uden A, Landin LA. Pain drawing and myelography in sciatic pain. Clin Orthop 1987; 216:124–130.

van Akkerveeken PF. On pain patterns of patients with lumbar nerve root entrapment. Neuro-Orthopedics 1993; 14:81–102.

Vucetic N, Maattanen H, Svensson O. Pain and pathology in lumbar disc hernia. Clin Orthop 1995; 320:65–72.

Weinreb JC, Wolbarsht LB, Cohen JM, Brown CEL, Maravilla KR. Prevalence of lumbosacral intervertebral disk abnormalities on MR images in pregnant and asymptomatic nonpregnant women. Radiology 1989; 170:125–128.

Weishaupt D, Zanetti M, Hodler J, Boos N. MR imaging of the lumbar spine: prevalence of intervertebral disk extrusion and sequestration, nerve root compression, end plate abnormalities, and osteoarthritis of the facet joints in asymptomatic volunteers. Radiology 1998; 209:661–666.

Wiesel SW, Tsourmas N, Feffer HL, Critrin CM, Patronas N. A study of computer-assisted tomography: I. The incidence of positive CAT scans in an asymptomatic group of patients. Spine 1984; 9:549–551.

Disc Degeneration and Internal Disc Disruption

Aprill C, Bogduk N. High-intensity zone: a diagnostic sign of painful lumbar disc on magnetic resonance imaging. Br J Radiol 1992; 65:361–369.

Bangert BA, Modic MT, Ross JS, Obuchowski NA, Perl J, Ruggieri PM, Masaryk TJ. Hyperintense disks on T1-weighted MR images: correlation with calcification. Radiology 1995; 195:437–443.

Boden SD, Riew KD, Yamaguchi K, Branch TP, Schellinger D, Wiesel SW. Orientation of the lumbar facet joints: association with degenerative disc disease. J Bone Joint Surg Am 1996; 78:403–411.

Bogduk N. Clinical Anatomy of the Lumbar Spine, 3rd ed. New York, Churchill Livingstone, 1997.

Brightbill TC, Pile N, Eichelberger RP, Whitman M. Normal magnetic resonance imaging and abnormal discography in lumbar disc disruption. Spine 1994; 19:1075–1077.

Buirski G. Magnetic resonance signal patterns of lumbar discs in patients with low back pain: a prospective study with discographic correlation. Spine 1992; 17:1199–1204.

Butler D, Trafimow JH, Andersson GBJ, McNeill TW, Huckman MS. Disc degenerate before facets. Spine 1990; 15:111–113.

Carragee EJ, Paragioudakis SJ, Khurana S. Lumbar high-intensity zone and discography in subjects without low back problems. Spine 2000; 25:2987–2992.

Carragee EJ, Tanner CM, Yang B, Brito JL, Truong T. False-positive findings on lumbar discography: reliability of subjective concordance assessment during provocative disc injection. Spine 1999; 24:2542–2547.

de Roos A, Kressel H, Spritzer C, Dalinka M. MR imaging of marrow changes adjacent to end plates in degenerative lumbar disk disease. AJR Am J Roentgenol 1987; 149:531–534.

Fardon DF, Herzog RJ, Mink JH, Simmons JD, Kahonovitz N, Haldeman S. Nomenclature of lumbar disc disorders. In Garfin SR, Vaccaro AR (eds). Orthopaedic Knowledge Update: Spine. Abstract presented at the American Academy of Orthopaedic Surgeons, Rosemont, IL, 1997, pp A3–A14.

Farfan HF, Sullivan JD. The relation of facet orientation to intervertebral disc failure. Can J Surg 1967; 10:179–185.

Feffer HD. Treatment of low back and sciatic pain by the injection of hydrocortisone into degenerated intervertebral discs. J Bone Joint Surg Am 1956; 38:585–592.

Feffer HD. Therapeutic intradiscal hydrocortisone: a long-term study. Clin Orthop 1969; 67:100–104.

Frymoyer JW, Selby DK. Segmental instability: rationale for treatment. Spine 1985; 20:280–286.

Gill K, Blumenthal SL. Functional results after anterior lumbar fusion at L5–S1 in patients with normal and abnormal MRI scans. Spine 1992; 17:940–942.

Graham CE. Chemonucleolysis: a double-blind study comparing chemonucleolysis with intra-discal hydrocortisone. Med J Aust 1985; 142:461–462.

Grenier N, Grossmas RI, Schiebler ML, Yeager BA, Goldberg HI, Kressel HY. Degenerative lumbar disk disease: pitfalls and usefulness of MR imaging in detection of vacuum phenomenon. Radiology 1987; 164:861–865.

Horton WC, Daftari TK. Which disc as visualized by magnetic resonance is actually a source of pain? A correlation between magnetic resonance imaging and discography. Spine 1992; 17:S164–S171.

Ito M, Incorvaia KM, Yu SF, Fredrickson BE, Yuan HA, Rosenbaum AE. Predictive signs of discogenic lumbar pain on magnetic resonance imaging with discographic correlation. Spine 1998; 23:1252–1260.

Jackson RP. Lumbar discography. Semin Spine Surg 1997; 9:51–56.

Kirkaldy-Willis WH, Farfan HF. Instability of the lumbar spine. Clin Orthop 1982; 165:110–123.

Kuslich SD, Ulstrom CL, Griffith SL, Ahern JW, Dowdle JD. The Bagby and Kuslich method of lumbar interbody fusion: history, techniques, and 2-year follow-up results of a United States prospective, multicenter trial. Spine 1998; 23:1267–1279.

Leao L. Intradiscal injection of hydrocortisone and prednisolone in the treatment of low back pain. Rheumatism 1960; 16:72–77.

Luoma K, Vehmas T, Riihimaki H, Raininko R. Disc height and signal intensity of the nucleus pulposus on magnetic resonance imaging as indicators of lumbar disc degeneration. Spine 2001; 26:680–686.

Milette PC, Fontaine S, Lepanto L, Cardinal E, Breton G. Differentiating lumbar disc protrusions, disc bulges, and discs with normal contour but abnormal signal intensity. Spine 1999; 24:44–53.

Modic MT, Masaryk TJ, Ross JS, Carter JR. Imaging of degenerative disk disease. Radiology 1988a; 168:177–186.

Modic MT, Steinberg PM, Ross JS, Masaryk TJ, Carter JR. Degenerative disk disease: assessment of changes in vertebral body marrow with MR imaging. Radiology 1988b; 166:193–199.

Moneta GB, Videman T, Kalvanto K, Aprill C, Spivey M, Vanharanta H, Sachs BL, Guyer RD, Hochschuler SH, Raschbaum RF. Reported pain during lumbar discography as a function of anular ruptures and disc degeneration: a re-analysis of 833 discograms. Spine 1994; 19:1968–1974.

Muggleton JM, Kondracki M, Allen R. Spinal fusion for lumbar instability: does it have a scientific basis? J Spinal Disord 2000; 13:200–204.

Muhle C, Wiskirchen J, Weinert D, Falliner A, Wesner F, Brinkmann G, Heller M. Biomechanical aspects of the subarachnoid space and cervical cord in healthy individuals examined with kinematic magnetic resonance imaging. Spine 1998; 23:556–567.

Noren R, Trafimow J, Andersson GBJ, Huckman MS. The role of facet joint tropism and facet angle in disc degeneration. Spine 1991; 16:530–532.

Osti OL, Fraser RD. MRI and discography of annular tears and intervertebral disc degeneration: a prospective clinical comparison. J Bone Joint Surg Br 1992; 74:431–435.

Rankine JJ, Fortune DG, Hutchinson CE, Hughes DG, Main CJ. Pain drawings in the assessment of nerve root compression: a comparative study with lumbar spine magnetic resonance imaging. Spine 1998; 23:1668–1676.

Ray CD. Threaded titanium cages for lumbar interbody fusions. Spine 1997; 22:667–679.

Resnick D. Degenerative disease of the vertebral column. Radiology 1985; 156:3–14.

Ricketson R, Simmons JW, Hauser BO. The prolapsed intervertebral disc: the high-intensity zone with discography correlation. Spine 1996; 21:2758–2762.

Ross JS, Modic MT, Masaryk TJ. Tears of the anulus fibrosus: assessment with Gd-DTPA-enhanced MR imaging. AJR 1990; 154:159–162.

Saal JS, Saal JA. Management of chronic discogenic low back pain with a thermal intradiscal catheter: a preliminary report. Spine 2000; 25:382–388.

Saifuddin A, Braithwaite I, White J, Taylor BA, Renton P. The value of lumbar spine magnetic resonance imaging in the demonstration of anular tears. Spine 1998; 23:453–457.

Sandhu HS, Sanchez-Caso LP, Parvataneni HK, Cammisa FP Jr, Girardi FP, Ghelman B. Association between findings of provocative discography and vertebral endplate signal changes as seen on MRI. J Spinal Disord 2000; 13:438–443.

Sato H, Kikuchi S. The natural history of radiographic instability of the lumbar spine. Spine 1993; 18:2075–2079.

Schellhas KP, Poillei SR, Gundry CR, Heithoff KB. Lumbar disc high-intensity zone: correlation with magnetic resonance imaging and discography. Spine 1996; 21:79–86.

Schmid MR, Stucki G, Duewell S, Wildermuth S, Romanowski B, Hodler J. Changes in cross-sectional measurements of the spinal canal and intervertebral foramina as a function of body position: in vivo studies on an open-configuration MR system. AJR Am J Roentgenol 1999; 172:1095–1102.

Schwarzer AC, Aprill CN, Derby R, Fortin J, Kine G, Bogduk N. The prevalence and clinical features of internal disc disruption in patients with chronic low back pain. Spine 1995; 20:1878–1883.

Sether LA, Yu S, Haughton VM, Fischer ME. Intervertebral disk: normal age-related changes in MR signal intensity. Radiology 1990; 177:385–388.

Simmons JW, McMillin JN, Emery SF, Kimmich SJ. Intradiscal steroids: a prospective double-blind study. Spine 1992; 17:S172–S175.

Smith MT, Hurwitz EL, Solsbert D, Rubinstein D, Corenman DS, Dwyer AP, Kleiner J. Interobserver reliability of detecting lumbar intervertebral disc high-intensity zone on magnetic resonance and association of high-intensity zone with pain and anular disruption. Spine 1998; 23:2074–2080.

Stabler A, Weiss M, Scheidler J, Krodel A, Seiderer M, Reiser M. Degenerative disk vascularization on MRI: correlation with clinical and histopathologic findings. Skeletal Radiol 1996; 25:119–126.

Stadnik TW, Lee RR, Coen HL, Neirynck EC, Buisseret TS, Osteaux MJC. Annular tears and disk herniation: prevalence and contrast enhancement on MR images in the absence of low back pain or sciatica. Radiology 1998; 206:49–55.

Waddell G. The Back Pain Revolution. New York, Churchill Livingstone, 1998.

Weishaupt D, Schmid MR, Zanetti M, Boos N, Romanowski B, Kissling R, Dvorak J, Hodler J. Positional MR imaging of the lumbar spine: does it demonstrate nerve root compromise not visible at conventional MR imaging? Radiology 2000; 215:247–253.

Weishaupt D, Zanetti M, Hodler J, Min K, Fuchs B, Pfirrmann CWA, Boos N. Painful lumbar disk derangement: relevance of endplate abnormalities at MR imaging. Radiology 2001; 218:420–427.

Wilkinson HA, Schuman N. Intradiscal corticosteroids in the treatment of lumbar and cervical disc problems. Spine 1980; 5:385–389.

Willen J, Danielson B. The diagnostic effect from axial loading of the lumbar spine during computed tomography and magnetic resonance imaging in patients with degenerative disorders. Spine 2001; 2607–2614.

Yong-Hing K, Kirkaldy-Willis WH. The pathophysiology of degenerative disease of the lumbar spine. Orthop Clin North Am 1983; 14:491–504.

Yu S, Haughton VM, Sether LA, Wagner M. Comparison of MR and diskography in detecting radial tears of the anulus: a postmortem study. AJNR Am J Neuroradiol 1989; 10:1077–1081.

Disc Herniation

Ahn UM, Ahn NU, Buchowski MJ, Garrett ES, Sieber AN, Kostiuk JP. Cauda equina syndrome secondary to lumbar disc herniation: a meta-analysis of surgical outcomes. Spine 2000; 25:1515–1522.

Alexiadou-Rudolf C, Ernestus RI, Nanassis K, Lanfermann H, Klug N. Acute nontraumatic spinal epidural hematomas: an important differential diagnosis in spinal emergencies. Spine 1998; 23:1810–1823.

Atlas SJ, Keller RB, Robson D, Deyo RA, Singer DE. Surgical and nonsurgical management of lumbar spinal stenosis: 4-year outcomes from the Maine lumbar spine study. Spine 2001; 25:556–562.

Beattie PF, Meyers SP, Stratford P, Millard RW, Hollenberg GM. Associations between patient report of symptoms and anatomic impairment visible on lumbar magnetic resonance imaging. Spine 2000; 25:819–828.

Bessette L, Liang MH, Lew RA, Weinstein JN. Classics in spine surgery literature revisited. Spine 1996; 21:259–263.

Boden SD, Davis DO, Dina TS, Patronas NJ, Wiesel SW. Abnormal magnetic resonance scans of the lumbar spine in asymptomatic subjects. J Bone Joint Surg Am 1990a; 72:402–408.

Boden SD, McCowin PR, Davis DO, Dina TS, Mark AS, Wiesel S. Abnormal magnetic resonance scans of the cervical spine in asymptomatic subjects. J Bone Joint Surg Am 1990b; 72:1178–1184.

Bogduk N. Clinical Anatomy of the Lumbar Spine. 3rd Edition. Churchill Livingstone 3rd ed., New York, 1997.

Boos N, Rieder R, Schade V. The diagnostic accuracy of magnetic resonance imaging, work perception, and psychosocial factors in identifying symptomatic disc herniations. Spine 1998; 20:2613–2625.

Bozzao A, Gallucci M, Masciocchi C, Aprile I, Barile A, Passariello R. Lumbar disc herniation: MR imaging assessment of natural history in patients treated without surgery. Radiology 1992; 185:135–141.

Chiba K, Toyama Y, Matsumoto M, Maruiwa H, Watanabe M, Nishizawa T. Intraspinal cyst communicating with the intervertebral disc in the lumbar spine: discal cyst. Spine 2001; 26:2112–2118.

Crisi G, Carpeggiani P, Trevisan C. Gadolinium-enhanced nerve roots in lumbar disk herniation. AJNR Am J Neuroradiol 1993; 14:1379–1392.

Debois V, Herz R, Berghmans D, Hermans B, Herregodts P. Soft cervical disc herniation: influence of cervical spinal canal measurements on development of neurologic symptoms. Spine 1999; 24:1996–2002.

Fardon DF, Herzog RJ, Mink JH, Simmons JD, Kahonovitz N, Haldeman S. Nomenclature of lumbar disc disorders. In Garfin SR, Vaccaro AR (eds). Orthopedic Knowledge Update: Spine. Abstract presented at the American Academy of Orthopaedic Surgeons, Rosemont IL, 1997, pp A3–A14.

Fardon D, Pinkerton S, Balderston R, Garfin S, Nasca R, Salib R. Terms used for diagnosis by English-speaking spine surgeons. Spine 1993; 18:274–277.

Franson RC, Saal JS, Saal JA. Human disc phospholipase A_2 is inflammatory. Spine 1992; 17(Suppl):S129–S132.

Furusawa N, Baba H, Miyoshi N, Maezawa Y, Uchida K, Kokubo Y, Fukuda M. Herniation of cervical intervertebral disc: immunohistochemical examination and measurement of nitric oxide production. Spine 2001; 26:1110–1116.

Garfin SR, Rydevik BL, Brown RA. Compressive neuropathy of spinal nerve roots: a mechanical or biological problem? Spine 1991; 16:162–166.

Georgy BA, Snow RD, Hesselink JR. MR imaging of spinal nerve roots: techniques, enhancement patterns, and imaging findings. AJR Am J Roentgenol 1996; 166:173–179.

Glickstein MF, Burke L, Kressel HY. Magnetic resonance demonstration of hyperintense herniated discs and extruded disc fragments. Skeletal Radiol 1989; 18:527–530.

Gronblad M, Virri J, Seitsalo S, Habtemariam A, Karaharju E. Inflammatory cells, motor weakness, and straight leg raising in transligamentous disc herniations. Spine 2000; 25:2803–2807.

Gronblad M, Virri J, Tolonen J, Seitsalo S, Kaapa E, Kankare J, Myllynen P, Karaharju EO. A controlled immunohistochemical study of inflammatory cells in disc herniation tissue. Spine 1994; 19:2744–2751.

Gundry CR, Heithoff KB. Epidural hematoma of the lumbar spine: 18 surgically confirmed cases. Radiology 1993; 187:427–431.

Habtemariam A, Gronblad M, Virri J, Seitsalo S, Karaharju E. A comparative immunohistochemical study of inflammatory cells in acute-stage and chronic-stage disc herniations. Spine 1998; 23:2159–2166.

Haijiao W, Koti M, Smith FW, Wardlaw D. Diagnosis of lumbosacral nerve root anomalies by magnetic resonance imaging. J Spinal Disord 2001; 14:143–149.

Harrington JF, Messier AA, Bereiter D, Barnes B, Epstein MH. Herniated lumbar disc material as a source of free glutamate available to affect pain signals through the dorsal root ganglion. Spine 2000; 25:929–936.

Heithoff KB, Ray CD, Schellhas KP, Fritts HM. CT and MRI of lateral entrapment syndromes. Spine Update 1987

Hurme M, Alaranta H. Factors predicting the result of surgery for lumbar intervertebral disc herniation. Spine 1987; 12:933–938.

Igarashi T, Kikuchi S, Subayev V, Myers RR. Exogenous tumor necrosis factor-alpha mimics nucleus pulposus-induced neuropathology: molecular, histologic, and behavioral comparison in rats. Spine 2000; 25:2975–2980.

Jensen MC, Brant-Zawadski MN, Obuchowski N, Modic MT, Malkasian D, Ross J. Magnetic resonance imaging of the lumbar spine in people without back pain. N Engl J Med 1994; 331:69–73.

Kang JD, Georgescu HI, McIntyre-Larkin L, Stefanovic-Racic M, Donaldson WF, Eans CH. Herniated lumbar intervertebral discs spontaneously produce matrix metalloproteinases, nitric oxide, interleukin-6, and prostaglandin E_2. Spine 1996; 21:271–277.

Kayama S, Olmarker K, Larsson K, Sjogren-Jansson E, Lindahl A, Rydevik B. Cultured, autologous nucleus pulposus cells induce functional changes in spinal nerve roots. Spine 1998; 23:2155–2158.

Kobayashi S, Yoshizawa H, Hachiya Y, Ukai T, Morita T. Vasogenic edema induced by compression injury to the spinal nerve root: distribution of intravenously injected protein tracers and gadolinium-enhanced magnetic resonance imaging. Spine 1993; 18:1410–1424.

Lee HM, Weinstein JN, Meller ST, Hayashi N, Spratt KF, Gebhart GF. The role of steroids and their effects on phospholipase A_2: an animal model of radiculopathy. Spine 1998; 23:1191–1196.

Masaryk TJ, Ross JS, Modic MT, Boumphrey F, Bohlman H, Wilber G. High-resolution MR imaging of sequestered lumbar intervertebral disks. AJR Am J Roentgenol 1988; 150:1155–1162.

Matsumoto M, Fujimura Y, Suzuki N, Nishi Y, Nakamura M, Yabe Y, Shiga H. MRI of the cervical intervertebral discs in asymptomatic patients. J Bone Joint Surg Br 1998; 80:19–24.

McCarron RF, Wimpee MW, Hudkins PG, Laros GS. The inflammatory effect of nucleus pulposus: a possible element in the pathogenesis of low-back pain. Spine 1987; 12:760–761.

McNeill TW, Andersson GBJ, Schell B, Sinkora G, Nelson J, Lavender SA. Epidural administration of methylprednisolone and morphine for pain after a spinal operation. J Bone Joint Surg 1995; 77A: 1814–1817.

Mercer S, Bogduk N. The ligaments and anulus fibrosus of human adult cervical intervertebral dics. Spine 1999; 24:619–628.

Milette PC, Fontaine S, Lepanto L, Cardinal E, Breton G. Differentiating lumbar disc protrusions, disc bulges, and discs with normal contour but abnormal signal intensity. Spine 1999; 24:44–53.

Mixter WJ, Barr JS. Rupture of the intervertebral disc with involvement of the spinal canal. N Engl J Med 1934; 211:210–214.

Mochica K, Kormori H, Okawa A, Muneta T, Haro H, Shinomiya K. Regression of cervical disc herniation observed on magnetic resonance images. Spine 1998; 23:990–997.

Modic MT. Degenerative disorders of the spine. In Modic MT, Masaryk TJ, Ross JS (eds). Magnetic Resonance Imaging of the Spine, 2nd ed. St. Louis, Mosby, 1994.

Olmarker K, Larsson K. Tumor necrosis factor-alpha and nucleus pulposus–induced nerve root injury. Spine 1998; 23:2538–2544.

Olmarker K, Rydevik B. Single- versus double-level nerve root compression. Clin Orthop 1992; 279:35–39.

Olmarker K, Rydevik B, Nordborg C. Autologous nucleus pulposus induces neurophysiologic and histologic changes in porcine cauda equina nerve roots. Spine 1993; 18:1425–1432.

Ozaktay AC, Kallakuri S, Cavanaugh JM. Phospholipase A_2 sensitivity of the dorsal root and dorsal root ganglion. Spine 1998; 23:1297–1306.

Porter RW, Ward D. Cauda equina dysfunction: the significance of two-level pathology. Spine 1992; 17:9–15.

Roberts S, Caterson B, Menage, J, Evans EH, Jaffray DC, Eisenstein SM. Matrix metalloproteinases and aggrecanase: their role in disorders of the human intervertebral disc. Spine 2000; 25:3005–3013.

Saal JS. The role of inflammation in lumbar pain. Spine 1995; 20:1821–1827.

Saal JS, Franson RC, Dobrow R, Saal JA, White AH, Goldthwaite N. High levels of inflammatory phospholipase A_2 activity in lumbar disc herniations. Spine 1990; 15:674–679.

Schellinger D, Manz JH, Vidic B, Patronas NJ, Deveikis JP, Muraki AS, Abdullah DC. Disk fragment migration. Radiology 1990; 175:831–836.

Schmid MR, Stucki G, Duewell S, Wildermuth S, Romanowski B, Hodler J. Changes in cross-sectional measurements of the spinal canal and intervertebral foramina as a function of body position: in vivo studies on an open-configuration MR system. AJR Am J Roentgenol 1999; 172:1095–1102.

Shapiro S. Medical realities of cauda equina syndrome secondary to lumbar disc herniation. Spine 2000; 25:348–352.

Spangfort EV. The lumbar disc herniation: a computer-aided analysis of 2504 operations. Acta Orthop Scand Suppl 1972; 142:1–95.

Spengler DM, Freeman CW. Patient selection for lumbar discectomy: an objective approach. Spine 1979; 4:129–134.

Stadnik TW, Lee RR, Coen HL, Neirynck EC, Buisseret TS, Osteaux MJC. Annular tears and disk herniation: prevalence and contrast enhancement on MR images in the absence of low back pain or sciatica. Radiology 1998; 206:49–55.

Tamburrelli F, Leone A, Pitta L. A rare cause of lumbar radiculopathy: spinal gas collection. J Spinal Disord 2000; 13:451–454.

Teplick JG, Haskin ME. Spontaneous regression of herniated nucleus pulposus. AJR Am J Roentgenol 1985; 145:371–375.

Willen 2001 (see above in Disc Degeneration).

Watanabe N, Ogura T, Kimori K, Hase H, Hirasawa Y. Epidural hematoma of the lumbar spine, simulating extruded lumbar disk herniation: clinical, discographic, and enhanced magnetic resonance imaging features. Spine 1997; 22:105–109.

Weber H. Lumbar disc herniation: a controlled, prospective study with ten years of observation. Spine 1983; 8:131–139.

Weishaupt D, Schmid MR, Zanetti M, Boos N, Romanowski B, Kissling R, Dvorak J, Hodler J. Positional MR imaging of the lumbar spine: does it demonstrate nerve root compromise not visible at conventional MR imaging? Radiology 2000; 215:247–253.

Weishaupt D, Zanetti M, Hodler J, Boos N. MR imaging of the lumbar spine: prevalence of intervertebral disk extrusion and sequestration, nerve root compression, end plate abnormalities, and osteoarthritis of the facet joints in asymptomatic volunteers. Radiology 1998; 209:661–666.

White JG, Strait TA, Binkley JR, Hunter SE. Surgical treatment of 63 cases of conjoined nerve roots. J Neurosurg 1982; 56:114–117.

Wiltse LL, Fonseca AS, Amster J, Dimartino P, Ravessoud FA. Relationship of the dura, Hofmann's ligaments, Batson's plexus, and a fibrovascular membrane lying on the posterior surface of the vertebral bodies and attaching to the deep layer of the posterior longitudinal ligament: an anatomical, radiologic, and clinical study. Spine 1993; 18:1030–1043.

Yasuma T, Koh S, Okamura T, Yamauachi Y. Histologic changes in aging lumbar intervertebral discs: their role in protrusions and prolapses. J Bone Joint Surg Am 1990; 72:220–229.

Yu S, Haughton VM, Sether LA, Wagner M. Comparison of MR and diskography in detecting radial tears of the anulus: a postmortem study. AJNR Am J Neuroradiol 1989; 10:1077–1081.

Spinal Stenosis

Amundsen T, Weber H, Lilleas F, Nordal HJ, Abdelnoor M, Magnaes B. Lumbar spinal stenosis: clinical and radiographic features. Spine 1995; 10:1178–1186.

Arnoldi CC, Brodsky AE, Cauchoix J, et al. Lumbar spinal stenosis and nerve root entrapment syndromes. Clin Orthop 1976; 115:2–3.

Atlas SJ, Keller RB, Robson D, Deyo RA, Singer DE. Surgical and nonsurgical management of lumbar spinal stenosis. Spine 2000; 25:556–562.

Bolender NF, Schonstrom NSR, Spengler DM. Role of computed tomography and myelography in the diagnosis of central spinal stenosis. J Bone Joint Surg 1985; 67–A:240–246.

Drew B, Bhandari M, Kulkarni AV, Louw D, Reddy K, Dunlop B. Reliability in grading severity of lumbar spinal stenosis. J Spinal Disord 2000; 13:253–258.

Ferrante FM. Epidural steroids in the management of spinal stenosis. Semin Spine Surg 1989; 1:177–181.

Garfin SR, Rydevik BL, Brown RA. Compressive neuropathy of spinal nerve roots: a mechanical or biological problem? Spine 1991; 16:162–166.

Grob D, Humke T, Dvorak J. Degenerative lumbar spinal stenosis: decompression with and without arthrodesis. J Bone Joint Surg 1995; 77A:1036–1041.

Grobler LJ, Robertson PA, Novotny JE, Pope MH. Etiology of spondylolisthesis: assessment of the role played by lumbar facet joint morphology. Spine 1993; 18:80–91.

Heithoff KB, Ray CD, Schellhas KP, Fritts HM. CT and MRI of lateral entrapment syndromes. Spine Update 1987.

Herkowitz HN, Garfin SR. Decompressive surgery for spinal stenosis. Semin Spine Surg 1989; 1:163–167.

Iguchi T, Kurihara A, Nakayama J, Sato K, Kurosaka M, Yamasaki K. Minimum 10-year outcome of decompressive laminectomy for degenerative lumbar spinal stenosis. Spine 2000; 25:1754–1759.

Jenis LG, An HS. Lumbar foraminal stenosis. Spine 2000; 25:389–394.

Johnsson KE, Rosen I, Uden A. The natural course of lumbar spinal stenosis. Acta Orthop Scand (Suppl 251) 1993; 64:67–68.

Kaiser JA, Holland BA. Imaging of the cervical spine. Spine 1998; 23:2701–2712.

Kameyama T, Ando T, Yanagi T, Yasui K, Sobue G. Cervical spondylotic amyotrophy: magnetic resonance imaging demonstration of intrinsic cord pathology. Spine 1998; 23:448–452.

Kauppila LI, Eustace S, Kiel DP, Felson DT, Wright AM. Degenerative displacement of lumbar vertebrae: a 25 year follow-up study in Framingham. Spine 1998; 17:1868–1874.

Krauss WE, Ebersold MJ, Quast LM. Cervical spondylotic myelopathy: surgical indications and technique. Contemp Spine Surg 2000; 1:15–19.

Macnab I. Spondylolisthesis with an intact neural arch–the so-called pseudo-spondylolisthesis. J Bone Joint Surg Br 1950; 32:325–333.

Matsunaga S, Sakou T, Morizone Y, Masuda A, Demirtas AM. Natural history of degenerative spondylolisthesis: pathogenesis and natural course of the slippage. Spine 1990; 15:1204–1210.

McCullough JA. Microdecompression and uninstrumented single-level fusion for spinal canal stenosis with degenerative spondylolysthesis. Spine 1998; 23:2243–2252.

McNeill TW, Andersson GBJ, Schell B, Sinkora G, Nelson J, Lavender SA. Epidural administration of methylprednisolone and morphine for pain after a spinal operation. J Bone Joint Surg Am 1995; 77:1814–1817.

Moller H, Hedlund R. Surgery versus conservative management in adult isthmic spondylolisthesis: a prospective randomized study: I. Spine 2000; 25:1711–1715.

Morio Y, Teshima R, Nagashima H, Nawata K, Yamasaki D, Nanjo Y. Correlation between operative outcomes of cervical compression myelopathy and MRI of the spinal cord. Spine 2001; 26:1238–1245.

Nagaosa Y, Kikuchi S, Hasue M, Sato S. Pathoanatomic mechanisms of degenerative spondylolisthesis: a radiographic study. Spine 1998; 23:1447–1451.

Newman PH. The etiology of spondylolisthesis. J Bone Joint Surg Br 1955; 45:39–59.

Nurick S. The natural history and the results of surgical treatment of the spinal cord disorder associated with cervical spondylosis. Brain 1972; 95:101–108.

Okada Y, Ikata T, Katoh S, Yamada H. Morphologic analysis of the cervical spinal cord, dural tube, and spinal canal by magnetic resonance imaging in normal adults and patients with cervical spondylotic myelopathy. Spine 1994; 19:2331–2335.

Olmarker K, Rydevik B. Single- versus double-level nerve root compression. Clin Orthop 1992; 279:35–39.

Ono K, Ebara S, Fuji T, Yonenobu K, Fujiwara K, Yamashita K. Myelopathy hand: new clinical signs of cervical cord damage. J Bone Joint Surg 1987; 69B:215–219.

Porter RW. Spinal stenosis and neurogenic claudication. Spine 1996; 21:2046–2052.

Porter RW, Ward D. Cauda equina dysfunction: the significance of two-level pathology. Spine 1992; 17:9–15.

Postacchini F. Lumbar Spine Stenosis. New York, Springer-Verlag, 1989.

Rosenberg NJ. Degenerative spondylolisthesis: predisposing factors. J Bone Joint Surg Am 1975; 57:467–474.

Sampath P, Bendebba M, Davis JD, Ducker TB. Outcome of patients treated for cervical myelopathy: a prospective, multicenter trial with independent clinical review. Spine 2000; 25:670–676.

Schonstrom NSR, Bolender NF, Spengler DM. The pathomorphology of spinal stenosis as seen on CT scans of the lumbar spine. Spine 1985; 10:806–811.

Simotas AC, Dorey FJ, Hansraj KK, Cammisa F. Nonoperative treatment for lumbar spinal stenosis: clinical and outcome results and a 3-year survivorship analysis. Spine 2000; 25:197–204.

St. Amour TE, Hodges SC, Laakman RW, Tarnas DE. Osteomyelitis of the spine. In St. Amour TE, Hodges SC, Laakman RW, Tarnas DE (eds). MRI of the Spine. New York, Raven Press, 1994.

Takahashi K, Miyazaki T, Takino T, Matsui T, Tomita K. Epidural pressure measurements: relationship between epidural pressure and posture in patients with lumbar spinal stenosis. Spine 1995; 20:650–653.

Takahashi M, Yamashita Y, Sakamoto Y, Kojima R. Chronic cervical cord compression: clinical significance of increased signal intensity on MR images. Radiology 1989; 173:219–224.

Turner JA, Ersek M, Herron L, Deyo R. Surgery for lumbar spinal stenosis: attempted meta-analysis of the literature. Spine 1992; 17:1–8.

Verbiest H. Neurogenic intermittent claudication in cases with absolute and relative stenosis of the lumbar vertebral canal (ASLC and RSLC), in cases with narrow lumbar intervertebral foramina, and in cases with both entities. Clin Neurosurg 1973; 20:204–214.

Verbiest H. Stenosis of the lumbar vertebral canal and sciatica. Neurosurg Rev 1980; 3:75–89.

Vogt MT, Rubin D, Valentin SR, Palermo L, Donaldson WF III, Nevitt M, Cauley JA. Lumbar olisthesis and lower back pain symptoms in elderly white women: the study of osteoporotic fractures. Spine 1998; 23:2640–2647.

Wada E, Ohmura M, Yonenobu K. Intramedullary changes of the spinal cord in cervical spondylotic myelopathy. Spine 1995; 20:2226–2232.

Wada E, Yonenobu K, Suzuki S, Kanazawa A, Ochi T. Can intramedullary signal change on magnetic resonance imaging predict surgical outcome in cervical spondylotic myelopathy? Spine 1999; 24:455–462.

Weisz GM, Lee P. Spinal canal stenosis–concept of spinal reserve capacity: radiologic measurements and clinical applications. Clin Orthop 1983; 179:134–140.

Wiltse LL, Guyer RD, Spencer CW, Glenn WV, Porter IS. Alar transverse process compression of the L5 spinal nerve: the far-out syndrome. Spine 1984; 9:31–41.

Yoshida M, Shima K, Taniguchi Y, Tamaki T, Tanaka T. Hypertrophied ligamentum flavum in lumbar spinal canal stenosis: pathogenesis and morphologic and immunohistochemical observation. Spine 1992; 11:1353–1360.

Yousem DM, Atlas SW, Goldberg HI, Grossman RI. Degenerative narrowing of the cervical spine neural foramina: evaluation with high-resolution 3D FT gradient-echo MR imaging. AJNR Am J Neuroradiol 1991; 156:229–236.

Facet Joint Disease

Abdullah AF, Chambers TW, Daut DP. Lumbar nerve root compression by synovial cysts of the ligamentum flavum. J Neurosurg 1984; 60:617–620.

Aksoy FG, Gomori JM. Symptomatic cervical synovial cyst associated with an os odontoideum diagnosed by magnetic resonance imaging. Spine 2000; 25:1300–1302.

Apostolaki E, Davies AM, Evans N, Cassar-Pullicino VN. MR imaging of lumbar facet joint synovial cysts. Eur Radiol 2000; 10:615–623.

Awwad EE, Martin DS, Smith KR, Bucholz RD. MR imaging of lumbar juxtaarticular cysts. J Comput Tomogr 1990; 14:415–417.

Beks JWF. Kissing spines: fact or fancy? Acta Neurochirurgica 1989, 100:134–135.

Bjorkengren AG, Kurz LT, Resnich D, Sartorius DJ, Garfin SR. Symptomatic intraspinal synovial cysts: opacification and treatment by percutaneous injection. AJR Am J Roentgenol 1987; 149:105–107.

Boden SD, Riew KD, Yamaguichi K, Branch TP, Schellinger D, Wiesel SW. Orientation of the lumbar facet joints: association with degenerative disc disease. J Bone Joint Surg Am 1996; 78:403–411.

Butler D, Trafimow JH, Andersson GBJ, McNeill TW, Huckman MS. Disc degenerate before facets. Spine 1990; 15:111–113.

Carette S, Marcoux S, Truchon R, Grondin C, Gagnon J, Allard Y, Latulippe M. A controlled trial of corticosteroid injections into facet joints for chronic low back pain. N Engl J Med 1991; 325:1002–1007.

Chang H, Park JB, Kim KW. Synovial cyst of the transverse ligament of the atlas in a patient with os odontoideum and atlantoaxial instability. Spine 2000; 25:741–744.

Dreyfuss P, Halbrook B, Pauza K, Joshi A, Mclarty J, Bogduk N. Efficacy and validity of radiofrequency neurotomy for chronic lumbar zygapophysial joint pain. Spine 2000; 25:1270–1277.

Dwyer AB, Aprill C, Bogduk N. Cervical zygapophyseal joint pain patterns: I. A study in normal volunteers. Spine 1990; 15:453–457.

El-Khoury GY, Renfrew DL. Percutaneous procedures for the diagnosis and treatment of lower back pain: diskography, facet joint injection, and epidural injection. AJR Am J Roentgenol 1991; 157:685–691.

Farfan HF, Sullivan JD. The relation of facet orientation to intervertebral disc failure. Can J Surg 1967; 10:179–185.

Fujiwara A, Lim TH, An HS, Tanaka N, Jeon CH, Andersson GBJ, Haughton VM. The effect of disc degeneration and facet joint osteoarthritis on the segmental flexibility of the lumbar spine. Spine 2000a; 25:3036–3044.

Fujiwara A, Tamai K, An HS, Kurihashi A, Lim TH, Yoshida H, Saotome K. The relationship between disc degeneration, facet joint osteoarthritis, and stability of the degenerative lumbar spine. J Spinal Disord 2000b; 13:444–450.

Grogan J, Nowicki BH, Schmidt TA, Haughton VM. Lumbar facet joint tropism does not accelerate degeneration of the facet joints. AJNR Am J Neuroradiol 1997; 18:1325–1329.

Hanakita J, Suwa H, Ohta F, Nishi S, Sakaida H, Iihara K. Neuroradiological examination of thoracic radiculo-myelopathy due to ossification of the ligamentum flavum. Neuroradiology 1990; 32:38–42.

Howington JU, Connolly ES, Voorhies RM. Intraspinal synovial cysts: ten-year experience at the Ochsner Clinic. J Neurosurg 1999; 91(2 suppl):193–199.

Howling SJ, Kessel D. Case report: acute radiculopathy due to a haemorrhagic lumbar synovial cyst. Clin Radiol 1997; 52:73–74.

Hsu KY, Zucherman JF, Shea WJ, Jeffrey RA. Lumbar intraspinal synovial and ganglion cysts (facet cysts): ten-year experience in evaluation and treatment. Spine 1995; 20:80–89.

Jackson DE, Atlas SW, Mani JR, Norman D. Intraspinal synovial cysts: MR imaging. Radiology 1989; 170:527–530.

Jackson RP, Jacobs RR, Montesano PX. Facet joint injection in low back pain: a prospective statistical study. Spine 1988; 13:966–971.

Jonsson B, Tufvesson A, Stromqvist B. Lumbar nerve root compression by intraspinal synovial cysts: report of eight cases. Acta Orthop Scand 1999; 70:203–206.

Kaplan M, Dreyfuss P, Halbrook B, Bogduk N. The ability of lumbar medial branch blocks to anesthetize the zygapophyseal joint: a physiologic challenge. Spine 1998; 23:1847–1852.

Kellgren JH. On the distribution of pain arising from deep somatic structures with charts of segmental pain areas. Clin Sci 1939; 4L:35–46.

Khoury GM, Shimkin PM, Kleinman GM, Mastroianni PP, Nijensohn DE. Computed tomography and magnetic resonance imaging findings of pigmented villonodular synovitis of the spine. Spine 1991; 16:1236–1237.

Kirkaldy-Willis WH, Farfan HF. Instability of the lumbar spine. Clin Ortho Rel Res 1982; 165:110–123.

Kurz LT, Garfin SR, Unger AS, Thorne RP, Rothman RH. Intraspinal synovial cyst causing sciatica. J Bone Joint Surg Am 1985; 67:865–871.

Kuslich SD, Ulstrom CL, Michael CJ. The tissue of origin of low back pain and sciatica: a report of pain response to tissue stimulation during operations on the lumbar spine using local anesthesia. Orthop Clin North Am 1991; 22:181–187.

Lippitt AB. The facet joint and its role in spine pain: management with facet joint injections. Spine 1984; 7:746–750.

Liu SS, Williams KD, Drayer BP, Spetzler RF, Sonntag VKH. Synovial cysts of the lumbosacral spine: diagnosis by MR imaging. AJR Am J Roentgenol 1990; 154:163–166.

Lynn B, Watkins RG, Williams LA. Acute traumatic myelopathy secondary to a thoracic cyst in a professional football player. Spine 2000; 25:1593–1595.

Lyons MK, Atkinson JL, Wharen RE, Deen HG, Zimmerman RS, Lemens SM. Surgical evaluation and management of lumbar synovial cysts: the Mayo Clinic experience. J Neurosurg 2000; 93(1 suppl):53–57.

Modic MT, Ross JS, Obuchowski NA, Browning KH, Cianflocco AJ, Mazanec DJ. Contrast-enhanced MR imaging in acute lumbar radiculopathy: a pilot study of the natural history. Radiology 1995; 195:429–435.

Noren R, Trafimow J, Andersson GBJ, Huckman MS. The role of facet joint tropism and facet angle in disc degeneration. Spine 1991; 16:530–532.

Okada K, Oka S, Tohge K, Ono K, Yonenobu K, Hosoya T. Thoracic myelopathy caused by ossification of the ligamentum flavum: clinicopathologic study and surgical treatment. Spine 1991; 16:280–287.

Onofrio BM, Mih AD. Synovial cysts of the spine. Neurosurgery 1988; 22:642–647.

Parlier-Cuau C, Wybier M, Nizard R, Champsaur P, Le Hir P, Laredo JD. Symptomatic lumbar facet joint synovial cysts: clinical assessment of facet joint steroid injection after 1 and 6 months and long-term follow-up in 30 patients. Radiology 1999; 210:509–513.

Resnick D, Niwayama G. Degenerative disease of the spine. In Resnick D (ed). Diagnosis of Bone and Joint Disorders, 3rd ed. Philadelphia, WB Saunders, 1995.

Revel M, Poiraudeau S, Auleley GR, Payan C, Denke A, Nguyen M, Chevrot A, Fermanian J. Capacity of the clinical picture to characterize low back pain relieved by facet joint anesthesia: proposed criteria to identify patients with painful facet joints. Spine 1998; 23:1972–1977.

Sabo RA, Tracy PT, Weinger JM. A series of 60 juxtafacet cysts: clinical presentation, the role of spinal instability, and treatment. J Neurosurg 1996; 85:560–565.

Schwarzer AC, Aprill CN, Derby R, Fortin J, Kine G, Bogduk N. Clinical features of patients with pain stemming from the lumbar zygapophyseal joints: is the lumbar facet syndrome a clinical entity? Spine 1994; 19:1132–1137.

Schwarzer AC, Wang SC, O'Driscoll D, Harrington T, Bogduk N, Laurent R. The ability of computed tomography to identify a painful zygapophyseal joint in patients with chronic low back pain. Spine 1995; 20:907–912.

Silbergleit R, Gebarski SS, Brunberg JA, McGillicudy J, Blaivas M. Lumbar synovial cysts: correlation of myelographic, CT, MR, and pathologic findings. AJR Am J Neuroradiol 1990; 11:777–779.

St. Amour TE, Hodges SC, Laakman RW, Tarnas DE. Cervical spine. In St. Amour TE, Hodges SC, Laakman RW, Tarnas DE (eds). MRI of the Spine. New York, Raven Press, 1994.

Stoodley MA, Jones NR, Scott G. Cervical and thoracic juxtafacet cysts causing neurologic deficits. Spine 2000; 25:970–973.

Sugimura H, Kakitsubata Y, Suzuki Y, Kakitsubata S, Tamura S, Uwada O, Kodama T, Yano T, Watanabe K. MRI of ossification of ligamentum flavum. J Comput Tomogr 1992; 16:73–76.

van Kleef M, Barendse GA, Kessels A, Voets HM, Wever WEJ, de Lange S. Randomized trial of radiofrequency lumbar facet denervation for chronic low back pain. Spine 1999; 24:1937–1942.

van Oostenbrugge RJ, Herpers MJ, de Kruijk JR. Spinal cord compression caused by unusual location and extension of ossified ligamenta flava in a Caucasian male. Spine 1999; 24:486–488.

Wang AM, Haykal HA, Lin JCT, Lee JH. Synovial cysts of the lumbar spine: CT evaluation. Comput Radiol 1987; 11:253–257.

Woodring JH, Goldstein SJ. Fractures of the articular processes of the cervical spine. AJR Am J Roentgenol 1982; 139:341–344.

Yong-Hing K, Kirkaldy-Willis WH. The pathophysiology of degenerative disease of the lumbar spine. Orthop Clin North Am 1983; 14:491–504.

Yuh WTC, Drew JM, Weinstein JN, McGuire CW, Moore TE, Kathol MH, El-Khoury GY. Intraspinal synovial cysts: magnetic resonance evaluation. Spine 1991; 16:740–745.

Scheuermann's Disease, Thoracolumbar Osteochondrosis, and Juvenile Discogenic Disease

Alexander CJ. Scheuermann's disease: a traumatic spondylodystrophy? Skeletal Radiol 1977; 1:209–221.

Aufdermaur M. Juvenile kyphosis (Scheuermann's disease): radiography, histology, and pathogenesis. Clin Orthop 1981; 14:166–174.

Blumenthal SL, Roach J, Herring JA. Lumbar Scheuermann's: a clinical series and classification. Spine 1987; 12:929–932.

Cleveland RH, Delong GR. The relationship of juvenile lumbar disc disease and Scheuermann's disease. Pediatr Radiol 1981; 10:161–164.

Dorland's Illustrated Medical Dictionary, 28th ed. Philadelphia, WB Saunders, 1994.

Fahey V, Opeskin K, Silberstein M, Anderson R, Briggs C. The pathogenesis of Schmorl's nodes in relation to acute trauma: an autopsy study. Spine 1998; 23:2272–2275.

Greene TL, Hensinger RN, Hunter LY. Back pain and vertebral changes simulating Scheuermann's disease. J Pediatr Orthop 1985; 5:1–7.

Hafner RHV. Localised osteochondritis (Scheuermann's disease). J Bone Joint Surg Br 1952; 34:38–40.

Heithoff KB, Gundry CR, Burton CV, Winter RB. Juvenile discogenic disease. Spine 1994; 19:335–340.

Jensen MC, Brant-Zawadski MN, Obuchowski N, Modic MT, Malkasian D, Ross J. Magnetic resonance imaging of the lumbar spine in people without back pain. N Engl J Med 1994; 331:69–73.

Lowe TG. Scheuermann disease. J Bone Joint Surg Am 1990; 72:940–945.

McCall IW, Park WM, O'Brien JP, Seal V. Acute traumatic intraosseous disc herniation. Spine 1985; 10:134–137.

Milsom C, Wishart P. Spondylolisthesis: a radiological survey of 118 cases. N Z Med J 1961; 60:306–311.

Ogilvie JW, Sherman J. Spondylolysis in Scheuermann's disease. Spine 1987; 12:251–253.

Paajanen H, Alanen A, Erkintalo M, Salminen JJ, Katevuo K. Disc degeneration in Scheuermann disease. Skeletal Radiol 1989; 18:523–526.

Paassilta P, Lohiniva J, Goring HHH, Perala M, Raina SS, Karppinen J, Hakala M, Palm T, Kroger H, Kaitila I, Vanharanta H, Ott J, Ala-Kokko L. Identification of a novel common genetic risk factor for lumbar disk disease. JAMA 2001; 285:1843–1849.

Resnick D. Osteochondroses and osteonecrosis. In Resnick D (ed). Diagnosis of Bone and Joint Disorders, 3rd ed. Philadelphia, WB Saunders, 1995.

Salminen JJ, Erkintalo MO, Pentti J, Okasanen A, Kormano MJU. Recurrent low back pain and early disc degeneration in the young. Spine 1999; 24:1316–1321.

Scoles PV, Latimer BM, DiGiovanni BF, Vargo E, Bauza S, Jellema LM. Vertebral alterations in Scheuermann's kyphosis. Spine 1991; 16:509–515.

Soderberg L, Andren L. Disc degeneration and lumbago-ischias. Acta Orthopaedica Scand 1955; 25:137–148.

Stabler A, Belan M, Weiss M, Gartner C, Brossmann J, Reiser MF. MR imaging of enhancing intraosseous disk herniation (Schmorl's nodes). AJR Am J Roentgenol 1997; 168:933–938.

Swischuk LE, John SD, Allbery S. Disk degenerative disease in childhood–Scheuermann's disease, Schmorl's nodes, and the limbus vertebra: MRI findings in 12 patients. Pediatr Radiol 1998; 28:334–338.

Tallroth K, Schlenzka D. Spinal stenosis subsequent to juvenile lumbar osteochondrosis. Skeletal Radiol 1990; 19:203–205.

Walters G, Coumas JM, Akins CM, Ragland RL. Magnetic resonance imaging of acute symptomatic Schmorl's node formation. Pediatr Emerg Care 1991; 7:294–296.

Wassman K. Kyphosis juvenilis Scheuermann: an occupational disorder. Acta Orthop 1946; 21:65–74.

Wood KB, Schellhas KP, Garvey TA, Aeppli D. Thoracic discography in healthy individuals: a controlled prospective study of magnetic resonance imaging and discography in asymptomatic and symptomatic individuals. Spine 1999; 24:1548–1555

3 Imaging of the Postoperative Spine

DONALD L. RENFREW • MICHAEL MACMILLAN • KENNETH B. HEITHOFF

Although 80% to 90% of patients who have had a discectomy (Davis 1994, Findlay 1998, Frymoyer 1988) and 70% to 90% of patients who have had fusion surgery (Brantigan 2000, Brodsky 1989, Gill 1992, Hutter 1983, Kuslich 1998, Ray 1997) do well following surgery with improvement or elimination of symptoms, some patients return for imaging because of persistent or recurrent symptoms. Radiologists' perceptions of the success of back surgery may be biased because they will see virtually all of these patients (some several times) while infrequently hearing of the many successful procedures. There are several possible causes of persistent or recurrent back and leg pain following surgery, and these causes need to be considered when reviewing postoperative images. In addition, the clinical scenario of the postoperative patient is, if anything, more important than it is in evaluating preoperative pain, because the temporal course of the pain following surgery may allow differentiation between a surgical complication, failure to address the patient's problem at surgery, recurrence of the patient's problem, or a new problem that has transpired or worsened since surgery (Federowicz 1991, Kostiuk 1997).

Spine surgeons not only perform a wide variety of surgical procedures on patients but also refine these procedures and develop new procedures on an ongoing basis. At the same time, other procedures fall from favor, but the patients treated with these procedures return for imaging, often decades later. In an ideal world, the radiologist would have full knowledge of the exact surgical technique employed on a patient undergoing imaging, including actual observation of one or more of the procedures. This ideal is unattainable, and the radiologist may be presented with what is, to the radiologist, a novel surgical technique. Consultation with the surgeon performing the technique will no doubt increase the radiologist's knowledge base and may well lead to an improved interpretation of the images. In those instances when this is not possible, and as a general rule for all surgical procedures, the radiologist needs to apply certain basic principles when analyzing the postoperative spine. This chapter lists, explains, and illustrates those principles.

Brief Review of Surgical Procedures

As noted earlier, surgeons continue to develop an ever-changing array of procedures to treat spine disorders. Given the rapid expansion within this field, no book can describe all surgical procedures (or, therefore, all possible postoperative imaging findings). It is possible, however, to categorize most surgical procedures as follows:

1. Procedures to reduce or eliminate disc herniations. As noted in Chapter 2, disc herniations may produce symptoms through chemical irritation, mechanical impingement, or a combination of both. Surgical options include automated percutaneous discectomy (Davis 1991), interlaminar discectomy (performed with or without bone removal) (Fig. 3–1) (Findlay 1998), and transforaminal discectomy (Mathews 1996).
2. Procedures to reduce stenosis. In these procedures, the surgeon decreases compression of neural tissue viaremoval of a portion of the confining structure. Decompression of spinal cord stenosis is usually produced by removing portions of the posterior elements (Fig. 3–2). In the cervical spine, vertebrectomy can achieve spinal canal and foraminal decompression (Fig. 3–3). Lateral decompression is achieved by removing the medial portion of the superior facet. Decompressive surgery is often accompanied by fusion surgery (see later) (Fig. 3–4). Although most decompressions are done on an elective basis to reduce degenerative stenosis, more urgent decompressions may be performed in cases of fractures with displaced fragments, hematomas and abscesses, and as part of tumor surgery, where progressive neurologic deficits are occurring.
3. Procedures to fuse motion segments.
   a. A fundamental assumption of orthopedic surgery is that joints immobilized through solid bony union do not cause pain. Therefore, fusion of symptomatic facet joints will eliminate facet joint pain, and fusion of the intervertebral disc will eliminate pain caused by intervertebral segmental instability (Kirkaldy-Willis 1982, Langrana 1993). Surgeons have employed a myriad of techniques to produce fusion. These techniques rely

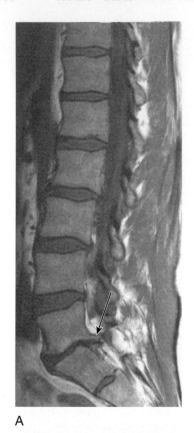

A

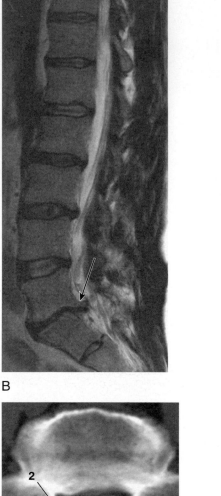

B

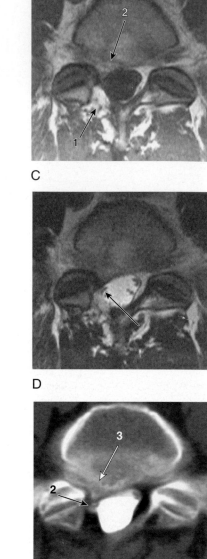

C

D

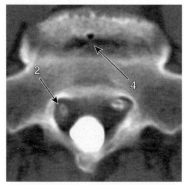

E

F

G

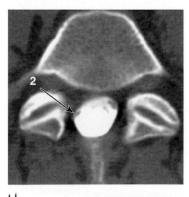

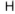

H

FIGURE 3–1

Postoperative discectomy patient with osteophyte formation along the disc margin and accompanying neural displacement. A 46-year-old man with low back pain and right leg pain for several years following remote laminectomy. *A,* Sagittal T1WI shows marked L5–S1 disc narrowing and osteophyte formation projecting off the posterior aspect of the inferior L5 vertebral body *(arrow). B,* Sagittal T2WI shows multilevel degenerative disc disease, including L2–3 mild loss of disc height and hydration, L3–4 mild loss of disc height and hydration along with degenerative disc bulging, and L5–S1 severe loss of disc height and hydration with subchondral Modic Type II degenerative changes. At the L5–S1 level, an osteophyte projects from the posteroinferior vertebral body margin *(arrow). C,* Axial T1WI just above the level of the L5–S1 intervertebral disc shows a right laminectomy posteriorly *(arrow 1)* and a right paracentral and subarticular disc contour abnormality isointense with adjacent bone *(arrow 2). D,* Axial T2WI shows similar findings to *C,* but with better demonstration of the displaced traversing S1 nerve root *(arrow). E–H,* Sequential CT-myelogram images from just below to just above the L5–S1 disc demonstrate a right S1 laminectomy defect *(arrow 1).* Below the level of the disc, the S1 nerve root *(arrow 2)* demonstrates an approximately normal position, whereas at the level of the disc there is considerable displacement of the root by osteophytic spurring along the dorsal disc margin *(arrow 3).* There is a vacuum phenomenon of the intervertebral disc *(arrow 4)* secondary to degenerative disc disease. This complicated case emphasizes the difficult problem of evaluating the postoperative patient. The large disc contour abnormality seen on the MRI appeared to represent mostly bone, but the referring surgeon requested the myelogram to evaluate the relative contributions of bone and soft tissue to the mass effect. Virtually no soft tissue is present, but the S1 nerve root is nonetheless significantly displaced from its normal location. On the other hand, the lamina has been removed and there is no compression of S1. The consensus of orthopedic and neurosurgical opinion was that the patient would not benefit from further surgery at this time.

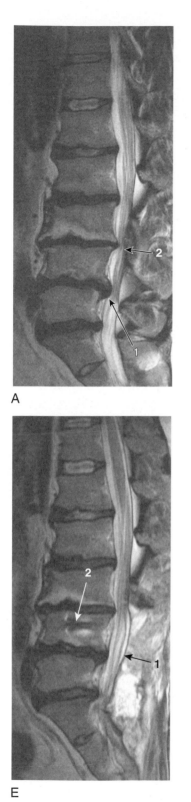

A

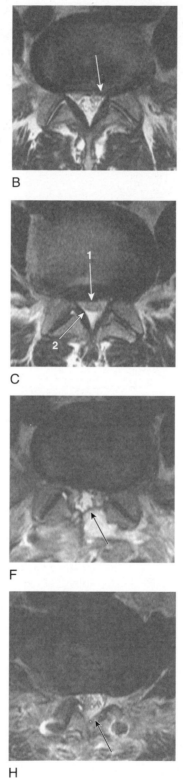

B

C

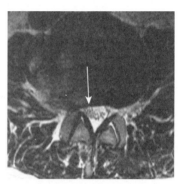

D

F

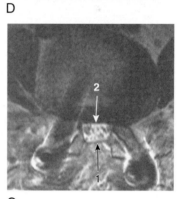

G

E

H

FIGURE 3–2

Preoperative and postoperative MRI demonstrating lessening stenosis following decompression surgery. A 36-year-old man with chronic low back and bilateral leg pain. *A,* Sagittal T2WI demonstrates reversal of normal lumbar lordosis with multilevel degenerative changes, including L1–2 and L5–S1 moderate loss of disc height and hydration and L2–3, L3–4, and L4–5 severe loss of disc height and hydration. There is multilevel Schmorl's node formation and anterior osteophytic spurring, and the patient meets the criteria of juvenile discogenic disease (see Chapter 2). There is a 6-mm, caudally dissecting disc extrusion at L4–5 *(arrow 1)*, contributing to severe central spinal canal stenosis, and there is osteophytic spurring and degenerative disc bulging contributing to moderate subarticular recess stenosis at L3–4 *(arrow 2)* (because of scoliosis, the L3–4 level is imaged in the right parasagittal plane on this image). *B,* Axial T2WI at the L5–S1 level shows degenerative disc bulging with left subarticular recess stenosis *(arrow)*. *C,* Axial T2WI just below the L4–5 disc shows the caudally dissecting component of the disc extrusion *(arrow 1)* and severe spinal canal narrowing *(arrow 2)*. *D,* Axial T2WI at the L3–4 disc shows moderate right-sided spinal canal and subarticular recess stenosis from degenerative disc bulging and osteophyte formation *(arrow)*. *E,* Sagittal T2WI following multilevel decompression/fusion surgery again demonstrates multilevel degenerative changes. Posterior decompression has been performed *(arrow 1)* with reduction of spinal canal narrowing. There is metallic artifact from a pedicle screw within the L4 vertebral body *(arrow 2)*. *F,* Axial T2WI at the L5–S1 level (compare with *B*) demonstrates posterior decompression *(arrow)* with lessened stenosis. *G,* Axial T2WI just below the L4–5 level (compare with *C*) demonstrates removal of posterior elements *(arrow 1)* and removal of disc herniation material *(arrow 2)* with lessened stenosis. *H,* Axial T2WI at the L3–4 level demonstrates removal of posterior elements *(arrow)* with lessened stenosis.

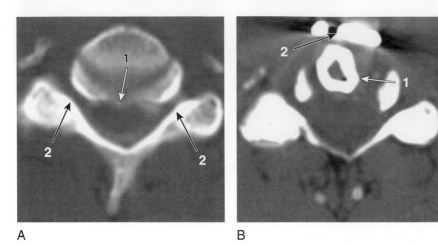

A   B

FIGURE 3–3

Cervical vertebrectomy to reduce stenosis. A 44-year-old woman with neck and bilateral arm and hand pain with multilevel degenerative disc disease and both spinal canal and foraminal stenosis. *A,* Axial 3-mm CT slice through the C4–5 disc performed after myelography. There is effacement of contrast anterior and posterior to the cord, and a small midline osteophyte (*arrow 1*) indents the ventral aspect of the spinal cord and worsens spinal canal stenosis. There is also bilateral foraminal stenosis (*arrows 2*) (note some volume averaging on this 3-mm slice with the C5 pedicle on the left side). The patient had similar degenerative changes at C3–4, C5–6, and C6–7 (not shown). *B,* Axial 1-mm CT slice through the C4–5 disc following vertebral body resection with placement of a tubular bony strut graft (*arrow 1*) and anterior metallic plate (*arrow 2*). Although performed without myelographic contrast, this study demonstrates definite lessening of the spinal canal stenosis with less impressive reduction of foraminal stenosis.

on a combination of metallic fixation devices and bone graft material (Figs. 3–4 to 3–7). Because of its inevitable material fatigue, any metallic device may fail with time. Living tissue such as bone, on the other hand, can produce fusion able to withstand ongoing, variable stress (Figs. 3–7 to 3–9). Bone graft material may be harvested from the patient for an *autograft*, or taken from a bank of tissue from other individuals for an *allograft*. Autograft is generally preferable with higher rates of incorporation and fusion in posterior surgery (Kostiuk 1997). Structural allografts are useful as anterior struts.

b. Progressive deformity may produce symptoms. Such deformity may be predominantly in the sagittal plane (e.g., painful juvenile kyphosis, degenerative spondylolisthesis), in the coronal plane (idiopathic scoliosis), or a combination of both (degenerative rotoscoliosis). Fusion surgery in these cases may either reduce the deformity or prevent progression of deformity.

c. Surgery may be performed to stabilize a fractured vertebra (or vertebrae).

4. Procedures to remove tumors. In the case of soft tissue masses, tumor removal may be accomplished with little or no bone removal. For bony lesions, or for large soft tissue tumors within the spinal canal or occupying a foramen, removal of bone with or without a fusion is often necessary.

Although such a classification is helpful, some procedures do not fit into this scheme. For example, intradiscal electrothermal treatment may work by shrinking collagen along an annular fissure of the disc or coagulating nociceptive fibers in the disc annulus (Karasek 2000, Saal 2000a, Saal 2000b). Misplacement of the heating catheter in this procedure could result in neural damage. As another example, percutaneous vertebroplasty involves injection of the vertebrae with barium-impregnated methyl methacrylate (Barr 2000, Cyteval 1999, Gangi 1998). Kyphoplasty involves injection of barium-impregnated methyl methacrylate after attempted reduction of kyphosis through expanding a balloon in a collapsed vertebral body

(Fig. 3–10). Causes of pain following these procedures include complications of the procedures themselves (e.g., leakage of cement, rib fractures (Fig. 3–11), and adjacent segment fractures (Fig. 3–12).

Imaging of Postoperative Patients

PLAIN FILMS

Patients who have had prior spine surgery usually have postoperative plain films taken. In patients who have undergone fusion surgery, plain films allow evaluation of hardware migration, breakage, and loosening. Comparison of flexion-extension films allows evaluation of excessive motion not only at the fusion site but also at adjacent segments. Note, however, that plain films have generally demonstrated limited accuracy in the evaluation of postoperative patients when compared with computed tomography (CT) (Farber 1995, Frymoyer 1979, Laasonen 1989, Lang 1988, Zinreich 1990).

COMPUTED TOMOGRAPHY

CT scanning is generally superior to plain film evaluation in assessment of non-union (Frymoyer 1979, Laasonen 1989, Lang 1988, Zinreich 1990), pedicle screw misplacement (Farber 1995, Schwarzenbach 1997), and stenosis (Lang 1988, Zinreich 1990).

In the lumbar spine, we routinely use 3-mm scan thickness at 2-mm intervals through the fused area with sagittal and curved coronal reconstructions. If the patient has anterior interbody fusion, we obtain 1-mm slices at 1-mm intervals through the fusion device to better assess the critical interface between the device and the native bone. The lumbar spine above the fusion is scanned at 3-mm thickness to at least the L3 pedicle, followed by 5-mm thickness to the T12 pedicle (or higher if there are obvious abnormalities on the scout radiograph).

In the cervical spine, we routinely use 1-mm slices at 1-mm intervals through levels of fusion with 3-mm slices through the remainder of the cervical spine, with sagittal

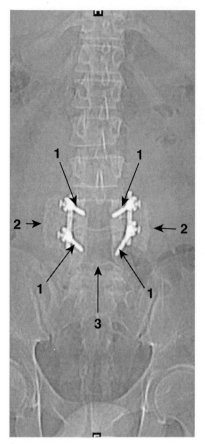

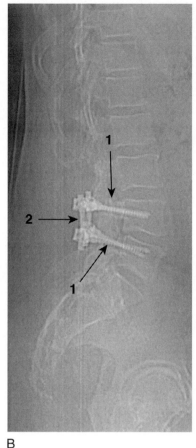

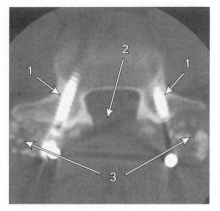

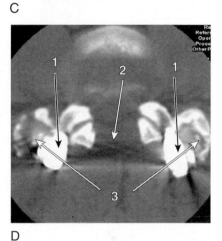

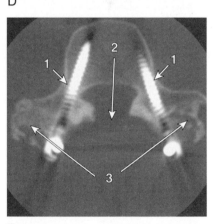

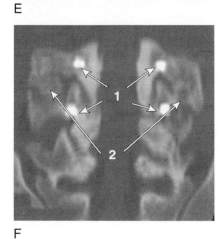

A   B   C

D

E

F

FIGURE 3–4

Lumbar decompression/fusion surgery. A 45-year-old man after fusion at L4–5 with bilateral pedicle screws, dorsal interconnecting hardware, and intertransverse process fusion as well as dorsal decompression. *A,* Anteroposterior scout view for CT study shows pedicle screws (*arrows 1*) and fusion bone (*arrows 2*) as well as dorsal decompression (*arrow 3*). *B,* Lateral scout view for CT study also demonstrates pedicle screws (*arrows 1*) and dorsal interconnecting rods (*arrow 2*). *C,* Axial study through the L5 pedicle level shows bilateral pedicle screws (*arrows 1*) without loosening, fracture, or migration. The screws are not imaged on a single axial study owing to obliquity with respect to the scan plane. Note changes of dorsal decompression (*arrow 2*) and bone graft material posterolaterally (*arrow 3*). *D,* Axial study through the L4–5 disc level shows posterolateral interconnecting rods (*arrows 1*), dorsal decompression (*arrow 2*), dorsolateral fusion graft (*arrow 3*), and no evidence of recurrent or residual spinal canal stenosis or disc extrusion. *E,* Axial study through the L4 pedicles demonstrates, as at the L5 level, pedicle screws (*arrows 1*) without loosening, fracture, or migration, dorsal decompression (*arrow 2*), and dorsolateral fusion graft material (*arrow 3*). *F,* Curved coronal reconstruction shows the pedicle screws (*arrows 1*) and lateral graft material (*arrows 2*). Note that the solidity of the graft is difficult to evaluate on a single image, and integration of findings on sequential axial studies as well as sagittal and curved coronal reconstructions is often required to fully evaluate whether a fusion is solid or not. In this patient, when all studies were reviewed, fusion was definitely present.

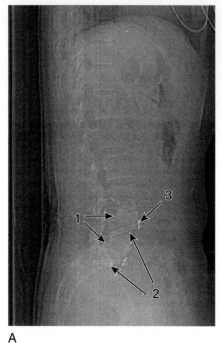

A

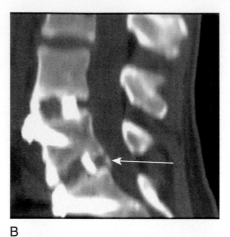

B

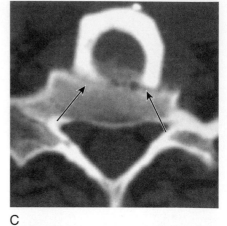

C

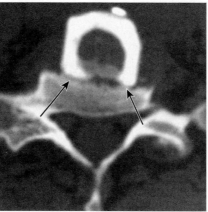

D

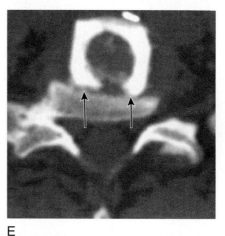

E

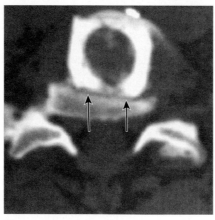

F

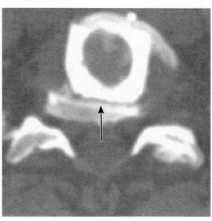

G

FIGURE 3–5

Interbody fusion surgery performed with femoral ring allografts. A 34-year-old woman with low back pain and left leg pain 6 months following L4–5 and L5–S1 fusion surgery. *A,* Lateral scout digital radiograph demonstrates femoral ring allografts at the L4–5 and L5–S1 levels *(arrows 1)* with associated hardware consisting of screws into the L5 and S1 vertebral bodies *(arrows 2).* There are washers on the anterior aspects of the screws, as best seen at L4–5 *(arrow 3).* *B,* Sagittal reconstruction view shows portions of the hardware as well as the disc fusion material. There is ossification along the posterior disc margin at L5–S1 from either a calcified herniated disc or remote, calcified apophyseal avulsion injury *(arrow).* *C–G,* Sequential inferior-to-superior 1-mm axial slices through the L5–S1 disc demonstrate lucency along the posterior, inferior margin separating the femoral ring allograft and native S1 vertebral segment *(arrows),* consistent with possible pseudarthrosis.

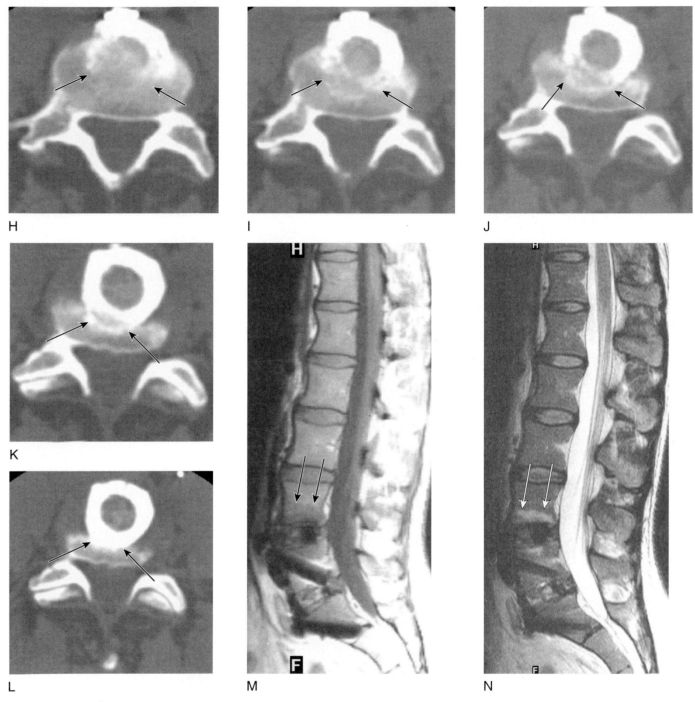

FIGURE 3–5 *(continued)*

H–L, Sequential inferior-to-superior 1-mm axial slices through a comparable region of the L4–5 disc demonstrate no such lucency separating the femoral ring allograft and the adjacent L5 vertebral body *(arrows)*; rather, there is smooth transition without an interface between these structures, consistent with solid union at this level. *M,* Sagittal T1WI obtained 6 months later shows mild T1 prolongation of subchondral marrow *(arrows)*. *N,* Sagittal T2WI shows T2 prolongation *(arrows)*. The subchondral changes at L4–5 favor a lack of functional union at this level. No neural compression or other cause of radicular pain was identified in this patient. Possible causes of the patient's ongoing back and leg pain include continued motion at the L4–5 level, adjacent segment disease, and facet arthropathy.

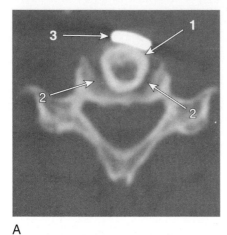

A

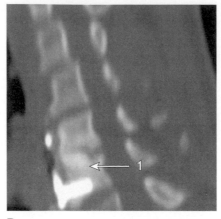

B

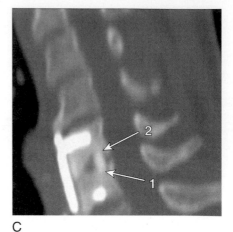

C

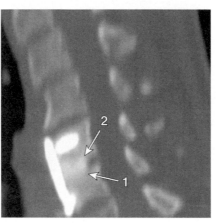

D

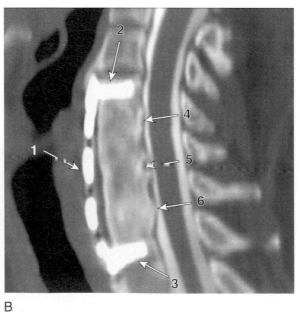

E

FIGURE 3–6

Anterior cervical discectomy and fusion with anterior hardware and interbody graft material. A 40-year-old patient with persistent neck and bilateral shoulder pain following fusion surgery at C5–6. Plain films (not shown) demonstrated apparent lucency along the superior margin of the graft. *A,* Axial 1-mm CT scan through the C6 pedicle level shows resection of the anterior portion of the vertebral body and placement of a tubular bone graft *(arrow 1).* Note the lucency along the margins of the tubular bone graft lateral and posterior margins *(arrows 2),* which is a normal postoperative finding that does not indicate loosening. There is an anterior plate *(arrow 3)* (fixed by screws into the ventral aspects of C5 and C6) in place as well. *B–E,* Sagittal reconstructions demonstrate incorporation of the tubular graft into the subjacent C6 *(arrow 1)* and suprajacent C5 *(arrow 2)* levels, an appearance that was confirmed on sequential axial 1-mm slices. The findings are those of a solid union at the level of the surgery.

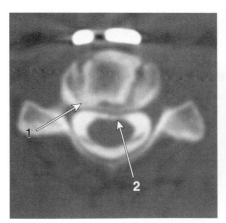

A

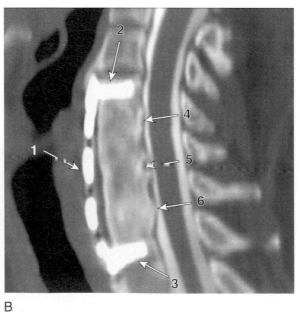

B

FIGURE 3–7

Multilevel cervical fusion with solid incorporation of bony grafts. A 44-year-old woman with neck and arm pain after fusion surgery. *A,* Axial 1-mm CT scan through the C6 vertebra shows incorporation of tubular bony graft along its right posterolateral aspect *(arrow 1).* There is partial effacement of ventral cerebrospinal fluid secondary to osteophytic spurring along the residual (fused) C5–6 vertebral disc *(arrow 2). B,* Sagittal reconstruction shows an anterior plate *(arrow 1),* proximal *(arrow 2)* and distal *(arrow 3)* screws, and elimination of the C4–5 *(arrow 4),* C5–6 *(arrow 5),* and C6–7 *(arrow 6)* intervertebral discs with continuous bony union. No adjacent segment disc extrusion or severe spinal canal stenosis was identified. Note that the graft in this case is much more mature than that seen in Figure 3–3.

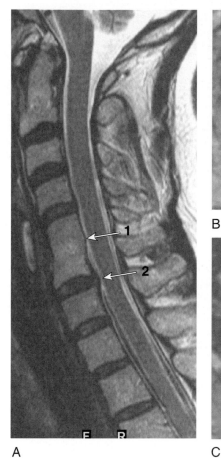

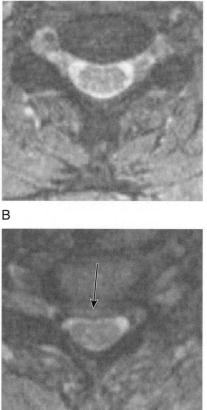

A   B   C

FIGURE 3–8

Remodeling at fusion level with bone replacing disc. A 51-year-old woman who underwent a cervical fusion (without hardware) 20 years prior to this MRI. She was virtually symptom free until 2 months prior to the examination, at which time she developed right arm pain and numbness. *A,* Sagittal T2WI demonstrates an inherently small spinal canal on a congenital/developmental basis with anteroposterior (AP) measurements in the 11- to 13-mm range from C3 to C7. There is complete elimination of the C5–6 intervertebral disc (*arrow 1*) with solid union of the C5 and C6 vertebral bodies. At the inferior adjacent segment (C6–7), there is a disc protrusion (*arrow 2*) with resultant indentation of the anterior aspect of the spinal cord. *B,* Axial gradient-recalled echo (GRE) T2WI at the level of the former C5–6 disc demonstrates mild spinal canal narrowing but no cord flattening and widely patent neural foramina. *C,* Axial GRE T2WI at the inferior adjacent segment (C6–7) level demonstrates a small disc protrusion with moderate spinal canal stenosis and mild AP cord indentation. The AP measurement of the spinal canal is 9.8 mm. A metallic device with no living graft material would be unlikely to have lasted 20 years, but the patient's biologic fusion mass demonstrates solid union and no evidence of complication.

and curved coronal reconstructions. Myelography may be performed in conjunction with CT if, as is frequently the case, stenosis is a clinical consideration

NUCLEAR MEDICINE

Bone scans usually demonstrate increased radiotracer localization at postoperative levels for many years following surgery. As is the case with degenerative changes in the spine, single photon-emission computed tomography images better localize abnormalities. Bone scans are generally most helpful in a negative manner: lack of increased radiotracer localization is generally taken to be a sign that no significant abnormality is present. Increased radiotracer localization may indicate any of several processes (e.g., pseudarthrosis, fusion, degenerative change).

MAGNETIC RESONANCE IMAGING

Magnetic resonance imaging (MRI) is the study of choice for evaluation of recurrent disc herniation. Although the literature is replete with references advocating routine administration of contrast material in patients undergoing imaging for recurrent or new symptoms following discectomy (Cavanaugh 1993, Hueftle 1988, Ross 1990), we have found that routine administration is unnecessary (Mullin 2000). Our routine for evaluation of the postoperative spine is the same as for our evaluation of degenerative disease (see earlier).

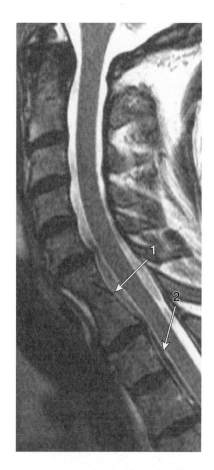

FIGURE 3–9

Remodeling at fusion level with bone replacing disc. A 55-year-old patient after cervical fusion more than 20 years earlier. Sagittal T2WI demonstrates marked narrowing of the C6–7 level along with elimination of the intervertebral disc (*arrow 1*). Such an "hourglass" appearance is more characteristic of congenital/developmental anomaly rather than surgery but, in some long-standing cases, postoperative fusion may have this appearance, which is a manifestation of ongoing biologic activity at the fusion level. Also note anterior flow void ventral to the spinal cord on this fast spin-echo T2WI (*arrow 2*).

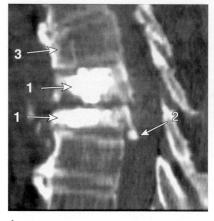

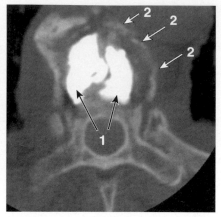

A   B

FIGURE 3–10

Kyphoplasty. A 69-year-old man with benign osteoporotic vertebral compression fractures after a two-level kyphoplasty. *A,* Sagittal reconstruction CT study demonstrating adjacent segment compression deformities with barium-impregnated methyl methacrylate (*arrows 1*). The lower margin of the lower vertebra is posteriorly displaced, narrowing the spinal canal to approximately 7 mm (*arrow 2*). There is wedging of the next superior vertebral body as well (*arrow 3*). *B,* Axial study through the pedicles of the lower vertebra demonstrates two nodes of barium (*arrows 1*) and centripetal displacement of vertebral fracture fragments (*arrows 2*). Note that there is no extravasation of contrast material nor, at least at this level, any spinal canal narrowing.

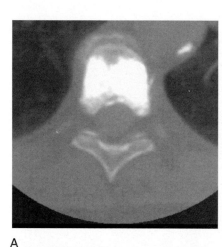

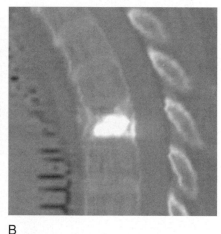

A   B

FIGURE 3–11

Rib fracture accompanying vertebroplasty. A 66-year-old man with continued pain following T7 vertebroplasty. *A,* Axial CT study at the vertebral level demonstrates barium-impregnated methyl methacrylate within the vertebral body without evidence of extravasation. *B,* Sagittal reconstruction again demonstrates barium-impregnated methyl methacrylate within T7 without evidence of extravasation. *C,* Axial image through the level of the T8 ribs demonstrates a healing left rib fracture (*arrow*). *D,* Axial image through the level of the T9 ribs demonstrates a healing left rib fracture at this level as well (*arrow*). The patient had additional fractures of the T7 and T10 ribs (not shown). Patients undergoing vertebroplasty for osteoporosis may already have rib fractures as a concomitant cause of pain at the time of vertebroplasty, or they may develop fractures at the time of the procedure.

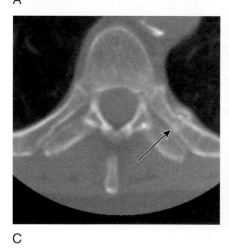

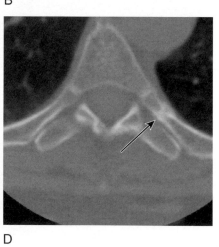

C   D

MRI may be helpful in the evaluation of postfusion patients, even when metallic devices are in place (Rupp 1996). Titanium generally causes minimal local field inhomogeneity, and spin-echo and fast spin-echo sequences are not drastically degraded (Rudisch 1998).

Postoperative Discectomy

Most discectomies are done for leg pain, and 85% to 90% of these procedures are successful (Davis 1994, Findlay 1998,

Frymoyer 1988) In patients who return for imaging following discectomy, evaluation of imaging findings should be done with knowledge of the clinical course of events (Federowicz 1991, Kostiuk 1997). For the purposes of the following discussion, we assume that patients have undergone discectomy for a disc herniation identified on a preoperative study and that the patient had either exclusively leg symptoms or a combination of back and leg symptoms prior to surgery. We divide our discussion to address the four most frequently encountered clinical scenarios in patients who have pain following discectomy.

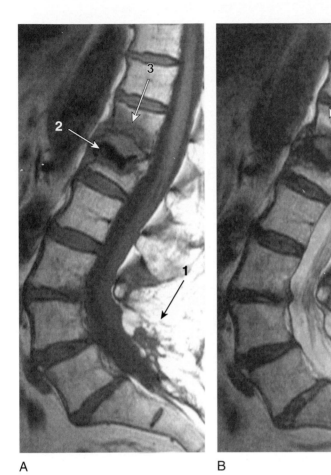

A   B

FIGURE 3–12

Vertebroplasty with adjacent segment fracture. A 78-year-old woman with multilevel degenerative changes of the spine who had had prior lower lumbar spinal fusion surgery and who had a painful osteoporotic compression fracture of L1. This was successfully treated with vertebroplasty with reduction of pain and return to activity. *A,* Sagittal T1WI demonstrates accentuation of lumbar lordosis, postoperative changes of the lower lumbar spine (*arrow 1*), and barium within the superior aspect of the deformed L1 vertebral body (*arrow 2*). There is a broad, band-like focus of T1 prolongation within the T12 vertebral body (*arrow 3*). *B,* Sagittal T2WI demonstrates T2 prolongation in the T12 vertebral body (*arrow*) corresponding to the T1 prolongation seen in *A* and diagnostic of an acute or subacute compression deformity. The patient was successfully treated with an additional vertebroplasty.

1. The patient continues to have the same symptoms after surgery (without any change in the character of the symptoms).
2. The patient has improvement of symptoms after surgery, with later recurrence of identical symptoms.
3. The patient has improvement of leg symptoms with ongoing back pain.
4. The patient has improvement of symptoms after surgery, with later development of new and different symptoms.

CLINICAL SCENARIO 1: THE PATIENT CONTINUES TO HAVE THE SAME SYMPTOMS AFTER SURGERY

Some patients undergo discectomy only to have no relief of symptoms with the procedure. Assuming that the surgery was performed at the correct level and on the correct side, the main possibilities are that there was (1) an incomplete resection of disc material; (2) an early-onset complication (e.g., hematoma or infection) with irritation of the nerve root and symptoms; (3) a combination of foraminal stenosis and surgical nerve root irritation that has caused previously minimally symptomatic spinal stenosis to become clinically manifest (Heithoff 1987); (4) an ongoing nerve root inflammation of unknown cause that is producing symptoms despite adequate surgery. See Figure 3–A for an algorithm for postoperative discectomy.

No good test exists to evaluate whether surgery has removed sufficient disc material in the immediate postoperative period (Boden 1992, Deutsch 1993, Dina 1995, Montaldi 1988, St. Amour 1994, Tullberg 1993). MRI done in the immediate postoperative period on patients *with relief of symptoms following surgery* shows extensive soft tissue material at the operative site (Boden 1992, Deutsch 1993, Dina 1995); thus, there is a great deal of overlap of imaging findings in those patients with (Fig. 3–13) and without (Fig. 3–14) persistence of symptoms following surgery. MRI may be reassuring in a negative manner: if there is very little or no residual material at the operative site, then residual disc herniation is unlikely to represent the cause of ongoing symptoms (Fig. 3–15). However, ascribing symptoms to apparent residual disc material at the level of the lesion soon after surgery must be done with caution since "residual disc herniation" may be seen in patients without symptoms (Fig. 3–14). Unless another prior postoperative study demonstrates less material at the level of the operation, reports of MRI done within 6 months of discectomy should explicitly note that evaluation of the level of surgery for residual and recurrent disc herniation is problematic. Regardless of the status of the operated level, other sources of the patient's persistent symptoms should be sought. In cases after the 6-month period, or in those cases where a prior (but still postoperative) study is available, diagnosis is easier (Fig. 3–16).

Although postoperative MRI may be of little use in the diagnosis of residual disc herniation in the immediate postoperative period, such studies may nicely demonstrate complications of surgery. Complications of disc surgery include hematoma and infection. Large fluid col-

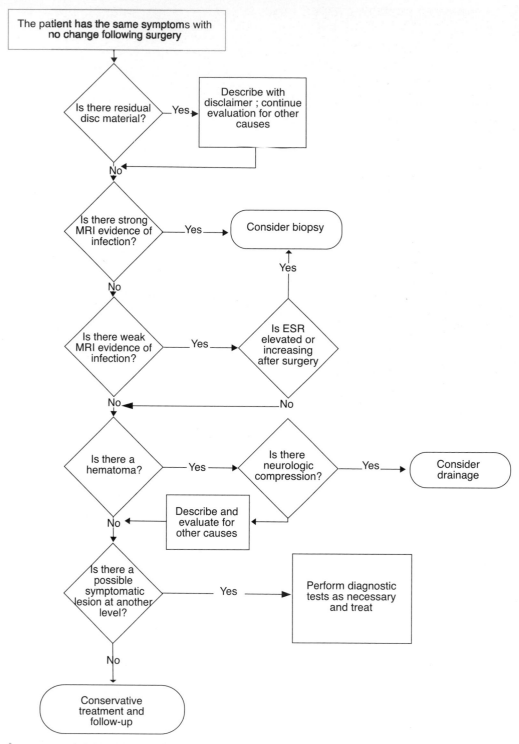

FIGURE 3–A

FIGURE 3–A

Algorithm for postoperative period after discectomy. ESR, erythrocyte sedimentation rate.

A

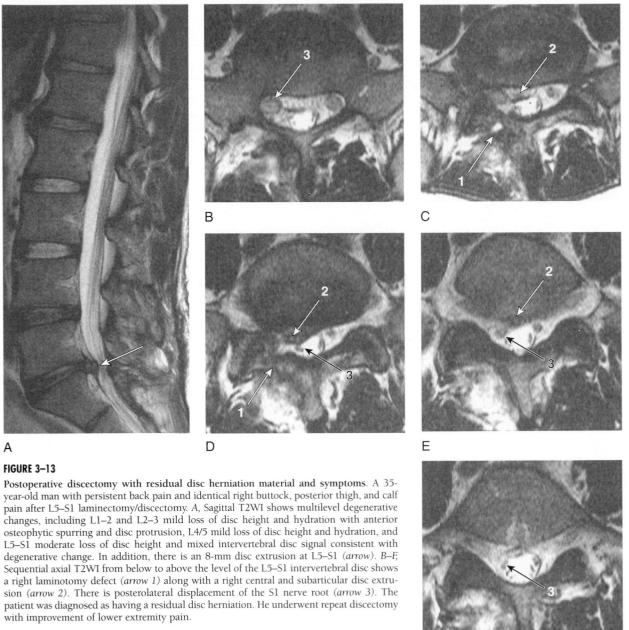

FIGURE 3–13

Postoperative discectomy with residual disc herniation material and symptoms. A 35-year-old man with persistent back pain and identical right buttock, posterior thigh, and calf pain after L5–S1 laminectomy/discectomy. *A,* Sagittal T2WI shows multilevel degenerative changes, including L1–2 and L2–3 mild loss of disc height and hydration with anterior osteophytic spurring and disc protrusion, L4/5 mild loss of disc height and hydration, and L5–S1 moderate loss of disc height and mixed intervertebral disc signal consistent with degenerative change. In addition, there is an 8-mm disc extrusion at L5–S1 *(arrow)*. *B–F,* Sequential axial T2WI from below to above the level of the L5–S1 intervertebral disc shows a right laminotomy defect *(arrow 1)* along with a right central and subarticular disc extrusion *(arrow 2)*. There is posterolateral displacement of the S1 nerve root *(arrow 3)*. The patient was diagnosed as having a residual disc herniation. He underwent repeat discectomy with improvement of lower extremity pain.

lections within the spinal canal or intervertebral nerve root canals in the absence of an elevated white blood cell count, fever, and normal (or normalizing) erythrocyte sedimentation rate (ESR) should be suspected to represent hematomas. If these collections are producing symptoms, drainage should be considered. Abnormalities within the disc itself may represent infection. However, there is overlap between the imaging findings of infection, degenerative disc disease, and postoperative changes of the disc. For a full discussion, see Chapter 6. Briefly, intense increased signal on T2-weighted image (T2WI), particularly if accompanied by fluid collections within the epidural space or paraspinal region and/or erosions of the vertebral end

plates, should be strongly suspected to be infection, and biopsy should be considered. Less dramatic imaging findings, with minimal increased signal intensity of the disc, questionable end-plate erosions, and no associated fluid collection may represent infection but may also be seen with degenerative changes, or represent typical postoperative findings (Fig. 3–17) (Bircher 1988, Fouquet 1992, Grane 1998, Post 1990, Ross 1996, Sharif 1992). Serial evaluation of serum ESR and C-reactive protein represents a valuable tool in differentiating these processes (Bircher 1988, Jonsson 1991).

To evaluate whether surgery was done at the wrong location, it is first necessary to establish that the surgical proce-

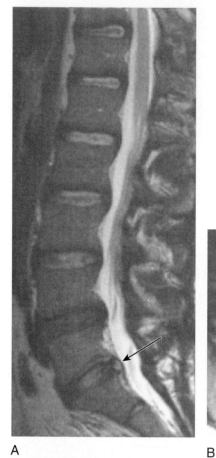

A

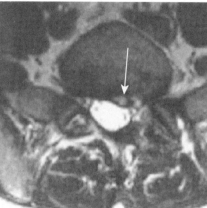

B

FIGURE 3–14

Postoperative discectomy with residual disc herniation material but no symptoms. A 38-year-old man who underwent surgery at L5–S1 for low back, left buttock, and posterior thigh and calf pain. The patient was completely relieved of pain following surgery, and the MRI study was done as part of a research study. A, Sagittal T2WI following surgery demonstrates a 6.4-mm caudally dissecting disc extrusion (arrow). B, Axial T2WI shows the left central disc extrusion (arrow) with displacement and compression of the left S1 nerve root. The degree of mass effect and neural compression was similar to the patient's preoperative study (not shown), despite the fact that the patient was symptom free following surgery.

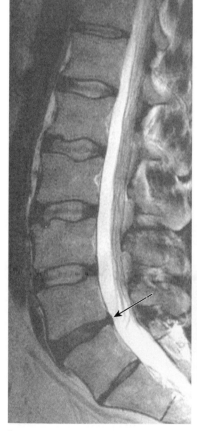

A

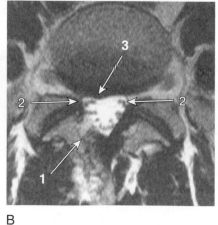

B

FIGURE 3–15

Postoperative discectomy MRI showing complete removal of disc material. A 44-year-old man with right low back and leg pain following remote discectomy. A, Sagittal T2WI demonstrates transitional anatomy with a relatively well-developed S1–2 disc, L5–S1 moderate loss of disc height and hydration, and multilevel Schmorl nodes. The posterior disc contour at L5–S1 is essentially straight, with only 1 to 2 mm of bulging (arrow). B, Axial T2WI at the level of the L5–S1 disc demonstrates a right laminotomy defect (arrow). The traversing S1 nerve roots are symmetric, with no displacement or compression of the right S1 nerve roots (arrows 2). A small undulation along the right paracentral aspect of the disc remains from prior discectomy (arrow 3). This appearance excludes the possibility of recurrent disc herniation as the cause of the patient's symptoms.

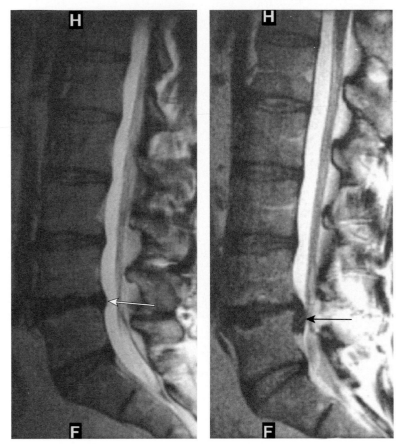

A   B

FIGURE 3–16

Recurrent disc herniation with a prior (but also postoperative) study available to prove that the herniated material is new. A 53-year-old man with low back pain. *A,* Sagittal T2WI (done after surgery) demonstrates multilevel degenerative disc disease with mild dehydration of all visualized discs. In addition, at the L4–5 level, which had undergone prior discectomy, there is not only moderate loss of disc height and hydration, Schmorl's node formation, and subchondral Modic Type I degenerative change (there was T1 prolongation on the T1WI), but there is also 3.3-mm disc protrusion *(arrow).* Subsequently, the patient developed left leg pain. *B,* Sagittal T2WI acquired 15 months after *A* demonstrates a 6.3-mm anteroposterior dimension caudally dissecting disc extrusion *(arrow)* at the same level. This set of studies demonstrates a change at a postoperative level diagnostic of recurrent disc herniation.

dure was actually performed at the level and on the side of what was taken to be the symptom-producing lesion. Assuming that this was done, the principles of Chapter 2 should be applied: a pain diagram should be reviewed along with other sources of information about the character of the patient's pain, and each segment of the spine should be evaluated for sources of nerve root, ganglionic, or spinal nerve irritation. Sources of nerve irritation other than the removed disc must be sought. The symptom-producing lesion may be above the level of the resected disc. Tumors of the cauda equina or disc herniations in the high lumbar or lower thoracic spine may produce lower lumbar radicular pain (see Chapter 4). Subarticular recess stenosis or a synovial cyst one level (or rarely two levels) above a resected foraminal or extraforaminal disc extrusion may be responsible for leg symptoms (Fig. 3–18). Alternately, the lesion may be below the level of the resected disc. A foraminal or extraforaminal (far lateral) disc extrusion may produce symptoms that are falsely attributed to a subarticular disc herniation at the next higher level. Tumors along the course of peripheral nerves may occasionally cause radicular symptoms (Bickels 1999) (see Chapter 4). Because of overlap within dermatomes (see Chapter 2, "Pain and Pain Diagrams") (Bogduk 1997, van Akkerveeken 1993a), sources of irritation of the nerve roots proximal and distal to the root originally assumed to be the symptom producer should also be sought. In these cases, ancillary studies such as nerve blocks may be beneficial in confirming the symptomatic nature of an alternate lesion (El-Khoury 1991, Link

1998, van Akkerveeken 1993b). Such blocks may occasionally be therapeutic, but a second surgery may be necessary for discovered alternative pathology.

In many patients with failed surgery, there is coexistent foraminal stenosis (Heithoff 1987) (Fig. 3–19). At least three mechanisms may cause persistent radicular symptoms in a patient with a disc herniation and spinal stenosis compressing the same nerve root. The foraminal stenosis may have been the sole original cause of the patient's radiculopathy. The foraminal stenosis may also represent the second location of narrowing along the course of a nerve and thus cause venous congestion and resultant radiculopathy (Olmarker 1992, Porter 1992). Finally, the nerve root may develop postoperative swelling following discectomy, converting a previously asymptomatic stenosis into a symptomatic stenosis (Heithoff 1987). Such patients may benefit from transforaminal epidural steroid injection, which decreases inflammation and swelling and may allow recovery without further surgery (Link 1998). If conservative measures are not successful, surgery should be considered in patients with foraminal stenosis who have persistent pain following discectomy.

Occasionally, patients with persistent pain following surgery have gas collections that demonstrate a confusing appearance on MR imaging. The nature of such lesions is obvious if CT is performed (Fig. 3–20). Symptoms have been attributed to such gas collections (associated with degenerative disc disease) in patients who have not undergone surgery (Tamburrelli 2000).

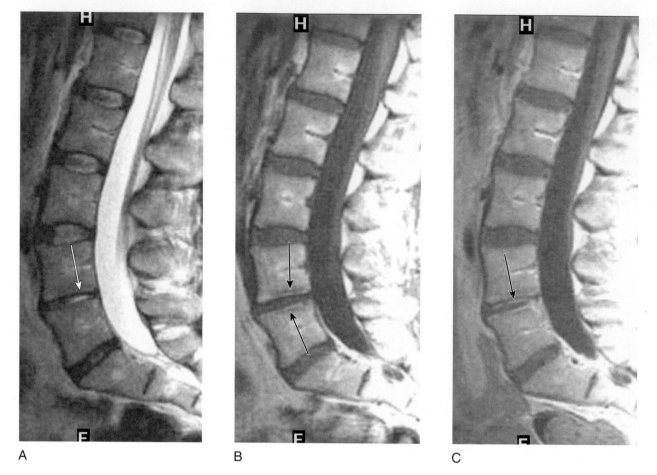

A   B   C

FIGURE 3–17

Postoperative "mechanical discitis" mimicking infectious spondylitis. A 40-year-old woman after L4–5 discectomy with ongoing low back pain. *A,* Sagittal T2WI shows severe loss of disc height and hydration at L5–S1 and severe loss of disc height but T2 prolongation at the L4–5 level *(arrow)*. *B,* Sagittal T1WI confirms loss of disc height at L4–5 and also demonstrates linear areas of T1 prolongation along the disc *(arrows)*. *C,* Sagittal T1WI following contrast agent injection demonstrates linear contrast enhancement along the disc margins. The patient's erythrocyte sedimentation rate and C-reactive protein level were normal, and she was afebrile. The findings are typical of "mechanical discitis," which is sometimes seen following discectomy.

CLINICAL SCENARIO 2: THE PATIENT HAS IMPROVEMENT OF SYMPTOMS AFTER SURGERY, WITH LATER RECURRENCE OF IDENTICAL SYMPTOMS

The fact that patients are generally at rest and on analgesic medication in the immediate postoperative period complicates evaluation, because some pain relief actually secondary to these factors may be attributed to surgery. If the patient has relief of symptoms outlasting the postoperative medications, with recurrence of identical symptoms later, the main suspicion will be for recurrent disc herniation (Figs. 3–16, 3–21, and 3–22). Relief of symptoms following surgery strongly supports ascribing the patient's symptoms to the disc (van Akkerveeken 1993a). As noted earlier under Clinical Scenario 1, MRI of patients in the postoperative period may demonstrate either little change or worsening in the morphologic appearance at the operated level, even in patients who are doing well clinically. These imaging findings generally slowly resolve in the 4 to 6 months following surgery. If a patient has recurrence of symptoms and an MRI examination showing significant mass effect 6 months or more after surgery, the overwhelming likelihood is that there has been a recurrent disc herni-

ation that may well require repeat discectomy for resolution (Federowicz 1991). As noted earlier, we do not believe that it is necessary to administer contrast agent to differentiate recurrent disc herniation from scar (Mullin 2000); however, if a contrast agent is administered, contrast enhancement of a single nerve root may correspond to active neural pathology (Jinkins 1993).

Approximately 6% of patients undergoing discectomy may suffer recurrent disc herniations, and although most of these occur within the first year, recurrence may take place even after 20 years (Davis 1994). Success following reoperation on these patients is comparable to the initial procedure (Suk 2001).

Although the overwhelming likelihood for the cause of symptoms in this clinical scenario is recurrent disc herniation, other lesions may occasionally cause recurrence of symptoms. As noted earlier, lesions involving the nerve root proximal to the level of the original disc herniation, and the nerve root, ganglion, or spinal nerve distal to the level of the disc herniation, may cause pain in the same location. Occasionally, such proximal or distal lesions, by chance, occur along the same nerve root at a different time, causing

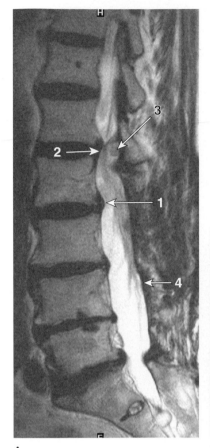

A   B

FIGURE 3–18

Persistent leg pain following multilevel decompression/ fusion secondary to a synovial cyst superior to the level of surgery. An 82-year-old man with multilevel fusion/decompression from L5–S1 through L2–3 with persistent anterior thigh pain on the right. *A*, Sagittal T2WI shows multilevel degenerative disc disease with severe dehydration at all levels and severe loss of disc height at L5–S1, L4–5, and L3–4. At T12–L1 there is mild loss of disc height. At L2–3 there is moderate loss of disc height and a 3.9-mm cranially dissecting relatively flat disc extrusion (*arrow 1*). At L1–2, there is a 4.7-mm cranially dissecting disc extrusion (*arrow 2*). In addition, there is an ill-defined lesion in the posterior spinal canal (*arrow 3*). Posterior resection changes are seen in the lower lumbar spine (*arrow 4*). *B*, There is bilateral mild degenerative change of the facet joints with associated joint effusions (*arrows 1*). Furthermore, there is a right synovial cyst (*arrow 2*) measuring 8.7 mm at its widest point, with associated severe right subarticular recess stenosis. This cyst underwent percutaneous fluoroscopically directed rupture, resulting in immediate alleviation of the patient's thigh pain.

recurrence of the same symptoms by virtue of compression of the same nerve root, although the cause, level, and time of compression are different.

Delayed complications of discectomy are uncommon, with hematomas and infections occurring in the immediate postoperative period. Authorities have debated whether scar tissue directly causes pain (Barbara 1978, Benoist 1980, Bryant 1983, Keller 1978, Ray 1987, Yong-Hing 1980) or not (Braun 1984, Cervellini 1988, Cooper 1991; Montaldi 1988, Tullberg 1993). Ross and associates (1996), in a multicenter, prospective study, found a statistically significant association between the presence of extensive peridural scar and recurrent radicular pain; however, they also found that the vast majority of patients with extensive scar formation actually did not have radicular pain. Regardless of whether scar tissue is painful, resection of scar tissue in postoperative patients with recurrent symptoms usually does not result in significant improvement of symptoms (Benoist 1980, Law 1978).

CLINICAL SCENARIO 3: THE PATIENT HAS IMPROVEMENT OF LEG SYMPTOMS WITH ONGOING BACK PAIN

Most surgeons warn their patients prior to surgery that their leg symptoms may improve but their back pain may not be relieved, and this situation is often regarded as the normal course of events. Most surgeons manage this residual back pain with conservative measures. For patients with severe and disabling back pain, coexisting internal disc disruption (see Chapter 2) should be suspected as a cause of backache. In some cases, such severe and disabling pain requires evaluation for possible fusion.

CLINICAL SCENARIO 4: THE PATIENT HAS IMPROVEMENT OF SYMPTOMS AFTER SURGERY, WITH LATER DEVELOPMENT OF DIFFERENT SYMPTOMS

In most cases in which the patient's original symptoms have been improved with delayed development of different symptoms, discectomy will be regarded as a success. These patients have usually developed collateral disease elsewhere in the spine (Figs. 3–23 and 3–24). Residual and recurrent disc abnormalities at the site of prior surgery should be noted, but patient symptoms should not be ascribed to such abnormalities: recurrent disc herniation should cause recurrence of similar symptoms. Evaluation of the non-operated segments of the spine follows the principles elucidated in Chapter 2.

A few miscellaneous entities may result in new symptoms following discectomy. On occasion, patients with

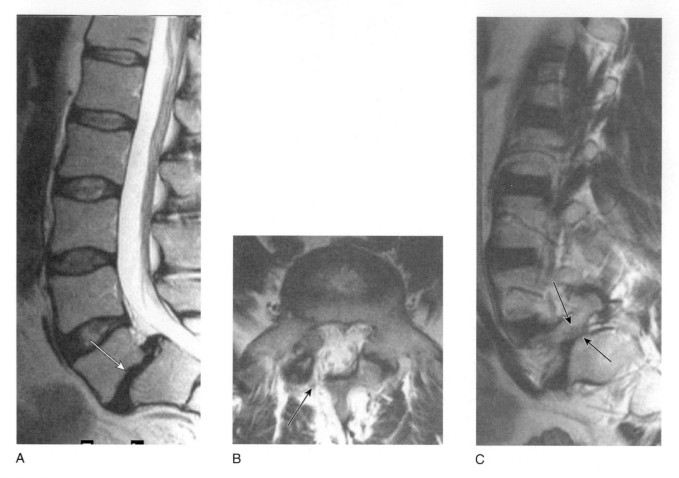

A   B   C

FIGURE 3–19

Foraminal stenosis causing persistent radicular pain following laminectomy and discectomy. A 49-year-old man with right leg pain and right lower extremity pain. The patient had a laminectomy and discectomy with limited, transient relief of leg pain. *A,* Sagittal T2WI shows 35% lytic spondylolisthesis at L5–S1 with associated severe loss of disc height and hydration *(arrow). B,* Axial T2WI shows a right S1 laminectomy defect *(arrow). C,* Right parasagittal T2WI at the level of the foramina shows severe up-down foraminal stenosis at L5–S1 *(arrows),* with associated severe L5 ganglionic flattening.

dural tears develop new radicular symptoms shortly after surgery because of herniation of nerve roots into the dural defect (Fig. 3–25). Of course, dural tears may also result in cerebrospinal fluid (CSF) leaks and headaches (Fig. 3–26). Another lesion that may lead to new back or leg pain in a patient who has undergone laminectomy and facetectomy is a postoperative fracture of the lumbar articular process (Rothman 1985). Such fractures are suggested by asymmetric widening of the inferior aspect of the facet joints on axial imaging and are ideally demonstrated by sagittal and coronal reconstructions with CT. Rothman and colleagues (1985) have speculated that such fractures most likely occur through a weakened articular process when the patient returns to an upright position following surgery.

Postoperative Decompression or Fusion

In appropriately selected patients, fusion for segmental spinal instability has a success rate approaching that of discectomy (Brantigan 2000, Hutter 1983, Gill 1992, Kuslich 1998, Ray 1997, Zdeblick 1993), and most patients undergoing simultaneous decompression and fusion for stenosis do well (Turner 1992). However, success of such procedures is not universal, and many patients will return for postoperative imaging. Although clinical evaluation and imaging interpretation of the nonoperated spine may be extremely demanding and postdiscectomy patients present their own special challenges, the most difficult patient for both the surgeon and the radiologist to evaluate is probably the one who has had a fusion procedure. Several factors, as follows, contribute to this difficulty:

1. Fusions of the lumbar or cervical spine are often done for central low back (or neck) pain secondary to segmental spinal instability. The likelihood of misdiagnosis and performing the wrong procedure is greater than that associated with performing discectomy for radicular pain.
2. Fusions are technically more demanding than discectomy. Insertion of multiple lumbar pedicle screws with dorsal interconnecting rods and bone graft material is an arduous, multistep process that may result in any of multiple complications. Resection of most of three or four cervical vertebrae with interposition of a tubular strut graft and placement of a spanning plate affixed with screws is also technically challenging.

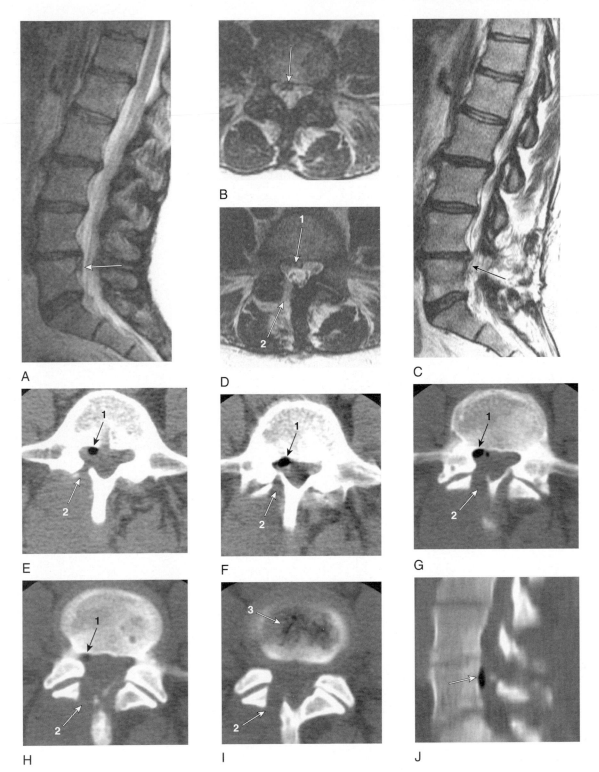

FIGURE 3–20

Gas collection mimicking residual/recurrent disc material on MRI. A 52-year-old woman with low back and right "hip," lateral thigh, and lateral calf pain. *A,* Right parasagittal T2WI done prior to surgery demonstrates multilevel degenerative disc disease with mild disc dehydration and Schmorl's node formation at T12–L1, Schmorl's node formation at L1–2, mild loss of disc height and moderate dehydration with a cranially and caudally dissecting disc extrusion at L2–3, preservation of disc height and hydration at L3–4, and moderate disc dehydration at L5–S1. At L4–5, there is moderate loss of disc height and hydration as well as a caudally dissecting disc extrusion *(arrow)*. *B,* Axial T2WI at the level of the L5 pedicles demonstrates a right central disc extrusion *(arrow)*. The patient underwent an L4–5 laminectomy and discectomy, with partial, transient relief of symptoms. *C,* Right parasagittal proton density–weighted image (PDWI) following surgery shows posterior postoperative changes and a focus of decreased signal intensity along the dorsal vertebral margin, in the region previously occupied by the caudally dissecting disc extrusion *(arrow)*. *D,* Axial PDWI at the level of the L5 pedicle following surgery shows heterogeneous material of intermediate and markedly decreased signal intensity along the dorsal vertebral body and in the lateral recess medial to the L5 pedicle *(arrow 1)*. Note changes of laminectomy *(arrow 2)*. *E–I,* Sequential inferior-to-superior axial CT studies from the L5 pedicle to the L4–5 disc demonstrate a right paracentral, caudally dissecting gas collection *(arrows 1)*. Note posterior laminectomy defect *(arrows 2)* and vacuum phenomenon *(arrow 3)*. *J,* Sagittal reconstruction CT shows gas along the posterior border of the L5 vertebral body *(arrow)*.

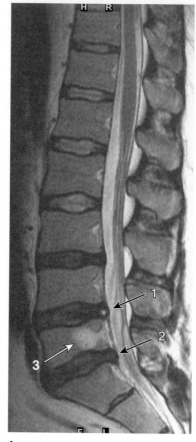

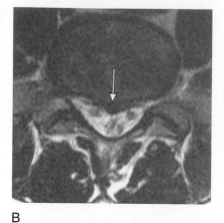

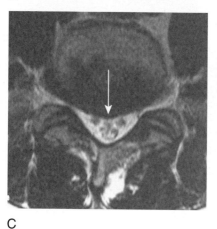

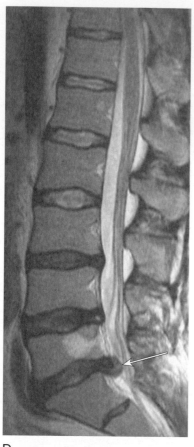

A

B

C

D

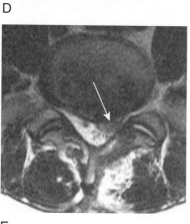

E

FIGURE 3–21

Recurrent disc herniation. A 29-year-old man with central low back pain and left leg pain that was better following surgery but then recurred, with return of identical leg pain and new back pain. Recurrent disc extrusion is larger and has more mass effect than original. *A,* Preoperative sagittal T2WI shows multilevel degenerative disc disease. The T11–12 through L2–3 discs demonstrate preserved disc height and hydration but also undulation of vertebral marginal contour. L3–4 demonstrates preservation of disc height with mild disc dehydration and minimal degenerative disc bulging. L4–5 demonstrates mild disc dehydration and a 3.1-mm disc protrusion with accompanying T2 prolongation along the dorsal disc margin (*arrow 1*). L5–S1 demonstrates mild disc dehydration and a 6.6-mm disc protrusion (*arrow 2*). Incidentally noted is a 13-mm L5 hemangioma (*arrow 3*). *B* and *C,* Preoperative, sequential inferior-to-superior axial T2WIs at the level of the L5–S1 disc show a central disc protrusion (*arrow*) without contact or displacement of the S1 nerve roots. Pain was relieved by surgery, with sudden recurrence of identical symptoms 7 weeks later. *D,* Sagittal T2WI following return of symptoms (which had been relieved following surgery) demonstrates a much more abnormal appearance at L5–S1, with the heterogeneous disc extrusion measuring 11.8 mm in anteroposterior dimension (*arrow*). *E,* Axial T2WI following surgery demonstrates a left central disc extrusion (*arrow*) with posterior displacement and compression of the left S1 nerve root. Although still within the 6-month period when there may be a considerable residual mass effect following surgery, the marked increase in size of the disc contour abnormality (compared to the preoperative examination) combined with the typical history is diagnostic of recurrent disc herniation.

3. Placement of hardware inevitably degrades image quality and evaluation of remaining anatomy. Although the imaging algorithms on newer CT scanners and use of titanium and other nonsteel alloys (Rupp 1996, Weiner 1998) significantly decrease streak artifacts, evaluation of tissue adjacent to implants remains challenging. MRI through the levels of fusion is often uninterpretable, and CT scanning (even when performed with intrathecal contrast) may not reveal sufficient detail to fully evaluate small structures such as the neural foramina.

4. Patients treated with fusion surgery are more likely to have multilevel spinal disease, complicating preoperative diagnosis, surgical planning, and postoperative evaluation.

5. The postoperative recuperation from fusion surgery far exceeds that of discectomy, and distinguishing between

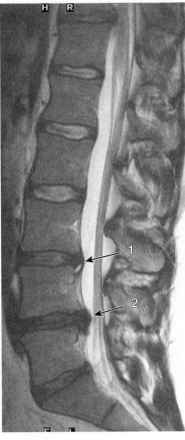

A

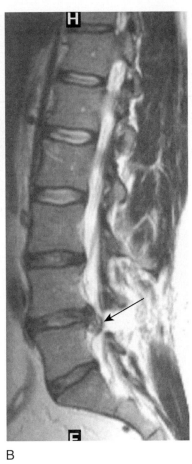

B

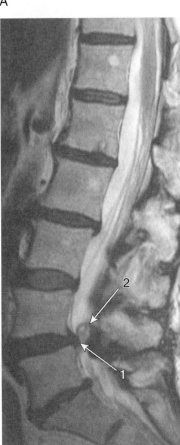

A

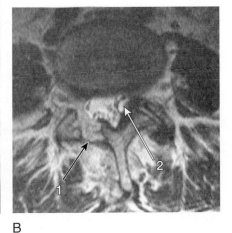

B

FIGURE 3–22

Recurrent disc herniation. A 32-year-old man with chronic low back pain and recent onset of right leg pain, numbness, and tingling. *A,* Preoperative sagittal T2WI shows multilevel degenerative changes, with moderate loss of disc height and hydration at L5–S1, L4–5, L3–4, and T11–12. In addition, the patient has an L3–4 disc protrusion with accompanying T2 prolongation (high-intensity zone) (*arrow 1*) and an 8-mm caudal dissection disc extrusion at L4–5 (*arrow 2*). The patient underwent laminectomy with complete relief of leg symptoms for 3 weeks. Following a single sneeze, the patient had recurrence of his preoperative symptoms. *B,* Postoperative sagittal T2WI following return of symptoms demonstrates enlargement of the L4–5 disc extrusion (*arrow*). Note the posterior postoperative changes. As in the prior case, the history is typical for recurrent disc herniation, with increased mass effect at the level of the abnormality securing the diagnosis.

FIGURE 3–23

Development of new and different symptoms following surgery secondary to additional pathology. A 75-year-old woman with a remote history of right leg pain relieved following a right L4–5 laminectomy and discectomy. The patient had no right leg pain at the time of this MRI but rather had low back and left "hip," lateral thigh, and calf pain. *A,* Sagittal T2WI shows multilevel degenerative disc disease, including T12–L1 anterior osteophyte formation, L1–2 moderate loss of disc height and hydration and anterior osteophyte formation, L2–3 mild loss of disc height, moderate disc dehydration, and an anterior disc extrusion, L3–4 mild disc dehydration, and L5–S1 severe loss of disc height and severe disc dehydration and degenerative disc bulging. At the L4–5 level, there is 5% degenerative spondylolisthesis, a 4.3-mm disc protrusion (*arrow 1*), and an 8-mm synovial cyst (*arrow 2*). *B,* Axial T2WI at the level of the L4–5 disc shows a right laminectomy defect (*arrow 1*) without residual or recurrent stenosis or right-sided disc extrusion or neural compression. On the left side, there is severe facet arthropathy and a synovial cyst (*arrow 2*) contributing to severe subarticular recess narrowing and compression of the traversing L5 nerve root.

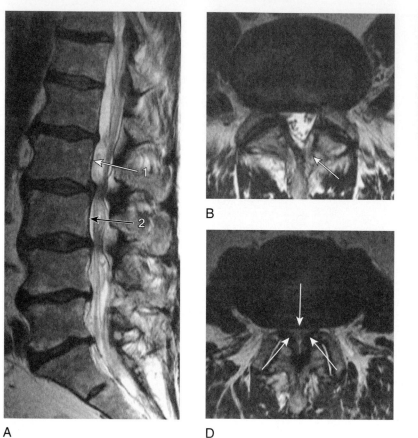

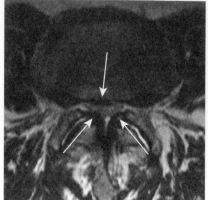

A

B

C

D

FIGURE 3–24

Development of new and different symptoms following surgery secondary to additional pathology. A 78-year-old man who had undergone an L4–5 laminotomy/discectomy for left leg pain 10 years earlier with excellent relief of pain. The patient returned with new and different bilateral "hip" and leg pain. *A*, Sagittal T2WI shows multilevel degenerative disc disease with L1–2 mild loss of disc height and hydration and degenerative disc bulging, L2–3 mild loss of disc height and disc hydration, degenerative disc bulging, and minimal degenerative spondylolisthesis *(arrow 1)*, L3–4 mild disc dehydration and minimal degenerative spondylolisthesis *(arrow 2)*, L4–5 severe loss of disc height and hydration, Modic Type II subchondral marrow changes, degenerative disc bulging, and mild retrolisthesis, and L5–S1 severe loss of disc height and hydration, Modic Type II subchondral marrow changes, and degenerative disc bulging. *B*, Axial T2WI at the level of the L4–5 disc shows minimal changes of posterior tissues at the side of the patient's prior left laminotomy *(arrow)*. There is degenerative disc bulging without residual or recurrent disc herniation. *C*, Axial T2WI at the level of the L3–4 disc shows bilateral severe facet arthropathy. The patient has severe spinal canal stenosis and a trefoil appearance of the spinal canal *(arrows)*. *D*, Axial T2WI at the L2–3 level shows bilateral severe facet arthropathy. As at the L3–4 level, but even more severe at this level, there is central spinal canal stenosis and a trefoil appearance of the spinal canal *(arrows)*. This patient had severe, multilevel spinal canal and subarticular recess stenosis accounting for symptoms.

a difficult postoperative recovery and a new problem or complication of surgery can be challenging.

In patients who return for imaging following decompression/fusion surgery, as in the case with discectomy, evaluation of imaging findings should be done with knowledge of the clinical course of symptoms (Kostiuk 1997). As with our discussion of discectomy, we direct our discussion to the most frequently encountered clinical scenarios in patients who have pain following decompression/fusion surgery. Note that some of these scenarios differ from the scenarios most frequently encountered following discectomy:

1. The patient wakes up after surgery with new and different symptoms.
2. The patient continues to have the same symptoms following surgery with no change in the character of the symptoms.
3. The patient improves after surgery, with later recurrence of identical symptoms.
4. The patient improves after surgery, with later development of new and different symptoms.

CLINICAL SCENARIO 1: THE PATIENT WAKES UP FROM SURGERY WITH NEW AND DIFFERENT SYMPTOMS

New symptoms on wakening from surgery may indicate a surgical complication and usually result in immediate imaging if the symptoms are significant. Of course, pain from the surgical site is to be expected, and pain from a bone graft harvest site (if performed) frequently exceeds the pain of the area of primary surgery (Kostiuk 1997). Other symptoms may be categorized as radiculopathy/radicular pain, myelopathy, cauda equina syndrome, and pain disproportionate or of a differing character than that expected in the normal postoperative course of events.

Causes of radiculopathy/radicular pain include injury of a nerve root, ganglion, or segmental nerve at the time of surgery from, for example, instrument manipulation. Such damage may be accompanied by a hematoma or seroma but may also cause no imaging features. If the surgeon has placed pedicle screws, careful evaluation of the margins of all screws should be performed: penetration of the medial margin may result in damage to the nerve root in the lateral

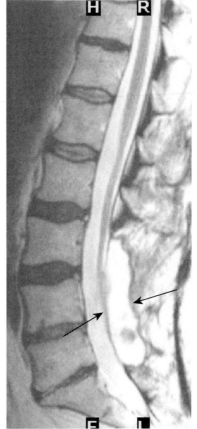

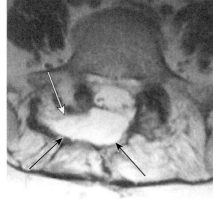

A   B

FIGURE 3–25

Development of new and different symptoms following surgery secondary to unusual operative complication. A 54-year-old woman after posterior decompression/fusion of L3–4 through L5–S1. Two days after surgery, the patient had an onset of left hip, lateral thigh, and lateral calf pain that she had never had before. *A*, Sagittal T2WI demonstrates multilevel degenerative changes, including T11–12 moderate loss of disc height and severe disc dehydration, L2–3 mild disc dehydration with a posterior focus of T2 prolongation (high-intensity zone), L3–4 mild loss of disc height, L4–5 moderate loss of disc height and apparently normal signal intensity, and L5–S1 severe loss of disc height with mixed intervertebral disc signal consistent with degeneration. The disc signal intensity at L4–5, although apparently normal compared to the T12–L1 level, is not normal considering the loss of disc height but represents degenerative change. There is also multilevel posterior decompression and a large fluid collection (*arrows*) dorsal to the thecal sac. *B*, Axial T2WI at the level of the L5 pedicle shows dorsal decompression and a dorsal fluid collection (*arrows*). At repeat surgery, a small dural rent was found with the left L5 nerve root herniated into the defect. This was reduced and repaired, and the patient had an uneventful recovery.

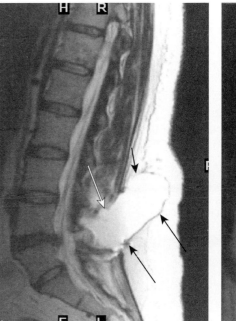

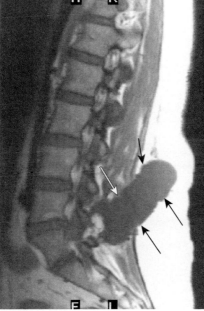

A   B

FIGURE 3–26

Development of new and different symptoms following surgery secondary to unusual operative complication. A 37-year-old patient who underwent discectomy had low back and leg pain with subsequent development of back pain at the level of the incision, as well as incisional bulging and headache. *A*, Sagittal T2WI with contrast and brightness set to optimally demonstrate the patient's large fluid collection (*arrows*) extending from the operative site into the dorsal subcutaneous fat. There is also moderate L4–5 disc dehydration. *B*, Sagittal T1WI confirms T1 prolongation of the lesion (*arrows*), consistent with a fluid collection. Along with the axial studies (not shown), the findings are diagnostic of cerebrospinal fluid leak. The patient underwent repair of a dural tear with relief of back pain and headaches.

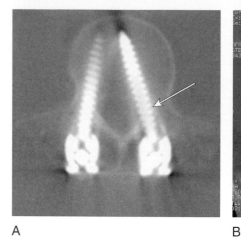

A

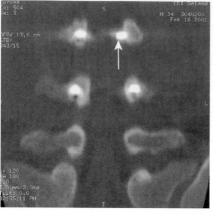

B

FIGURE 3–27

New radicular pain following surgery secondary to screw placement. A 34-year-old patient with fusion surgery and new onset of left hip and anterior thigh pain immediately following surgery. *A,* Axial CT at the level of the L3 pedicles demonstrates broach of the medial aspect of the L3 pedicle by the pedicle screw (*arrow*). Streak artifact obscures fine detail. *B,* Coronal reconstructions at the level of the pedicle demonstrates medial broach of the L3 pedicle by the screw at this level. Note that although the nerve roots cannot be directly visualized on this nonmyelographic study, the position of the screw would definitely bring it into contact with the preganglionic L3 nerve root in the lateral recess.

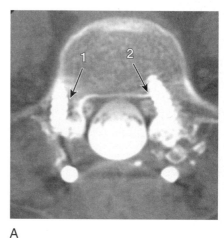

A

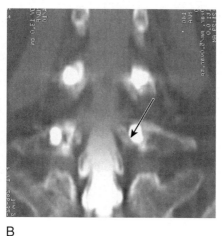

B

FIGURE 3–28

New radicular pain following surgery secondary to screw placement. A 71-year-old woman after fusion/decompression surgery with new onset of left lower extremity pain after surgery. *A,* Axial CT-myelogram through the level of the L5 pedicles shows posterior decompression and bone graft material, as well as bilateral L5 pedicle screws. The right pedicle screw is in the lateral aspect of the pedicle, well away from the medial pedicle margin (*arrow 1*). The left screw is medially located and broaches the medial cortex (*arrow 2*), with the screw margin directly adjacent to the L5 nerve root sleeve. *B,* Curved coronal CT reconstruction following myelography again demonstrates the medial location of the L5 pedicle screw with contact of the left L5 nerve root sleeve (*arrow*). The patient's hardware was subsequently removed, with reduction of symptoms.

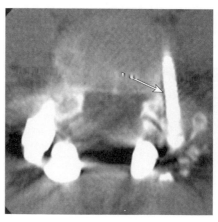

A

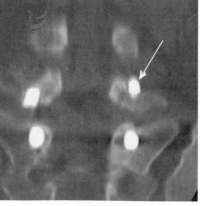

B

FIGURE 3–29

New radicular pain following surgery secondary to screw placement. A 40-year-old woman who underwent posterior decompression/fusion surgery. The patient's large size complicated surgery, and it was recognized at the time of surgery that the left L5 pedicle screw was not in ideal location. The patient woke up from surgery with new left leg pain and dysesthesias. *A,* Axial CT study at the L5 pedicle level shows the left pedicle screw (*arrow*) lateral to the pedicle, in a location to contact and distort the L4 ventral ramus. *B,* Curved coronal CT reconstruction demonstrates the left L5 pedicle screw (*arrow*) lateral to the pedicle.

recess (Figs. 3–27 and 3–28); penetration of the inferior margin may cause nerve root or ganglionic damage (Esses 1993, Farber 1995, Odgers 1996, Sjostrom 1993, Wiesner 2000); penetration of the lateral pedicle margin may result in contact of the postganglionic ventral ramus of the spinal nerve (Fig. 3–29); and penetration of the lateral vertebral body margin at L2 or higher may result in aortic erosion (Sjostrom 1993). Similarly, lateral mass and pedicle screws placed in the cervical spine may enter the neural foramen and cause neural impingement or damage (Abumi 2000, Karasick 1997). Note, however, that simply because the screw enters the neural foramen, radiculopa-

thy is not necessarily inevitable: there is a reserve space that may measure up to 4 mm between the cortical edge of the pedicle and the position of the passing nerve root (Gertzbein 1990). Lateral placement of interbody fusion cages may cause extraforaminal impingement of a segmental nerve with radicular symptoms (Fig. 3–30) (Taylor 2001), and even central placement of cages or other fusion devices may force disc material through the posterior margin of the disc, producing a disc herniation with accompanying radiculopathy/radicular pain (McAfee 1999). Similarly, cervical fusion may result in displacement of material from the disc into the central spinal canal or

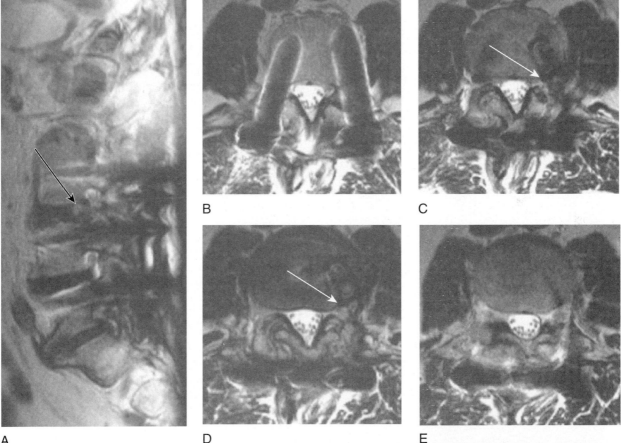

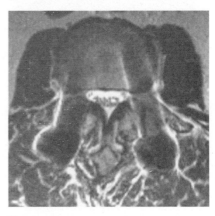

FIGURE 3–30

New radicular pain following surgery secondary to interbody fusion cage placement. A 60-year-old man who underwent spine surgery for central back pain. Following surgery, the patient developed new left anterior thigh and groin pain. *A,* Left parasagittal T2WI demonstrates artifact from pedicle screws at L3, L4, and L5. Along the dorsolateral disc margin at L3–4, the edge of an interbody fusion cage is seen *(arrow). B–F,* Sequential inferior to superior axial T2WI through the L3–4 disc demonstrates pedicle screws at L4 and L3. The interbody fusion cage, placed transforaminally from a left-sided approach, minimally broaches the posterolateral margin of the disc and vertebral bodies *(arrows)* and contacts the exiting L3 ganglion.

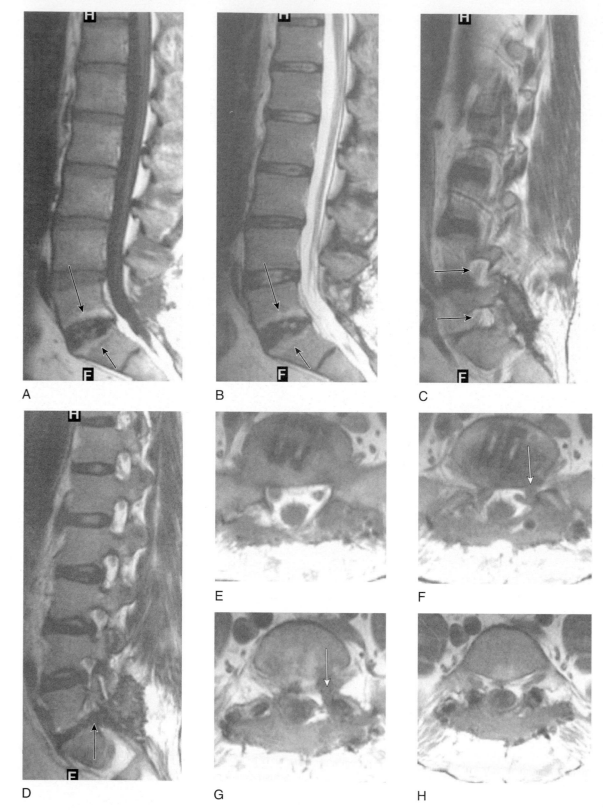

FIGURE 3–31

Radicular pain caused by placement of graft material. A 40-year-old man after posterior decompression/reconstruction and anterior fusion surgery at L5–S1. The patient had an onset of left leg pain following his latest surgery. *A,* Sagittal T1WI demonstrates an abnormal appearance from interbody fusion devices. There is also T1 shortening along the margins of the L5–S1 disc *(arrows),* consistent with functional union across this level. Note posterior post-operative changes. *B,* Sagittal T2WI shows mild loss of disc height and mild disc dehydration at L2–3 and L3–4. At L5–S1, there is abnormal disc signal because of fusion devices and subchondral T2 prolongation *(arrows),* consistent with Modic Type II changes and functional stability at this level. *C,* Right parasagittal T2WI demonstrates widely patent right L4–5 and L5–S1 foramina *(arrows). D,* Left parasagittal T2WI demonstrates narrowing of the L5–S1 foramen by material with T1 prolongation *(arrow). E–H,* Sequential inferior-to-superior T1WIs through the L5–S1 disc demonstrates anterior interbody carbon fiber fusion cages (with little attendant artifact) and, as on the parasagittal images, material demonstrating T1 prolongation *(arrow).*

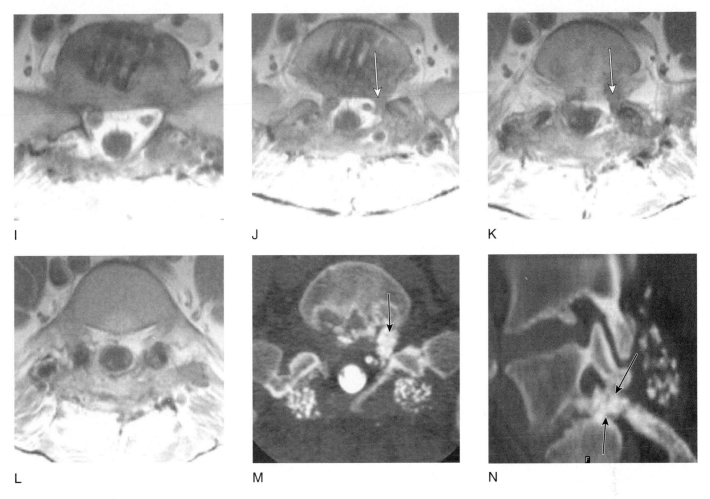

FIGURE 3–31 *(continued)*

I–L, Sequential inferior-to-superior T1WIs following contrast through the L5–S1 disc. The material in the foramen does not demonstrate any contrast enhancement *(arrows).* The abnormal signal intensity minimally distorts both the exiting L5 and traversing S1 nerve roots but does not have imaging characteristics of recurrent disc herniation or scar formation. The material demonstrated T2 shortening on axial T2WI (not shown). Because of persistent left leg pain, a CT-myelogram was done. *M,* Axial CT done at the L4–5 disc level demonstrates graft material not only dorsolaterally, but within the left foramen *(arrow). N,* Sagittal reconstruction view demonstrates graft material filling the inferior aspect of the neural foramen. The CT study provided important additional information regarding the cause of the abnormal signal intensity encountered on the MRI.

neural foramen (Karasick 1997). Graft material may also produce neural irritation or compression if it is placed in or migrates to sensitive areas (Fig. 3–31).

Myelopathy rarely results from direct injury at the time of surgery, because the cord is seldom approached in spine surgery except when tumor removal demands such an approach. Cervical or thoracic surgery may lead to myelopathy by displacing adjacent tissue into the cord or by precipitating an epidural hematoma or abscess that causes cord compression (Karasick 1997). Hardware misplacement may result in cord injury. Ischemic damage to the cord, either from hypotension during the procedure or damage to arterial feeders, may produce myelopathy. Cauda equina syndrome shares clinical features and causes with myelopathy.

Pain disproportionate or differing in character from that expected in the normal postoperative course of events is difficult to evaluate. Unless severe and persistent, such pain is likely to be ascribed to surgery or the events surrounding surgery. The same structures that may produce pain when

stimulated in volunteers (Bogduk 1997, Kellgren 1939, McCall 1979), including the disc margin, facet joints, dura, and spinal ligaments and musculature, frequently undergo much more sustained and vigorous stimulation during surgery, so ascribing most new or disproportionate pain to such manipulations is reasonable. If imaging reveals a large focal fluid collection, symptoms may be ascribed to this abnormality, and drainage of the collection may be considered.

CLINICAL SCENARIO 2: THE PATIENT CONTINUES TO HAVE THE SAME SYMPTOMS AFTER SURGERY, WITH NO CHANGE IN THE CHARACTER OF THE SYMPTOMS

Because the recuperation from fusion surgery may take several weeks if not months, patients are often not considered failures until at least 1 or 2 years later (Flynn 1979, Kostiuk 1997). Until this long period has passed, it may be assumed that the fusion is undergoing incorporation and that pain may remit. At some point, however, three possibilities must be considered: (1) continued pain from other

TABLE 3–1. Imaging Findings of Pseudarthrosis

Finding	Comments
Lucency around hardware	Lucency adjacent to pedicle screws, bone dowels, and interbody fusion cages should never be visualized. Lucency adjacent to bone grafts (e.g., fibular strut grafts of the cervical spine, iliac crest grafts in the cervical spine, and femoral ring allografts in the lumbar spine) may exist along the sides of the grafts, but the ends should be closely applied or incorporated into the adjacent structures.
Gas in fused structure	A vacuum phenomenon within a supposedly fused disc or facet is generally taken as a sign of motion in this structure, which should not persist following fusion.
Motion at the level	This is best evaluated by the method of stereophotogrammetry, which requires implantation of metallic beads and subsequent flexion/extension stereo films (a research technique). Flexion/extension plain films are relatively insensitive, and most imaging is performed in a single position, making evaluation of motion at the fusion site impossible.
Gap in bone graft	This usually occurs in the transverse plane and may be better visualized on coronal or sagittal reconstructions.

joints at the same motion segment, (2) operation on the wrong level, and (3) pseudarthrosis.

Since a three-joint complex comprises each level of the spine, pain emanating from a given level may come from any of the three joints. Although anterior fusion generally reduces movement through the level sufficiently to eliminate pain from the facet joints, such is not always the case (Frymoyer 1985). Patients who have undergone anterior interbody fusion with persistent pain may be evaluated with either intra-articular facet injections or facet joint blocks, followed by rhizotomy or posterior fusion as necessary. Patients who have undergone posterior fusion with persistent pain may be suffering from ongoing discogenic pain secondary to "chemical sensitivity" and require discography for evaluation, followed by anterior disc resection and fusion (Derby 1999).

As noted earlier, many fusions are done for internal disruption, and there is the possibility of fusing the wrong levels or an insufficient number of levels. As a first step, review of preoperative studies to check if levels adjacent to the fused levels may be a cause of pain should be performed. Discography of levels adjacent to the level of the

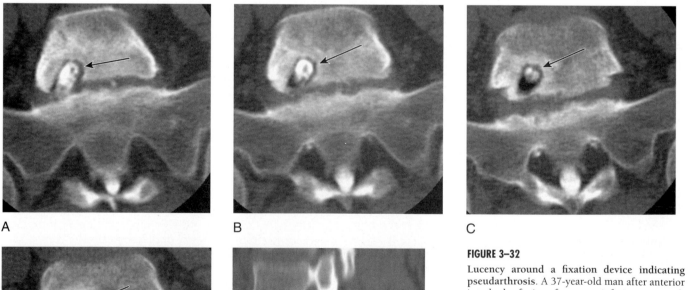

A   B   C

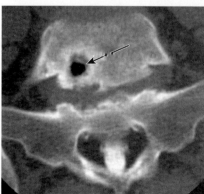

D   E

FIGURE 3–32

Lucency around a fixation device indicating pseudarthrosis. A 37-year-old man after anterior interbody fusion from an inferior approach for lytic spondylolisthesis with low back pain. *A–D,* Sequential inferior to superior axial CT studies. The scan plane is oblique with respect to the disc, so that S1 is posterior and L5 anterior. There is a screw that has adjacent lucency and even a vacuum phenomenon along its margin in the L5 vertebral body (*arrows*) diagnostic of motion at this level. *E,* Sagittal reconstruction through the screw confirms lucency around the margin of the screw (*arrow*).

fusion (which may have been done prior to surgery) may be helpful.

Pseudarthrosis occurs when the intended fusion fails to transpire and may or may not be associated with ongoing pain (Kim 1992, Laasonen 1989). Imaging findings of pseudarthrosis (Table 3–1) may be gross or subtle (Laasonen 1989). Imaging findings include lucency around implanted hardware, which indicates movement at the interface between the hardware and the adjacent bone. In the peripheral skeleton, surgeons place implanted joint prostheses into a reamed cavity; marginal lucency of 1 to 3 mm may be expected and does not necessarily indicate loosening unless it progresses on serial films. In the spine, however, pedicle screws, interbody fusion cages, and bone dowels should fit with no intervening tissue and with no perimetallic lucency. Any lucency along these structures can be a sign of pseudarthrosis (Figs. 3–32 to 3–37). Note, however, that beam hardening along the metal-bone interface may make evaluation of this interface difficult.

In addition, we have found that lucency along the margins of fusion cages is an insensitive indicator of pseudarthrosis and have encountered several cases wherein high-quality thin-cut CT scans have failed to demonstrate pseudarthrosis that was evident at surgery (Heithoff 1999). Indirect signs of pseudarthrosis include persistent gas within a supposedly fused disc or facet joint (Fig. 3–38) and motion through the fused level. Usually, imaging is not able to evaluate for motion because scans are obtained in only one position. Some advocate placement of bone graft material away from the edge of the metallic fusion device to allow better plain film (and CT) evaluation of fusion status (Eck 2000).

Pseudarthrosis through a bone graft of the spine usually occurs in the transverse plane (Kostiuk 1997). This complicates evaluation of CT studies, since abnormalities in the plane of acquisition are more difficult to evaluate. Obtaining axial images with thin slices and reformatting the data in the coronal and sagittal plane may considerably assist evaluation of the fusion mass. The coronal or sagittal reconstructions may much better demonstrate a transverse gap within the fusion mass that is more difficult to appreciate on only the axial studies (Kostiuk 1997, Lang 1988) (Figs. 3–39 to 3–41). In some cases, extensive resorption of

graft material results in scant material remaining at the time of imaging (Fig. 3–42). In other cases, a thin undulate plane separates two relatively large masses of bone, and diagnosis depends on evaluation of not only the original axial plane images but also the sagittal and coronal reconstructions. In "plate-type" pseudarthrosis, graft material coalesces but will not unite with the underlying native bone (Kostiuk 1997) (Fig. 3–38).

CT evaluates the *structural* integrity of a fusion, that is, whether there is a firm attachment of unbroken bone crossing the fusion site (Laasonen 1989, Lang 1990). Despite an apparent lack of structural integrity, a fusion may still have *functional* integrity, wherein the levels intended to be fused move as a single unit (Lang 1990). Traditionally, evaluation of functional integrity relied on flexion/extension plain films. Lang and coworkers (1990) found that MR may reliably evaluate the postfusion site for functional integrity: patients with functional integrity of a fusion have Modic Type II (fatty) degenerative changes along the margins of the fusion (Figs. 3–31 and 3–43); whereas patients without fusion have Modic Type I (fluid/inflammatory) changes along the margins of the fusion (Fig. 3–5).

Pseudarthrosis should not necessarily be taken as the sole or main cause of symptoms in patients following fusion surgery. Many patients with a pseudarthrosis are symptom free (DePalma 1968, Flynn 1979, Frymoyer 1979, Rothman 1975, St. Amour 1994), so other causes of new symptoms in the postfusion patient should also be sought. Conversely, it is theorized that some patients may continue to have discogenic pain despite solid dorsal or lateral fusion (Derby 1999, Weatherley 1986) (Fig. 3–44) and may require an anterior fusion as a supplement to posterior fusion to alleviate pain.

CLINICAL SCENARIO 3: THE PATIENT IMPROVES AFTER SURGERY, WITH LATER RECURRENCE OF IDENTICAL SYMPTOMS

Analogous to the situation with discectomy, improvement following fusion surgery may be taken as one of the best indicators that the preoperative diagnosis was correct and that surgery was (at least temporarily) successful. Indeed, unlike the case of discectomy (where no "trial surgery" can

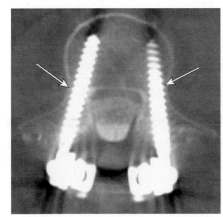 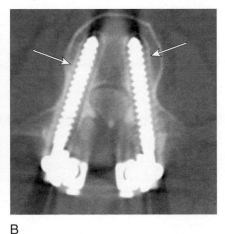

A   B

FIGURE 3–33

Lucency around pedicular screws indicating pseudarthrosis. A 77-year-old woman after L3 through S1 decompression/fusion surgery with ongoing low back pain following surgery. *A,* Axial CT-myelogram at the L4 level demonstrates posterior decompression with no residual or recurrent spinal canal stenosis. There are bilateral L4 pedicle screws without evidence of loosening, fracture, or migration (*arrows*). Note the lack of any lucency between the screws and the adjacent vertebral body trabecular bone. *B,* Axial CT-myelogram through the level of the L3 pedicles demonstrates bilateral pedicle screws, with lucency surrounding the screws indicating lack of solid union.

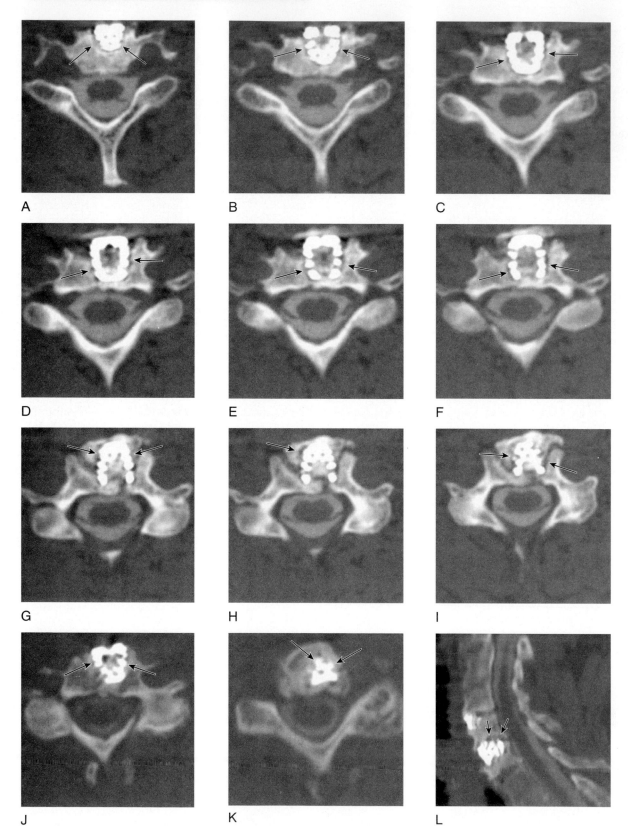

FIGURE 3–34

Lucency around interbody fusion cages indicating pseudarthrosis. A 63-year-old man after C4–5 and C5–6 anterior interbody fusion with titanium cages. *A–I,* Sequential 1-mm CT-myelogram studies slightly oblique to the C5–6 disc space demonstrate lucency surrounding the interbody fusion cage along both its inferior (adjacent to C6) and superior (adjacent to C5) levels *(arrows),* consistent with pseudarthrosis. These fusion cages should have no lucency around them. *J,* Axial CT-myelogram at the inferior aspect of the patient's C4–5 cage demonstrates no lucency along the cage–vertebral body margin *(arrows),* arguing against pseudarthrosis at this level. *K,* Axial CT-myelogram at the superior aspect of the patient's C4–5 cage demonstrates no lucency along this margin *(arrows)* of the cage, either. *L,* Sagittal reconstruction demonstrates lucency along the C5–6 cage margins *(arrows).* This reconstruction view is through the lateral aspect of the C4–5 cage owing to patient scoliosis and obliquity.

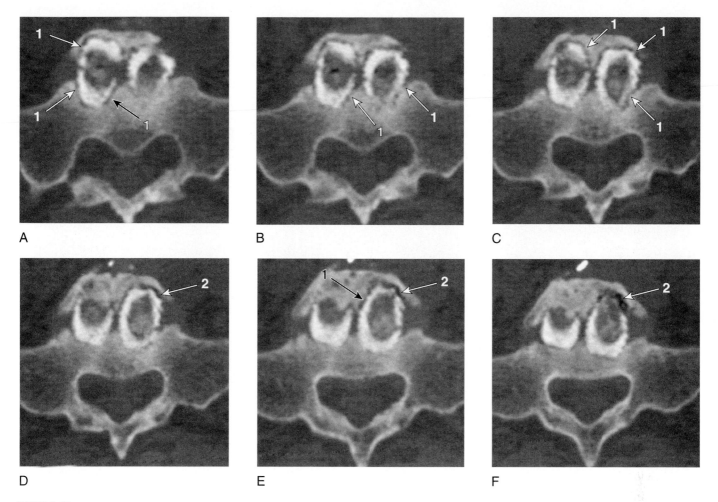

FIGURE 3–35

Lucency around bone dowel grafts indicating pseudarthrosis. A 40-year-old woman after L5–S1 fusion with bone dowels and persistent central low back pain. *A–F,* Sequential 1-mm cuts obliquely angled through the L5–S1 intervertebral disc demonstrates that there is lucency around the margins of the bone dowels *(arrows 1)*; this is more prominent along the graft-L5 interface than along the graft-S1 interface. Some gas outlines the superior margin of the left cage *(arrows 2)*, which is another sign of loosening.

be performed), trials of fusion with external fixators have been used as a predictor of the response to fusion surgery (Bednar 1996, Esses 1989, Jeanneret 1994, Soini 1993, van der Schaaf 1999). In some studies, success of such a trial of fixation has reliably predicted success of fusion surgery. In a patient who has undergone fusion surgery and obtained good but transient pain relief, the main possibilities to consider include development of pseudarthrosis and adjacent segment degeneration with development of the same symptoms.

Some patients with pseudarthrosis never obtain relief from pain (see earlier), whereas others may obtain temporary relief with redevelopment of symptoms. Note that in cases where symptoms have relented but then returned, a solid fusion may undergo traumatic fracture or displacement, either through the bone graft or at the hardware-graft interface (Fig. 3–45). In other patients, the hardware may temporarily alleviate pain but then fail (Fig. 3–46). Fusion masses may be both more fragile than native bone and also subjected to additional stresses because of lack of normal motion through the fused segments. The frequency of adja-

cent segment degeneration is controversial: it is widely held that fusion surgery hastens degeneration of adjacent levels (Langrana 1993), but Hambly and associates (1998) published a study stating that adjacent segments were at no greater risk for degeneration because of fusion. Adjacent segment degenerative disc and facet disease may reproduce the patient's original preoperative symptoms (Fig. 3–47).

CLINICAL SCENARIO 4: THE PATIENT IMPROVES AFTER SURGERY AND LATER DEVELOPS NEW AND DIFFERENT SYMPTOMS

New and different symptoms following treatment with fusion implies that fusion has succeeded but that another problem has arisen. For the purposes of our discussion, we divide such problems into those related to the surgery and those independent of the surgery.

Regarding problems related to surgery, adjacent segment degeneration may cause recurrence of similar symptoms (see earlier) or development of new symptoms. Assessment of degenerative changes such as loss of disc height or -

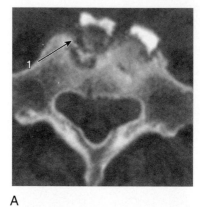

A

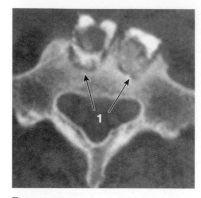

B

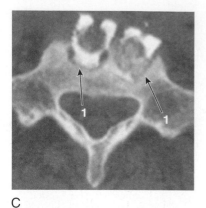

C

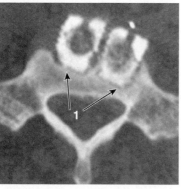

D

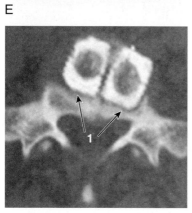

E

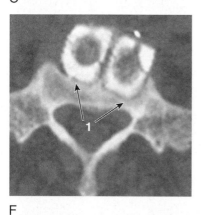

F

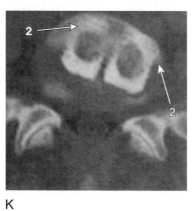

G

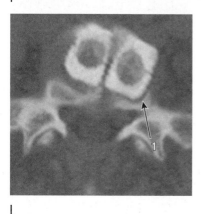

H

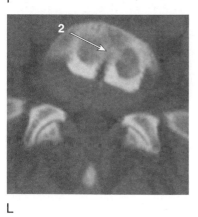

I

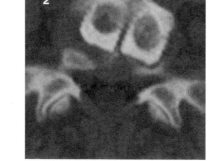

J

K

L

FIGURE 3–36

Lucency along one side of bone dowel grafts indicating pseudarthrosis. A 37-year-old woman with persistent low back pain after L5–S1 fusion with bone dowel grafts. *A–P,* Sequential 1-mm CT scans through the L5–S1 level demonstrates bilateral lucencies along the graft-S1 interface *(arrows 1)* but solid incorporation along the graft-L5 interface *(arrows 2).*

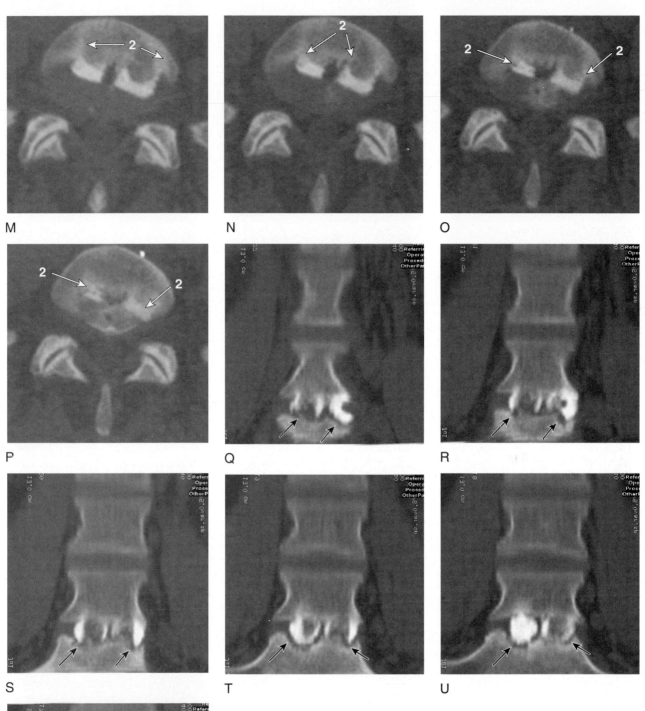

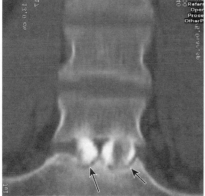

FIGURE 3–36 (*continued*)

Q–V, Coronal CT reconstructions confirm lucency along the inferior graft-S1 interface (*arrows*). Note that the curved coronal reconstructions are often more helpful in evaluating the interface between the graft and vertebral body than sagittal reconstructions.

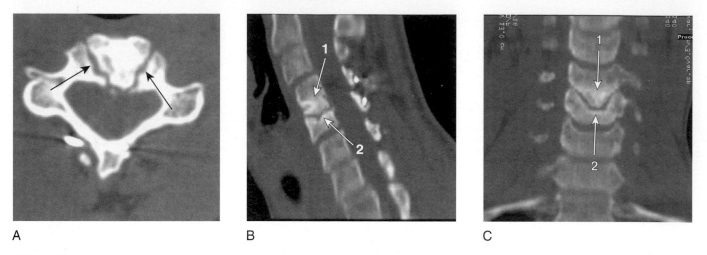

A   B   C

FIGURE 3–37

Lucency around bone graft indicating pseudarthrosis. A 39-year-old woman after C4–5 anterior cervical discectomy with fusion surgery. The patient has had chronic neck pain following cervical fusion surgery. *A*, Axial 1-mm slice through the lower aspect of the graft at C5 demonstrates lucency *(arrows)* along the graft-C5 margin. *B*, Sagittal reconstruction demonstrates graft incorporation into the C4 vertebral body above *(arrow 1)* but not the C5 level below *(arrow 2)*. There is also a posterior fixation wire in place. *C*, Coronal reconstruction also shows incorporation into C4 above *(arrow 1)* but not into C5 below *(arrow 2)*.

hydration and facet arthropathy should be performed. Comparison with preoperative studies may reveal progression or new-onset degenerative changes that might account for patient symptoms (Figs. 3–47 and 3–48). Delayed disc herniation following successful fusion, either at the level of fusion or at the adjacent or at a more remote segment, may or may not be related to the original surgery (Figs. 3–47, 3–49, and 3–50). Whether related to the fusion surgery or not, symptomatic disc herniation in a postfusion patient is certainly one of the most straightforward problems to address. Additional problems related to surgery include development (or redevelopment) of stenosis, delayed hardware complications, pseudomeningocele, and arachnoiditis.

With dorsal fusion (a surgery now rarely performed), eventual spinal canal stenosis through the level of the fusion often occurred (Lehmann 1987, Quencer 1978, Rothman 1975). Dorsolateral fusion with central decompression and intertransverse process fusion (the replacement for simple dorsal fusion) infrequently results in stenosis through the levels of fusion but may be associated with symptomatic adjacent segment stenosis as a delayed complication (Fig. 3–51), as can also be seen in patients who have undergone dorsal fusion (Fig. 3–52). Those patients undergoing their initial decompression and fusion surgery for stenosis are at greater risk for adjacent segment stenosis than those undergoing fusion for internal derangement.

Regarding delayed hardware complications, narrowing of the spinal canal caused by hardware at the time of surgery may only become symptomatic later, perhaps as the result of a second site of narrowing developing along the same nerve root (Olmarker 1992, Porter 1992) (Fig. 3–53). Other delayed complications of hardware include fatigue fracture and displacement of hardware (Fig. 3–54). Fracture and displacement of hardware may not require corrective surgery if they do not result in irritation of soft tissues or if they are not accompanied by symptomatic fracture through bony fusion.

Pseudomeningoceles presumably form from defects in the dura and may be either asymptomatic or cause headaches, back pain, or radiculopathy (St. Amour 1994, Teplick 1983). MRI demonstrates a collection of CSF signal intensity adjacent to the central spinal canal, usually posterior and in the midline (Fig. 3–55). CT-myelogram examination may demonstrate contrast material within the pseudomeningocele (Fig. 3–56). Radicular pain may follow from herniation of a nerve root into the pseudomeningocele (Fig. 3–25) or from adhesions along the course of the nerve root adjacent to the meningocele (St. Amour 1994). Such adhesions, of course, may form without a pseudomeningocele in arachnoiditis.

MRI demonstrates a spectrum of findings in arachnoiditis, consistent with the variable clinical findings (Guyer 1989). Although it is discussed here as a postoperative complication, arachnoiditis has many causes, including trauma, infection, intrathecal hemorrhage, myelography, and even disc herniation and stenosis (Burton 1978, St. Amour 1994). Arachnoiditis should not necessarily be attributed to surgery in patients who have several of these risk factors. MR findings of minimal arachnoiditis include clumping of nerve roots together within the thecal sac or adherence of one or a few nerve roots to the walls of the spinal canal (Fig. 3–57). Moderate cases show clumping and peripheralization of several nerve roots (Fig. 3–58), whereas in severe cases there is an "empty canal" sign because the nerve roots are plastered along the sides of the thecal sac (Fig. 3–59). In some cases the thecal sac collapses, and it is difficult to identify any CSF within the central spinal canal at the afflicted levels. In some patients, a syrinx may accompany arachnoiditis (St. Amour 1994). In others, calcification or even ossification may occur (Fig. 3–60) (Frizzell 2001, Ng 1996). Treatment of arachnoiditis is difficult and the prognosis is generally poor, with little relief

Text continued on page 167

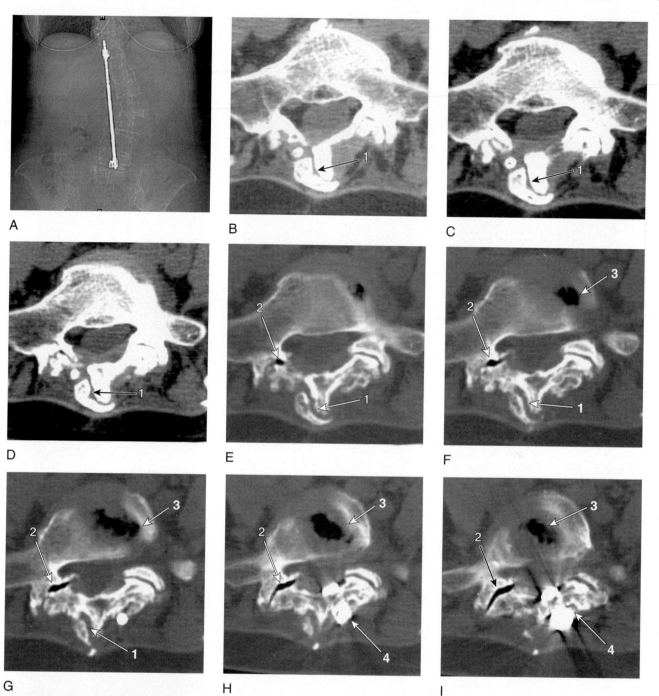

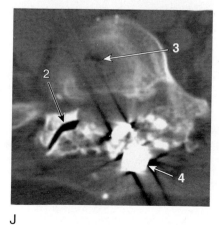

FIGURE 3–38

Vacuum phenomenon of a disc with plate-type pseudarthrosis. A 54-year-old woman after remote posterior multilevel fusion for scoliosis with central low back pain. *A*, Anteroposterior scout view demonstrates scoliosis convex to the left at the L2–3 level. A Harrington rod connects laminar hooks at the T11 level above and L5 level below. *B–J*, Sequential axial 3-mm CT images through the L5–S1 level demonstrates posterior bone graft material separated from the posterior elements of S1 (*arrow 1*), consistent with plate-type pseudarthrosis. There is a vacuum phenomenon of the right facet joint (*arrow 2*) and of the intervertebral disc (*arrow 3*) indicating motion and pseudarthrosis at this level. The laminar hook arches over the left L5 level (*arrow 4*). Higher levels (not shown) were solidly fused.

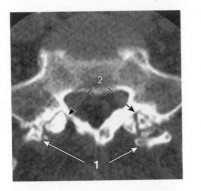
A

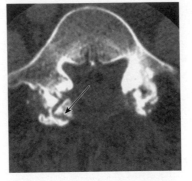
B

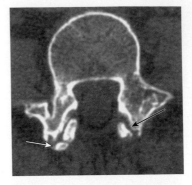
C

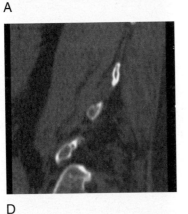
D

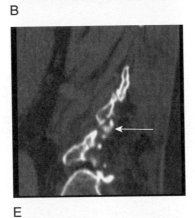
E

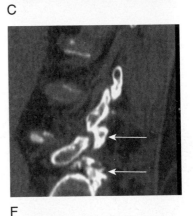
F

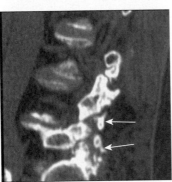
G

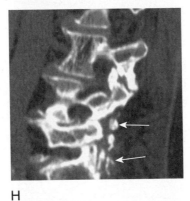
H

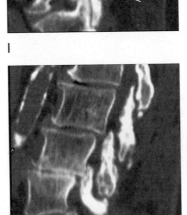
I

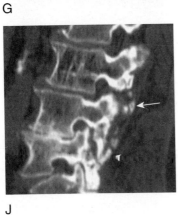

J

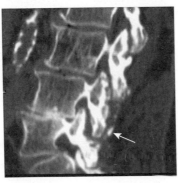

K

L

FIGURE 3–39

Pseudarthrosis better seen on reconstruction views. A 71-year-old woman after multilevel decompression/fusion surgery with persistent back pain. Axial CT included from the sacrum through the L2 level, with a total of 118 1-mm slices obtained, along with sagittal and coronal reconstructions. *A,* Axial CT at the S1 pedicle level demonstrates dorsolateral fusion graft material *(arrows 1)* but no firm incorporation into the underlying S1 lamina *(arrows 2). B,* Axial CT at the L5 pedicle level demonstrates dorsal decompression and dorsolateral fusion material. No definite incorporation of the fusion material and the L4 inferior articular process is present *(arrow). C,* Axial CT at the L4 pedicle level again demonstrates posterolateral fusion material without definite incorporation *(arrows). D–L,* Sequential right parasagittal CT reconstructions demonstrate a moderate amount of laterally placed bone graft material *(arrows),* but no firm union crossing the different levels is present. Left parasagittal images (not shown) showed similar findings.

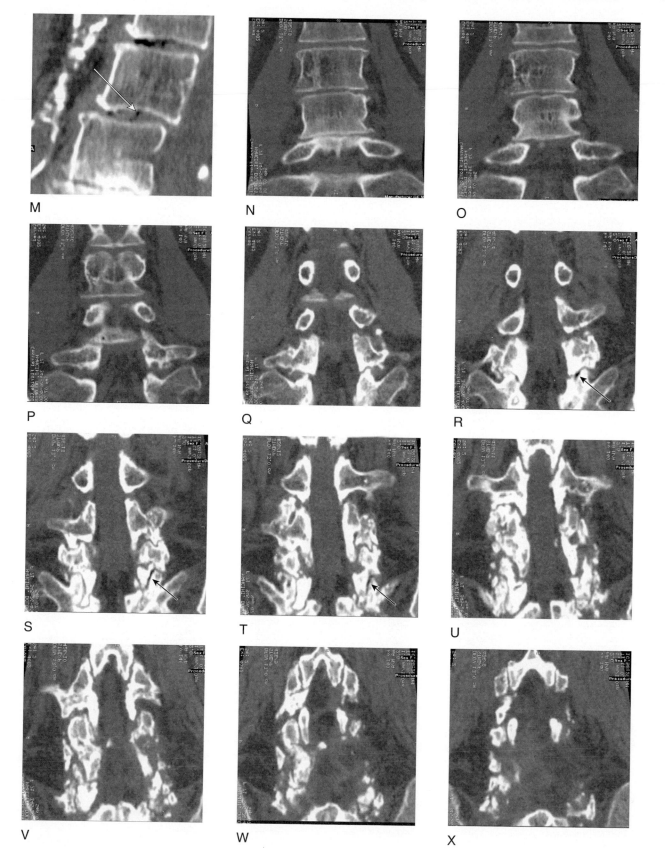

FIGURE 3–39 *(continued)*

M, Midline sagittal CT reconstruction demonstrates retrolisthesis of L4 on L5 and a vacuum phenomenon of the L3–4 intervertebral disc *(arrow),* consistent with pseudarthrosis. *N–X,* Sequential anterior-to-posterior curved coronal reconstructions demonstrate dorsolateral graft material, but there is no union crossing between the levels at L3–4, L4–5, or L5–S1. There is a vacuum phenomenon on the left at the L5–S1 level *(arrow).* The findings are those of pseudarthrosis.

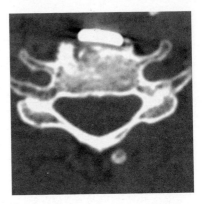

A

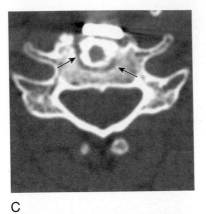

B

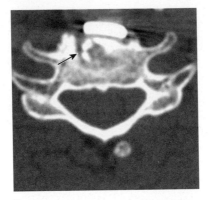

C

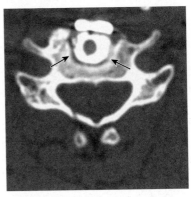

D

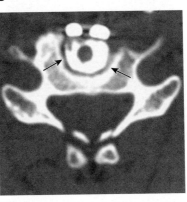

E

F

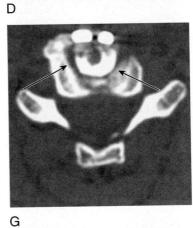

G

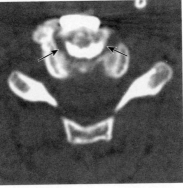

H

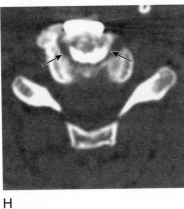

I

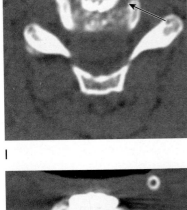

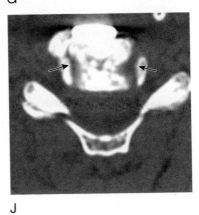

J

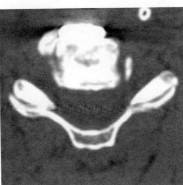

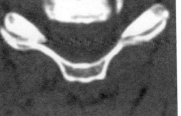

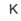

K

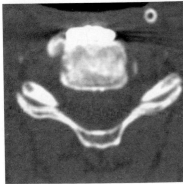

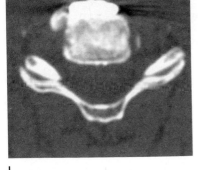

L

FIGURE 3–40

Pseudarthrosis better seen on reconstruction views. A 54-year-old man after ACDF at C4–5 with persistent neck pain. *A–L*, Sequential 1-mm axial CT images through the C4–5 level demonstrate an anterior plate and bone graft in place. The lucencies along the lateral margins of the bone graft are expected and not a sign of pseudarthrosis (*arrows*). The upper and lower margins appear to blend relatively smoothly into the adjacent vertebral bodies on the axial studies.

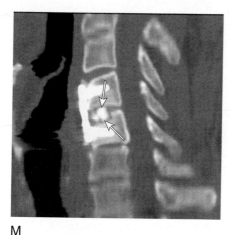

M

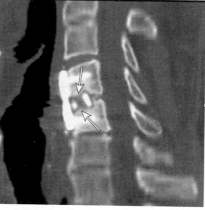

N

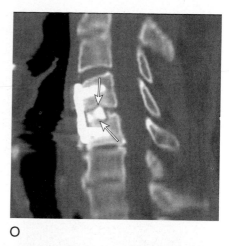

O

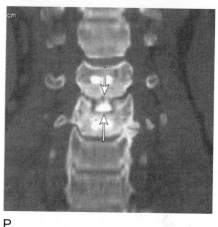

P

FIGURE 3–40 *(continued)*

M–O, Sequential right-to-left sagittal reconstructions demonstrate lucency *(arrows)* along the inferior and superior aspects of the bone graft at the C4–5 level, consistent with pseudarthrosis. *P,* Curved coronal reconstruction through the C4–5 level also shows lucency along the margins of the graft *(arrows),* consistent with pseudarthrosis. This examination demonstrates the difficulty in judging fusion on only axial images.

of symptoms with either time or specific therapy (Federowicz 1991, Guyer 1989).

Patients who have had improvement following fusion surgery may also develop new and different symptoms at another level for totally unrelated, but additional, disease: fusion surgery at one level does not confer immunity from spinal disease at other levels. Whether one of the processes listed earlier has been identified in the postoperative patient or not, the remaining levels of the spine should be evaluated for symptom-producing lesions. Such evaluation should follow the principles described in Chapter 2.

Reporting Postoperative Imaging Studies

In interpretation of postoperative images, the clinical context (as outlined in this chapter) should be kept in mind, and the reader should also keep in mind the following questions during interpretation:

1. Has the surgery been a success?
   a. Was the disc herniation removed?
   b. Was decompression accomplished?
   c. Has fusion been achieved?
2. Was there a complication of surgery?
   a. Was there hardware misplacement?
   b. Is there evidence of infection?
   c. Are there findings to suggest that surgery was performed on the wrong level?
3. Has the patient had interval development of additional pathology?

In general, for the body of the report it is easiest to follow a level-by-level approach similar to that outlined in Chapter 2. The same multiple considerations at each level (such as disc height, hydration, and contour; stenosis of the central, subarticular, and foraminal aspects of the disc margin; facet arthropathy) must be addressed. In addition to these features, postoperative changes must be noted. These include surgical removal of bone (e.g., laminotomy, laminectomy, facetectomy, and vertebrectomy) and soft tissue (e.g., discectomy), and addition of surgically placed devices (e.g., interbody fusion cages, pedicle screws with posterior interconnecting hardware, and fixation wires) or material (e.g., bone graft and barium-impregnated methyl methacrylate). The status of any attempted fusion should be evaluated; usually, MRI does not allow assessment of fusion unless the fusion is unquestionably solid (and the result of a remote procedure). CT evaluation may need to rely not only on axial images but on sagittal and coronal reconstruction views. In dorsolateral fusions of the lumbar spine, bone should join adjacent transverse processes and the facet joints are usually fused. In anterior cervical fusions, bone graft should be incorporated along its proxi-

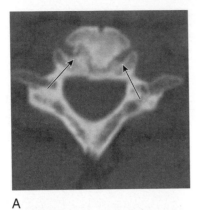

A

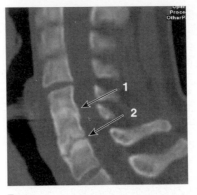

B

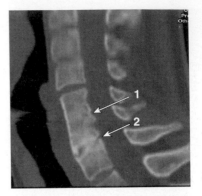

C

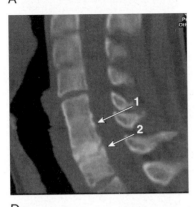

D

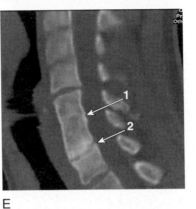

E

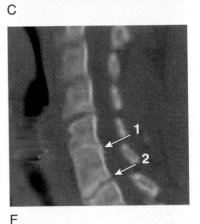

F

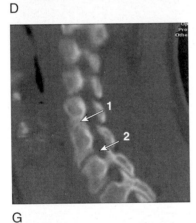

G

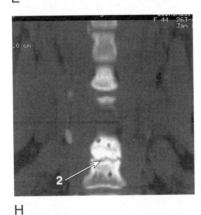

H

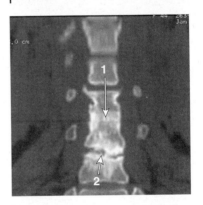

I

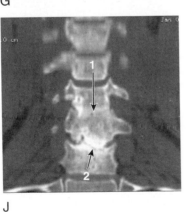

J

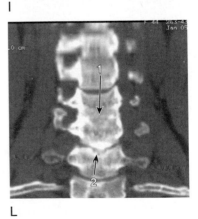

K

L

FIGURE 3–41

Pseudarthrosis better seen on reconstruction views. A 44-year-old woman after C5–6 and C6–7 fusion with persistent neck pain. *A*, Axial CT at the C6–7 level demonstrates a curved interface between the bottom of C6 and top of C7 (*arrows*), suggesting pseudarthrosis but difficult to evaluate on axial studies. *B–G*, Sequential right-to-left sagittal CT reconstructions demonstrate solid union at the C5–6 level (*arrow 1*) but lucency along the interface between C6 and C7 (*arrow 2*). *H–L*, Sequential anterior-to-posterior curved coronal CT reconstructions also show solid union at the C5–6 level (*arrow 1*) with lucency between C6 and C7 (*arrow 2*). In such cases where the pseudarthrosis margin is complex, it is helpful to have all three imaging planes for analysis.

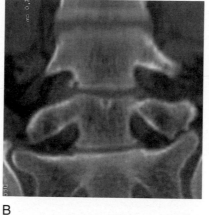

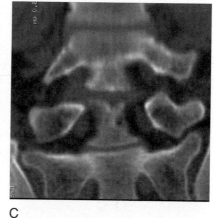

A   B   C

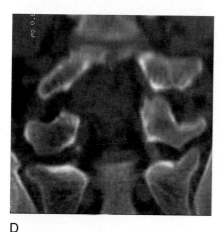

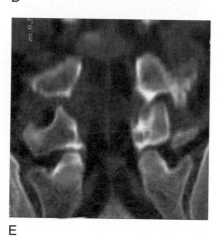

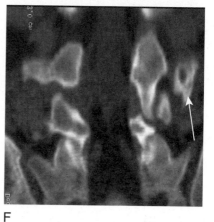

D   E   F

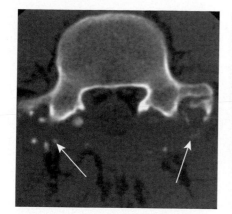

G

FIGURE 3–42

Resorption of graft material with little graft material remaining. A 36-year-old man after L4–5 decompression/fusion surgery. *A,* Axial 1-mm CT image at the L4 pedicle level demonstrates dorsal decompression with scant dorsolateral fusion material *(arrows). B–L,* Sequential anterior-to-posterior curved coronal reconstructions demonstrate scant fusion material *(arrows)* along the lateral aspects of the L4 and L5 transverse processes without any union.

mal and distal margins, although incorporation along the midsection may take considerable time, and lack of such incorporation does not imply pseudarthrosis. Interbody fusion cages and pedicle screws should have no intervening lucency between the device and adjacent bone, whereas small gaps between fixation plates and underlying bone do not necessarily indicate pseudarthrosis. Postoperative abnormalities of soft tissue (e.g., hematoma, pseudomeningocele, and arachnoidal adhesions) should be noted.

To provide a helpful conclusion, possible diagnoses must be considered in the context of the clinical symptoms, as outlined in this chapter. Identical imaging findings may

have vastly different implications for patient management, depending on the time from surgery, the patient's present symptoms, and the course of the patient's symptoms. An MRI demonstrating a disc extrusion at an operated level may be a normal postoperative finding in a patient who has had elimination of pain with surgery (Fig. 3–14); the same finding in the context of persistent and unchanged symptoms may indicate unsuccessful surgery with residual disc herniation (Fig. 3–13); and the same finding in a patient who has had a period of complete pain relief followed by recurrence of symptoms likely represents a recurrent disc herniation (Fig. 3–22).

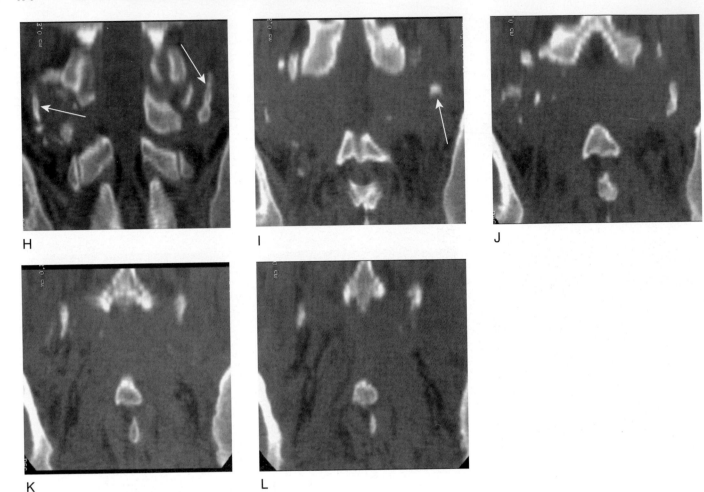

FIGURE 3–42   (*continued*)

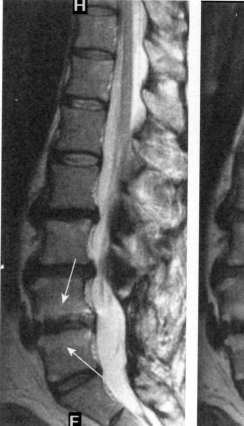

A   B

FIGURE 3–43

Functional integrity of fusion with Modic Type II subchondral changes. A 51-year-old woman after L4–5 anterior interbody fusion with posterior decompression. *A,* Sagittal T2WI shows multilevel degenerative changes, including L2–3 mild loss of disc height and moderate disc dehydration, L3–4 mild loss of disc height and moderate disc dehydration with degenerative disc bulging and retrolisthesis of L3 on L4, and L5–S1 mild disc dehydration and degenerative disc bulging. At the L4–5 level, there is posterior decompression and the intervertebral disc has a fusion device in place. The subchondral marrow demonstrates mild T2 prolongation *(arrows)*. *B,* Sagittal T1WI shows T1 shortening along the vertebral body margins *(arrows)*, indicating Modic Type II changes. Such changes are consistent with functional integrity of the L4–5 fusion.

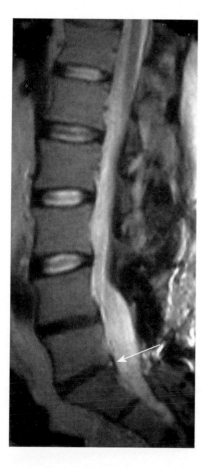

FIGURE 3–44

Discogenic pain despite dorsal fusion. A 44-year-old man with persistent low back pain following decompression/fusion at L4/5 and L5/S1. Sagittal T2WI demonstrates posterior postoperative changes. There is severe loss of disc height and disc dehydration at both L4–5 and L5–S1. Furthermore, there is T2 prolongation in the dorsal disc margin at the L5–S1 level *(arrow)*. The patient underwent L3–4, L4–5, and L5–S1 discography; he had no pain on intranuclear injection at L3–4 or L4–5 but intense concordant pain on injection at the L5–S1 level despite solid dorsolateral fusion.

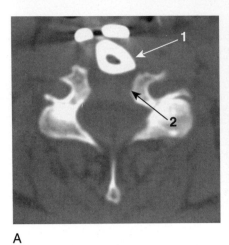

A

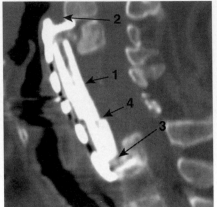

B

FIGURE 3–45

Solid fusion with relief of pain, followed by traumatic failure with redevelopment of symptoms. A 73-year-old woman with rheumatoid arthritis after several total joint replacement surgeries and multilevel fusion/decompression with a bony strut graft of the cervical spine. The patient had prolonged, excellent relief of neck pain with sudden return of pain after a fall. *A,* CT scan at the C5 pedicle level demonstrates anterior displacement of the tubular bony strut graft (*arrow 1*) from the vertebrectomy defect (*arrow 2*) designed to house the graft. *B,* Sagittal reconstruction demonstrates anterior displacement of the tubular bony strut graft (*arrow 1*) from its appropriate position. There is displacement of the superior margin of the plate from the C2 vertebra superiorly (*arrow 2*) and similar displacement inferiorly at C7 (*arrow 3*). Note that the apparent discontinuity of the graft (*arrow 4*) is a result of patient motion in the middle of the study: the graft itself was intact but displaced. Previous postoperative studies done prior to the patient's fall (not shown) demonstrated a more appropriate position of the patient's graft.

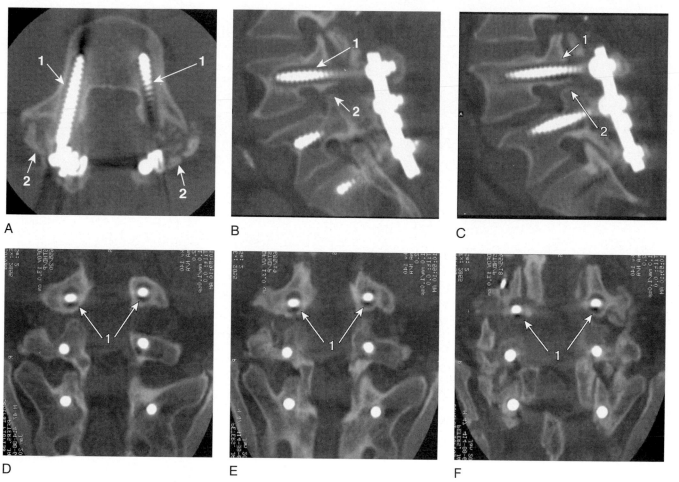

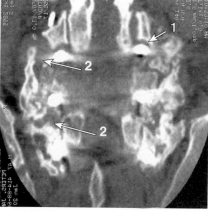

FIGURE 3–46

Temporary relief of pain following fusion with return of pain after fusion failure. A 47-year-old man who underwent L4–5 and L5–S1 fusion/decompression surgery with 18 months of excellent pain relief, followed by return of low back pain. *A,* Axial 1-mm CT study at the L4 pedicle level shows bilateral loosening of the L4 pedicle screws *(arrows 1).* There is lateral fusion material, but this is not consolidated into a single fusion mass or incorporated into the underlying bone *(arrows 2). B,* Right CT reconstruction at the level of the L4 pedicle demonstrates lucency around the pedicle screw consistent with loosening *(arrow 1).* There is a gap of fusion material *(arrow 2)* consistent with pseudarthrosis. *C,* Left parasagittal CT reconstruction shows similar findings on the left side with lucency around the L4 pedicle screw *(arrow 1)* and a gap in the fusion material *(arrow 2).* *(continued)*

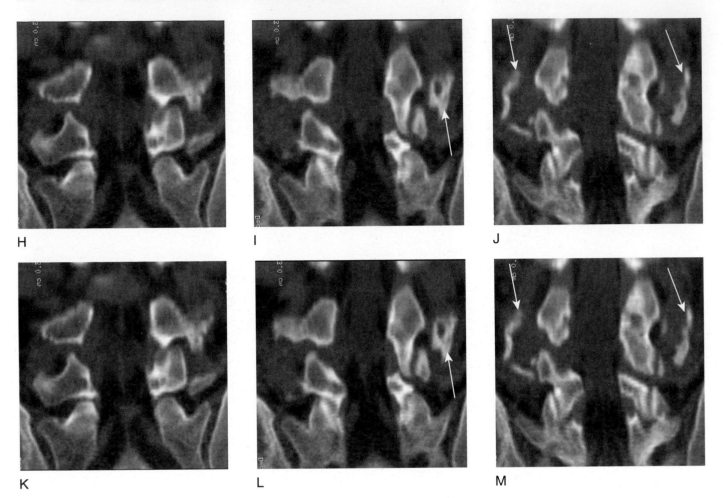

FIGURE 3–46 *(continued)*

D–M, Sequential anterior-to-posterior curved coronal reconstructions demonstrate bilateral L4 pedicle screw loosening *(arrows 1)* and no connection between the fusion mass along the L4 lateral transverse processes/facet joints *(arrows 2).* There is a component of platelike pseudarthrosis here, with a solid unit of incorporated graft rising from the L5 transverse processes posterolaterally, but not incorporated into the L4 transverse processes. It is likely that this patient was pain free as long as the L4 pedicle screws held the L4–5 segment motionless, but the lack of solid dorsolateral fusion eventually resulted in motion around the L4 screws and return of pain.

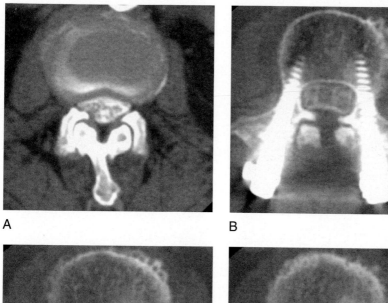

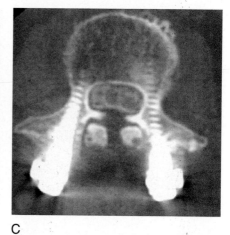

A

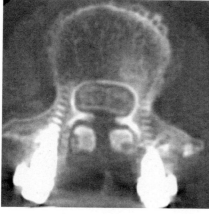

B

C

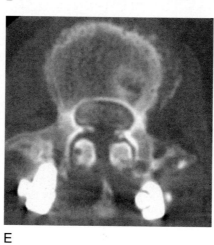

D

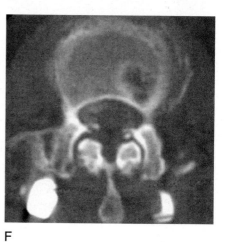

E

F

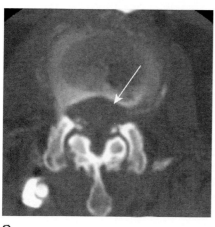

G

FIGURE 3–47

Successful fusion with adjacent segment degenerative changes with return of pain. A 76-year-old woman with low back pain and bilateral leg weakness. *A,* Axial CT-myelogram done through the L1–2 level prior to surgery demonstrates degenerative disc bulging, moderate facet arthropathy, and mild spinal canal stenosis. The patient had multilevel lower lumbar stenosis (not shown). The patient underwent L2 through S1 fusion/decompression surgery with bilateral L2, L3, L4, L5, and S1 pedicle screws and dorsolateral hardware. The patient's preoperative low back and leg symptoms were relieved for several months following surgery, with a return of low back pain and bilateral leg weakness. *(continued)*

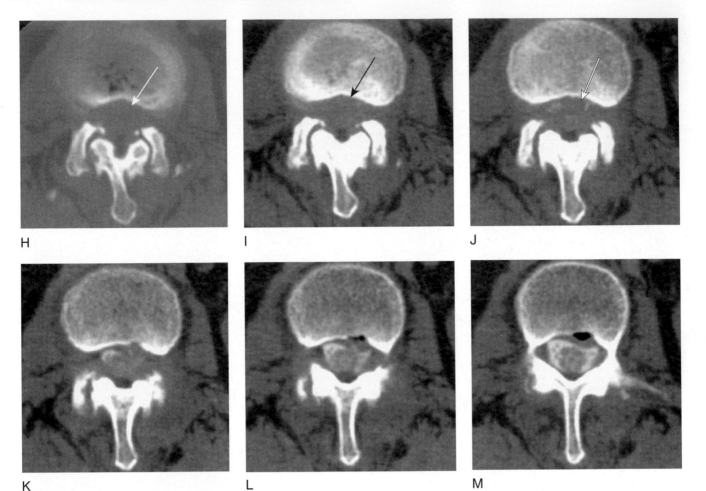

H   I   J

K   L   M

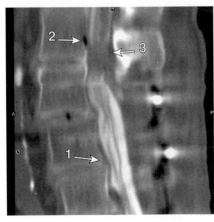

N

FIGURE 3–47 *(continued)*

B–M, Axial 3-mm CT studies done from the L2 through the bottom of the L1 pedicle. Through the level of the disc, there is severe constriction of the contrast column with severe spinal canal stenosis and attenuation of the contrast column *(arrow)* from a combination of disc bulging and facet arthropathy. There is gas within the L1–2 disc and also along the posterior margin of the L1 vertebral body. (The patient's myelogram was performed through the laminectomy defect at L4. This gas was not injected by the radiologist.) Above the level of the disc, there is an anterior indentation of the contrast column indicating an extruded disc herniation. This disc herniation combines with degenerative disc bulging and facet arthropathy to cause severe spinal canal narrowing at the level of the disc. *N,* Sagittal reconstruction showing multilevel degenerative changes including L3–4 minimal (<5%) degenerative spondylolisthesis with disc narrowing *(arrow 1),* L2–3 disc narrowing with a vacuum phenomenon and 5% spondylolisthesis, and L1–2 intervertebral disc narrowing. Gas is seen dorsal to the L1 vertebral body *(arrow 2),* and there is complete attenuation of the contrast column at the L1–2 level *(arrow 3).* This patient's recurrence of symptoms was secondary to L1–2 stenosis exacerbated by a disc herniation that occurred following her surgery.

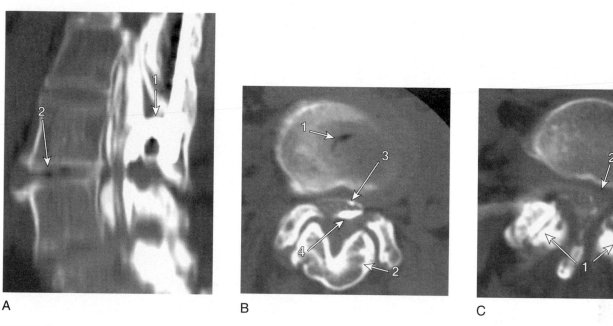

A   B   C

FIGURE 3–48

Back pain from adjacent segment degeneration. A 47-year-old woman who underwent remote multilevel fusion surgery for scoliosis, including dorsal rod placement and dorsal fusion to the posterior elements of L3. *A*, Sagittal reconstruction view demonstrates multilevel postoperative and degenerative changes. There is a Harrington rod with a laminar hook *(arrow 1)* over the lamina at L3 with solid dorsal fusion to this point. At L3–4 (the inferior junction level from the fusion), there is disc narrowing, a vacuum phenomenon *(arrow 2)*, and degenerative disc bulging and osteophytic spurring. At L4–5, there is degenerative spondylolisthesis of approximately 10% with disc narrowing. At L5–S1 (imperfectly seen secondary to obliquity of the scan plane), there is disc narrowing as well. *B*, CT at the L3–4 level shows a vacuum phenomenon *(arrow 1)* along with degenerative disc bulging. A fusion mass is incorporated into the posterior elements of L3 *(arrow 2)* (this scan is below the level of the laminar hook seen in *A*). There is severe spinal canal stenosis with attenuation of the contrast column around the nerve roots *(arrow 3)*. Some pooling of contrast material mimics an epidural injection posteriorly along the left margin of the thecal sac *(arrow 4)*, but this contrast was seen to be continuous with similar-appearing (dense) intrathecal contrast at other levels. *C*, CT at the L4–5 level demonstrates degenerative disc bulging and some volume averaging secondary to degenerative spondylolisthesis, along with bilateral severe facet arthropathy *(arrows 1)*. There is severe spinal canal and subarticular recess narrowing (left *[arrow 2]* > right).

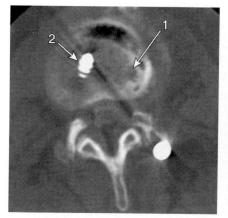

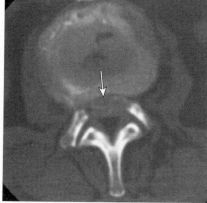

A   B

FIGURE 3–49

Delayed disc herniation at another level following successful fusion. A 60-year-old woman after L3–4 through L5–S1 dorsal decompression and posterolateral fusion with pedicle screws and dorsal interconnecting hardware. She now has had increased leg weakness and pain in the right back radiating into the iliac crest. *A*, CT-myelogram at the L2–3 level (the superior junctional level next to the fusion) demonstrates degenerative changes, including degenerative bulging and "pitting" *(arrow 1)* along the end plate of the disc. There is moderate spinal canal stenosis. Note also that one of the pedicle screw tips *(arrow 2)* is superiorly placed into and through the intervertebral disc. *B*, CT-myelogram at the L1–2 level shows a right central 5.1-mm disc extrusion *(arrow)* (demonstrating cranial and caudal dissection on adjacent images), along with degenerative changes of the intervertebral disc, including a vacuum phenomenon and degenerative disc bulging. There is severe right and moderate left spinal canal narrowing.

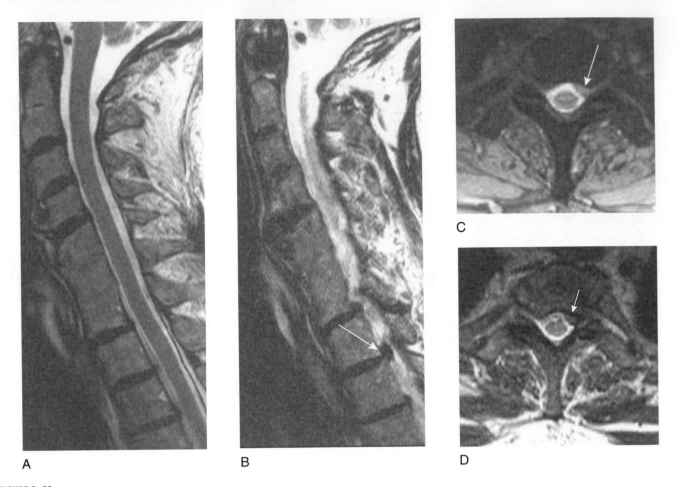

A   B   C   D

FIGURE 3–50

Delayed disc herniation at another level following successful fusion. A 70-year-old man, after remote C5–6 and C6–7 anterior cervical discectomy with fusion, had many years of good pain relief. He subsequently developed new-onset neck and left arm pain following a motor vehicle accident. *A,* Sagittal fast spin-echo (FSE) T2WI shows multilevel degenerative and postoperative changes, including C5–6 and C6–7 fusion and degenerative bulging of C7–T1 through T2–3. *B,* Parasagittal left T2WI shows degenerative disc bulging at C7–T1 and a 4.7-mm cranially and caudally dissecting disc extrusion at T1–2 *(arrow).* *C,* Axial gradient-recalled echo T2WI at the T1–2 level confirms the left central and foraminal disc extrusion *(arrow)* with compression of the exiting T1 nerve. *D,* Axial FSE T2WI at the T1–2 level also shows the left central and foraminal disc extrusion *(arrow).*

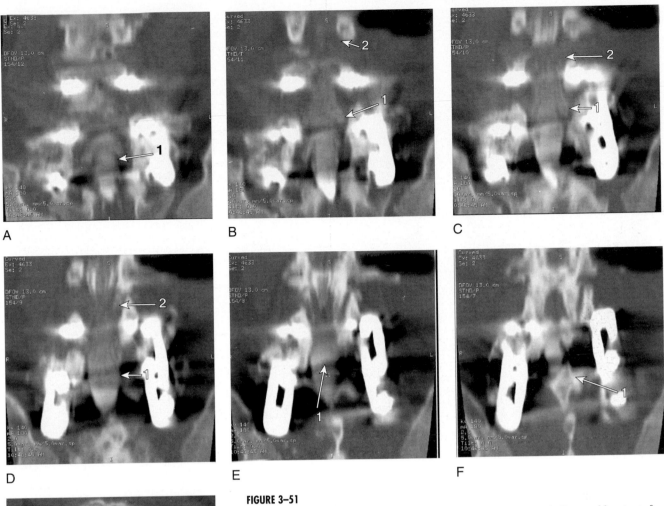

A   B   C

D   E   F

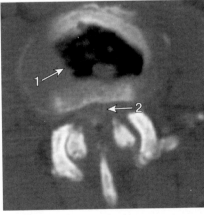

G

FIGURE 3–51

Successful fusion surgery followed by adjacent segment stenosis. A 63-year-old patient after remote L4–S1 intertransverse process fusion with plates and bone graft with low back and left thigh pain. *A–F,* Sequential anterior-to-posterior curved coronal CT-myelogram reconstructions. There is adequate dimension of the lower spinal canal (*arrow 1*) but narrowing of the spinal canal at the superior adjacent segment (L3–4 level) (*arrow 2*). *G,* Axial CT-myelogram at the L3–4 level demonstrates a vacuum disc phenomenon (*arrow 1*) and spinal canal stenosis with attenuation of the contrast column (*arrow 2*) from a combination of degenerative disc bulging and facet arthropathy.

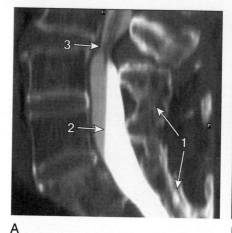

A

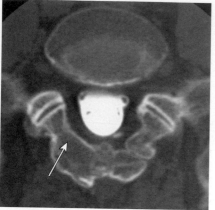

B

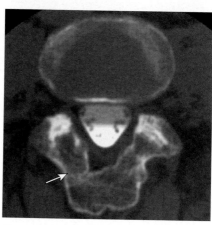

C

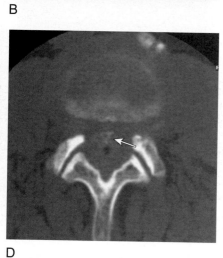

D

FIGURE 3–52

Successful fusion surgery followed by adjacent segment stenosis. A 67-year-old man after remote dorsal fusion from L4 through the sacrum. The patient developed right hip and leg pain. *A,* Sagittal reconstruction view from CT-myelogram shows solid L4 through sacral fusion bone *(arrow 1)* and a widely patent spinal canal through these levels (note layering of contrast material in the spinal canal *[arrow 2]*). At the L3–4 level (the superior junctional level of the fusion), there is degenerative disc bulging and severe spinal canal stenosis *(arrow 3)*. *B,* CT-myelogram at the L5–S1 level shows a widely patent spinal canal and solid dorsal fusion mass *(arrow)*. There is posterolateral fusion of the facet joints. *C,* CT-myelogram at the L4–5 level, as at the L5–S1 level, shows a widely patent spinal canal with solid dorsal fusion *(arrow)* and fusion of the facet joints. *D,* CT-myelogram at the L3–4 level shows degenerative disc bulging and moderate facet arthropathy resulting in severe spinal canal stenosis with a paucity of cerebrospinal fluid around the traversing nerve roots *(arrow)*.

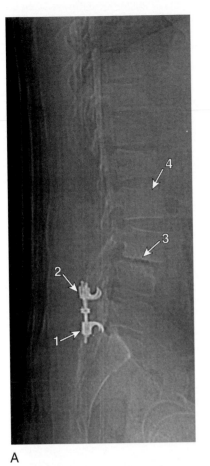

A

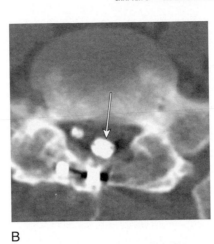

B

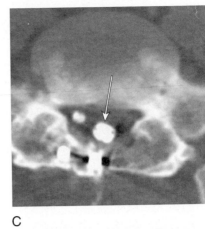

C

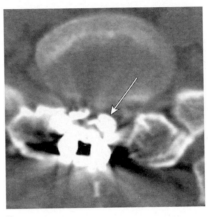

D

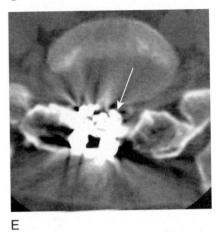

E

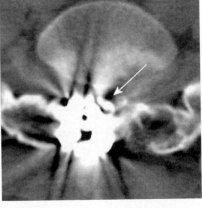

F

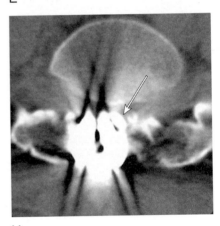

G

H

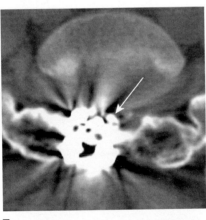

I

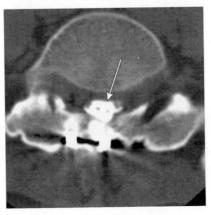

J

FIGURE 3–53 *See legend on next page*

(continued)

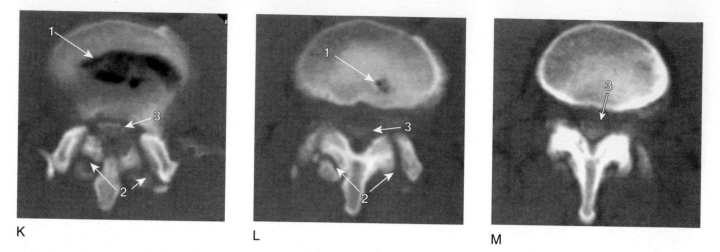

K   L   M

FIGURE 3–53 (continued)

Delayed stenosis from dorsal hardware. A 43-year-old man who had undergone remote posterior fusion with instrumentation at the L5–S1 level. The patient now has symptoms of low back pain with lower extremity pain on ambulation. *A,* Lateral scout digital radiograph from CT-myelogram study demonstrates posterior hardware with two sets of paired laminar hooks; the lower set is over the S1 laminae (*arrow 1*) and the upper set beneath the L4 laminae (*arrow 2*). There is L3–4 degenerative disc narrowing with a vacuum phenomenon (*arrow 3*) and 15% degenerative spondylolisthesis, and wedging of L1 (*arrow 4*). *B–J,* Selected (every other) sequential 3-mm CT-myelogram images from below to above the L5–S1 intervertebral disc demonstrate solid dorsal fusion, posterior instrumentation, and severe spinal canal stenosis, particularly at the level of the laminar hooks (*arrow*). *K–M,* CT-myelogram images through the L3–4 (superior adjacent segment) demonstrate degenerative disc disease with a vacuum phenomenon (*arrow 1*) and disc bulging combining with severe facet arthropathy (*arrows 2*) and degenerative spondylolisthesis to produce severe spinal canal and subarticular recess stenosis (*arrow 3*). The patient tolerated the spinal canal stenosis at L5–S1 relatively well until development of stenosis at L3–4.

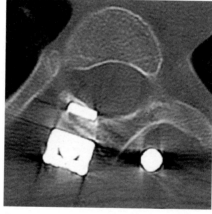

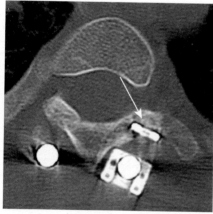

A   B

FIGURE 3–54

Migration of hardware. A 16-year-old boy who underwent scoliosis correction surgery and developed upper left back pain. *A,* Axial CT at T6 demonstrates a right laminar hook in appropriate position. *B,* Axial CT at T4 demonstrates the left transverse process hook to be posterior to the transverse process (*arrow*) rather than engaging it. A similar state of affairs existed on the left at the T8 level.

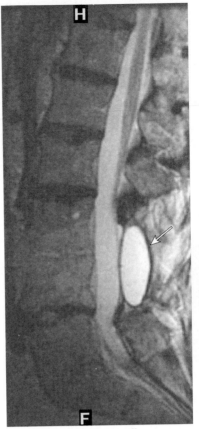

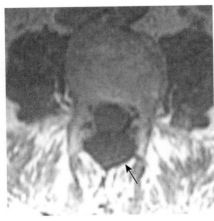

A

B

FIGURE 3–55

Pseudomeningocele. A 69-year-old man after L3–4 fusion/decompression with central low back pain. *A,* Sagittal T2WI shows multilevel postoperative and degenerative changes, including T12–L1 mild loss of disc height and severe disc dehydration, L1–2 mild loss of disc height and moderate disc dehydration, L2–3 moderate loss of disc height and severe disc dehydration, L3–4 fusion, L4–5 moderate loss of disc height and mixed intervertebral disc signal consistent with degenerative changes, and L5–S1 severe loss of disc height and severe disc dehydration. In addition, there is an oblong, smoothly marginated focus of T2 prolongation posterior to the L3 and L4 vertebral bodies measuring 53 × 18 mm *(arrow). B,* Axial T1WI at the fused L3–4 level demonstrates the lesion behind the thecal sac demonstrating T1 prolongation *(arrow).* The signal intensity follows that of cerebrospinal fluid. It was believed that the patient's pain was unlikely to have arisen from the pseudomeningocele, and he underwent bilateral L4, L5, and S1 medial branch blocks followed by rhizotomy, resulting in long-lasting pain relief.

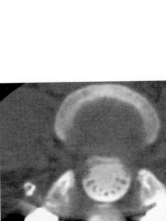

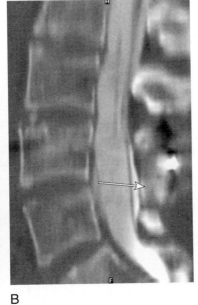

A

B

FIGURE 3–56

Pseudomeningocele. A 43-year-old woman after posterior L4–5 decompression/fusion with persistent central low back pain. *A,* CT-myelogram at the L4–5 level shows posterior decompression and posterolateral hardware. No residual central spinal canal stenosis or disc extrusion is identified. Posterior to the thecal sac, there is contrast density within the soft tissues *(arrow)* secondary to pseudomeningocele formation. *B,* Sagittal reconstruction demonstrates a posterior interconnecting rod at the L4–5 disc level and remaining posterior elements at L5, with contrast material posterior to the thecal sac at the L4 and L5 levels *(arrow).*

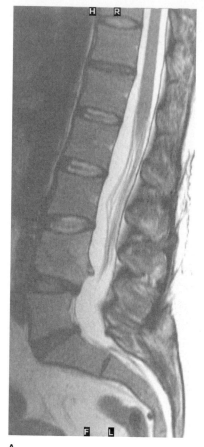

A

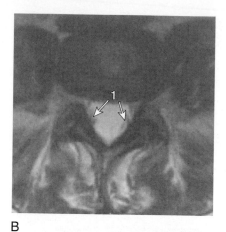

B

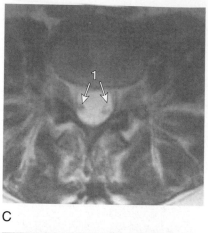

C

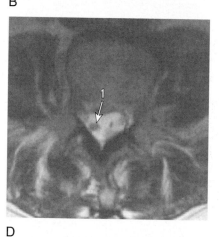

D

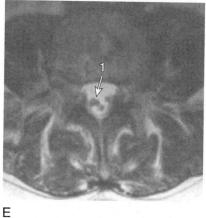

E

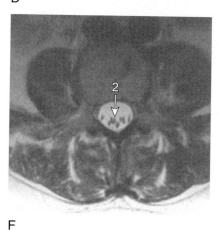

F

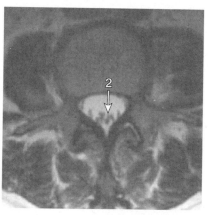

G

FIGURE 3–57

Arachnoiditis. A 40-year-old woman after L4–5 fusion with mid and lower back pain and bilateral lower extremity weakness, tingling, and numbness. *A,* Sagittal T2WI shows multilevel degenerative and postoperative changes, including T12–L1 moderate loss of disc height and hydration, L3–4 fusion (note the bony spur projecting along the dorsal fusion margin), L4–5 moderate disc dehydration with retrolisthesis, and L5–S1 mild loss of disc height and severe disc dehydration with degenerative disc bulging. *B–G,* Sequential axial T2WI from the L4–5 disc to the L3 pedicle. Distally, there is a clumped and peripheralized appearance of the nerve roots (*arrows 1*), whereas more proximally there is an even and symmetric distribution (*arrows 2*).

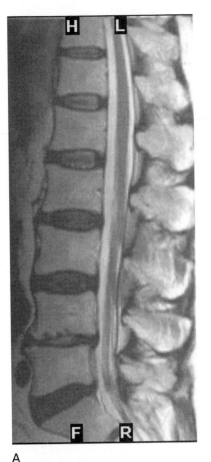

A

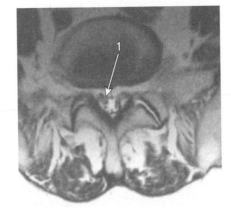

B

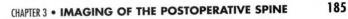

C

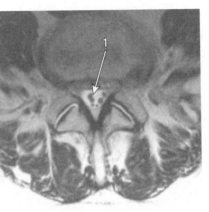

D

E

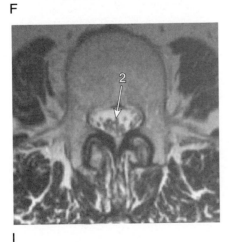

F

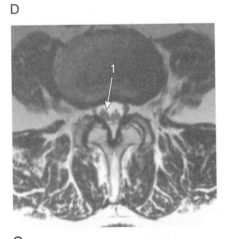

G

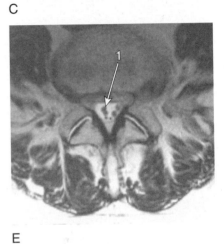

H

I

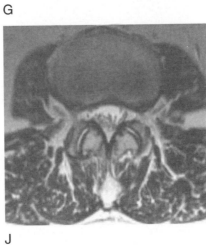

J

FIGURE 3–58

Arachnoiditis. A 72-year-old man with low back pain and bilateral calf and heel pain. *A,* Sagittal T2WI shows multilevel degenerative changes of the spine including L1–2 mild disc dehydration, L2–3 and L3–4 moderate disc dehydration, L4–5 severe loss of disc height and disc dehydration along with anterior osteophyte formation and retrolisthesis of L4 on L5, and L5–S1 moderate disc dehydration. *B–J,* Sequential inferior-to-superior, selected (every other) 4-mm cuts from the L5–1 to the L3–4 disc. Inferior cuts demonstrate clumping and peripheralization of the nerve roots (*arrow 1*), whereas at the more superior levels there is much less clumping of the nerve roots (*arrow 2*).

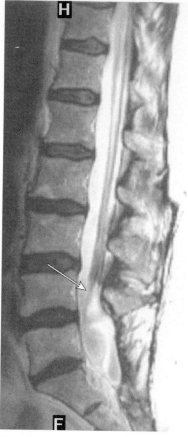

A

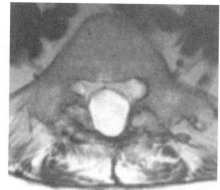

B

FIGURE 3–59

Arachnoiditis. A 64-year-old woman after L4–5 and L5–S1 decompression fusion and new left leg pain. *A,* Sagittal T2WI shows multilevel degenerative and postoperative changes including T12–L1 and L1–2 mild disc dehydration, L2–3 moderate disc dehydration with anterior subchondral degenerative changes, L3–4 moderate disc dehydration, L4–5 moderate disc dehydration with posterior decompression, and L5–S1 moderate loss of disc height and severe disc dehydration. Note that the nerve roots appear to course anteriorly in the lower thecal sac *(arrow).* Flow artifact creates some inhomogeneity of signal intensity within the lower thecal sac. *B,* Axial T2WI at the L5 pedicle level shows changes of posterior decompression with fused facet joints. Note the "empty" appearance of the thecal sac secondary to the nerve roots' adherence to the margins of the spinal canal.

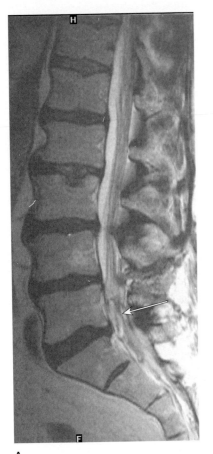

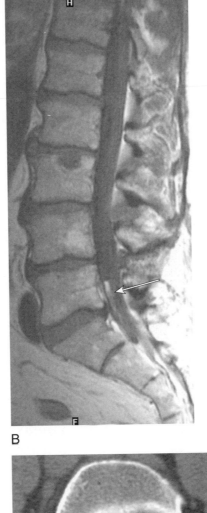

A

B

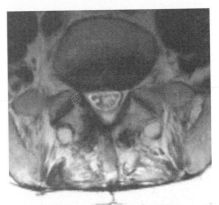

C

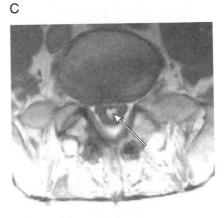

D

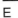

E

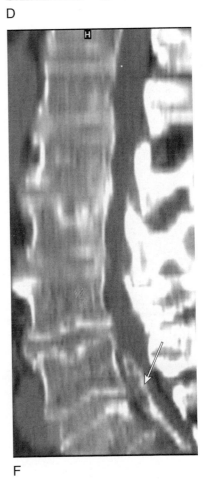

F

FIGURE 3–60

Arachnoiditis ossificans. A 70-year-old man after remote posterior decompression/fusion surgery at L4–5 with low back and bilateral hip and leg pain and foot tingling. *A,* Sagittal T2WI shows multilevel degenerative and postoperative changes including T12–L1 mild loss of disc height and hydration with Schmorl's nodes, L1–2 mild loss of disc height and moderate disc dehydration, L2–3 moderate loss of disc height with heterogeneous disc signal with Schmorl's nodes, L3–4 moderate loss of disc height with severe disc dehydration with degenerative disc bulging and central spinal canal narrowing, L4–5 moderate loss of disc height with severe disc dehydration and posterior postoperative changes, and L5–S1 mild loss of disc height with severe disc dehydration. Note the unusual appearance of nerve roots within the thecal sac and the subtle oblong lesion posterior to the L5 and S1 vertebral bodies *(arrow)*. *B,* Sagittal T1WI shows that the lesion *(arrow)* demonstrates T1 shortening, consistent with fat. *C,* Axial T2WI at the L5–S1 disc level shows a lack of the usual even distribution of nerve roots within the central thecal sac. *D,* Axial T1WI at the L5–S1 disc level shows a central 7-mm focus of T1 shortening *(arrow)*, again consistent with fat. *E,* Axial CT scan just below the L5–S1 disc shows dense calcification/ossification *(arrow)* in the same region as the lesion seen on the axial MRI studies, with a small focus of internal decreased attenuation consistent with fat. Note right posterior postoperative changes. *F,* Sagittal reconstruction CT study shows calcification *(arrow)* corresponding to the lesion that shows T1 and T2 prolongation on the other images. The findings are consistent with calcification/ossification of the thecal sac secondary to arachnoiditis, with conversion of the central portion of the calcified lesion to fat.

References

Abumi K, Shono Y, Ito M, Taneichi H, Kotani Y, Kaneda K. Complications of pedicle screw fixation in reconstructive spine surgery of the cervical spine. Spine 2000; 25:962–969.

Barbera J, Gonzolez J, Esquerdo J, Broseta J, Barcia-Salorio JL. Prophylaxis of the laminectomy membrane: an experimental study in dogs. Neurosurg 1978; 49:419–424.

Barr JD, Barr MS, Lemley TJ, McCann RM. Percutaneous vertebroplasty for pain relief and spinal stabilization. Spine 2000; 25:923–928.

Bednar DA, Raducan V. External spinal skeletal fixation in the management of back pain. Clin Orthop 1996; 322:131–145.

Benoist M, Ficat C, Baraf P, Cauchoix J. Postoperative lumbar epiduro-arachnoiditis: diagnostic and therapeutic aspects. Spine 1980; 5:432–436.

Bickels J, Kahanovitz N, Rubert CK, Henshaw RM, Moss DP, Meller I, Malawer MM. Extraspinal bone and soft-tissue tumors as a cause of sciatica: clinical diagnosis and recommendations. Analysis of 32 cases. Spine 1999; 24:1611–1616.

Bircher MD, Tasker T, Crawshaw C, Mulholland RC. Discitis following lumbar surgery. Spine 1988; 13:98–102.

Boden SD, Davis DO, Dina TS, Parker CP, O'Malley S, Sunner JL, Wiesel SW. Contrast-enhanced MR imaging performed after successful lumbar disk surgery: prospective study. Radiology 1992; 182:59–64.

Bodguk N. Clinical Anatomy of the Lumbar Spine. (3rd Edition). New York, Churchill Livingstone, 1997.

Brantigan JW, Steffee AD, Lewis ML, Quinn LM, Persenaire JM. Lumbar interbody fusion using the Brantigan I/F cage for posterior lumbar interbody fusion and the variable pedicle screw placement system: two-year results from a Food and Drug Administration investigational device exemption clinical trial. Spine 2000; 25:1437–1446.

Braun IF, Lin JP, Benjamin MV, Kricheff II. Computed tomography of the asymptomatic postsurgical lumbar spine: analysis of the physiologic scar. AJR Am J Roentgenol 1984; 142:149–152.

Brodsky AE, Hendricks RL, Dhalil MA, Darden BV, Brotzman TT. Segmental ("floating") lumbar spine fusions. Spine 1989; 14:447–450.

Bryant MS, Bremer AM, Nguyen TQ. Autogenic fat transplants in the epidural space in routine lumbar spine surgery. Neurosurgery 1983; 13:367–370.

Burton CV. Lumbosacral arachnoiditis. Spine 1978; 3:24–30.

Cavanagh S, Stevens J, Johnson JR. High-resolution MRI in the investigation of recurrent pain after lumbar discectomy. J Bone Joint Surg Br 1993; 75:524–528.

Cervellini P, Curri D, Volpin L, Bernardi L, Pinna V, Benedetti A. Computed tomography of epidural fibrosis after discectomy: a comparison between symptomatic and asymptomatic patients. Neurosurgery 1988; 23:710–713.

Cooper RG, Mitchell WS, Illingworth KJ, Forbes W, Gillespie JE, Jayson MIV. The role of epidural fibrosis and defective fibrinolysis in the persistence of postlaminectomy back pain. Spine 1991; 16:1044–1048.

Cyteval C, Sarrabere MPB, Roux JO, Thomas E, Jorgensen C, Blotman F, Sany J, Taourel P. Acute osteoporotic vertebral collapse: open study on percutaneous injection of acrylic surgical cement in 20 patients. AJR Am J Roentgenol 1999; 173:1685–1690.

Davis GW, Onik G, Helms C. Automated percutaneous diskectomy. Spine 1991; 16:359–363.

Davis RA. A long-term outcome analysis of 984 surgically treated herniated lumbar discs. J Neurosurg 1994; 80:415–421.

DePalma AF, Rothman RH. The nature of pseudarthrosis. Clin Orthop 1968; 59:113–118.

Derby R, Howard HW, Grant JM, Lettice JJ, Peteghem PKV, Ryan DP. The ability of pressure-controlled discography to predict surgical and nonsurgical outcomes. Spine 1999; 24:364–372.

Deutsch AL, Howard M, Dawson EG, Goldstein TB, Mink JH, Zeegen EH, Delamarter RB. Lumbar spine following successful surgical discectomy: magnetic resonance imaging features and implications. Spine 1993; 18.1054–1060.

Dina TS, Boden SD, Davis DO. Lumbar spine after surgery for herniated disk: imaging findings in the early postoperative period. AJR Am J Roentgenol 1995; 164:665–671.

Eck KR, Lenke LG, Bridwell KH, Gilula LA, Lashgari CJ, Riew KD. Radiographic assessment of anterior titanium mesh cages. J Spinal Disord 2000; 13:501–510.

El-Khoury GY, Renfrew DL. Percutaneous procedures for the diagnosis and treatment of lower back pain: diskography, facet-joint injection, and epidural injection. AJR Am J Roentgenol 1991; 157:685–691.

Esses SI, Botsford DJ, Kostuik JP. The role of external spinal skeletal fixation in the assessment of low back disorders. Spine 1989; 14:594–601.

Esses SI, Sachs BL, Dreyzin V. Complications associated with the technique of pedicle screw fixation: a selected survey of ABS members. Spine 1993; 15:2231–2239.

Farber GL, Place HM, Mazur RA, Jones DEC, Damiano TR. Accuracy of pedicle screw placement in lumbar fusions by plain radiographs and computed tomography. Spine 1995; 13:1494–1499.

Federowicz SG, Wiesel SW. An algorithm for the multiply operated low back patient and treatment of operative complications. Semin Spine Surg 1991; 3:175–183.

Findlay GF, Hall BI, Musa BS, Oliveira MD, Fear SC. A 10-year follow-up of the outcome of lumbar microdiscectomy. Spine 1998; 23:1168–1171.

Flynn JC, Hoque A. Anterior fusion of the spine: end-result study with long-term follow-up. J Bone Joint Surg Am 1979; 61:1143–1150.

Fouquet B, Goupile P, Jattiot F, Cotty P, Lapierre F, Valat JP, Amouroux J, Benatre A. Discitis after lumbar disc surgery: features of "aseptic" and "septic" forms. Spine 1992; 17:356–358.

Frizzell B, Kaplan P, Dussault R, Sevick R. Arachnoiditis ossificans: MR imaging features in five patients. AJR Am J Roentgenol 2001; 177:461–464.

Frymoyer JW. Back pain and sciatica. N Engl J Med 1988; 318:291–300.

Frymoyer JW, Hanley EN, Howe J, Kuhlmann D, Matteri RE. A comparison of radiographic findings in fusion and nonfusion patients ten or more years following lumbar disc surgery. Spine 1979; 4:435–440.

Frymoyer JW, Selby DK. Segmental instability: rationale for treatment. Spine 1985; 20:280–286.

Gangi A, Dietemann JL, Mortazavi R, Pfleger D, Kauff C, Roy C. CT-guided interventional procedures for pain management in the lumbosacral spine. Radiographics 1998; 18:621–633.

Gertzbein SD, Robbins SE. Accuracy of pedicle screw placement in vivo. Spine 1990; 15:11–14.

Gill K, Blumenthal SL. Functional results after anterior lumbar fusion at L5–S1 in patients with normal and abnormal MRI scans. Spine 1992; 17:940–942.

Grane P, Josephsson A, Seferlis A, Tullberg T. Septic and aseptic postoperative discitis in the lumbar spine—evaluation by MR Imaging. Acta Radiol 1998; 39:108–115.

Guyer DW, Wiltse LL, Eskay ML, Guyer BH. The long-range prognosis of arachnoiditis. Spine 1989; 14:1332–1341.

Hambly MF, Wiltse LL, Raghavan N, Schneiderman G, Koenig C. The transition zone above a lumbosacral fusion. Spine 1998; 23:1785–1792.

Heithoff KB, Mullin WJ, Holte D, Renfrew DL, Gilbert TJ. The failure of radiographic detection of pseudoarthrosis in patients with titanium lumbar interbody fusion cages. Presented at the 26th Annual Meeting of The International Society for the Study of the Lumbar Spine, June 1999, Kona, Hawaii.

Heithoff KB, Ray CD, Schellhas KP, Fritts HM. CT and MRI of lateral entrapment syndromes. In Genant HK (ed). Spine Update 1987. Radiology Research and Education Foundation, San Francisco, CA, 1987.

Hueftle MG, Modic MT, Ross JS, Masaryk TJ, Carter JR, Wilber RG, Bohlman HH, Steinberg PM, Delamarter RB. Lumbar spine: postoperative MR imaging with Gd-DTPA. Radiology 1988; 167:817–824.

Hutter CG. Posterior intervertebral body fusion: a 25-year study. Clin Orthop 1983; 179:86–96.

Jeanneret B, Jovanovic M, Magerl F. Percutaneous diagnostic stabilization for low back pain: correlation with results after fusion operations. Clin Orthop 1994; 304:130–138.

Jinkins JR, Osborn AG, Garrett D, Hunt S, Story JL. Spinal nerve enhancement with Gd-DTPA: MR correlation with the postoperative lumbosacral spine. AJNR Am J Neuroradiol 1993; 14:383–394.

Jonsson B, Soderholm R, Stromqvist B. Erythrocyte sedimentation rate after lumbar spine surgery. Spine 1991; 16:1049–1050.

Karasek M, Bogduk N. Twelve-month follow-up of a controlled trial of intradiscal thermal annuloplasty for back pain due to internal disc disruption. Spine 2000; 25:2601–2607.

Karasick D, Schweitzer ME, Vaccaro AR. Complications of cervical spine fusion: imaging features. AJR 1997; 169:869–874.

Keller JT, Dunsker SB, McWhorter JM, Ongkiko CM, Saunders MC, Mayfield FH. The fate of autogenous grafts to the spinal dura: an experimental study. J Neurosurg 1978; 49:412–418.

Kellgren JH. On the distribution of pain arising from deep somatic structures with charts of segmental pain areas. Clin Sci 1939; 4L:35–46.

Kim SS, Michelsen CB. Revision surgery for failed back surgery syndrome. Spine 1992; 17:957–960.

Kirkaldy-Willis WH, Farfan HF. Instability of the lumbar spine. Clin Orthop 1982; 165:110–123.

Kostiuk JP. Failures after spine fusion. In Frymoyer JW (ed). The Adult Spine: Principles and Practice, 2nd ed. Philadelphia, Lippincott-Raven, 1997.

Kuslich SD, Ulstrom CL, Griffith SL, Ahern JW, Dowdle JD. The Bagby and Kuslich method of lumbar interbody fusion: history, techniques, and 2-year follow-up results of a United States prospective, multicenter trial. Spine 1998; 23:1267–1279.

Laasonen EM, Soini J. Low back pain after lumbar fusion: surgical and computed tomographic analysis. Spine 1989; 14:210–213.

Lang P, Chafetz N, Genant HK, Morris JM. Lumbar spine fusion: assessment of functional stability with magnetic resonance imaging. Spine 1990; 15:581–588.

Lang P, Genant HK, Chafetz N, Steiger P, Morris JM. Three-dimensional computed tomography and multiplanar reformations in the assessment of pseudarthrosis in posterior lumbar fusion patients. Spine 1988; 13:69–75.

Langrana NA, Hawkins MV, Zimmerman M, Lee CK, Parsons JR. Spinal fusions: past, present, and future. Semin Spine Surg 1993; 5:81–87.

Law JD, Lehman RAW, Kirsch WM. Reoperation after lumbar intervertebral disc surgery. J Neurosurg 1978; 48:259–263.

Lehmann TR, Spratt KF, Tozzi JE, Weinstein JN, Reinarz SJ, El-Khoury GY, Colby H. Long-term follow-up of lower lumbar spine fusion patients. Spine 1987; 12:97–104.

Link SC, El-Khoury GY, Guilford WB. Percutaneous epidural and nerve root block and percutaneous lumbar sympatholysis. Radiol Clin North Am 1998; 36:509–521.

Mathews HH. Transforaminal endoscopic microdiscectomy. Neurosurg Clin North Am 1996; 7:59–63.

McAfee PC, Cunningham BW, Lee GA, Orbegoso CM, Haggerty CJ, Fedder IL, Griffith SL. Revision strategies for salvaging or improving failed cylindrical cages. Spine 1999; 24:2147–2153.

McCall IW, Park WM, O'Brien JP. Induced pain referral from posterior lumbar elements in normal subjects. Spine 1979; 4:441–446.

Montaldi S, Fankhauser H, Schnyder P, de Tribolet N. Computed tomography of the postoperative intervertebral disc and lumbar spinal canal: investigation of 25 patients after successful operation for lumbar disc herniation. Neurosurgery 1988; 22:1014–1022.

Mullin WJ, Heithoff KB, Gilbert TJ, Renfrew DL. Magnetic resonance evaluation of recurrent disc herniation: is gadolinium necessary? Spine 2000; 25:1493–1499.

Ng P, Lorentz I, Soo US. Arachnoiditis ossificans of the cauda equina demonstrated on computed tomography scanogram: a case report. Spine 1996; 21:2504–2507.

Odgers CJ, Vaccaro AR, Pollack ME, Cotler JM. Accuracy of pedicle screw placement with the assistance of lateral plain radiography. J Spinal Disord 1996; 9:334–338.

Olmarker K, Rydevik B. Single- versus double-level nerve root compression: an experimental study on the porcine cauda equina with analyses of nerve impulse conduction properties. Clin Orthop 1992; 279:35–39.

Porter RW, Ward D. Cauda equina dysfunction: the significance of two-level pathology. Spine 1992; 17:9–15.

Post MJD, Sze G, Quencer RM, Eismont FJ, Green BA, Gahbauer H. Gadolinium-enhanced MR in spinal infection. J Comput Assist Tomogr 1990; 14:721–729.

Quencer RM, Murtagh FR, Post JD, Rosomoff HL, Stokes NA. Postoperative bony stenosis of the lumbar spinal canal: evaluation of 164 symptomatic patients with axial radiography. AJR Am J Roentgenol 1978; 131:1059–1064.

Ray CD. Threaded titanium cages for lumbar interbody fusions. Spine 1997; 22:667–679.

Ross JS, Masaryk TJ, Schrader M, Gentili A, Bohlman H, Modic MT. MR imaging of the postoperative lumbar spine: assessment with gadopentetate dimeglumine. AJR Am J Roentgenol 1990; 155:867–872.

Ross JS, Robertson JT, Frederickson RCA, Petrie JL, Obuchowski N, Modic MT, de Tribolet N. Association between peridural scar and recurrent radicular pain after lumbar discectomy: magnetic resonance evaluation. Neurosurgery 1996; 38:855–863.

Rothman RH, Booth R. Failures of spine fusion. Orthop Clin North Am 1975; 6:299–303.

Rothman SLG, Glenn WV, Kerber CW. Postoperative fractures of lumbar articular facets: occult cause of radiculopathy. AJR Am J Roentgenol 1985; 145:779–784.

Rudisch A, Kremser C, Peer S, Kathrein A, Judmaier W, Daniaux H. Metallic artifacts in magnetic resonance imaging of patients with spinal fusion: a comparison of implant materials and imaging sequences. Spine 1998; 23:692–699.

Rupp RE, Ebraheim NA, Wong FF. The value of magnetic resonance imaging of the postoperative spine with titanium implants: case report. J Spine Disord 1996; 9:342–346.

Saal JS, Saal JA. Intradiscal electrothermal treatment for chronic discogenic low back pain: a prospective outcome study with minimum 1-year follow-up. Spine 2000a; 25:2622–2627.

Saal JS, Saal JA. Management of chronic discogenic low back pain with a thermal intradiscal catheter: a preliminary report. Spine 2000b; 25:382–388.

Schwarzenbach O, Berlemann U, Jost B, Visarius H, Arm E, Langlotz F, Nolte LP, Ozdoba C. Accuracy of computer-assisted pedicle screw placement: an in vivo computed tomography analysis. Spine 1997; 22:452–458.

Sharif HS. Role of MR imaging in the management of spinal infections. AJR Am J Roentgenol 1992; 158:1333–1345.

Sjostrom L, Jacobsson O, Karlstrom G, Pech P, Rauschning W. CT analysis of pedicles and screw tracts after implant removal in thoracolumbar fractures. J Spinal Disord 1993; 6:225–231.

Soini J, Slatis P, Kannisto M, Sandelin J. External transpedicular fixation test of the lumbar spine correlates with the outcome of subsequent lumbar fusion. Clin Orthop 1993; 293:89–96.

St. Amour TE, Hodges SC, Laakman RW, Tamas DE (eds). MRI of the Spine. New York, Raven Press, 1994.

Suk K-S, Lee H-M, Moon S-H, Kim N-H. Recurrent lumbar disc herniation: results of operative management. Spine 2001; 26:672–676.

Tamburrelli F, Leone A, Pitta L. A rare cause of lumbar radiculopathy: spinal gas collection. J Spinal Disord 2000; 13:451–454.

Taylor BA, Vaccaro AR, Hilibrand AS, Zlotolow DA, Albert TJ. The risk of foraminal violation and nerve root impingement after anterior placement of lumbar interbody fusion cages. Spine 2001; 26:100–104.

Teplick JG, Peyster RG, Teplick SK, Goodman LR, Haskin ME. CT identification of postlaminectomy pseudomeningocele. AJR Am J Roentgenol 1983; 140:1203–1206.

Tullberg T, Rydberg J, Isacson J. Radiographic changes after lumbar discectomy: sequential enhanced computed tomography in relation to clinical observation. Spine 1993; 18:843–850.

Turner JA, Ersek M, Herron L, Deyo R. Surgery for lumbar spinal stenosis: attempted meta-analysis of the literature. Spine 1992; 17:1–8.

van Akkerveeken PF. On pain patterns of patients with lumbar nerve root entrapment. Neuroorthopedics 1993a; 14:81–102.

van Akkerveeken PF. The diagnostic value of nerve root sheath infiltration. Acta Orthop Scand (Suppl 251) 1993b; 64:61–63.

van der Schaaf DB, van Limbeek J, Pavlov PW. Temporary external transpedicular fixation of the lumbosacral spine. Spine 1999; 24:481–485.

Weatherley CR, Prickett CF, O'Brien JP. Discogenic pain persisting despite solid posterior fusion. J Bone Joint Surg Br 1986; 38:142–143.

Weiner BK, Fraser RD. Lumbar interbody cages. Spine 1998; 23:634–640.

Wiesner L, Kothe R, Schulitz KP, Ruther W. Clinical evaluation and computed tomography scan analysis of screw tracts after percutaneous insertion of pedicle screws in the lumbar spine. Spine 2000; 25:615–621.

Yong-Hing K, Reilly J, de Korompay V, Kirkaldy-Willis WH.
    Prevention of nerve root adhesions after laminectomy. Spine 1980;
    5:59–64.
Zdeblick TA. A prospective, randomized study of lumbar fusion:
    preliminary results. Spine 1993; 18:983–991.

Zinreich SJ, Long DM, Davis R, Quinn CB, McAfee PC, Wang H.
    Three-dimensional CT imaging in postsurgical "failed back"
    syndrome. J Comput Assist Tomogr 1990; 14:574–580.

4 Imaging of Spine Tumors

DONALD L. RENFREW • SANJAY SALUJA • MICHAEL W. HAYT

Definitions

Textbooks (Cassidy 1997, Heller 1997, Masaryk 1994, Osborn 1994, Ross 2000, St. Amour 1994) typically divide tumors of the spine into compartments originally defined by the myelographic appearance of the lesion (Shapiro 1984). Although myelography has been supplanted by magnetic resonance imaging (MRI) (supplemented where necessary by computed tomography [CT] or CT-myelography), the classification system remains. The three compartments provided by this classification system are (1) intramedullary, (2) intradural-extramedullary (IDEM), and extramedullary. *Intramedullary* tumors are tumors of the spinal cord; *IDEM* tumors are tumors within the dura but not arising within the spinal cord; and *extramedullary* tumors arise outside the dura. All three categories contain not only several histolog-

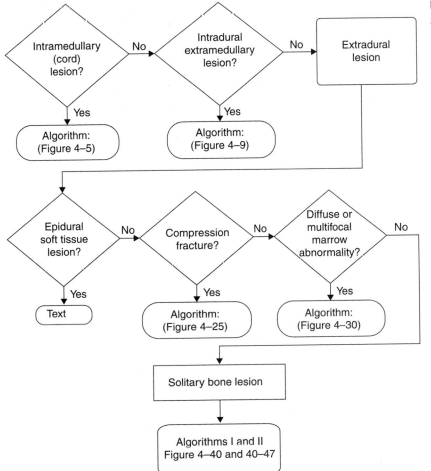

FIGURE 4–1

Algorithm for spine tumor on MRI.

ic types of tumor but also many tumor mimics. The first step in tumor evaluation requires placing the lesion into one of the three categories (Fig. 4–1). We subdivide the "extramedullary" category into epidural soft tissue lesions, compression fractures, diffuse and multifocal marrow abnormalities, and solitary bone lesions. Some tumors may not fit neatly into these categories, either because they involve more than one compartment or because it is sometimes more difficult to differentiate intradural and extradural processes with MRI than it is with myelography (which was the imaging modality for which the compartmentalization scheme was devised). It may be necessary to base the categorization of lesions on where the tumors appear centered or to consider both IDEM and extradural processes for a given lesion.

Imaging

Although the initial radiographic categorization of tumors was by myelography, this test is now infrequently performed for the primary evaluation of suspected tumors. Furthermore, many tumors are discovered when imaging the spine for nonspecific symptoms of pain or radiculopathy, and this imaging is usually done with MRI. Therefore, at least the initial study will be done using the imaging protocols for evaluation of these clinical symptoms (usually designed to detect degenerative processes).

PLAIN FILMS

Plain films show intramedullary and IDEM tumors only in those cases with associated bone expansion or erosion (Cassidy 1997), which usually occurs late in the disease process. Plain films may allow tissue characterization in certain highly typical bone lesions (e.g., hemangiomas) but are often insensitive, nonspecific, and of little diagnostic utility.

MAGNETIC RESONANCE IMAGING

MRI is the study of choice for evaluation of tumors of the spine, and often no other studies are necessary (Heller 1997, Masaryk 1991, Smoker 1987, Sze 1991). Contrast-enhanced studies assist in determining tumor extent, differentiating tumor from peritumoral edema and cysts, evaluating involvement of dura and other important structures, and detecting possible additional lesions (Heller 1997, Parizel 1989, Ross 2000). Therefore, the minimum evaluation should include axial and sagittal precontrast and postcontrast T1- (T1WI) and T2-weighted images (T2WI). Coronal examinations may be helpful in some cases, particularly in laterally located or multilevel lesions. The dynamics of contrast enhancement have been studied, and, generally, imaging at a routine time following injection of contrast agent (0 to 30 minutes) will allow adequate characterization of most lesions, although delayed imaging of certain necrotic tumors may be useful (Sze 1989).

COMPUTED TOMOGRAPHY

In primary and metastatic extramedullary (bone) tumors of the spine, CT scanning often provides important additional information to MRI, including the extent of cortical bone destruction and calcified tumor matrix (Beltran 1987). Additional characterization of the lesion may allow a specific diagnosis to be rendered (e.g., hemangioma, osteoid osteoma) or at least rated as highly likely (e.g., osteoblastoma, aneurysmal bone cyst). Thin cuts (3-mm slices at 2-mm intervals or 1-mm contiguous slices) allow sagittal and coronal reconstructions; these should be obtained whenever possible in any bone tumor to allow better lesion characterization.

NUCLEAR MEDICINE

Bone scintigraphy serves two functions in imaging of tumors in the spine. Perhaps the more important function is to allow a widespread search for additional lesions (Frank 1990). This provides both staging and often a biopsy site more amenable to safe and easy access than the spine (Heller 1997). Bone scintigraphy may also be helpful in evaluation of a lesion of questionable significance on plain films, CT, or MRI. If such a lesion demonstrates no abnormality on nuclear medicine, it may be assumed to be "benign" or "inactive." Although this is not an unreasonable approach when the prior probability of disease is low, nuclear medicine may be falsely negative: highly aggressive lesions, multiple myeloma, and leukemia (Boriani 1997b) are notorious for showing no bone scan abnormality despite histologically confirmed tumor. MRI is more sensitive in the detection of tumor in the spine than bone scintigraphy, provided the area with the tumor is scanned (Algra 1991, Colletti 1991, Frank 1990, Kostiuk 1997); of course, one cannot screen the entire skeleton with MRI as one can with a nuclear medicine study.

[18]F-fluorodeoxyglucose (FDG) positron-emission tomography (PET) is revolutionizing oncologic imaging, and Daldrup-Link and associates (2001) have recently reported that FDG PET is superior to both skeletal scintigraphy *and* MRI in detection of bone marrow metastases.

Intramedullary (Cord) Lesions

To cut to the chase, there is usually no way to tell on imaging whether a cord tumor is an astrocytoma (Fig. 4–2), an ependymoma (Fig. 4–3), or one of several less frequently seen primary cord tumors (Fig. 4–4) (Bourgouin 1998, Cassidy 1997, Ross 2000) (Table 4–1). Furthermore, different grades of astrocytoma have different prognoses and require different treatment, but the grade cannot be determined preoperatively (Cassidy 1997, Ross 2000). A definite diagnosis requires biopsy, and whether the radiologist is correct or incorrect in predicting the cell type is of no material consequence to either the patient or the surgeon. Therefore, the role of the radiologist is not to provide a particular histologic diagnosis but rather (to the extent possible) tell whether the biopsy is genuinely indicated and to provide the surgeon with the pertinent anatomic features of the tumor. This will allow biopsy (and resection, if warranted by histologic examination) to proceed with the least possible difficulty.

The surgeon ultimately decides whether the biopsy is genuinely indicated, but the radiologist may be of great

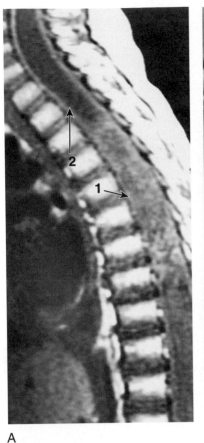

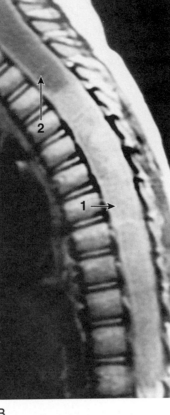

A   B

FIGURE 4–2

Intramedullary tumor with nonspecific imaging features. A 4-year-old boy with new-onset weakness of both upper and lower extremities. *A,* Sagittal T1WI demonstrates extensive expansion of the spinal cord (*arrow 1*) with associated syrinx (*arrow 2*). *B,* Sagittal T1WI following contrast demonstrates the tumor (*arrow 1*) and syrinx (*arrow 2*). Histologic analysis revealed a low-grade astrocytoma.

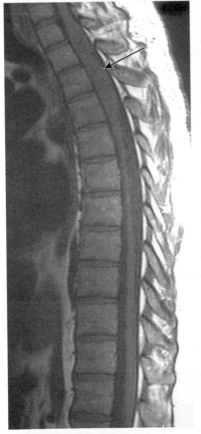

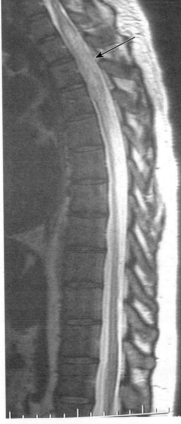

A   B

FIGURE 4–3

Intramedullary tumor with nonspecific imaging features. A 34-year-old man with lower extremity spasticity. *A,* Sagittal T1WI demonstrates fusiform enlargement of the thoracic spinal cord from T1 through T4 (*arrow*) with a diminished caliber below this level. *B,* Sagittal T2WI again demonstrates fusiform enlargement of the thoracic spinal cord from T1 through T4 (*arrow*), with inhomogeneous signal intensity within the abnormal area of the spinal cord. This imaging appearance is nonspecific, with the main considerations being primary spinal cord astrocytoma and ependymoma. Histologic evaluation revealed an ependymoma, although astrocytoma or any of several less likely tumors are possible on the basis of imaging alone.

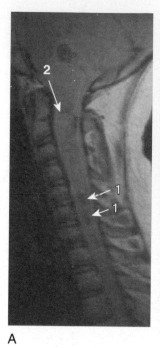

A

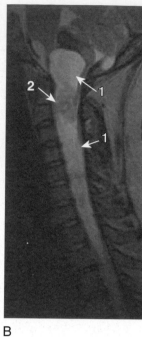

B

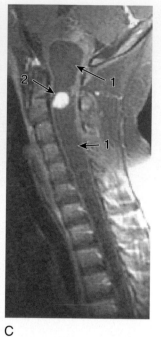

C

FIGURE 4–4

Intramedullary tumor with nonspecific imaging features. A 13-year-old boy with progressive right arm weakness and difficulty walking. *A,* Sagittal T1WI demonstrates a lesion of the cervical cord, with foci of T1 prolongation (*arrows 1*) and a nodular, isointense mass (*arrow 2*). *B,* Sagittal T2WI demonstrates syringobulbia (*arrows 1*) and again shows the cervical cord mass (*arrow 2*). *C,* Sagittal T1WI following contrast administration demonstrates syringobulbia (*arrows 1*) and intense contrast enhancement of the mass (*arrow 2*). Histology revealed a ganglioglioma of the cervical cord.

TABLE 4–1. Intramedullary Lesions

Intramedullary Lesion	Differential Diagnosis

Solitary
    (Bourgouin 1998, Cassidy 1997,
    Masaryk 1994, Parizel 1989)
	Tumor
	    Astrocytoma
	    Ependymoma
	    Hemangioblastoma
	    Lipoma
	    Dermoid
	    Teratoma
	    Primitive neuroectodermal
	    Ganglioglioma
	    Primary cord lymphoma
	    Primary cord melanoma
	    Cavernous hemangioma
	    Metastatic deposit
	Tumor mimics
	    Vascular malformation
	    Demyelinating disease (multiple sclerosis, ADEM)
	    Vasculitis
	    Transverse myelitis
	    Radiation myelitis
	    Infarction
	    Syringomyelia from arachnoiditis
	    Sarcoidosis
	    Fungus
	    Parasites
	    Immune-mediated and idiopathic myelitis

Multiple	Tumor
	    "Drop mets"
	    Hematogenous mets
	    Granulomatous disease
	    Demyelinating disease

ADEM, acute disseminated encephalomyelitis; mets, metastasis.

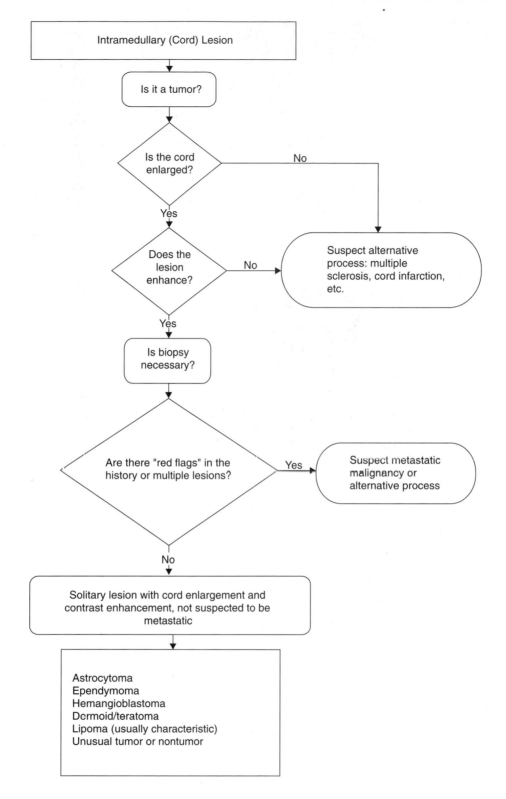

FIGURE 4–5

Algorithm of an intramedullary (cord) lesion.

assistance by evaluating the lesion for those features that may obviate a biopsy (Fig. 4–5). The first step in evaluation is to determine whether the lesion really is a tumor. Several processes may superficially (or not so superficially) resemble a tumor but usually do not require biopsy to establish the diagnosis (see Table 4–1). These include multiple sclerosis, sarcoidosis, vasculitis, radiation myelitis, vascular malformations, and cord infarction (see Chapter 9) (Bourgouin 1998, Cassidy 1997, Ross 2000). In cases of genuine cord tumor, the cord is almost always enlarged, and

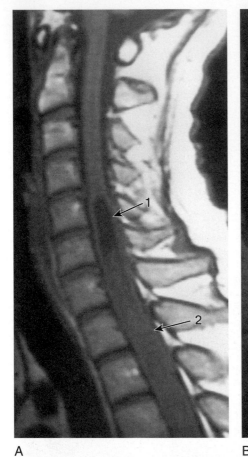

A

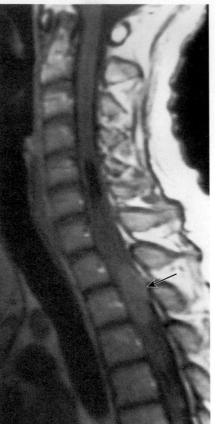

B

FIGURE 4–6

Intramedullary metastasis. A 31-year-old man previously treated for medulloblastoma now presenting with cervical pain and upper extremity sensory changes. *A*, Sagittal T1WI demonstrates a focus of T1 prolongation (*arrow 1*) posterior to the C5 and C6 vertebral bodies with expansion of the cord below this level (*arrow 2*). *B*, Sagittal T1WI following contrast administration demonstrates an oblong area of contrast enhancement centered at the T1 level (*arrow*).

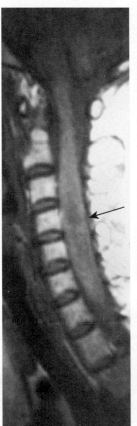

A

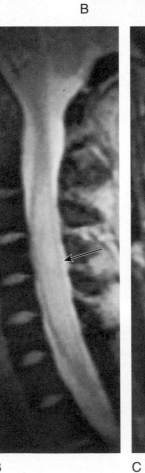

B

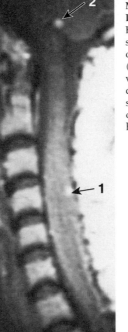

C

FIGURE 4–7

Multiple hemangioblastomas in a patient with Von Hippel-Lindau syndrome. A 9-year-old boy with known Von Hippel-Lindau syndrome presenting with upper cervical spine myelopathy. *A*, Sagittal T1WI demonstrates expansion of the cervical spinal cord with central T1 prolongation (*arrow*). *B*, Sagittal T2WI also shows expansion of the cord with T2 prolongation. *C*, Sagittal postcontrast T1WI demonstrates punctate areas of enhancement along the pial surface of the cord at the C4 level (*arrow 1*) and at the level of the cervicomedullary junction (*arrow 2*), consistent with hemangioblastomas.

the lesion almost always demonstrates contrast enhancement. The absence of either of these two features should cause the radiologist to review the available history, obtain additional history, and suggest the possibility of an alternative diagnosis (Cassidy 1997, Ross 2000, Sze 1988). If multiple sclerosis is a possibility, imaging of the remainder of the cord and brain should be done to look for additional characteristic lesions, and cerebrospinal fluid (CSF) analysis for oligoclonal bands should be performed. Benign syrinx does not require biopsy, and the cervicomedullary junction should be included in evaluation of a suspected syrinx to determine if a Chiari malformation is present (Cassidy 1997). Contrast-enhanced examination is necessary in the evaluation of any syrinx, because enhancement of any portion of the syrinx wall may indicate an otherwise occult tumor. Note that although the absence of contrast enhancement in an intramedullary lesion argues strongly *against* tumor, the presence of contrast enhancement does not necessarily *imply* tumor: multiple sclerosis, granulomatous disease, myelitis, sarcoidosis, and infarction are among the many nonmalignant causes of abnormal cord enhancement (Bourgouin 1998).

If the lesion does indeed demonstrate strong imaging features of being a tumor, it may still not require biopsy. Cord metastases, although once considered rare, are being seen with greater frequency, probably because of a combination of more widespread imaging capabilities and increased survivorship with tumor (Fig. 4–6) (Cassidy 1997, Ross 2000). The most frequently seen primary sites generating cord metastases include the lung, breast, and kidney. Generally speaking, a patient with a known tumor outside the cord and a cord lesion more likely has a metastatic cord deposit than a second primary. If a tissue diagnosis of metastatic tumor is required, other locations for tumor should be sought with a physical examination, and, if necessary, a chest/abdomen/pelvis CT and a bone scan. Considering the technical factors and attendant morbidity of spinal cord biopsy, almost any other site in the body is preferable.

Some patients may have certain "red flags" in the history suggesting metastatic malignancy (Waddell 1998). These include constant, progressive, nonmechanical pain; unexplained weight loss; and a previous history of carcinoma. Often, relatives or a primary care physician will note that the patient does not "seem right." Although any individual with a cord tumor (metastatic or not) may also manifest these symptoms, the symptoms should suggest the possibility of metastatic disease. A thorough review of systems may uncover symptoms of a lung, gastrointestinal, or urinary tract malignancy (Heller 1997). Specific symptoms (e.g., hemoptysis) should trigger appropriate additional testing (e.g., chest plain films and/or CT). If the patient manifests no particular symptoms but is still believed likely to have an extraspinal primary malignancy, a chest/abdomen/pelvis CT may disclose characteristic abnormalities in many individuals (Rougraff 1993). In men, prostate examination and prostate-specific antigen (PSA) determination, and in women, breast examination and mammography help diagnose (or exclude) two common primary malignancies.

The study disclosing the cord tumor should be carefully examined for any additional lesions of either the intra-

medullary or IDEM variety. The presence of multiple lesions makes metastatic deposit more likely not only from sources outside the neuraxis but also "drop metastases" from a primary brain tumor. The brain and remainder of the cord should be imaged in any patient with more than one cord lesion to see if lesions characteristic of primary brain malignancy, phakomatoses (Fig. 4–7), or granulomatous disease are present. Discovery of multiple lesions usually either provides a diagnosis or at least an alternative method of diagnosis (e.g., CSF tap) instead of cord biopsy. Of course, a family history of phakomatosis should be sought in any patient with a central nervous system tumor.

To review, after taking these steps to eliminate what does *not* need to undergo biopsy, we are left with a solitary lesion that enlarges the spinal cord and demonstrates contrast enhancement in a patient who is relatively unlikely to have a primary tumor elsewhere. We emphasize that the differential diagnosis at this point still includes astrocytoma (both low and high grade), ependymoma, hemangioblastoma, dermoids, teratomas, and cavernous angiomas (Cassidy 1997, Parizel 1989, Ross 2000). In addition to these benign and malignant primary tumors, metastatic disease and an unusual presentation of non-neoplastic disease are also still possibilities. Preoperatively, features that the radiologist should mention that will help the surgeon include the size and levels of the tumor (so that an appropriate laminectomy may be performed for lesion access) and the presence of any associated cyst or syrinx (so that surgical drainage of these may be planned). If the lesion is likely to represent a hemangioblastoma (a densely enhancing solitary tumor nodule within a cavity occupied at least partially by feeding vessels), this should be specifically noted, because biopsy and central debulking of the lesion may be relatively contraindicated (Baker 2000, Cassidy 1997). Gross and histologic examination at the time of surgery is necessary to determine the possibility of resection and grade of malignancy. Generally, the surgeon will attempt removal of low-grade astrocytomas and ependymomas, and these lesions have a relatively good prognosis, whereas high-grade astrocytomas carry a poor prognosis regardless of treatment (Cassidy 1997).

Intradural-Extramedullary (IDEM) Lesions

As is the case with intramedullary (cord) lesions, MRI features of intradural-extramedullary (IDEM) tumors generally do not allow tissue characterization (Fig. 4–8). The eventual histologic diagnosis is in the hands of the neurosurgeon and pathologist. Also, as in the case of cord lesions, the radiologist may be of benefit by ensuring that a biopsy is indeed necessary and in characterizing the lesion to the extent possible with existing imaging technology (Fig. 4–9).

IDEM metastases (as cord metastases) will probably be seen with greater frequency in the years to come owing to widespread imaging and increased survivorship among cancer patients. Metastatic deposit should be considered the most likely cause of an IDEM lesion in a patient with a known primary malignancy, and the same work-up considerations noted earlier in the evaluation of patients with intramedullary lesions apply to patients with IDEM lesions:

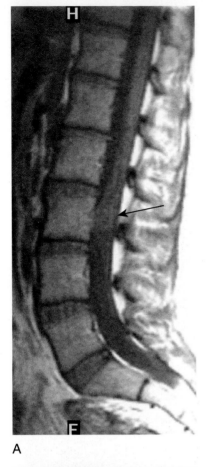

A

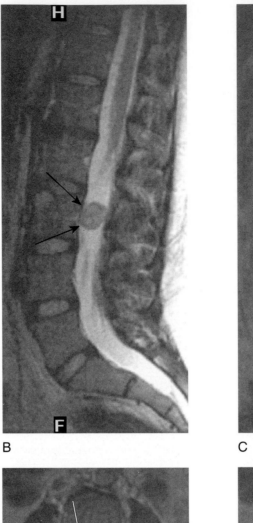

B

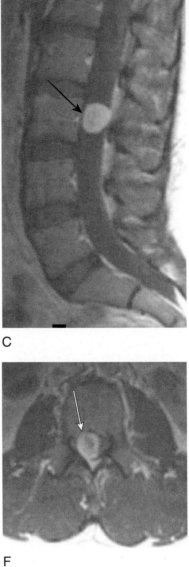

C

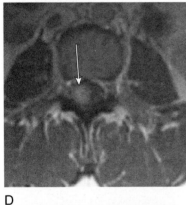

D

E

F

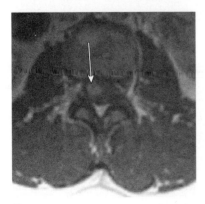

G

FIGURE 4–8

Intradural extramedullary tumor: schwannoma. A 23-year-old woman with chronic low back and right leg pain. *A*, Sagittal T1WI demonstrates a 16 × 14-mm oval lesion within the spinal canal at the L3 level with intermediate signal intensity *(arrow)*. *B*, Sagittal T2WI demonstrates the lesion; note the acute angle formed by cerebrospinal fluid invaginating along the lesion margins *(arrows)*, typical of an intradural, extramedullary lesion. *C*, Sagittal T1WI following contrast enhancement demonstrates the lesion *(arrow)*; there is intense contrast enhancement, with much greater lesion conspicuity than on precontrast images. *D–G*, Sequential axial post-contrast T1WI demonstrates the slightly eccentric position of the lesion within the spinal canal. There is intense contrast enhancement, particularly along the periphery of the lesion. At surgery, a schwannoma was removed.

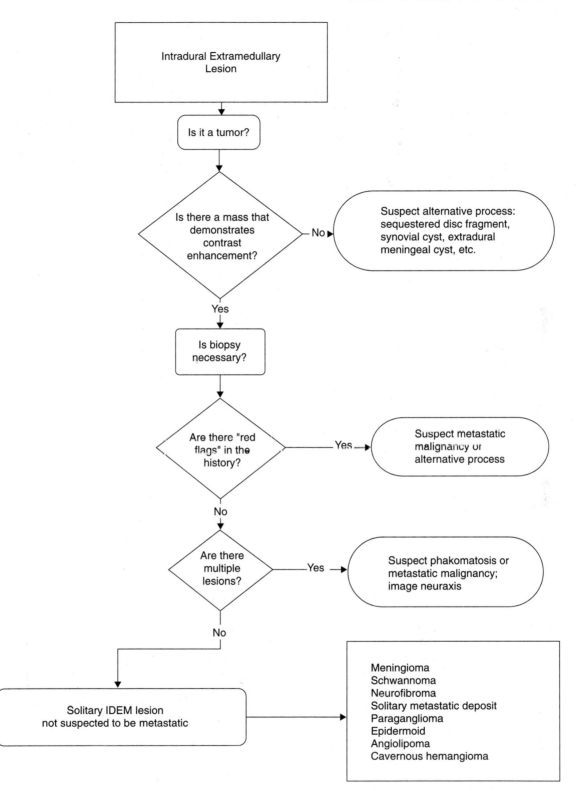

FIGURE 4–9

Algorithm of an intradural extramedullary (IDEM) lesion.

a review of systems for suspicious findings (hemoptysis, hematuria, hematochezia, unexplained lumps) and possibly a chest/abdomen/pelvis CT scan, supplemented by mammography in women and PSA and digital prostatic examination in men (Heller 1997).

IDEM lesions present with multiple abnormalities more frequently than do cord lesions, since the primary phakomatosis, neurofibromatosis I, will demonstrate multiple neurofibromas (Fig. 4–10) (Egelhoff 1992, Ross 2000). Multiple lesions usually represent neurofibromas, multiple

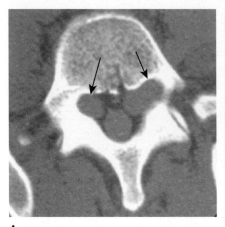

A

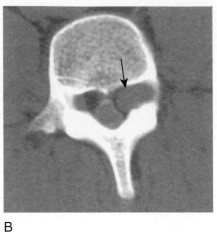

B

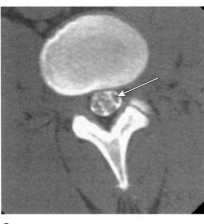

C

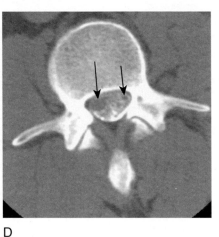

D

FIGURE 4–10

Multiple intradural-extramedullary lesions in neuro-fibromatosis. A 44-year-old man with low back and bilateral thigh and leg pain. The patient had a pacer in place because of a congenital heart abnormality and was thus not a candidate for MRI. *A–D,* Selected 3-mm CT-myelogram images demonstrate multiple intradural-extramedullary lesions *(arrows).* There is associated bone remodeling and complete block of contrast flow, so that the lower images demonstrate no intrathecal contrast.

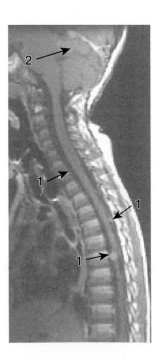

FIGURE 4–11

Drop mets from myxopapillary ependymoma. A 3-year-old girl seen by pediatric oncologists for palliative spinal radiation therapy with known metastatic disease. Sagittal T1WI following contrast shows multiple intradural-extramedullary lesions *(arrows 1)* representing "drop mets" from a primary tumor of the brain *(arrow 2).*

metastatic deposits, or (less likely) granulomatous tissue. If a lesion typical of hemangioblastoma (a densely enhancing solitary tumor nodule within a cavity occupied at least partially by feeding vessels) is found, examination of the brain should be performed to search for additional hemangioblastomas (and make the presumptive diagnosis of Von Hippel-Lindau syndrome) (Fig. 4–7) (Ross 2000). Malignant cells from primary brain tumors may seed the CSF and cause "drop mets," which are typically IDEM lesions (Fig. 4–11).

If there is diffuse enhancement of the dura, with or without nodularity, then the differential diagnosis includes leptomeningeal carcinomatosis (either from hematogenous or brain lesions) (Fig. 4–12), superficial siderosis from repeated intrathecal bleeding, granulomatous disease, and myelomatous meningitis (Table 4–2). The histologic diagnosis cannot be provided with MRI, but evaluation of CSF is diagnostic in most cases (Ross 2000). Multiple accompanying vertebral compression fractures suggests myelomatous meningitis (Quint 1995)

If non-neoplastic lesions, metastatic deposit, and multiple lesions have been excluded, this still leaves several histologic varieties of both benign and malignant lesions in the differential diagnosis. In general terms, a solitary IDEM tumor of the thoracic spine is most likely a meningioma (Fig. 4–13), a solitary nerve sheath tumor a schwannoma, and a solitary lesion in the lumbar spinal cord a myxopapillary ependymoma (Fig. 4–14), but these rules are only generalizations (Fig. 4–15). We reiterate that the neurosurgeon and the pathologist will provide the ultimate diagnosis (Fig. 4–16). Although malignant IDEM tumors are typically bigger and demonstrate more poorly defined margins than benign IDEM tumors, overlap in imaging findings prevents differentiation by imaging characteristics (Ross 2000). Therefore, as with cord lesions, the surgeon must obtain a biopsy of the lesion to establish a diagnosis. Fortunately, most of these lesions are benign and can be resected, and the patient outcome is frequently good with improved (or at least maintained) neurologic function and decreased pain (Cassidy 1997). The radiologist must provide the surgeon with the exact, correct level of the lesion. Remember that the surgeon is generally limited to fluoroscopic capabilities for localization in the operating room, so specific note of any transitional features of anatomy and double-checking the involved level are crucial. If the IDEM is of the dumbbell variety, with a portion in the spinal canal but another portion through the neural foramen, note the size of the extraforaminal component with respect to the associated foramen: the surgeon usually chooses to sacrifice the facet joint (and plan for fusion surgery if in the lumbar or cervical spine) if the lesion cannot be delivered through the foramen from a posterior approach (Cassidy 1997).

Tumor mimics with IDEM lesions rather than cord lesions (Table 4–2) include sequestered disc herniations (see Chapter 2), extradural meningeal cysts, nerve root sleeve diverticula, and vascular malformations (see Chapter 9). Sequestered disc herniations, extradural meningeal cysts, and nerve root sleeve diverticula generally do not enhance with contrast material, and vascular malformations often have a typical "bag-of-worms" appearance on imaging.

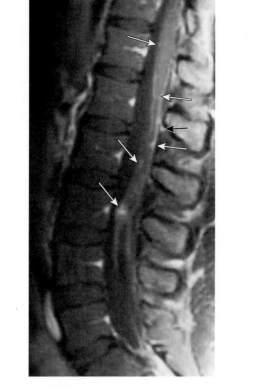

FIGURE 4–12

Multiple intradural-extramedullary lesions from metastatic disease. Sagittal T1WI following contrast enhancement demonstrates multiple, variably sized enhancing nodules of the meninges (arrows), as well as generalized leptomeningeal enhancement. The patient had diffuse leptomeningeal melanoma metastases.

TABLE 4–2. Intradural-Extramedullary Lesions

Intradural-Extramedullary Lesion	Differential Diagnosis

Single
(Cassidy 1997, Parizel 1989)
	Tumor
	  Meningioma
	  Schwannoma (neuroma, neurinoma, neurilemmoma)
	  Neurofibroma
	  Metastatic deposit
	  Paraganglioma
	  Epidermoid
	  Angiolipoma
	  Cavernous hemangioma (Carlier 2000)
	  Ependymoma (Duffau 2000)
	Tumor mimics
	  Sequestered disc herniation
	  Meningeal cysts (Nabors 1988)
	  Vascular malformations

Multiple	Metastatic disease
	Phakomatosis
	  Neurofibromas in neurofibromatosis
	  Hemangioblastomas in Von Hippel-Lindau Syndrome
	Granulomatous disease

Diffusely enhancing dura	Leptomeningeal carcinomatosis Superficial siderosis Granulomatous disease Myelomatous meningitis (Quint 1995)

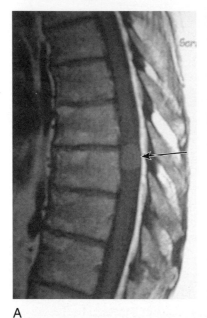

A

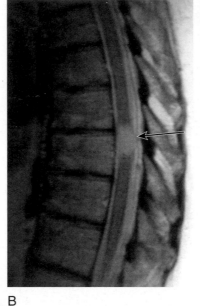

B

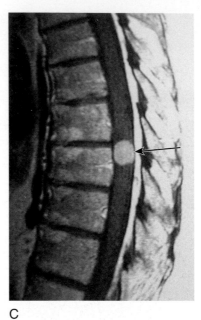

C

D

FIGURE 4–13

Solitary, intradural-extramedullary lesion of the thoracic spine: meningioma. A 57-year-old woman with mid back pain. *A,* Sagittal T1WI MRI demonstrates a 12 × 10-mm smoothly marginated lesion *(arrow)* within the spinal canal at the T8 level. *B,* Sagittal proton density images demonstrate T2 prolongation within the lesion *(arrow)*. *C,* Sagittal postcontrast MRI demonstrates uniform, intense contrast enhancement of the lesion *(arrow)*. *D,* Axial postcontrast images at the T7 pedicle level demonstrate the lesion *(arrow 1)* along the right side of the spinal canal, with marked compression of the spinal cord into a small crescent along the left side of the canal *(arrow 2)*. Histologic examination revealed a meningioma.

FIGURE 4–14

Intradural-extramedullary lesion of the upper lumbar spinal canal representing a myxopapillary ependymoma. A 7-year-old boy with back pain and increasing difficulty with ambulation over the past 2 months. *A,* Sagittal T2WI demonstrates a disrupted appearance of the conus medullaris nerve roots *(arrow 1)* and a large lesion with relatively uniform T2 prolongation filling the spinal canal from the mid L2 vertebral body inferiorly *(arrow 2)*. *B,* Sagittal T1WI following contrast administration demonstrates contrast enhancement of the lesion within the spinal canal *(arrow)*. *C,* Axial T1WI shows the lesion to fill the spinal canal. Because of T1 prolongation within the lesion, it resembles cerebrospinal fluid and is difficult to appreciate. *D,* Axial T1WI following contrast administration demonstrates the lesion much better, with intense contrast enhancement of much of the lesion *(arrow)*.

A

B

C

D

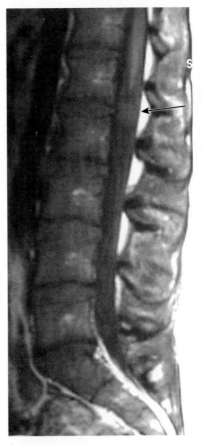

A

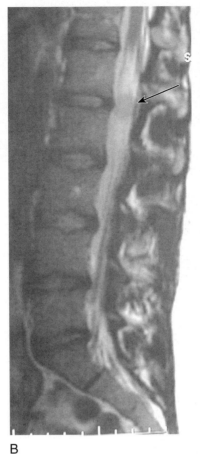

B

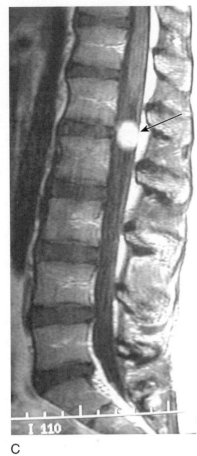

C

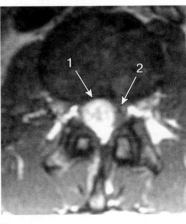

D

FIGURE 4–15

Solitary intramedullary-extradural lesion of the lumbar spinal canal. A 19-year-old man with low back pain radiating into the buttocks. *A,* Sagittal T1WI demonstrates a subtle round lesion of the cauda equina *(arrow)*. *B,* Sagittal T2WI shows the lesion to demonstrate intermediate signal intensity *(arrow)*. *C,* Sagittal T1WI following contrast enhancement demonstrates intense contrast enhancement of the lesion *(arrow)*. *D,* Axial T1WI following contrast enhancement demonstrates intense contrast enhancement of the lesion *(arrow 1)*. The spinal cord is compressed into a crescent on the left side of the spinal canal *(arrow 2)*. Histologic examination revealed a schwannoma.

Extradural Tumors

The nonspecific category of "extradural tumors" includes both epidural soft tissue masses and bone and joint lesions. Occasionally, nonspine bone and soft tissue tumors cause sciatica (Fig. 4–17) (Bickels 1999) or are seen at the margins of the spine examination (Fig. 4–18) (Olson 1994); for the most part, these lesions require separate imaging dedicated to the body part of origin, unless the examination provides complete characterization (Fig. 4–19).

For the purposes of our analysis, and with an eye to clinical use, we divide extradural lesions in the spine into the following categories: epidural soft tissue masses, compression fractures, marrow abnormality (diffuse or multifocal), and solitary bone lesions (Table 4–3 and Fig. 4–1).

EPIDURAL SOFT TISSUE MASSES

Myelography and CT-myelography, more so than MRI, allow more precise differentiation of epidural soft tissue masses and IDEM lesions since intradural lesions present as filling defects of the contrast column and epidural lesions indent the contrast column from outside. Differentiation of epidural soft tissue lesions and IDEM processes may be

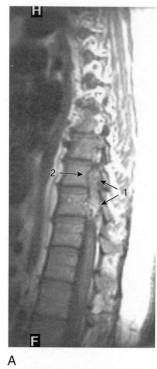

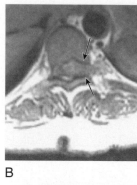

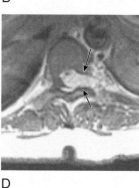

B

C

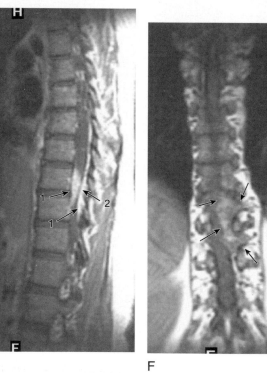

A

D

E

F

FIGURE 4–16

Intradural-extramedullary lesion. A 51-year-old patient with progressive lower extremity weakness. *A,* Left parasagittal T1WI demonstrates an inhomogeneous mass (*arrows 1*) with scalloping of the posterior aspect of the T9 vertebral body (*arrow 2*). Note areas of T1 prolongation. *B,* Axial T1WI at the level of the T9–10 neural foramen demonstrates the lesion expanding the foramen (*arrows*). *C,* Axial T2WI at the level of the T9–10 neural foramen demonstrates marked T2 prolongation of the lesion (*arrows*). *D,* Axial T1WI at the level of the T9–10 neural foramen following injection of contrast material demonstrates intense contrast enhancement of the lesion (*arrows*). *E,* Sagittal T1WI following contrast administration also demonstrates intense contrast enhancement of the lesion (*arrow 1*). The lesion extends up and down the epidural space at the T9 and T10 levels and displaces and compresses the spinal cord (*arrow 2*). *F,* Coronal T1WI following contrast administration demonstrates the lesion extending out the T8–9 and T9–10 neural foramina (*arrows*). Histologic examination revealed an angiolipoma, with lipid accounting for the T1 shortening seen on the precontrast T1WI.

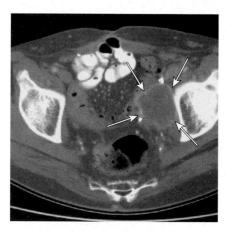

FIGURE 4–17

Pelvic tumor causing radicular pain. An 80-year-old man with left hip and lateral leg pain suggesting L5 radicular pain. The patient had a history of bladder cancer, and both a lumbar and pelvic CT were performed. *A,* Axial CT at the level of the mid pelvis demonstrates a 4.5-cm average diameter mass of the left pelvis with peripheral enhancement (*arrows*) consistent with necrotic metastatic disease.

more difficult with MRI. Extruded and sequestered disc fragments comprise many of the epidural soft tissue masses encountered in daily practice (see Chapter 2). Even when the disc of origin is not obvious and the lesion appears sizable relative to what would be expected based on visible disc pathology, a sequestered disc (with or without accompanying hematoma) is a far more likely diagnosis than a primary or metastatic epidural neoplasm. Synovial cysts of the facet joints (see Chapter 2) may also mimic epidural or intramedullary, extradural soft tissue tumors, but the loca-

tion of these lesions adjacent to degenerated facet joints usually makes diagnosis obvious (Fig. 4–20). Metastatic epidural tumors (Fig. 4–21) are most frequently seen with the same primary lesions as produce intramedullary and IDEM metastatic deposit: lung, breast, and kidney. Primary epidural soft tissue tumors include lymphoma (Fig. 4–22), hemangioma, angiolipoma (Fig. 4–23), extradural meningioma (Fig. 4–24), and neurofibroma (Fig. 4–10) (Boriani 1997b). Multiple lesions increase the likelihood of phakomatosis and metastatic deposit.

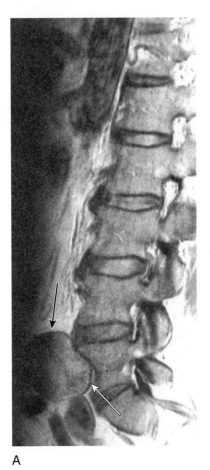

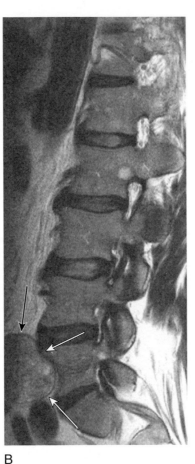

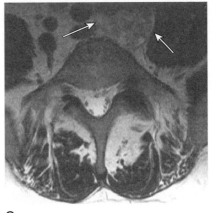

C

FIGURE 4–18

Serendipitously discovered retroperitoneal tumor. A 44-year-old man with low back and bilateral leg pain. *A*, Sagittal T1WI demonstrates a 4 × 3-cm lesion anterior to the L5 vertebral body with inhomogeneous signal intensity (*arrows*). *B*, Sagittal T2WI shows the lesion (*arrows*) to have mixed, predominantly slightly increased signal intensity. *C*, Axial T2WI demonstrates the lesion (*arrows*) between the L5 vertebral body and psoas muscle, displacing the psoas muscle anteriorly and toward the left. Histology of the lesion was a schwannoma.

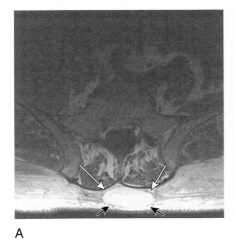

A

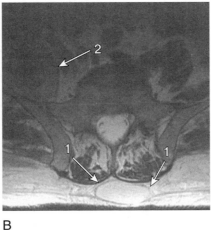

B

FIGURE 4–19

Lipoma of the dorsal subcutaneous tissues. An 82-year-old man with right lower extremity weakness (particularly right quadriceps weakness). *A*, Axial T1WI demonstrates a 48 × 22-mm lesion (*arrows*) with T1 shortening within the dorsal subcutaneous fat. *B*, Axial T2WI shows the same lesion (*arrows 1*) with signal intensity following the subcutaneous fat, slightly less pronounced on T2WI versus T1WI. The smooth margins of the lesion, along with the signal characteristics, are classic for a benign lipoma and require no further specific evaluation. Notice, however, that the patient has a 8 × 5-cm lesion of the right iliac fossa (*arrow 2*) (difficult to see on these images, which have been windowed and leveled for maximal visualization of the posterior subcutaneous fat). The patient was anticoagulated at the time of evaluation, and sequential follow-up CT scans demonstrated resolution of the lesion, consistent with a hematoma.

COMPRESSED VERTEBRAL BODY WITH ABNORMAL SIGNAL INTENSITY

Vertebral bodies demonstrating loss of height are almost always old wedge compression fractures and have the same marrow signal intensity as adjacent vertebrae (Fig. 4–25). These present no challenge to diagnosis, because if the marrow signal is the same as adjacent, normal levels, the likelihood of tumor is virtually nonexistent. At the other end of the spectrum, when the marrow is diffusely abnormal, and when there are multiple additional marrow abnormalities

seen at other levels on the same scan, the patient almost certainly has metastatic disease (Figs. 4–26 and 4–27). The difficulty comes in determining whether a single wedged vertebra demonstrating at least some abnormal marrow signal intensity represents an acute or subacute benign compression fracture or a fracture through tumor. Imaging features in this case may still be characteristic enough to allow treatment without biopsy. If the abnormal signal intensity of the marrow is confined to the vertebral body (and does not extend into the pedicles) and if the vertebral body has a combination of abnormal *and* normal signal intensity

TABLE 4–3. Extradural Lesions

Extradural Lesions	Differential Diagnosis

Epidural soft tissue lesion	Tumor
	   Hemangioma
	   Angiolipoma
	   Lipoma
	   Meningioma
	   Neurofibroma
	   Lymphoma
	   Metastatic deposit
	Tumor mimics
	   Extruded disc
	   Sequestered disc
	   Synovial cyst

Compressed vertebral body with abnormal signal intensity of marrow	Acute or subacute compression fracture, with or without osteoporosis Pathologic fracture through tumor
Diffusely abnormal marrow Multiple geographic lesions of marrow with T1 and T2 prolongation	Hemangiomas (atypical) Metastatic deposit Multiple myeloma Sarcoidosis (Fisher 1999)

T1 shortening	Myeloid depletion pattern
	   Radiation therapy
	   Chemotherapy

T1 shortening with isointensity on T2-weighted and STIR images	Reconversion Sclerotic metastatic deposit Leukemia Lymphoma Gaucher disease Myelofibrosis Infection (at levels other than discitis) (Stabler 2000)
T1 and T2 prolongation	Reconversion Metastatic deposit Multiple myeloma

Solitary bone or joint lesion	Characteristic tumor mimics
	   Paget's disease
	   Facet joint abnormality
	Characteristic benign tumors
	   Hemangioma
	   Osteoid osteoma
	Other lesions
	   Aneurysmal bone cyst
	   Osteoblastoma
	   Enchondroma
	   Eosinophilic granuloma
	   Osteosarcoma
	   Chondrosarcoma
	   Ewing's sarcoma
	   Chordoma
	   Solitary metastatic deposit
	   Lymphoma
	   Myeloma
	   Unusual presentations of meningioma

STIR, Short tau inversion recovery.

within it, with a linear interface between the abnormal and normal marrow, the overwhelming likelihood is that the patient has a benign compression fracture (Fig. 4–28) (An 1995, Baker 1990, Yuh 1989). Lack of contrast enhancement favors a benign fracture, but the presence of contrast enhancement may be seen in both fracture and tumor (An 1995, Heller 1997). If the findings favor a benign fracture,

a follow-up study may be obtained in 2 to 3 months. This should show a decrease in the amount of abnormal marrow and decreased contrast enhancement in a benign fracture (An 1995, Heller 1997). On the other hand, if the entire vertebral body has abnormal signal intensity, or if the abnormal signal intensity extends into the pedicles, or if there is marked contrast enhancement of the lesion, tumor

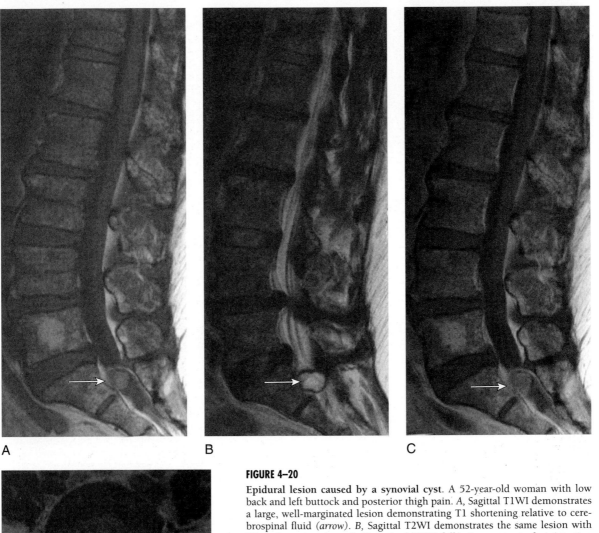

A   B   C

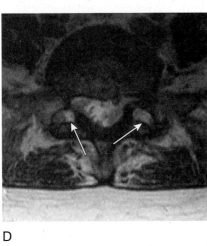

D

FIGURE 4–20

Epidural lesion caused by a synovial cyst. A 52-year-old woman with low back and left buttock and posterior thigh pain. *A*, Sagittal T1WI demonstrates a large, well-marginated lesion demonstrating T1 shortening relative to cerebrospinal fluid *(arrow)*. *B*, Sagittal T2WI demonstrates the same lesion with T2 prolongation *(arrow)*. *C*, Sagittal T1WI following contrast administration demonstrates no significant lesion enhancement *(arrow)*. *D*, Axial T2WI through the lower L5–S1 facet joints demonstrates bilateral large effusions *(arrows)*. The left effusion tracked directly into the large synovial cyst.

should be suspected and the patient should be evaluated for sources of primary tumor (Fig. 4–29) (An 1995, Baker 1990, Yuh 1989). CT of the spine may be of some benefit in problem cases: occasionally, frank cortical or cancellous bone destruction may strongly suggest a malignancy. In cases where tumor of the vertebrae is suspected but there is no known primary tumor, further examination would usually include a bone scan to search for additional possible metastatic deposits and a chest/abdomen/pelvis CT to evaluate possible primary tumors (Heller 1997, Rougraff 1993). Such scans may demonstrate the cause of metastatic deposit, but occasionally it is still necessary to obtain a biopsy of the vertebral lesion for histologic diagnosis.

A recent development that holds promise as a method of discriminating between benign and malignant tumors is diffusion-weighted images: there is strong signal attenuation in benign fractures, with minimal signal attenuation in fractures through tumor (Baur 1998, Spuentrup 2001).

DIFFUSE MARROW ABNORMALITY

The spine imager is an "accidental" marrow screener: as the site of a combination of hematopoietic (red) and inactive (yellow) marrow, the spine provides a window into a number of disease processes, many of which have overlapping findings and a confusing imaging appearance (Vogler

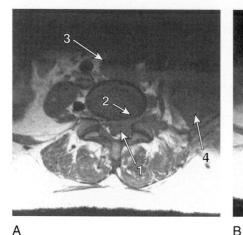
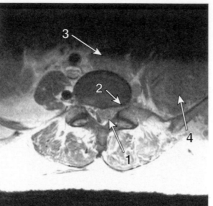

A   B

FIGURE 4–21

Epidural lesions from metastatic disease. A 63-year-old patient with known metastatic malignant melanoma and progressive lower extremity weakness. *A* and *B,* Axial precontrast and postcontrast T1WI at the level of the L4–5 disc demonstrates extensive metastatic deposit, including extensive epidural soft tissue abnormality (*arrow 1*) extending through the left neural foramen (*arrow 2*), anterior soft tissue abnormality adjacent to the vertebral body (*arrow 3*), and soft tissue lesions along the left side of the pelvis (*arrow 4*).

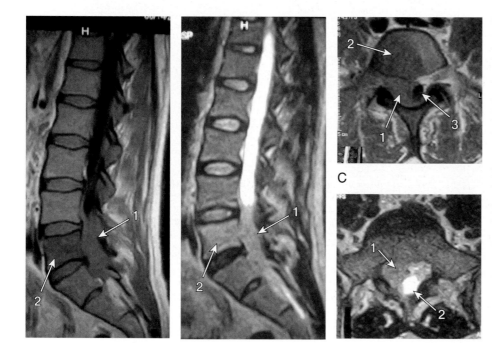

A   B   D

FIGURE 4–22

Epidural lesion in lymphoma. A 44-year-old man with low back pain and leg weakness. *A,* Sagittal T1WI demonstrates extensive epidural tumor in the lower thecal sac (*arrow 1*), as well as T1 prolongation of the L5 vertebral body (*arrow 2*). *B,* Sagittal T2WI again demonstrates abnormal epidural tissue filling the spinal canal from the L4–5 disc space inferiorly (*arrow 1*). The abnormal marrow in L5 is much less conspicuous on the T2WI (*arrow 2*). *C,* Axial T1WI demonstrates the epidural lymphoma (*arrow 1*) as well as T1 prolongation within the L5 vertebral body (*arrow 2*) secondary to tumor replacement of fat-containing marrow. The thecal sac (*arrow 3*) is displaced to the left and compressed by this epidural lesion. *D,* Axial T2WI demonstrates epidural tumor (*arrow 1*) and a posteriorly displaced and compressed thecal sac (*arrow 2*).

1988). Abnormal-appearing marrow does not necessarily imply tumor, but tumor is certainly one of the major concerns whenever diffusely abnormal marrow is encountered (Fig. 4–30).

Multiple, discrete lesions demonstrating geographic borders with T1 and T2 prolongation almost always represent metastatic disease (Figs. 4–26 and 4–31). Correlation with the clinical history and investigation with a review of systems, appropriate laboratory evaluation, and additional imaging as required usually result in a diagnosis without the necessity of a spine biopsy. Multiple myeloma and lymphoma (Fig. 4–32) (which are variably classified as primary or metastatic spine tumors [Kostiuk 1997]) share these imaging features, as do some nonmalignant processes such as sarcoidosis (Fig. 4–33) (Fisher 1999).

If there is diffuse T1 shortening (a predominantly fatty pattern), this virtually always represents a benign process. This "myeloid depletion" pattern may be seen as a consequence of radiation therapy (Figs. 4–28 and 4–34), chemotherapy, myelofibrosis (Fig. 4–35), or the predominantly fatty pattern seen in older patients (St. Amour 1994, Vogler 1988). Such a pattern is not indicative of metastatic deposit. Fatty marrow may also have a single or multifocal appearance that may accompany aging and degenerative changes (Hajek 1987) (Fig. 4–36) or present as a normal variant with fatty marrow along the basivertebral plexus (Fig. 4–37).

Diffuse T1 prolongation may be associated with less benign consequences. The first step is to define what constitutes genuine T1 prolongation. In older children and

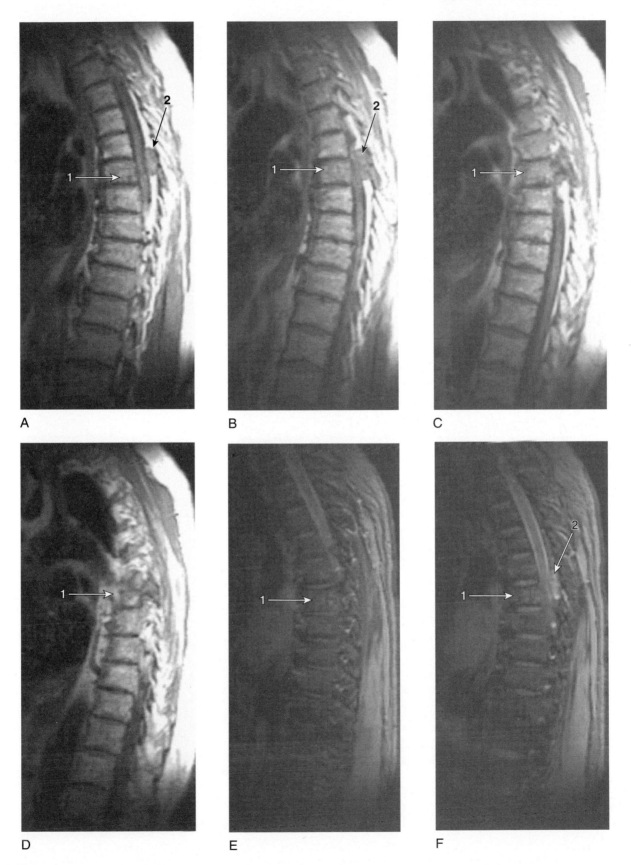

FIGURE 4–23

Epidural soft tissue lesion with a combined bony lesion representing an angiolipoma. A 65-year-old woman with an 18-month history of increasing leg numbness, tingling, and paresthesias. *A–D,* Sequential right-to-left T1WIs demonstrate an abnormal appearance of the T6 vertebral body *(arrow 1)* with a posterior epidural mass *(arrow 2)* and associated flattening of the spinal cord. *E–H,* Sequential right-to-left gradient-recalled echo T2WIs demonstrate T2 prolongation within the vertebral body *(arrow 1)* and lesion *(arrow 2)*. *I–N,* Sequential inferior-to-superior axial images through the T6 vertebral body

(continued)

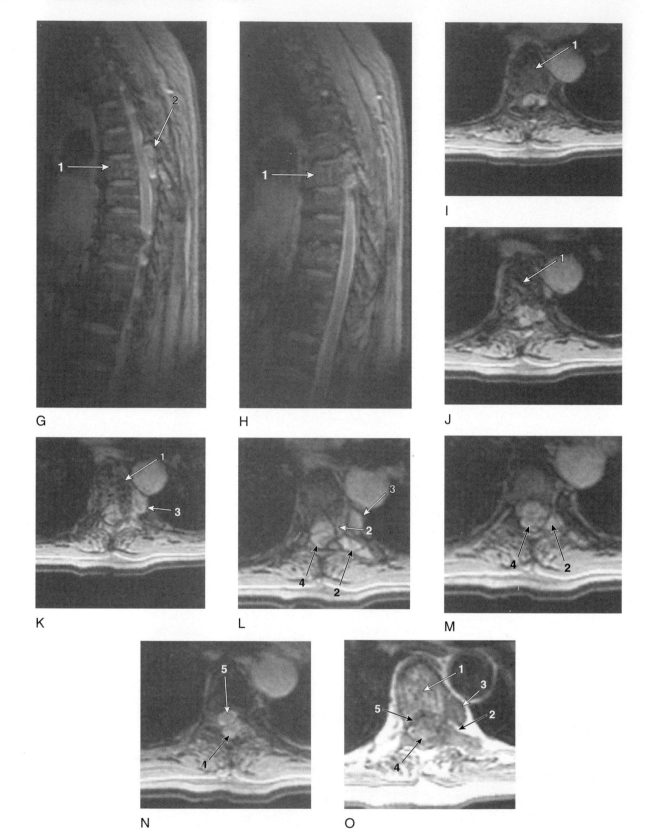

FIGURE 4–23 *(continued)*

including the lesion demonstrates a "salt-and-pepper" appearance of the vertebral body *(arrow 1)* along with abnormal marrow in the left pedicle and transverse process *(arrow 2)*, an extraspinal mass along the left side of the vertebral body *(arrow 3)*, and a posterior epidural mass *(arrow 4)*. The spinal cord *(arrow 5)* is displaced anteriorly and flattened. *O*, Axial T1WI at the T6 transverse process level again demonstrates the salt-and-pepper appearance of the vertebral body *(arrow 1)*, abnormal marrow in the transverse process *(arrow 2)*, an extraspinal mass along the vertebral body *(arrow 3)*, a posterior epidural mass *(arrow 4)*, and an anteriorly displaced and flatted spinal cord *(arrow 5)*. Histologic examination of the epidural component of the lesion revealed an angiolipoma.

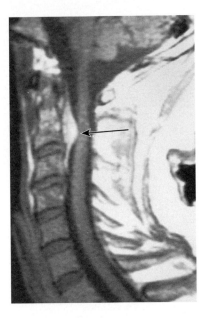

FIGURE 4–24

Extradural meningioma. A 39-year-old patient with neck pain. Sagittal T1WI following contrast enhancement demonstrates a fusiform anterior epidural mass behind the C2 vertebral body (*arrow*).

adults, the marrow should have greater signal intensity than the intervertebral disc on T1WI (St. Amour 1994, Vogler 1988); when the discs have relatively greater signal intensity than the marrow (the "bright disc" sign), this is abnormal (Fig. 4–31). This follows from the fact that fat comprises a significant amount of yellow marrow (80%). If the marrow is unequivocally decreased in signal intensity on T1WI, then the yellow marrow has been replaced, either by red marrow or other tissue. If the marrow shows no hyperintensity on T2WI and short tau inversion recovery (STIR) images, then tumor (although not entirely excluded) can be considered much less likely (Figs. 4–38 and 4–39). Conversion to red marrow (even if patchy and occasionally bizarre in appearance) is more likely than tumor. It may be prudent to screen the patient for anemia and renal disease with simple laboratory tests (Vogler 1988).

If the marrow demonstrates T1 and T2 prolongation, tumor is relatively more likely (Fig. 4–31). In these cases, pay special attention to detect any focal abnormalities (which would place the patient in the "multiple discrete abnormalities" category). If there are no discrete abnormalities, correlation with routine serum chemistries, a history of malignancy, and immunoelectrophoresis in the elderly (to evaluate for myeloma) may be appropriate.

SOLITARY BONE LESIONS

Application of an oncologic staging system, careful surgical planning, and the development and refinement of extensive surgical techniques (vertebrectomy, hemivertebrectomy, and posterior arch resection) have resulted in significant improvements in short- and long-term outcomes for patients with solitary spine tumors (Boriani 1997b). Imaging plays a key role in the diagnosis and surgical plan-

ning for these patients (Fig. 4–40). From the surgeon's perspective, the approach to primary bone tumors of the spine (which are rare compared to metastatic disease) involves three steps: "(1) achieve the diagnosis; (2), stage the lesion and decide the adequate margin; and (3), plan surgery according to these criteria" (Boriani 1997b). Diagnosis and management of primary spine neoplasms are exciting and rapidly evolving fields of knowledge. Recognizing that any attempt at a rigid algorithm for diagnosis and therapy may be overturned with next month's journal articles, we nonetheless attempt to provide an overview of how best to assist the spine surgeon to accomplish the three steps of diagnosis, lesion staging, and surgical planning.

First, we note that there are several generalizations that may be true but usually do not provide enough diagnostic power to affect patient management in a given instance. With respect to clinical history, patients with spine tumors usually present with back pain, with or without radicular symptoms. Of course, patients with degenerative processes present with the same complaints and thus this clinical presentation does not help much in the diagnosis of spine tumors. Patients with tumor have more constant, nonmechanical pain that is often worse at night (Boriani 1997b). Occasionally, however, patients with degenerative processes have a similar history, and since degenerative processes are literally thousands of times more common than tumors, a patient with unrelenting pain or night pain is more likely to have an uncommon presentation of degenerative disease instead of a common presentation of a tumor.

The age of the patient and location of the tumor provides a broad but not necessarily useful perspective. In patients younger than 21 years of age, most tumors will be benign, whereas in those older than 21 years, 70% will be malignant (Boriani 1997b). Posterior element tumors tend to be benign, whereas lesions of the vertebral body are more likely malignant. Again, these general rules do not actually help much in the evaluation of a given individual with a spine tumor, because therapy is aimed at specific cell types, and making this diagnosis requires either a highly characteristic radiographic appearance, biopsy result, or both.

In distinction to these generalities regarding spine tumors, the radiographic appearance of some spine lesions (e.g., hemangiomas, osteoid osteoma, and enostosis (bone island)) may be so characteristic that biopsy may not be required. In other cases (e.g., eosinophilic granuloma), although there is a characteristic radiographic appearance, biopsy will be necessary because of the small chance of an alternative diagnosis (with eosinophilic granuloma, the differential must include Ewing's sarcoma and unusual infection) and because tradition and convention dictate that histologic proof of the lesion be obtained prior to therapy (Boriani 1997b). On occasion, aneurysmal bone cysts demonstrate pathognomonic radiographic features, and in some cases selective arterial embolization may be based on clinical and radiographic features without the benefit of biopsy (Boriani 2001). Many lesions, however, have a nonspecific appearance at imaging and almost always require biopsy or go without a specific diagnosis. Even after biopsy, the diagnosis may be elusive (Kozlowski 1984). We now provide some guidelines regarding the various cell types and imaging appearance.

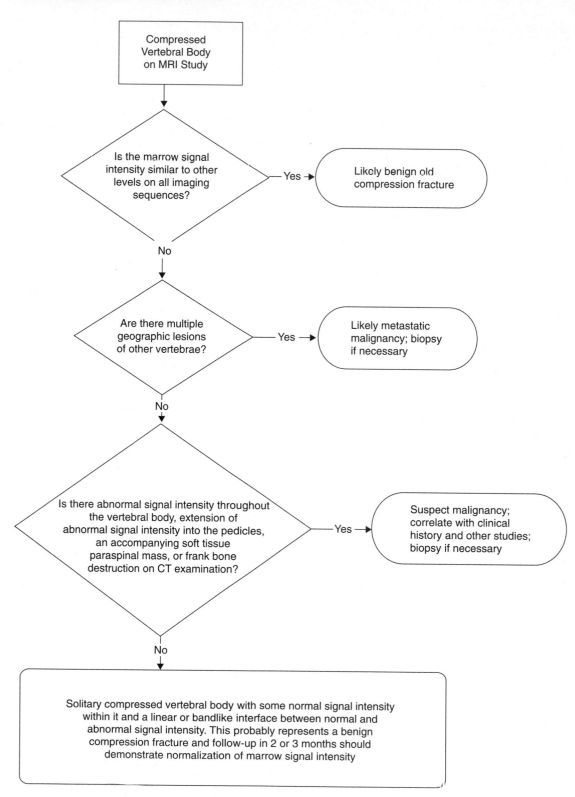

FIGURE 4–25

Algorithm of a compressed vertebral body.

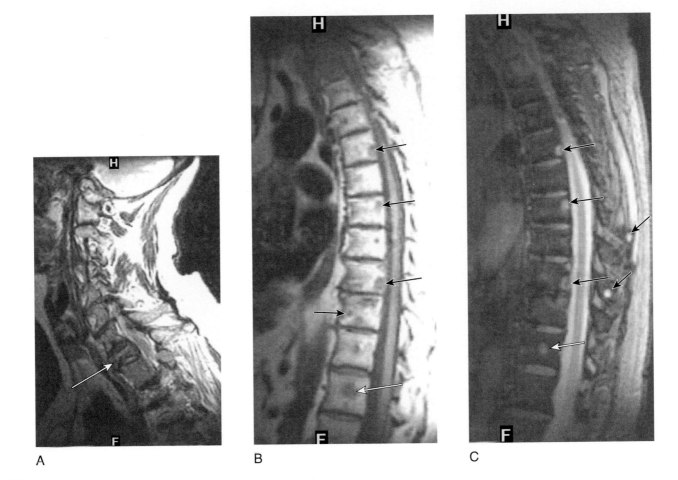

FIGURE 4–26

Compression fracture with obvious metastatic disease. A 78-year-old woman with breast cancer and multiple bone metastases. *A,* Sagittal T2WI through the cervical region demonstrates marked scoliosis and compression of the T1 vertebral body *(arrow).* Because of the scoliosis, it is somewhat difficult to appreciate the abnormal marrow of C7, T1, and T2. *B,* Sagittal T1WI of the thoracic spine demonstrates multiple, variably sized lesions *(arrows)* with extensive marrow abnormality seen in the T2 vertebral body at the top of the field. *C,* Sagittal gradient-recalled echo T2WI confirms multiple abnormalities *(arrows),* with variably sized foci of T2 prolongation scattered throughout the visualized marrow. Such multiple, variably sized lesions are highly characteristic of metastatic deposit.

Hemangioma

Hemangiomas are ubiquitous benign lesions that are so common that they are often not even mentioned in radiology reports. The typical MRI appearance includes T1 shortening and T2 prolongation because of adipose tissue within the lesion (Fig. 4–41) (Ross 1987), although some areas of many hemangiomas also show T1 and T2 prolongation because of extracellular fluid, particularly at the margin of the lesion. CT and MR imaging both typically demonstrate thickened trabeculae within the hemangioma (Fig. 4–42). When these imaging features are identified, biopsy is virtually never necessary and the diagnosis can be made with confidence on the imaging features alone.

Rarely, hemangiomas become symptomatic. Symptoms usually follow expansion of the bony cortex or soft tissue penetrating the cortex into the epidural space, with resultant neural compression (Fig. 4–43) (Laredo 1986). When this happens, the tissue outside the cortex will not share the characteristic imaging feature of containing fat (Ross 1987). However, the imaging appearance may still be specific enough to allow treatment without a histologic diagnosis: if

the intraosseous component of the lesion demonstrates classic findings of a hemangioma and treatment is necessary because of extraosseous expansion, angiography followed by embolotherapy (Laredo 1986) may be performed without biopsy. Alternately, the tumor may be ablated with an intralesion injection of ethanol (Doppman 2000). Surgical removal followed by radiotherapy may also be performed on lesions resulting in neurologic compromise (Lee 1999).

Osteoid Osteoma

Osteoid osteomas are small (<2 cm) lesions (Frassica 1996) that may be intensely painful. Given the typical clinical scenario of a young person with back pain worse at night and relieved by anti-inflammatory medication, and given typical imaging features on CT and a bone scan, treatment may be proceed without biopsy or at least combined with biopsy at a single setting. The MR appearance is not specific, with (generally speaking) T1 prolongation and T2 shortening (Fig. 4–44). The bone scan demonstrates intense, unifocal uptake at the site of the lesion. The CT scan shows a cen-

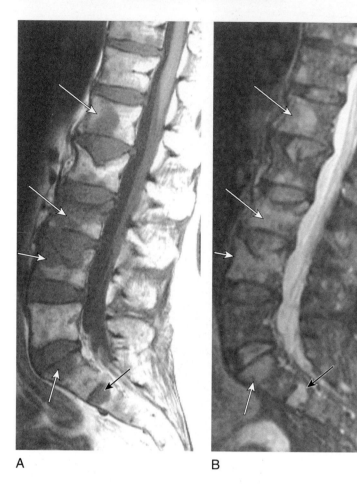

A   B

FIGURE 4–27

Compression fractures with obvious metastatic disease. A 68-year-old woman with low back and bilateral hip pain. *A,* Sagittal T1WI demonstrates multiple, variably sized foci of T1 prolongation scattered throughout the visualized marrow (*arrows*). There is deformity of L2, L3, and L4, with associated marrow abnormality at the L3 and L4 levels. *B,* Sagittal short tau inversion recovery (STIR) images demonstrate T2 prolongation within the marrow corresponding to areas of T1 prolongation seen in *A* (*arrows*). There is extensive T2 prolongation within the L3 and L4 vertebrae, but the marrow next to the superior margin of L2 is not as abnormal. The findings are characteristic of metastatic disease and associated pathologic fractures at L3 and L4; the L2 fracture may represent an older, compression fracture, but there is tumor in the inferior aspect of the L2 vertebral body as well.

tral nidus of increased density, surrounded by an area of relative lucency; this appearance, particularly in the appropriate clinical setting, makes the diagnosis a virtual certainty (Fig. 4–44). Painful scoliosis may accompany osteoid osteomas of the spine. When recognized, treatment options include conservative care with oral medications (Kneisl 1992), percutaneous excision, percutaneous thermal ablation (Cove 2000, Frassica 1996), and surgical excision (Frassica 1996).

Enostosis (Bone Island)

Enostoses (bone islands) are unresorbed cortical bone that are generally asymptomatic. Imaging findings include T1 prolongation and T2 shortening typical of cortical bone, and CT studies demonstrate marked density of the lesion. These lesions typically do not present any diagnostic challenge. Occasionally, sclerotic metastatic deposit may share some of the imaging characteristics, but the uniform cortical bone density seen on CT is quite specific (Fig. 4–45).

Lesions Suspicious for Metastatic Disease or Myeloma

Even with the specific efforts to recognize metastatic disease on the basis of characteristic imaging findings and attention to red flags in the clinical history applied to spine lesions (Fig. 4–1), metastatic disease will still probably account for the majority of bone lesions at this point in the work-up. Patients having lesions with imaging characteristics of metastatic disease, multiple myeloma, or plasmacytoma (a single focus of myelomatous tissue) should be fully evaluated for systemic tumor at this time (if they have not already been so evaluated). Characteristic imaging features of solitary metastatic deposit include a well-defined focus of T1 and T2 prolongation. CT findings include destruction of cancellous and cortical bone with little or no reactive bone formation. In such patients, additional imaging prior to biopsy may include a bone scan and chest/abdomen/pelvis CT scan to look for additional bony lesions and a solid source of tumor, respectively, supplemented by mammography in women and PSA with a digital rectal examination in men (Heller 1997, Rougraff 1993). Serum immunoelectrophoresis should be performed to evaluate for myeloma in patients older than 40 years of age. If all these studies turn up no primary tumor, biopsy will probably need to be performed. When performing percutaneous imaging-guided biopsy, the needle tract must be placed along a course so that it may be resected at the time of surgery if excision is done later.

Vertebra Plana

A special category of lesion is a "vertebra plana," or flat vertebral body. Such lesions typically represent eosinophilic granuloma (Fig. 4–46) but may also be secondary to Ewing's sarcoma and an unusual manifestation of infection, so biopsy is mandatory prior to treatment. Diagnosis of

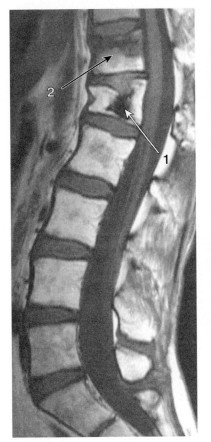

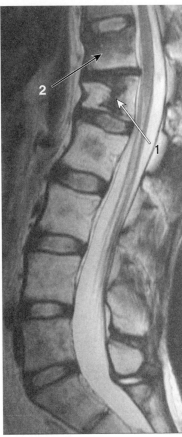

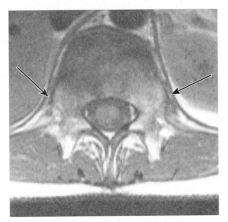

A

B

C

D

FIGURE 4–28

Acute benign compression fracture adjacent to a chronic abnormality. A 27-year-old woman with a history of childhood Ewing's sarcoma treated with radiation and chemotherapy. She suffered a sledding accident with acute back pain 3 weeks before the MRI was obtained. *A,* Sagittal T1WI shows compression of L1 with anterior wedging and central T1 prolongation (*arrow 1*). There is a myeloid depletion pattern, particularly within the marrow of the upper lumbar spine, from prior radiation therapy, with T1 shortening. The T12 vertebra demonstrates mild loss of height and a broad band of T1 prolongation along its superior margin (*arrow 2*). *B,* Sagittal T2WI shows T2 shortening at the L1 level (*arrow 1*) consistent with fibrosis or sclerosis given the findings on the T1WI. There is a broad band of T2 signal abnormality within the T12 vertebral body, with a well-defined, linear interface between the abnormal signal intensity in the upper vertebral body and the fatty signal intensity of the lower vertebral body (*arrow 2*). *C,* Axial T1WI at the T12 pedicle level shows that the T2 abnormality within the vertebral body does not extend into the pedicles. *D,* Planar bone scan demonstrates broad, bandlike activity within the T12 vertebral body (*arrow*), consistent with a healing fracture. The patient had sustained an acute fracture of T12 with a well-defined linear interface between the normal and abnormal marrow. The L1 changes are chronic and the result of remote chemotherapy and radiation therapy.

eosinophilic granuloma on frozen section at the time of needle biopsy, followed by intralesional instillation of steroids, has been recommended (Boriani 1997b). Infection obviously requires appropriate antibiotic therapy, with surgery as warranted (Hadjipavlou 2000), and Ewing's sarcoma usually requires excision, although results are often poor (Boriani 1997b).

Solitary Bone Lesion, Cell Type Unknown

At this point in the evaluation (Fig. 4–47), many histologic varieties of tumor remain in the differential diagnosis, including both benign and malignant conditions. Although specific imaging features may favor one diagnosis over another (Fig. 4–48), in most cases the only way to distinguish between these entities with enough diagnostic cer-

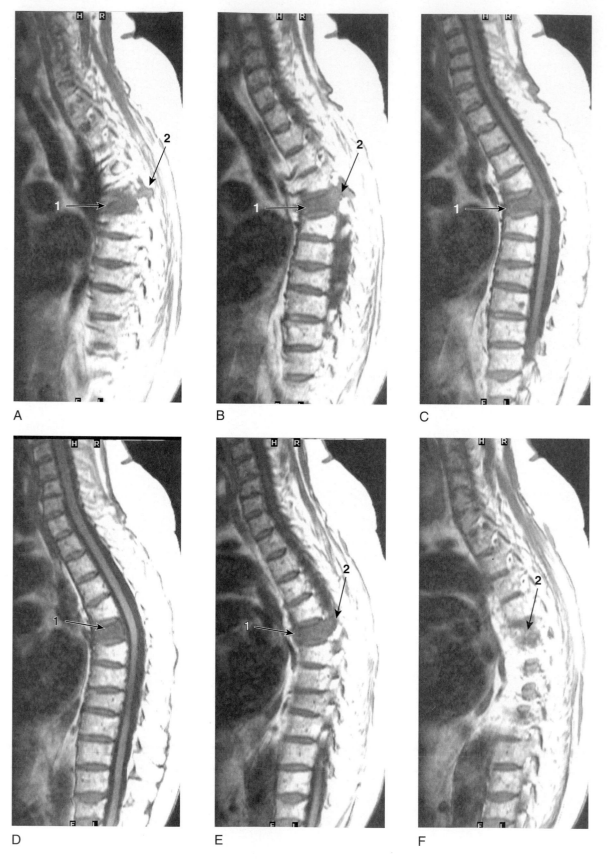

FIGURE 4–29

Acute and chronic benign osteoporotic fractures. A 78-year-old woman with a history of osteoporosis and upper mid back pain. *A–F,* Sequential sagittal T1WIs demonstrate a T5 compression *(arrows 1)* with 40% loss of height and uniform T1 prolongation that extends into the pedicles *(arrows 2)*. Note thoracic kyphosis, and compression deformity of multiple other vertebral bodies, including T4, T6, and T8. These levels demonstrate marrow signal intensity similar to other, noncompressed normal levels.

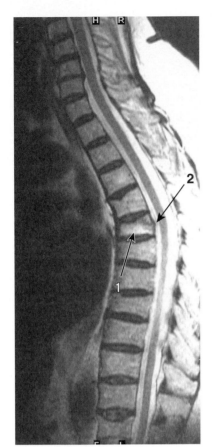

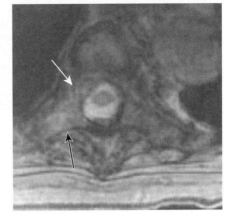

FIGURE 4–29 *(continued)*

G, Sagittal T2WI demonstrates T2 prolongation, particularly along the inferior aspect of the vertebral body *(arrow 1).* There are findings of middle column failure, with buckling of the dorsal cortex of T5 *(arrow 2). H,* Axial T1WI at the level of the T5 pedicles demonstrates T1 shortening of the right pedicle *(arrow 1)* extending into the base of the transverse process *(arrow 2). I,* Axial T2WI demonstrates T2 prolongation *(arrows)* corresponding to the T1 shortening seen in *H.* This patient had a simple osteoporotic compression fracture without tumor. The T4, T6, and T8 lesions all demonstrate characteristics of benign, chronic osteoporotic compression fractures with marrow signal intensity identical on all imaging sequences to other levels of normal height. The T5 level demonstrates a number of characteristics suggesting either an acute/subacute compression fracture or pathologic fracture including T1 and T2 prolongation, involvement of all the marrow at the level, a nonlinear configuration, and extension into the pedicle. An extensive work-up for malignancy was instituted that revealed no evidence of a primary tumor and the patient remains well 1 year later.

tainty to proceed with patient management is with a biopsy. Two steps precede the biopsy in most cases: (1) obtaining a bone scan and (2) obtaining any additional imaging necessary for surgical planning.

The bone scan allows assessment of any additional focus of abnormal radiotracer localization. This may point to a multifocal disease and obviate biopsy, at least of the spine. Whether there is activity at the site of the lesion itself does not matter: iso- or even decreased radiotracer localization may be seen in many cases of aggressive tumors, whereas increased activity is seen with such a wide variety of processes (e.g., benign and malignant tumors, degenerative joint disease, trauma, and infection) that it has little diagnostic value.

Current surgical planning for definitive treatment of primary spine tumors involves a surgical oncologic grading system known as the *WBB system* for its developers, Drs. James Weinstein, Stefano Boriani, and Roberto Biagini (Boriani 1997a, Boriani 1997b, Boriani 2000)). In this system, the spine is divided radially into 12 equal sections (like a clock face) with the spinous process in the 12 o'clock position. Within each section, five layers are recognized (from "outside in"): extraosseous soft tissues, superficial interosseous tissues, deep interosseous tissues, extradural extraosseous tissues, and intradural extraosseous tissues. This results in (12 × 5 =) 60 sectors at a given level of the spine. In general terms, vertebrectomy may be performed for resection of anterior tumors as long as only five sections are involved

(i.e., only one of the two pedicles has tumor within it). Hemivertebrectomy may be performed if tumor is confined to three sections (e.g., the lamina, transverse process, and pedicle) on one side of the spine. Resection of the posterior elements is possible if tumor is confined to the posterior tissues without involvement of the pedicles (involving up to six sections). Tumors extending into the dura or showing direct involvement of the cord require special consideration at surgery.

After completion of the bone scan and appropriate imaging to allow full staging of the tumor, the biopsy may be planned. Staging should precede biopsy, because in the event that definitive surgery is expected (pending appropriate histologic results), careful consideration must be given to the needle tract since it must be removed at the time of surgery (Weinstein 1987). When the tumor is too extensive to allow definitive surgery regardless of the tissue type, the biopsy tract may be placed with optimal patient comfort and technical ease in mind.

Reporting in Spine Tumors

The earlier discussions in this chapter review most of the necessary information to create a meaningful and concise report regarding tumors of the spine. In the body of the report, a description of the lesions should include their size, exact location, and imaging characteristics (i.e., T1 and T2

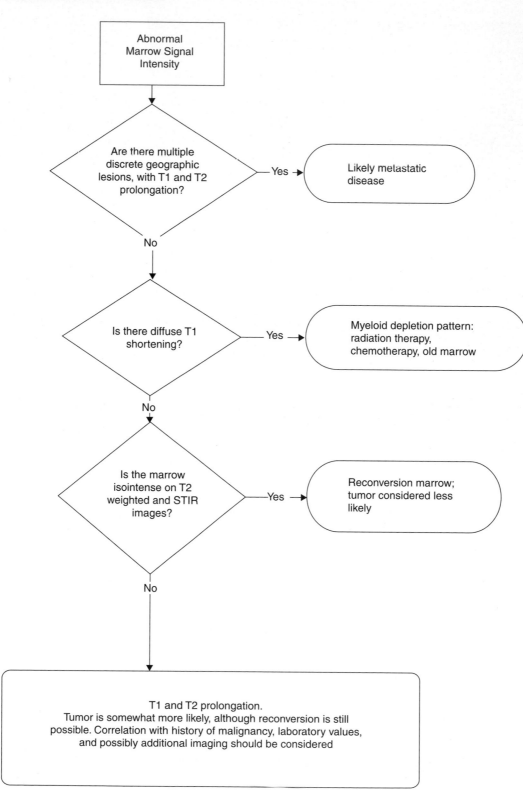

FIGURE 4–30

Algorithm of abnormal marrow signal intensity. STIR, short tau inversion recovery.

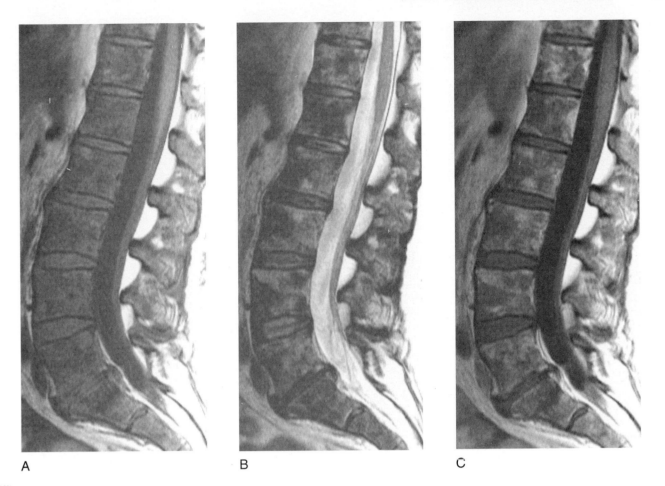

A   B   C

FIGURE 4–31

Diffuse abnormal marrow in metastatic disease. A 58-year-old patient with back pain and a history of metastatic breast cancer. *A,* Sagittal T1WI demonstrates the "bright discs" sign (with the signal intensity of the intervertebral discs exceeding that of the vertebral marrow on T1WI), along with multiple geographic areas of abnormal signal intensity. *B,* Sagittal T2WI shows diffuse marrow inhomogeneity. *C,* Sagittal T1WI after contrast injection demonstrates a mottled pattern with multiple geographic lesions. Such findings are highly characteristic of widespread metastatic disease.

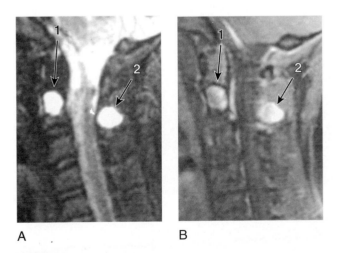

A   B

FIGURE 4–32

Hodgkin's lymphoma of the spine. *A,* Sagittal T2WI demonstrates foci of T2 prolongation within C2 vertebral body (*arrow 1*) and spinous process (*arrow 2*). *B,* Sagittal T1WI following contrast administration demonstrates contrast enhancement of the lesions within the C2 vertebral body (*arrow 1*) and spinous process (*arrow 2*).

shortening or prolongation on MRI examination). Special vigilance should be given to documentation of the level of the lesion and ensuring that any segmentation anomalies are explicitly noted, because imaging equipment available within the operating room (usually a C-arm fluoroscope) visualizes only the skeleton and does not directly demonstrate the tumor. The conclusion of the report should attempt to address three questions: (1) Is further imaging of the neuraxis necessary? (2) Is the lesion more likely a tumor or a tumor mimic? (3) What is (are) the most likely histology (-gies) of the lesion? Use of the principles delineated earlier will help in answering these questions. Note that often it is not possible to be certain of a specific histologic diagnosis and that biopsy will be necessary.

Conclusion

Most radiologists see few primary malignant spinal neoplasms in the course of their career. The greatest patient benefit most often results not from the ability of the radiol-

Text continued on page 230

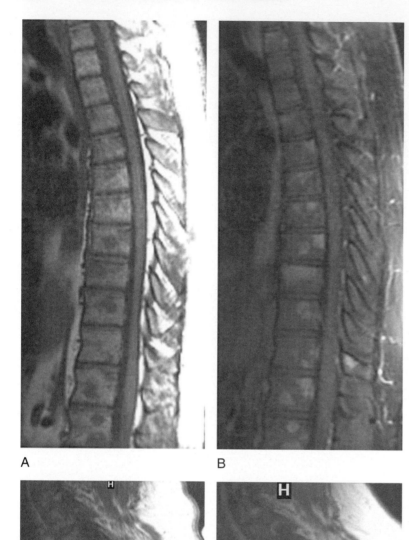

A

B

A

B

FIGURE 4–33

Diffuse abnormal marrow in sarcoidosis. A 29-year-old man with long-standing history of diffuse bony sarcoid. *A,* Sagittal T1WI demonstrates multiple, geographic lesions of marrow with T1 prolongation. *B,* Sagittal T2WI demonstrates T2 prolongation of the lesions. These lesions resemble metastatic deposits but are secondary to sarcoidosis.

FIGURE 4–34

Diffuse marrow abnormality, with both metastatic disease and myeloid depletion pattern following radiation therapy. A 55-year-old man with lung cancer. *A,* Sagittal T1WI demonstrates multiple, variably sized lesions with T1 prolongation *(arrows)* highly characteristic of metastatic disease. *B,* Sagittal T1WI 4 months later, following radiation therapy. Note the myeloid depletion pattern of T1 shortening in the T4 through T7 vertebrae *(arrows 1),* with extensive progression of marrow metastatic tumor elsewhere *(arrows 2).*

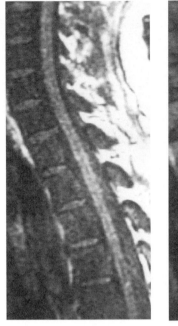
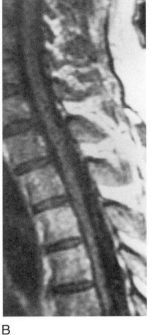

A   B

FIGURE 4–35

Myelofibrosis with myeloid depletion pattern. A 37-year-old patient with known myelofibrosis. *A,* Sagittal T1WI in a patient with myelofibrosis demonstrates T1 shortening of the upper thoracic vertebrae. The signal intensity of the marrow is so decreased that it is exceeded by the intervertebral discs and spinal cord. *B,* Sagittal T1WI following contrast demonstrates uniform contrast enhancement, with the marrow appearing hyperintense relative to the adjacent intervertebral discs.

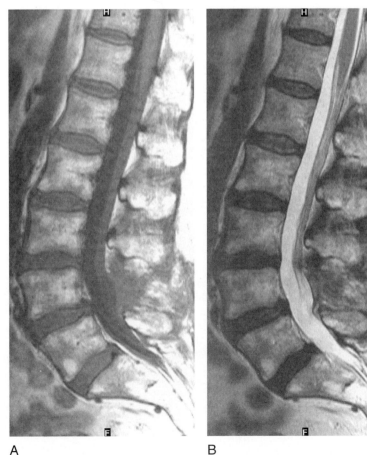

A   B

FIGURE 4–36

Diffuse abnormal marrow of aging. A 65-year-old woman with low back and leg pain after posterior decompression and discectomy at L4–5. *A,* Sagittal T1WI demonstrates multilevel signal intensity inhomogeneity within the lumbar vertebrae. The vertebrae demonstrate much greater signal intensity than the intervertebral discs, however. Postoperative changes are present posteriorly. *B,* Sagittal T2WI demonstrates an inhomogeneous pattern of marrow signal as well. There are areas of marrow that maintain moderate to increased signal intensity consistent with fat and other areas of isointensity consistent with fibrous tissue. No areas demonstrating matched T1 and T2 prolongation to suggest malignancy are identified. The patient had no known tumor, a negative review of systems, and a negative bone scan. The findings are typical of a mixed myeloid depletion pattern secondary to aging.

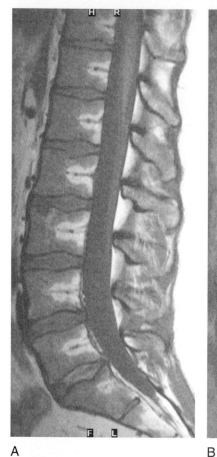

A

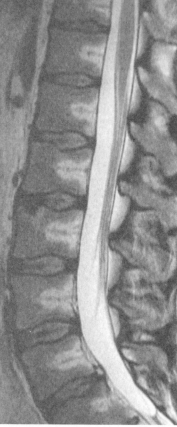

B

FIGURE 4–37

Normal variant, with fatty marrow along the basivertebral plexus. A 42-year-old woman after L5–S1 discectomy with recurrent low back and left leg pain. *A,* Sagittal T1WI demonstrates relatively striking T1 shortening along the basivertebral veins. *B,* Sagittal T2WI demonstrates T2 prolongation corresponding to the T1 shortening, consistent with fat. Also note the L3 limbus vertebrae and mild loss of disc height and hydration with postoperative changes along the posterior margin of the L5–S1 disc with a 3.5-mm disc contour abnormality. The marrow pattern is a benign variant.

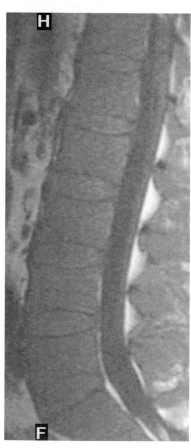

A

B

FIGURE 4–38

Abnormal marrow signal intensity with a reconversion pattern. A 60-year-old man with low back pain and acute myelogenous leukemia (in remission). *A,* Sagittal T1WI demonstrates diffusely abnormal marrow, with marrow signal intensity about the same as the intervertebral discs. *B,* Sagittal T2WI demonstrates decreased signal intensity of the marrow compared to the intervertebral discs. Note L4–5 disc dehydration with a small disc protrusion and associated focus of T2 prolongation and the L1–2 moderate disc dehydration and small cranially dissecting disc extrusion. The marrow pattern is typical of uniform reconversion to hematopoietic marrow.

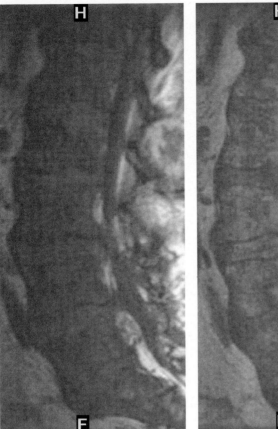

A   B

FIGURE 4–39

Abnormal marrow signal intensity with a reconversion pattern. A 70-year-old man with back pain and anemia. *A*, Sagittal T1WI shows the "bright discs" sign with greater signal intensity of the intervertebral discs than of the vertebral body marrow. *B*, Sagittal T2WI demonstrates no foci of T2 prolongation within the marrow. The patient had extensive multilevel degenerative change with central canal stenosis, with posterior decompression at L4. The pattern is that of reconversion of fatty to hematopoietic marrow. The lack of tissue contrast created by diminished marrow fat renders interpretation of spine MRI difficult.

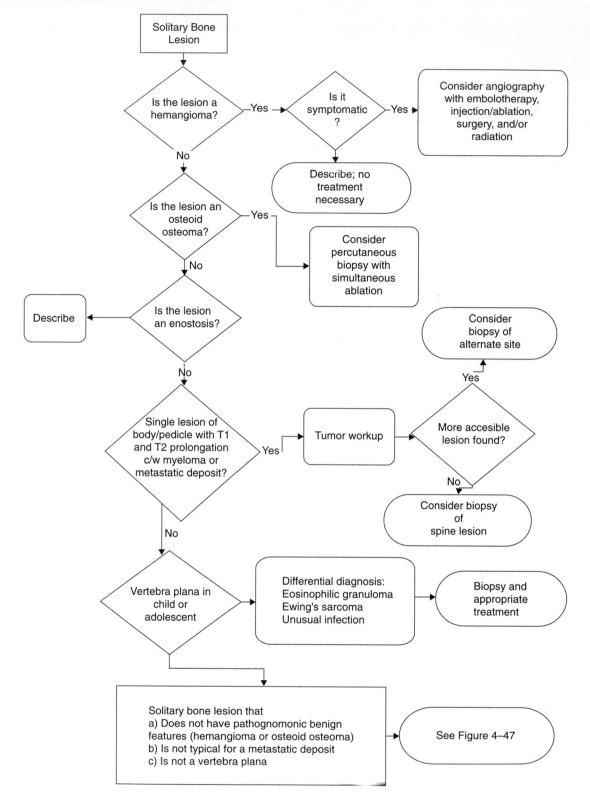

FIGURE 4–40

Algorithm of solitary bone lesion, part I (see Fig. 4–47 for part II).

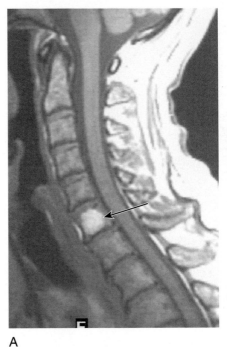

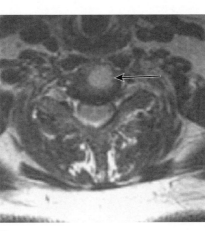

FIGURE 4–41

Asymptomatic hemangioma of the vertebral body. A 57-year-old woman with neck and left shoulder pain. *A,* Sagittal T1WI demonstrates a 12-mm focus of T1 shortening within the C5 vertebral body *(arrow). B,* Axial T2WI shows that the lesion *(arrow)* also demonstrates T2 prolongation. In addition, there are punctate areas of T2 shortening centrally within the lesion, characteristic of a hemangioma. The imaging findings are diagnostic of a hemangioma, and no further diagnostic studies are necessary to prove this.

A   B

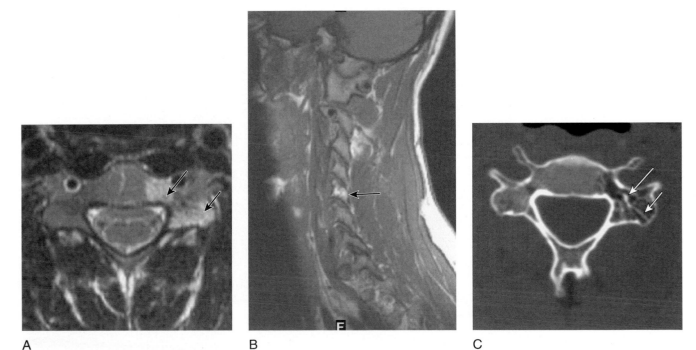

A   B   C

FIGURE 4–42

Asymptomatic hemangioma of the vertebral body, pedicle, and lateral mass. A 35-year-old man with left deltoid weakness. *A,* Axial T2WI at the C5 pedicle level demonstrates a lesion of the lateral vertebral body, pedicle, and lateral mass demonstrating predominantly T2 prolongation, with punctate foci of T2 shortening *(arrows). B,* Sagittal T1WI at the level of the C5 lateral mass demonstrates marked T1 shortening *(arrow)* with foci of T1 prolongation. *C,* Axial CT study demonstrates the lesion to have decreased attenuation consistent with fat accounting for T1 shortening and T2 relative prolongation, with thickened trabeculae *(arrows)* accounting for the punctate foci of T1 prolongation and T2 shortening seen on the MRI.

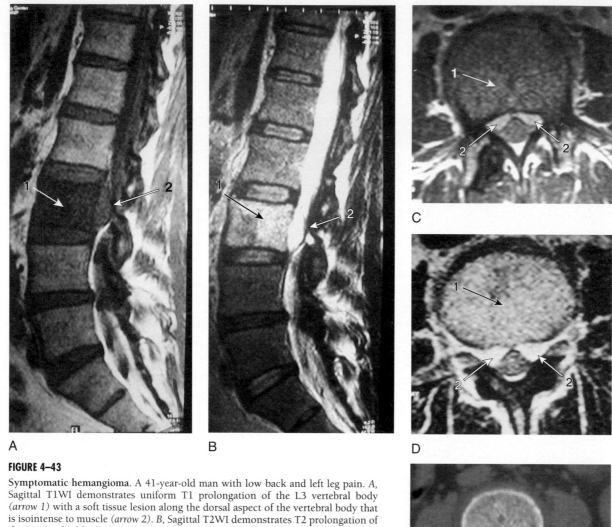

A B C

D E

FIGURE 4–43

Symptomatic hemangioma. A 41-year-old man with low back and left leg pain. *A,* Sagittal T1WI demonstrates uniform T1 prolongation of the L3 vertebral body (*arrow 1*) with a soft tissue lesion along the dorsal aspect of the vertebral body that is isointense to muscle (*arrow 2*). *B,* Sagittal T2WI demonstrates T2 prolongation of the L3 vertebral body (*arrow 1*) with even greater T2 prolongation in the posterior soft tissue mass (*arrow 2*). *C,* Axial T1WI at the level of the L3 pedicle demonstrates T1 prolongation of the vertebral body (*arrow 1*) with, again, greater signal intensity within the dorsal soft tissue mass (*arrow 2*). The dorsal soft tissue mass was located within the spinal canal and is tethered by the central septum. Note the accentuated trabecular pattern within the vertebral body. *D,* Axial T2WI demonstrates T2 prolongation within the vertebral body (*arrow 1*) and anterior spinal canal (*arrow 2*), along with trabecular accentuation. *E,* CT at the level of the L3 pedicle again shows accentuation of the trabeculae. Note that nearly any other process replacing the entire marrow space (as seen on the MRI) would be associated with more bone destruction.

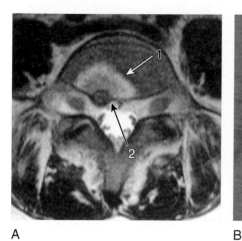

A

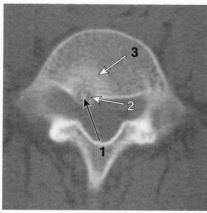

B

FIGURE 4–44

Osteoid osteoma. *A,* Axial T2WI demonstrates extensive T2 prolongation of the posterior vertebral body (*arrow 1*) with a focus of T2 shortening along the dorsal vertebral body margin (*arrow 2*). *B,* Axial CT demonstrates characteristic features of osteoid osteoma, with a "target" appearance: there is a central nidus of near-cortical bone density (*arrow 1*), surrounded by alternating areas of lucency and sclerosis (*arrow 2*). There is also reactive sclerosis in the posterior vertebral body (*arrow 3*), corresponding to the T2 prolongation of the posterior vertebral body seen on *A.* The MRI features are much less characteristic in this lesion than are the CT findings.

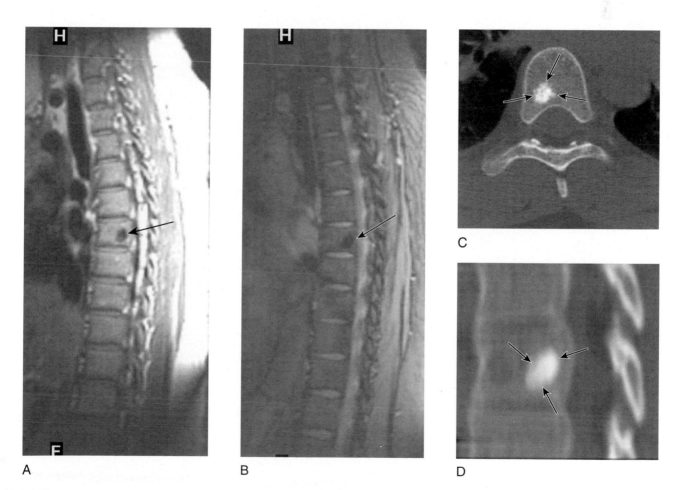

A   B   C

D

FIGURE 4–45

Enostosis (bone island). A 30-year-old woman with mid back pain. *A,* Sagittal T1WI demonstrates an 11 × 9-mm well-defined focus of T1 prolongation (*arrow*) within the T7 vertebral body. *B,* Sagittal T2WI shows the lesion (*arrow*) to have T2 shortening, with absent signal within its boundaries. *C,* A 3-mm CT scan at the mid T7 level shows the lesion to have cortical bone density with a feathered appearance to the margins (*arrows*) (such margins are typical of enostoses). *D,* Sagittal reconstruction CT demonstrates a well-defined sclerotic area (*arrows*) consistent of cortical bone. The imaging features are characteristic of an enostosis, and no further diagnostic or therapeutic maneuvers are necessary.

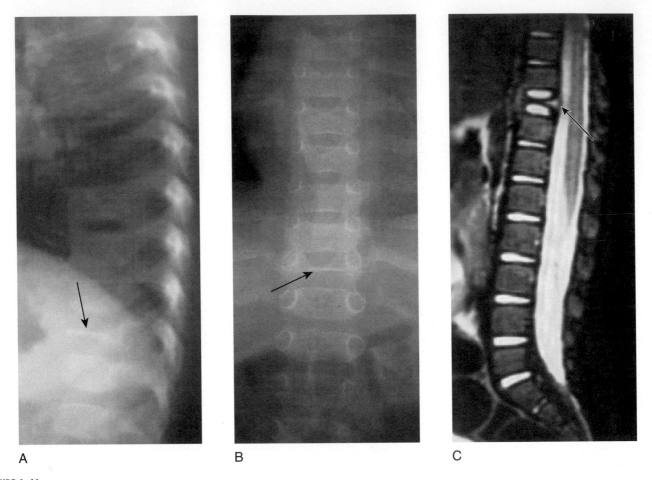

A   B   C

FIGURE 4–46

Vertebra plana from eosinophilic granuloma. A 1-year-old girl with orbital and left temporal soft tissue mass. *A,* Lateral plain film demonstrates vertebra plana at the T10 level *(arrow)*. *B,* Anteroposterior film also demonstrates vertebra plana at the T10 level *(arrow)*. *C,* Sagittal T2WI demonstrates marked loss of height at the T10 level *(arrow)*. Note the relative expansion of the T9–10 and T10–11 discs.

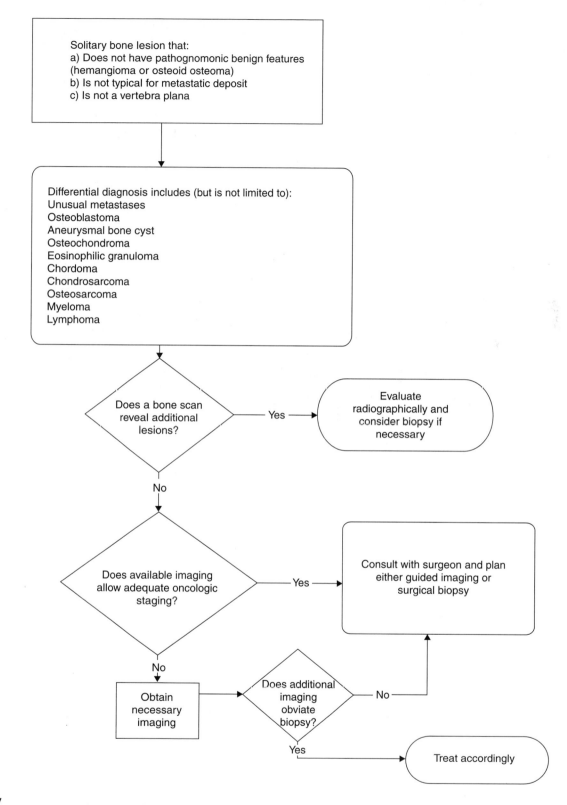

FIGURE 4–47

Algorithm of a solitary bone lesion, part II (see Fig. 4–40 for part I).

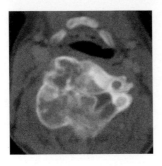

FIGURE 4–48

Osteoblastoma. A 16-year-old boy with progressive paraparesis and acute-onset quadriplegia. Axial CT scan shows extensive expansion of the right half of the C4 vertebral body with associated central spinal canal narrowing. The expansion of bone with a predominantly intact overlying cortex characteristic of a slow-growing lesion suggests osteoblastoma as the histologic diagnosis.

ogist to make a specific and correct histologic diagnosis but from the ability to analyze the case in such a manner as to prevent unnecessary biopsy and, if biopsy is found to be necessary, to assist planning an optimal biopsy. This requires not only analysis of features of the lesion on the imaging examination but also correlation with specific features of the patient's clinical history, physical examination, and laboratory data. An understanding of the surgeon's approach and, in particular, the relatively newly developed WBB surgical oncologic staging system will help the radiologist assist the spine surgeon. Familiarity with spine tumor mimics may prevent an unnecessary biopsy.

References

Algra PR, Bloem JL, Tissing H, Falke THM, Arndt JW, Verboom LJ. Detection of vertebral metastases: comparison between MR imaging and bone scintigraphy. Radiographics 1991; 11:219–232.

An HS, Andreshak TG, Nguyen C, Williams A, Daniels D. Can we distinguish between benign versus malignant compression fractures of the spine by magnetic resonance imaging? Spine 1995; 20:1776–1782.

Baker KB, Moran CJ, Wippold FJ, Smirniotopoulos JG, Rodriguez FJ, Meyers SP, Siegal TL. MR imaging of spinal hemangioblastoma. AJR Am J Roentgenol 2000; 174:377–382.

Baker LL, Goodman SB, Perkash I, Lane B, Enzman DR. Benign versus pathologic compression fractures of vertebral bodies: assessment with conventional spin-echo, chemical-shift, and STIR MR imaging. Radiology 1990; 174:495–502.

Baur A, Stabler A, Bruning R, Bartl R, Krodel A, Reiser M, Deimling M. Diffusion-weighted MR imaging of bone marrow: differentiation of benign versus pathologic compression fractures. Radiology 1998; 207:349–356.

Beltran J, Noto AM, Chakeres DW, Christoforidis AJ. Tumors of the osseous spine: staging with MR imaging versus CT. Radiology 1987; 162:565–569.

Bickels J, Kahanovitz N, Rubert CK, Henshaw RM, Moss DP, Meller I, Malawer MM. Extraspinal bone and soft-tissue tumors as a cause of sciatica—clinical diagnosis and recommendations: analysis of 32 cases. Spine 1999; 24:1611–1616.

Boriani S, Bandiera S, Biagini R, Picci P. Staging and treatment of primary spine tumors. Contemp Spine Surg 2000; 1:7–14.

Boriani S, De lure F, Campanacci L, Gasbarrini A, Bandiera S, Biagini R, Bertoni F, Picci P. Aneurysmal bone cyst of the mobile spine: report on 41 cases. Spine 2001; 26:27–35.

Boriani S, Weinstein JN, Biagini R. Primary bone tumors of the spine: terminology and surgical staging. Spine 1997a; 22:1036–1044.

Boriani S, Weinstein JN. Differential diagnosis and surgical treatment of primary benign and malignant spine neoplasms. In Frymoyer JW (ed). The Adult Spine: Principles and Practice, 2nd ed. Philadelphia, Lippincott-Raven, 1997b.

Bourgouin PM, Lesage J, Fontaine S, Konan A, Roy D, Bard C, Del Carpio O'Donovan R. A pattern approach to the differential diagnosis of intramedullary spinal cord lesions on MR imaging. AJR Am J Roentgenol 1998; 170:1645–1649.

Carlier R, Engerand S, Lamer S, Vallee C, Bussel B, Polivka M. Foraminal epidural extraosseous cavernous hemangioma of the cervical spine: a case report. Spine 2000; 25:629–631.

Cassidy JR, Ducker TB, Dienes EA. Intradural tumors. In Frymoyer JW (ed). The Adult Spine: Principles and Practice, 2nd ed. Philadelphia, Lippincott-Raven, 1997.

Colletti PM, Dang HT, Deseran MW, Kerr RM, Boswell WD, Ralls PW. Spinal MR imaging in suspected metastases: correlation with skeletal scintigraphy. Magn Reson Imaging 1991; 9:349–355.

Cove JA, Taminiau AH, Obermann WR, Vanderschueren GM. Osteoid osteoma of the spine treated with percutaneous computed tomography–guided thermocoagulation. Spine 2000; 25:1283–1286.

Daldrup-Link HE, Franzius C, Link TM, Laukamp D, Sciuk J, Jurgens H, Schober O, Rummeny EJ. Whole-body MR imaging for detection of bone metastases in children and young adults: comparison with skeletal scintigraphy and FDG PET. AJR Am J Roentgenol 2001; 177:229–236.

Doppman JL, Oldfield EH, Heiss JD. Symptomatic vertebral hemangiomas: treatment by means of direct intralesional injection of ethanol. Radiology 2000; 214:341–348.

Duffau H, Gazzaz M, Kujas M, Fohanno D. Primary intradural extraosseous ependymoma: case report and review of the literature. Spine 2000; 25:1993–1995.

Egelhoff JC, Bates DJ, Ross JS, Rothner AD, Cohen BH. Spinal MR findings in neurofibromatosis types 1 and 2. AJNR Am J Neuroradiol 1992; 13:1071–1077.

Fisher AJ, Gilula LA, Kyriakos M, Holzaepfel CD. MR imaging changes of lumbar vertebral sarcoidosis. AJR Am J Roentgenol 1999; 173:354–356.

Frank JA, Ling A, Patronas NJ, Carrasquillo JA, Horvath K, Hickey AM, Dwyer AJ. Detection of malignant bone tumors: MR imaging vs scintigraphy. AJR Am J Roentgenol 1990; 155:1043–1048.

Frassica FJ, Waltrip RL, Sponseller PD, Ma LD, McCarthy EF. Clinicopathologic features and treatment of osteoid osteoma and osteoblastoma in children and adolescents. Orthop Clin North Am 1996; 27:559–574.

Hadjipavlou AG, Mader JT, Necessary JT, Muffoletto AJ. Hematogenous pyogenic spinal infections and their surgical management. Spine 2000; 25:1668–1679.

Hajek PC, Baker LL, Goobar JE, Sartoris DJ, Hesselink JR, Haghighi P, Resnick D. Focal fat deposition in axial bone marrow: MR characteristics. Radiology 1987; 162:245–249.

Heller JG, Pedlow FX. Tumors of the spine. In Garfin SR, Vaccaro AR (eds). Orthopedic Knowledge Update: Spine. American Academy of Orthopedic Surgeons, Rosemonf, IL, 1997.

Kneisl JS, Simon MA. Medical management compared with operative treatment for osteoid osteoma. J Bone Joint Surg Am 1992; 74:179–185.

Kostiuk P. Differential diagnosis and surgical treatment of metastatic spinal tumors. In Frymoyer JW (ed). The Adult Spine: Principles and Practice, 2nd ed. Philadelphia, Lippincott-Raven, 1997.

Kozlowski K, Beluffi G, Masel J, Diard F, Ferrari-Ciboldi F, Le Dosseur P, Labatut J. Primary vertebral tumours in children: report of 20 cases with brief literature review. Pediatr Radiol 1984; 14:129–139.

Laredo JD, Reizine D, Bard M, Merland JJ. Vertebral hemangiomas: radiologic evaluation. Radiology 1986; 161:183–189.

Lee S, Hadlow AT. Extraosseous extension of vertebral hemangioma, a rare cause of spinal cord compression. Spine 1999; 24:2111–2114.

Masaryk TJ. Neoplastic disease of the spine. Radiol Clin North Am 1991; 29:829–845.

Masaryk TJ. Spinal tumors. In Modic MT, Masaryk TJ, Ross JS (eds). Magnetic Resonance Imaging of the Spine, 2nd ed. St. Louis, Mosby–Year Book, 1994.

Nabors MW, Pait TG, Byrd EB, Karim NO, Davis DO, Kobrine AI, Rizzoli HV. Updated assessment and current classification of spinal meningeal cysts. J Neurosurg 1988; 68:366–377.

Olson EM, Wong WHM, Hesselink JR. Extraspinal abnormalities detected on MR images of the spine. AJR Am J Roentgenol 1994; 162:679–684.

Osborn AG. Tumors, cysts, and tumorlike lesions of the spine and spinal cord. In Osborn AG. Diagnostic Neuroradiology. St. Louis, Mosby–Year Book, 1994.

Parizel PM, Baleriaux D, Rodesch G, Segebarth C, Lalmand B, Christophe C, Lemort C, Haesendonck P, Niendorf HP, Flament-Durand J, et al. Gd-DTPA–enhanced MR imaging of spinal tumors. AJR Am J Roentgenol 1989; 152:1087–1096.

Quint DJ, Levy R, Krauss JC. MR of myelomatous meningitis. AJNR Am J Neuroradiol 1995; 16:1316–1317.

Ross JS. MRI of the Spine. Philadelphia, Lippincott Williams & Wilkins, 2000.

Ross JS, Masaryk TJ, Modic MT, Carter JR, Mapstone T, Dengel FH. Vertebral hemangiomas: MR imaging. Radiology 1987; 165:165–169.

Rougraff BT, Kneisl JS, Simon MA. Skeletal metastases of unknown origin: a prospective study of a diagnostic strategy. J Bone Joint Surg Am 1993; 75:1276–1281.

Shapiro R. Myelography. Chicago, Year Book, 1984.

Smoker WRK, Godersky JC, Knutson RK, Keyes WD, Norman D, Bergman W. The role of MR imaging in evaluating metastatic spinal disease. AJR Am J Roentgenol 1987; 149:1241–1248.

Spuentrup E, Buecker A, Adam G, van Vaals JJ, Guenther RW. Diffusion-weighted MR imaging for differentiation of benign fracture edema and tumor infiltration of the vertebral body. AJR Am J Roentgenol 2001; 176:351–358.

St. Amour TE, Hodges SC, Laakman RW, Tamas DE. MRI of the Spine. New York, Raven Press, 1994.

Stabler A, Doma AB, Baur A, Kruger A, Reiser ME. Reactive bone marrow changes in infectious spondylitis: quantitative assessment with MR imaging. Radiology 2000; 217:863–868.

Sze G. Magnetic resonance imaging in the evaluation of spinal tumors. Cancer 1991; 67:1229–1241.

Sze G, Bravo S, Krol G. Spinal lesions: quantitative and qualitative temporal evolution of gadopentetate dimeglumine enhancement in MR imaging. Radiology 1989; 170:849–856.

Sze G, Krol G, Zimmerman RD, Deck MDF. Intramedullary disease of the spine: diagnosis using gadolinium-DTPA–enhanced MR imaging. AJR Am J Roentgenol 1988; 151:1193–1204.

Vogler JB, Murphy WA. Bone marrow imaging. Radiology 1988; 168:679–693.

Waddell G. The Back Pain Revolution. New York, Churchill Livingstone, 1998, p 12.

Weinstein JN, McLain RF. Primary tumors of the spine. Spine 1987; 12:843–851.

Yuh WTC, Zachar C, Barloon TJ, Sato Y, Sickels WJ, Hawes DR. Vertebral compression fractures: distinction between benign and malignant causes with MR imaging. Radiology 1989; 172:215–218.

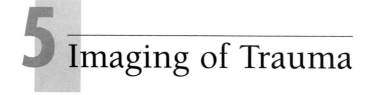

5 Imaging of Trauma

DONALD L. RENFREW • SANJAY SALUJA

Most texts and articles categorize fractures according to the mechanism of injury (e.g., flexion injuries, hyperextension injuries). Excellent textbooks (Daffner 1988, Harris 1987) and review articles (Berquist 1988) are available that outline this approach. This categorization is largely based on plain film analysis, supplemented by imaging when necessary. Here we list and illustrate imaging findings of trauma (emphasizing computed tomography [CT] and magnetic resonance imaging [MRI]) and provide a differential diagnosis of fracture findings. In addition, we review common clinical scenarios involving either acute or chronic trauma. In the discussion of these scenarios, we delineate what is important to include in the radiographic report of the traumatized patient. First, however, we briefly review the imaging of trauma.

Imaging of Trauma

There is ongoing controversy regarding optimal imaging of the acutely traumatized patient with possible cervical spine injury. Recommendations for evaluation include everything from a single cross-table lateral study to a minimum three-view cervical spine series (West 1997) to helical CT (Nunez 1998) to MRI (Katzberg 1999).

PLAIN FILMS

Although some emergency department physicians may think that there is a role for a single, lateral film to "screen" the cervical spine, such a limited examination will miss a significant number of fractures (Fig. 5–1) (West 1997). In most cases, a three-view (anteroposterior, lateral, and open mouth) series is considered the minimum standard, with oblique views when possible. If there is suspicion of instability, a repeat film 1 to 2 weeks after the initial study done with flexion-extension may be beneficial (Vandemark 1990).

COMPUTED TOMOGRAPHY

Performance of CT as a screening study in injured patients is an area of ongoing controversy. Some authors advocate routine use of helical CT in the evaluation of patients at risk of cervical spine fracture (Nunez 1996), whereas others have

found that screening CT provides little additional information compared with plain films (Acheson 1987, El-Khoury 1995, Eustace 2000, Vandemark 1990). Several series have demonstrated that CT may be positive when plain films are either unremarkable or minimally abnormal (Blacksin 1995, Lee 1982, Lee 1992, Nunez 1996, Woodring 1982). When CT is performed for a known injury, it is best to obtain 3-mm or finer cuts with reconstructions through the cervical spine. In cases where a single level is being evaluated, 1-mm axial cuts should probably be performed through the level and both adjacent segments. In many cases, fractures in the axial plane or complex fractures of the lateral masses are difficult to appreciate on axial studies, whereas coronal and sagittal reconstructions (obtained from overlapping axial thin slices) are of considerable additional benefit (Figs. 5–2 and 5–3) (Pech 1985, Shanmuganathan 1994).

MAGNETIC RESONANCE IMAGING

Although Katzberg and associates (1999) support a role for emergent use of screening MRI for trauma, MRI is generally reserved for evaluation of soft tissue injury in the subacute period (Klein 1999, Pettersson 1997). One exception to this rule may be evaluation of the spinal cord for hematoma versus edema. Hematomas of the spinal cord indicate a poor prognosis, whereas edema carries a much better prognosis and may be reversible (El-Khoury 1995, Flanders 1990, Kulkarni 1988) (Fig. 5–4).

NUCLEAR MEDICINE IMAGING

Generally speaking, bone scans demonstrate increased radiotracer localization from approximately 24 to 48 hours after fracture until at least 12 to 18 months later. A negative bone scan in this time interval effectively excludes fracture, but a positive bone scan is not characteristic, in that there are many causes of increased bone turnover (e.g., fracture, tumor, arthritis, infection).

Findings of Trauma

A summary of the imaging findings of post-traumatic abnormalities is found in Table 5–1.

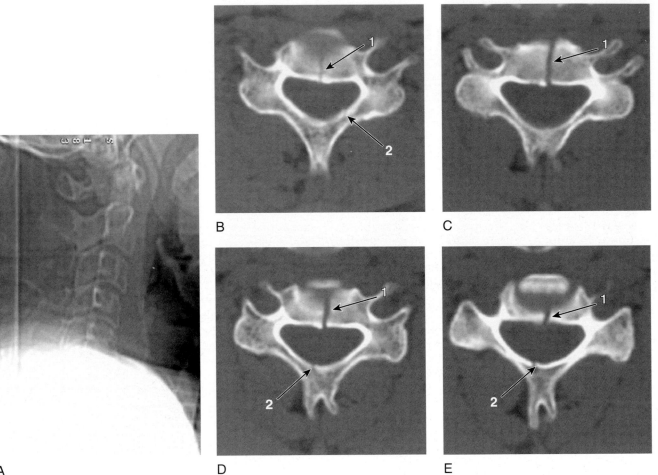

A

B

C

D

E

FIGURE 5–1

Cervical spine fracture impossible to identify on a lateral plain film examination but well seen on CT. A 41-year-old patient with persistent neck pain following trauma four days before CT study; initial plain films at an outside institution were interpreted as negative. *A,* Lateral scout view from CT examination demonstrates no obvious loss of vertebral body height or malalignment. *B,* 3 mm CT at the C5 level demonstrates a sagittal fracture line through the vertebral body with a *(arrow 1)* more subtle lesion of the left lamina *(arrow 2)* at the same level. *C–E,* Sequential inferior to superior 3 mm CT exams through the mid to upper C4 vertebral body demonstrate a sagittal fracture of the vertebral body *(arrow 1)* and a more subtle fracture of the right lamina *(arrow 2)* extending into the base of the spinous process.

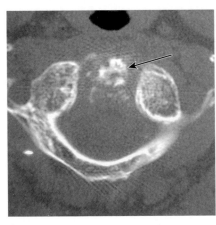

A

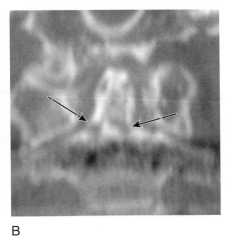

B

FIGURE 5–2

Base of dens fracture that is easier to appreciate on coronal reconstruction views than original axial CT images. An 85-year-old man with neck pain following trauma. *A,* Axial CT study at the base of the dens shows an irregular appearance with poorly defined margins *(arrow)*. *B,* Coronal reconstruction demonstrates a fracture through the base of the dens *(arrows)*. Fractures in same plane as the scan acquisition may be more easily visualized on reconstruction view.

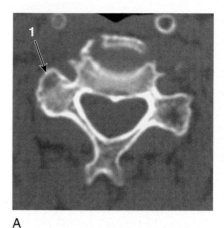

A

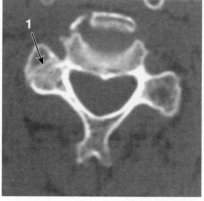

B

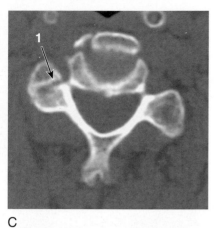

C

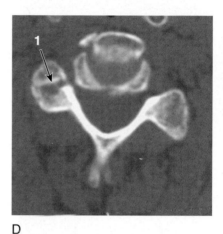

D

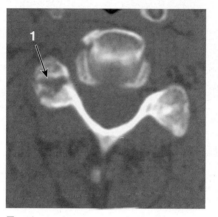

E

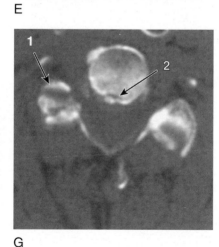

F

G

H

FIGURE 5–3

Lateral mass fracture that is easier to appreciate on sagittal reconstruction views than original axial CT images. A 60-year-old patient with neck pain following trauma. *A–G*, Sequential inferior-to-superior 1-mm CT slices from the C5 pedicle to the C4–5 disc level demonstrate an asymmetric appearance of the C5 right lateral mass, with lucencies in the mid-portion of the lateral mass (*arrow 1*). There is also a lucency through the posterior, inferior corner of C4 (*arrow 2*) along with spondylolisthesis. H, Sagittal reconstruction CT through the level of the right lateral mass demonstrates an abnormal configuration of the C5 lateral mass (*arrow 1*), with AP widening and a contour deformity along the superior margin secondary to fracture, and a fracture with posterior displacement of the inferoposterior tip of the C4 lateral mass (*arrow 2*).

INTERRUPTION OF CORTEX

Interruption of cortical bone is among the most clear-cut of all radiographic findings. Since "fracture" is defined as discontinuity of bone or cartilage, the presence of a discontinuous bony margin on a radiographic study strongly suggests fracture, particularly when seen on both sides of a tubular bone with an interposed gap. However, discontinuity of the bony cortex may be considerably more difficult to evaluate in a complex bone such as a vertebra. Although

fractures through the transverse process and spinous process (Fig. 5–5) are readily identified, these are relatively unimportant compared to other fractures that may result in neural compromise. These other fractures may manifest as discontinuities (occasionally subtle) of the bony cortex along the vertebral body margin (Figs. 5–1 and 5–6).

Although often indicating fracture, apparent discontinuity of the cortex of a bone may have several alternative explanations. On plain films, Mach lines (the result of collateral inhibition of cones in the retina along a sharply

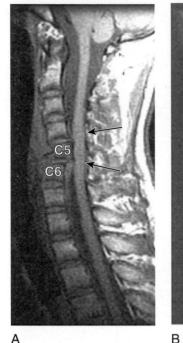
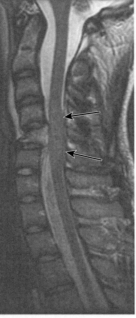

A B

FIGURE 5–4

Fracture with associated cord contusion. *A,* Sagittal T1WI demonstrates C5 wedging and retrolisthesis of C5 on C6. There is fusiform swelling of the cervical spinal cord centered at the C5 level *(arrows),* but no T1 prolongation within the cord is seen. *B,* Sagittal T2WI also demonstrates fusiform swelling of the spinal cord and mild T2 prolongation *(arrows).*

TABLE 5–1. Imaging Findings of Post-traumatic Abnormalities

Finding	Differential Diagnosis
Interruption of cortex	Fracture Mach lines Vascular channels Degenerative changes (with cysts) Overlapping structures Angulation of cut on CT Normal variants
Wedge deformity of vertebral body	Old or new compression fracture Normal variation, especially at C3 Scheuermann's disease Physiologic wedging at the thoracolumbar level Remodeling with osteoporosis
Abnormal bone fragment or contour abnormality	Displaced avulsion or burst fragment Un-united ossification center Osteophytic spurring Calcification of soft tissues
Abnormal alignment or position of bones	Fracture, dislocation, or subluxation Scoliosis Technique of examination (e.g., positioning so that cervical lordosis is lost) Degenerative change (e.g., degenerative spondylolisthesis) Lytic spondylolisthesis Scheuermann's disease
Vacuum phenomenon within the disc	Traumatic avulsion of Sharpey's fibers at margin of disc Traumatic central disc vacuum in fracture Degenerative disc disease with vacuum phenomenon
Gas or fluid within the vertebral body	Kummell's disease (avascular necrosis with vertebral body fracture) Acute fracture

Soft tissue abnormality	Hematoma
	  Post-traumatic
	  Spontaneous
	Retracted musculotendinous structure
	Directly visualized ligamentous or tendinous disruption
	Soft tissue tumor

defined dark-light interface) (Daffner 1988) give the false appearance of a fracture. Vascular channels may cause discontinuity not only in the long bones but also at the lumbar level on axial CT examinations (Fig. 5–7). Degenerative changes along the vertebral body margins may appear as discontinuities of cortex. Overlapping structures on plain films may be quite deceiving (Fig. 5–8), but CT and MR eliminate this problem since they are tomographic techniques. However, cuts across structures may give the appearance of a fracture where none exists. For example, an axial cut through a severely scoliotic spine may give the false impression of a sagittal fracture (Fig. 5–9) (Boechat 1987). It is therefore important to correlate images with scout views (for CT) and other planes (in MRI) for reference.

Interruption of cortex is usually less conspicuous on MRI than it is on plain films or CT but may be seen particularly if there is associated displacement of bone fragments (Figs. 5–6 and 5–10). Because of its high density, cortical bone appears as a bright white line on radiographs and CT. However, the lack of mobile protons results in a signal void within cortical bone on MRI, making bone contour (and any associated interruptions) difficult to see. Avulsion fractures in particular may be difficult to visualize, since they produce little corresponding marrow signal abnormality; on the other hand, compression injuries are often more conspicuous on MRI than on CT or plain films because of associated marrow signal change (Zanetti 2000).

WEDGE DEFORMITY OF VERTEBRAL BODY

Plain films may demonstrate wedging in acute fracture but also demonstrate virtually the same findings in chronic injury. Without old plain films for comparison, it is usually not possible to distinguish between acute and chronic wedge fractures of the vertebral bodies on plain films. CT for the most part shares this particular inadequacy with plain films, although "raw" fracture margins may be easier to demonstrate with CT (Figs. 5–7 and 5–11). Bone scans may provide some benefit, since they demonstrate a typical

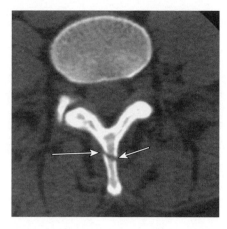

FIGURE 5–5

Spinous process fracture with obvious gap in the bone cortex. A 46-year-old woman after horseback riding injury with fall. Axial CT study through the lower aspect of the L4 vertebra demonstrates a minimally displaced fracture through the L4 spinous process. Note the obvious discontinuity of both cortices (*arrows*) and minimal leftward shift of the posterior fracture fragment.

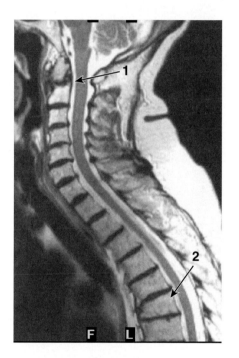

FIGURE 5–6

Discontinuity of bony cortex seen on MRI. A 70-year-old woman after MVA nine months prior to MRI; prior CT at another institution demonstrated an odontoid fracture. Sagittal T2WI demonstrates an odontoid fracture, with discontinuity of the posterior cortical margin (*arrow 1*) and anterior displacement of the inferior aspect of the fracture fragment relative to the underlying C2 vertebral body. There are multilevel degenerative changes of the cervical spine and there is wedging of the T6 (*arrow 2*) vertebral body; signal intensity is similar to other levels, indicating a chronic fracture.

configuration with a broad band of increased radiotracer localization in wedge fractures (Fig. 5–12). MRI typically demonstrates the abnormal configuration of the vertebral body, and in the case of a chronic fracture there will be marrow signal intensity similar to the other levels of the spine (Fig. 5–13). In the acute and subacute case, the mar-

row will demonstrate T1 and T2 prolongation (Fig. 5–14). Occasionally, there will be a band of decreased signal intensity that parallels the end plates of the vertebral body (Fig. 5–15). In most cases, the marrow demonstrates some normal signal intensity, either along the posterior superior and inferior margins or within the pedicles (Figs. 5–14 and 5–15) (An 1995, Yuh 1989). If no normal signal remains within the marrow, malignancy should be suspected with an associated pathologic fracture. For further discussion of differentiation of benign and malignant compression fractures, see Chapter 4.

Several other entities, in addition to acute and chronic fracture, may lead to wedge deformity of a vertebral body. Swischuk and associates (1993) note that vertebral bodies naturally progress from an oval shape to a wedge shape to a rectangular shape with age. Children may demonstrate the wedge configuration until relatively late in childhood, and a wedge deformity of C3 may be retained in adulthood. Scheuermann's disease may demonstrate wedging of one or more thoracic or upper lumbar vertebral bodies, usually with accompanying irregularity of the vertebral body margins (see Chapter 2). Chronic osteoporosis may lead to deformity of vertebral bodies with loss of height, possibly on a chronic basis and without a distinct or discrete fracture (Ryan 1994). In cases where plain films are equivocal, MR or nuclear medicine imaging may be helpful in determination of whether an abnormality represents an acute fracture: normal signal intensity within the marrow on MRI or lack of increased activity on the bone scan argues strongly against an acute fracture.

ABNORMAL BONE FRAGMENT OR CONTOUR ABNORMALITY

The complexity of shape of the vertebrae dictates that fractures may manifest as displaced fragments of bone rather than a simple cortical interruption (Daffner 1987). CT examination is an excellent method of detection of small, displaced bone fragments that are often difficult to appreciate on plain films. This ability proves particularly useful in evaluation of possible spinal canal fragments, which may be difficult or impossible to recognize on plain films but which may cause significant spinal canal narrowing and neural compression (Fig. 5–16). Similarly, CT greatly assists in evaluation of lateral mass fractures, which may be difficult or impossible to diagnose with plain films but which may account for persistent radiculopathy following trauma (Shanmuganathan 1994) (Fig. 5–17). MRI findings with small, displaced fragments, as noted earlier, tend to be more conspicuous in compression injuries than in avulsion injuries (Zanetti 2000).

Small fragments of bone or calcified tissue do not always represent fracture: un-united ossification centers may mimic fractures (Keats 1992). Osteophytes usually grow directly from the underlying cortical margin of bone, but occasionally degenerative calcifications begin in soft tissues a few millimeters from the cortical margin and mimic fracture fragments. Of course, osteophytes may also fracture, presenting a potentially confusing picture with an acute injury superimposed on chronic disease. In addition, remote fractures of the ring apophyses tend to heal with the appearance of osteophytes (Jonsson 1991). As with wedge deformities of

Text continued on page 242

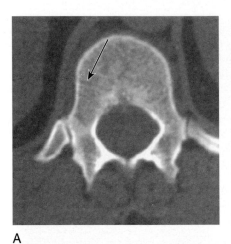

A

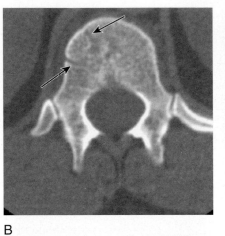

B

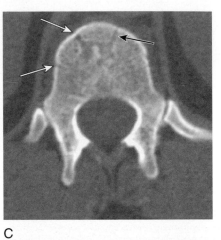

C

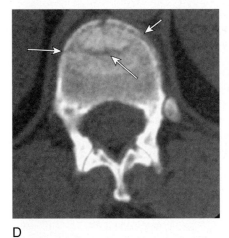

D

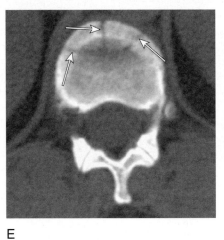

E

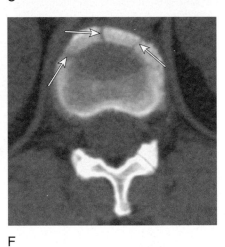

F

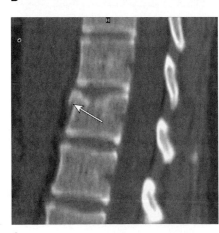

G

FIGURE 5–7

Fracture lines and vascular channels seen in the same patient. A 50-year-old woman with back pain following a fall. *A–C*, Sequential inferior to superior CT scans at the T12 pedicle level demonstrate vascular channels *(arrows)*. These channels have corticated margins and often lead to larger vascular channels. *D–F*, Sequential inferior-to-superior CT through the superior margin of the T12 vertebra with cortical discontinuities from fractures *(arrows)*. The fracture lines do not have corticated margins and are generally more sharply defined than vascular channels. *G*, Sagittal reconstruction demonstrates depression along the superior T12 vertebral margin and cortical discontinuity *(arrow)* along and anterior, superior aspect of the vertebral body. There is also slight wedging of T12, with loss of height of approximately 15%.

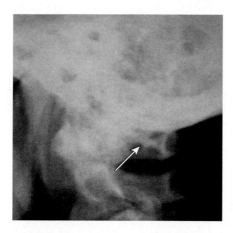

FIGURE 5–8

Overlapping structure on plain films resulting in an apparent fracture line. An 82-year-old man with neck and back pain and multilevel degenerative disease. Lateral plain film demonstrates apparent discontinuity of the posterior arch of C1 secondary to overlap of the skull base. CT examination (not shown) showed no abnormality of the C1 ring. Overlap of structures on plain films may frequently masquerade as fracture.

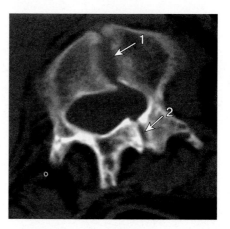

FIGURE 5–9

Simulated fracture in scoliosis secondary to obliquity of the spine with respect to the standard axial scan plane. An 84-year-old woman with low back pain after multilevel fusion surgery with severe scoliosis. Axial CT scan demonstrates apparent discontinuity of the vertebral body (*arrow 1*) and lamina (*arrow 2*). This appearance is caused by obliquity of the scan plane with respect to the spine.

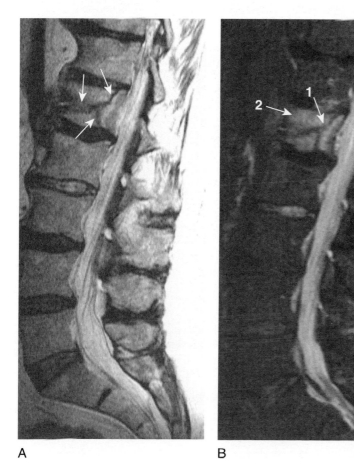

A   B

FIGURE 5–10

MRI of cortical (and cancellous bone) interruption. A 76-year-old man with back pain following a farming accident 1 week previously. *A,* Sagittal FSE T2WI demonstrates linear foci of decreased signal intensity along fracture lines within the L1 vertebral body (*arrows*). *B,* Sagittal STIR image also shows decreased signal intensity along the fracture lines (*arrow 1*), but also demonstrates T2 prolongation within the remaining marrow space of the vertebral body (*arrow 2*).

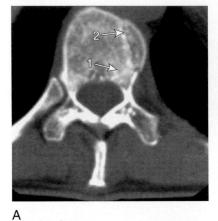
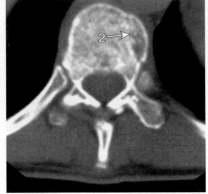
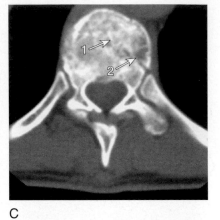

A   B   C

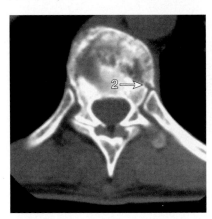
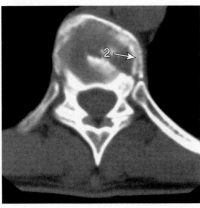
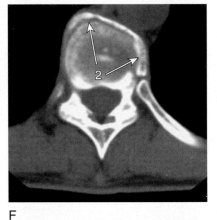

D   E   F

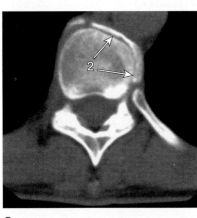
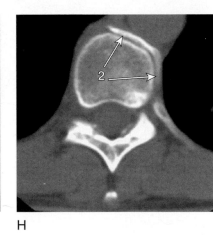
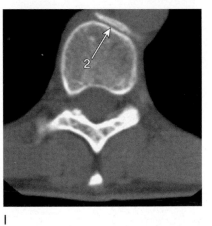

G   H   I

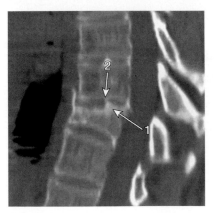

J

FIGURE 5–11

Comminuted, healing T10 compression fracture. A 45-year-old woman with a known T10 compression fracture sent for evaluation of fracture healing. *A–I*, Sequential 3-mm axial CT images from through the upper T10 vertebrae demonstrate a comminuted, healing fracture. Note the increased density of the vertebral body (*arrows 1*) consistent with fracture callus and the relatively smooth margins (*arrows 2*) of a healing fracture. *J*, Sagittal reconstruction CT demonstrating loss of 50% of the height of the vertebral body, sclerosis (*arrow 1*) and some fragmentation (*arrow 2*) along the anterior upper vertebral body.

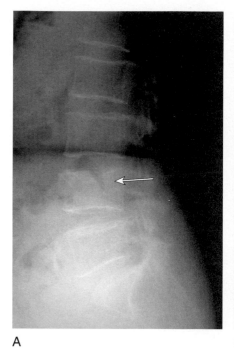

A

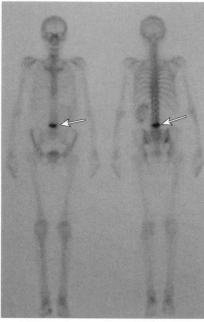

B

FIGURE 5–12

Wedge compression deformity with better dating of fracture on bone scintigraphy. A 65-year-old woman with low back pain. *A,* Lateral plain films demonstrate wedging of L4. It was not clear from the history and clinical findings whether this represented an acute or chronic fracture. *B,* Anterior and posterior bone scintigraphy studies demonstrate a broad, bandlike area of increased radiotracer localization (*arrows*), diagnostic of an L4 vertebral body fracture.

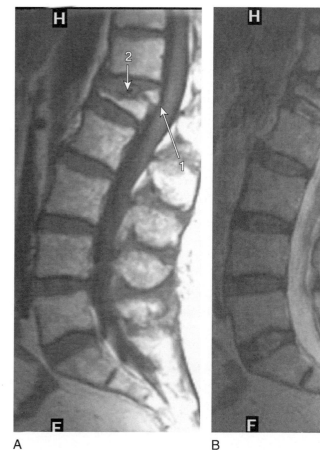

A

B

FIGURE 5–13

MRI of chronic L1 fracture. A 73-year-old woman with back pain and a history of remote fracture of the spine. *A,* Sagittal T1WI demonstrates 70% loss of height of the L1 vertebral body, with 6 mm of retropulsion of the posterior, superior cortex (*arrow 1*) consistent with middle column failure (a burst fracture) without associated neural compression. The marrow signal intensity within the abnormal vertebral body is similar or slightly increased compared to other levels (consistent with fatty replacement), with the exception of T1 prolongation along the superior vertebral body margin (*arrow 2*). *B,* Sagittal T2WI demonstrates similar signal intensity at the L1 and other levels, with some T2 shortening along the vertebral body margin (*arrow*). The findings are those of a chronic injury, with near isointensity of vertebral marrow signal, compared with adjacent level, and no paired T1/T2 prolongation.

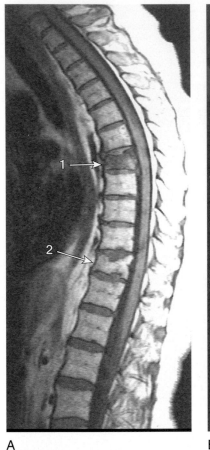

A

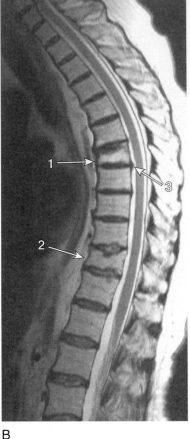

B

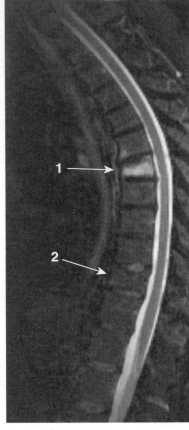

C

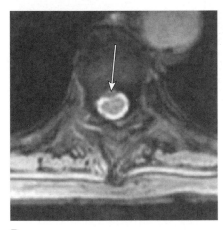

D

FIGURE 5–14

Chronic and acute wedge fractures of the spine. A 77-year-old woman with a known T11 compression fracture and new mid back pain. *A,* Sagittal T1WI demonstrates 30% loss of height of T7 *(arrow 1)* and 40% loss of height of T11 *(arrow 2)*. There is diffuse T1 prolongation at the T7 level, consistent with an acute or subacute fracture, whereas the marrow signal intensity of T11 is isointense with other levels, indicating chronic fracture. *B,* Sagittal FSE T2WI again demonstrates T7 *(arrow 1)* and T11 *(arrow 2)* loss of height. The T7 level demonstrates T2 prolongation, consistent with an acute or subacute fracture, whereas T11 shows isointensity consistent with a chronic injury. In addition, note the multilevel degenerative changes, including a 3.5-mm disc extrusion at the T7–8 level *(arrow 3)*. This may be an acute abnormality, accompanying the compression fracture. *C,* Sagittal GRE T2WI demonstrates conspicuous T2 prolongation of the T7 vertebral body *(arrow 1)*, with no such T2 prolongation at the T11 vertebral body *(arrow 2)*. *D,* Axial GRE T2WI at the T7–8 disc level demonstrates a 3.5-mm left central disc extrusion *(arrow)* with slight flattening of the thoracic spinal cord.

uncertain significance, additional imaging with a bone scan may provide important information and allow distinction between an acute fracture and a chronic degenerative process.

ABNORMAL ALIGNMENT OR POSITION OF BONES

Types of malalignment associated with fractures include accentuation of kyphosis (Figs. 5–11, 5–18, and 5–19) and lordosis as well as scoliosis and axial translation of one vertebra on the next. Abnormal alignment and position of bones may represent the result of fracture, dislocation or subluxation of a joint or joints, or both. Many rules have been generated for evaluation of plain films regarding the

typical distances between, for example, the pedicles, spinous processes, and intervertebral discs. Daffner (1988) has popularized a "rule of 2s." This rule states that 2 mm is the upper limit of normal for the interspinous or interlaminar space, atlantoaxial offset, anterolisthesis or retrolisthesis, and facet joint width. A distance of more than 2 mm for any of these should alert the physician that malalignment is present and a subtle fracture (which may not be directly perceptible on the radiographs) may be present.

Although malalignment may represent the effect of trauma, it has many other causes as well. A range of motion exists at each level of the spine, and this range is greater than "normal" in more or fewer individuals, depending on

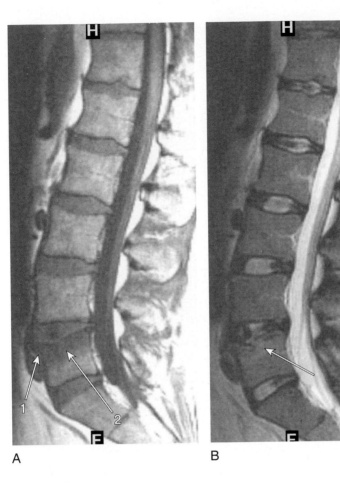

A   B

FIGURE 5–15

Acute L5 compression fracture with a sharp band of abnormal signal intensity within the vertebral body and remaining normal marrow at the level of the fracture. A 33-year-old man who had an injury 1 month prior to MR imaging. *A*, Sagittal T1WI demonstrates anterior wedging of L5 (*arrow 1*), along with a band of T1 prolongation. Note that the interface between this band and normal signal intensity in the more inferior aspect of the vertebral body is linear and well defined (*arrow 2*). *B*, Sagittal T2WI demonstrates corresponding T2 prolongation of the superior L5 vertebral body (*arrow*), consistent with an acute or subacute fracture, along with an abnormal contour of the superior vertebral margin.

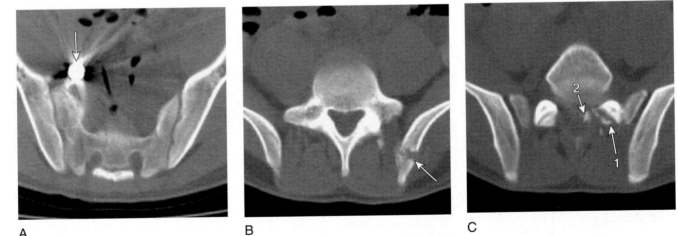

A   B   C

FIGURE 5–16

CT demonstrating spinal fragment not easily visualized on plain films. A 20-year-old patient after a gunshot wound. *A*, Axial CT shows bullet in pelvis (*arrow*). *B*, Axial CT at the L5 pedicle level shows a fracture of the iliac wing where the bullet crossed this structure (*arrow*). *C*, Axial CT at the L5–S1 disc level (superior to *A* but inferior to *B*) shows fracture of the L5 inferior articular process (*arrow 1*) with fragments carried into the canal medial to the L5–S1 facet joint (*arrow 2*). Such fragments of bone are not visualized on plain films.

where the cut-off is made within the normal population. Furthermore, some rules apply to only certain age groups: the predental distance in adults should not exceed 2 mm but may be up to 4 mm in children. Scoliosis is much more frequently idiopathic than post-traumatic, and spondylolisthesis is much more frequently degenerative or secondary to spondylolysis than it is to trauma. Accentuation of kyphosis may represent the result of either remodeling of the spine or multiple subclinical mild wedge fractures rather than an acute single-level compression fracture (Ryan 1994). Scheuermann's disease may result in wedging of multiple vertebral bodies with resultant kyphosis.

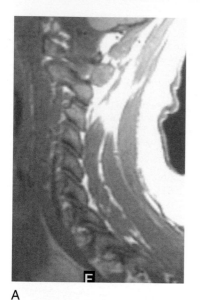

A

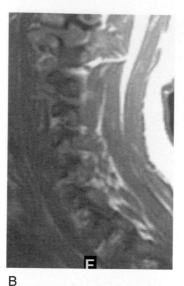

B

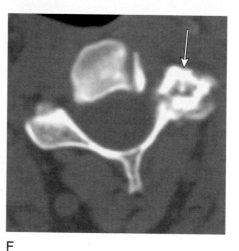

F

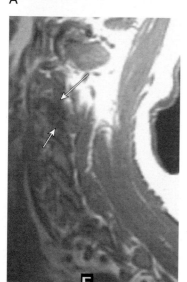

D

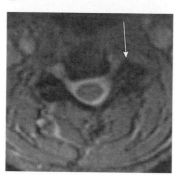

E

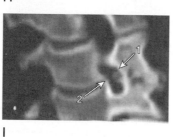

C

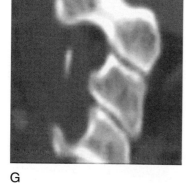

G

H

I

FIGURE 5–17

Subtle injury of the lateral mass documented by MRI and CT. A 45-year-old man after a motor vehicle accident (rear-ended with head turned to the left side) with plain films interpreted as normal at the time of the injury. The patient has persistent headaches, neck pain, and shoulder pain on the left side since the accident. *A,* Right parasagittal T1WI through the facet joints demonstrates a normal appearance of the right facet joints. *B–D,* Sequential left parasagittal T1WIs through the left facet joints demonstrates an abnormal appearance at the C3–4 level, with subchondral T1 shortening (*arrows*) and a deformed, widened appearance of the joint. *E,* Axial FSE T2WI at the C3–4 level demonstrates asymmetry of the lateral masses, with the left (*arrow*) being larger than the right. *F,* Axial image through the C3–4 lateral mass demonstrates overgrowth of the lateral mass (*arrow*) with bony contour abnormality consistent with a healing fracture and post-traumatic degenerative joint disease. *G,* Right parasagittal CT reconstruction demonstrates a normal appearance of the C2–3 and C3–4 facet joints. *H,* Left parasagittal CT reconstruction demonstrates a widened appearance of the C3–4 joint with irregular sclerosis and overgrowth of the inferior C3 (*arrow 1*) and superior C4 (*arrow 2*) lateral masses. *I,* Oblique coronal CT reconstruction through the right neural foramen demonstrates overgrowth of bone along the joint causing severe foraminal stenosis (*arrows*). The patient had good but transient relief of pain with intra-articular injection of steroids and anesthetic. The patient probably had an intra-articular injury at the time of the initial trauma, with subsequent degenerative changes of the facet joint that combined with overgrowth of the adjacent facet joints to produce foraminal stenosis.

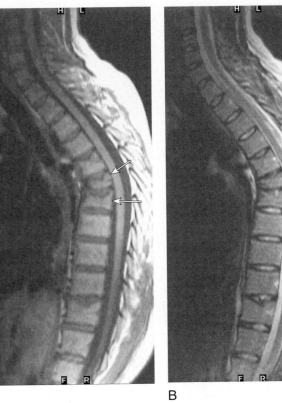

A

B

FIGURE 5–18

Accentuation of kyphosis secondary to deformity caused by fracture. A 23-year-old patient with trauma 3 months prior to imaging and who has ongoing upper mid back pain. *A*, Sagittal T1WI demonstrates wedge compression fractures of the T6 and T7 vertebral bodies (*arrows*) and associated accentuation of thoracic kyphosis. *B*, Sagittal T2WI again demonstrates accentuation of kyphosis. Note the Schmorl's node in the superior aspect of T11.

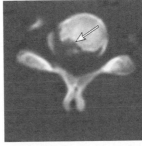

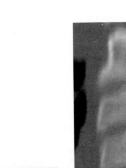

A

B

FIGURE 5–19

Abnormal alignment following fracture. A 15-year-old patient with neck pain and right arm numbness following trauma. *A*, Axial CT study through the inferior C5 vertebra demonstrates a fracture of the left posterior aspect (*arrow*). *B*, Sagittal reconstruction demonstrates abnormal alignment of the cervical spine, with focal kyphosis at C5–6 and 4 mm of traumatic spondylolisthesis (*arrow*).

As with other signs of fracture, CT may provide better detail and provide visualization of bone without overlapping structures, MRI allows evaluation of marrow signal intensity abnormalities that frequently accompany acute processes, and bone scans allow evaluation of increased bone turnover. Any of these three techniques may be helpful to determine whether malalignment is more likely acute (and more likely to require urgent therapy) or chronic.

VACUUM PHENOMENON WITHIN THE DISC

A vacuum phenomenon within a disc is an unusual manifestation of trauma (Edeiken-Monroe 1986, Harris 1987, Lafforgue 1994) (Fig. 5–20) and is far more frequently seen in degenerative disc disease. An exception to this rule is the small gas collection that may be seen along the margins of a disc in cases of avulsion of Sharpey's fibers (Fig. 5–21) (Finch 1996): such collections are virtually always post-traumatic rather than degenerative.

GAS OR FLUID WITHIN THE VERTEBRAL BODY

Gas within the vertebral body (as opposed to the intervertebral disc) is usually ascribed to ischemic necrosis of the vertebral body (Kummell's disease) (Figs. 5–22 and 5–23). This condition is thought to represent a post-traumatic collapse of the vertebral body. The primary trauma may be trivial and not remembered by the patient; ischemia and subsequent collapse may be delayed by days to weeks following the actual inciting event (El-Khoury 1993). The clinical importance is that such gas collections essentially

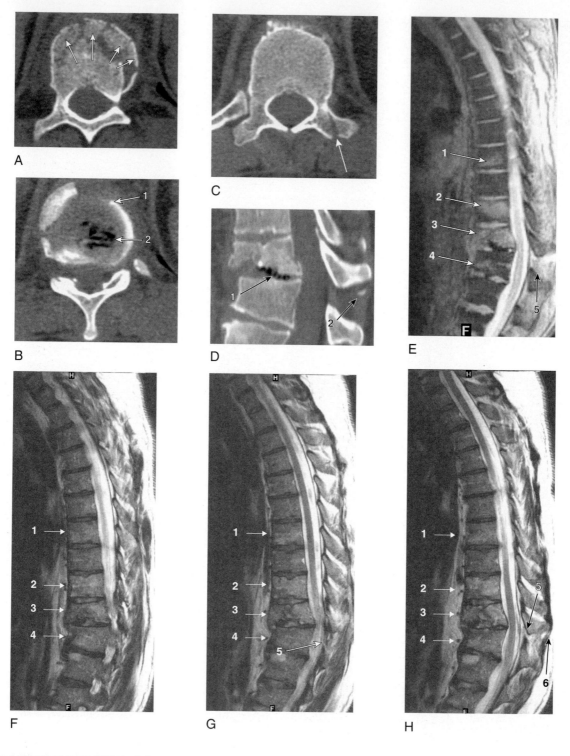

FIGURE 5–20

Multiple post-traumatic abnormalities including a vacuum phenomenon of a disc, ligamentous disruption, and raw fracture margins. A 43-year-old man after a fall from ladder with mid back pain. *A,* CT at the T10 vertebral body level demonstrates a comminuted vertebral body fracture with centripetal displacement of fracture fragments *(arrows)*. *B,* CT at the T10–11 disc level demonstrates fracture along the inferior aspect of the vertebral body *(arrow 1)* as well as a post-traumatic vacuum phenomenon of the intervertebral disc *(arrow 2)*. *C,* CT through the T11 level demonstrates a fracture through the base of the left transverse process *(arrow)*. Such a posterior fracture, particularly in conjunction with the comminuted T10 fracture at the level above, is an indication of severe trauma and potential instability. *D,* Sagittal reconstruction CT demonstrates wedging of the T10 and T11 vertebrae, as well as the post-traumatic vacuum phenomenon of the intervertebral disc *(arrow 1)*. Note the separation of the T10 and T11 spinous processes posteriorly, along with an avulsion fragment from the inferior aspect of the T10 spinous process *(arrow 2)*, indicating posterior ligamentous disruption. *E,* Sagittal GRE T2WI demonstrates abnormal signal intensity in the T7 *(arrow 1)*, T9 *(arrow 2)*, T10 *(arrow 3)*, and T11 *(arrow 4)* vertebral bodies, abnormal alignment at the T10–T11 level, and abnormal signal intensity between the spinous processes at the T10–11 level *(arrow 5)*. *F–H,* Sequential right parasagittal-to-sagittal T2WIs demonstrate T2 prolongation in the inferior aspect of T7 *(arrow 1)* and in T9 *(arrow 2)*, T10 *(arrow 3)*, and T11 *(arrow 4)* (although this is less conspicuous than on the STIR image). Again noted is accentuation of thoracic kyphosis and abnormal alignment at the T10/T11 level. The ligamentum flavum *(arrow 5)* and supraspinous ligament *(arrow 6)* appear discontinuous along the inferior aspect of the T10 spinous process. At surgery, there was complete disruption of all posterior ligamentous structures including the ligamentum flavum and supraspinatous ligament.

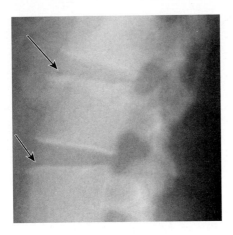

FIGURE 5–21

Small gas collections at the location of avulsion of Sharpey's fibers. A 26-year-old man with low back pain following a motor vehicle accident. Lateral plain film of the lumbar spine (cropped) demonstrates small gas collections along the anterior, inferior aspects of the L1–2 and L2–3 discs (*arrows*), consistent with soft tissue trauma and avulsion of Sharpey's fibers.

exclude malignancy as the cause of vertebral fracture (Bhalla 1998, Naul 1989). These gas collections may fill with fluid when the patient is undergoing MRI; such fluid collections typically demonstrate T1 and T2 prolongation (Naul 1989) (Fig. 5–24). However, acute trauma may produce similar fluid collections within the vertebral body (Le Hir 1999).

SOFT TISSUE ABNORMALITY

Plain films may demonstrate soft tissue abnormalities such as hematomas because of displacement of fat planes or normal air shadows. Soft tissue abnormalities are directly visualized on CT examination and even better seen on MRI study (Fig. 5–20) (Flanders 1990). MRI allows direct visu-

alization of the posterior longitudinal ligament, allowing evaluation of ligamentous disruption (Terk 1997). It also allows direct visualization of the spinal cord, allowing differentiation between hematoma and edema (Fig. 5–4) (El-Khoury 1995, Flanders 1990, Kulkarni 1988). Although soft tissue masses may be seen, for example, with tumor, this is usually not a difficult differentiation to make, because the clinical scenario is completely different. Lewis and associates (1990) presented a single case with widened prevertebral soft tissues on plain film mimicking prevertebral hematoma; the diagnosis of a widened prevertebral fat stripe was made with CT.

Clinical Scenarios and Reporting in Trauma

We review three scenarios with spine trauma: the acutely injured patient, the patient presenting in the subacute period with continued pain following injury, and the patient with a serendipitously discovered fracture on an imaging study performed where the pretest clinical suspicion of fracture is low.

ACUTE SPINE TRAUMA

The first step in the evaluation of acute spine trauma is to obtain plain films (Acheson 1987, El-Khoury 1995, Eustace 2000, Vandemark 1990) (Fig. 5–25). In many cases, these will completely characterize the injury and therapy may be based entirely on the plain film finding(s). If the plain films are negative, and if the clinical suspicion for fracture is low, then no other imaging studies need to be performed. Some authors (Vandemark 1990) recommend a delayed evaluation with flexion/extension plain films 10 to 14 days later to evaluate for possible ligamentous instability. Ronnen and colleagues (1996), however, found that a kyphotic angle seen on functional images typically did not indicate significant soft tissue abnormality but was secondary to hypermobility adjacent to a level with hypomobility produced by

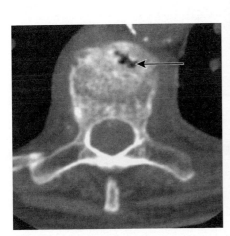

A

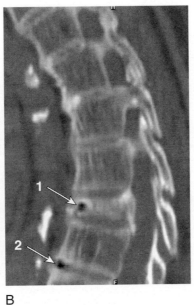

B

FIGURE 5–22

Kummell's disease (ischemic necrosis of the vertebral body). An 82-year-old woman with a known T8 compression fracture and ongoing back pain. *A,* CT at the T8 pedicle level demonstrates increased density of the vertebral body consistent with a healing fracture, and a small collection of gas in the anterior vertebral body (*arrow*). *B,* Sagittal reconstruction CT demonstrates loss of 70% of the height at the T8 level, along with gas within the vertebral body at T8 (*arrow 1*). Typical degenerative gas is seen at the T9–10 disc level (*arrow 2*).

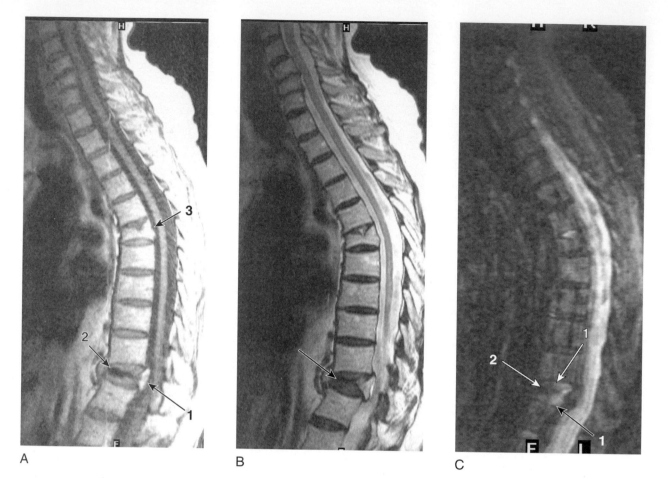

FIGURE 5–23

Kummell's disease (ischemic necrosis of the vertebral body). A 79-year-old woman with chronic back pain and no history of trauma. *A,* Sagittal T1WI demonstrates extensive abnormality at the T11 level including loss of height, middle column failure with retropulsion of the posterior aspect of the T11 vertebral body (*arrow 1*), and additional anteriorly displaced bone. Within the central portion of the vertebral body, there is a large area of T1 prolongation (*arrow 2*). Note also the T6 compression deformity (*arrow 3*) with marrow isointense to adjacent (normal) levels consistent with a benign, chronic compression fracture; there is associated accentuation of thoracic kyphosis at this level. *B,* Sagittal FSE T2WI demonstrates T1 shortening through much of the vertebral body (*arrow*), but particularly through the central portion of the vertebra, consistent with gas. T6 demonstrates isointensity relative to other, normal levels. *C,* Sagittal GRE T2WI demonstrates T2 prolongation along the superior and inferior margins of the vertebra (*arrows 1*) but T2 shortening in the central portion of the vertebra (*arrow 2*), again consistent with gas. This patient did not have any symptoms of myelopathy and the spinal canal was not significantly narrowed, despite the posterior displacement of the posterior T11 vertebral body.

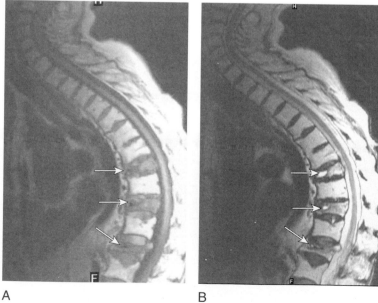

A   B

FIGURE 5–24

Kummell's disease (ischemic necrosis of the vertebral body). An 85-year-old woman with chronic back and leg pain. *A,* Sagittal T1WI demonstrates accentuation of thoracic kyphosis and cervical lordosis. T9, T11, and L1 demonstrate wedging and moderate T1 prolongation (*arrows*); within the T11 and L1 vertebral bodies are foci of pronounced T1 prolongation. There are additional wedged and deformed vertebral bodies with normal marrow consistent with old fractures. *B,* Sagittal T2WI demonstrates corresponding pronounced T2 prolongation within the T9, T11 and L1 vertebral bodies (*arrows*). Such collections represent fluid drawn into gas collections from Kummell's disease.

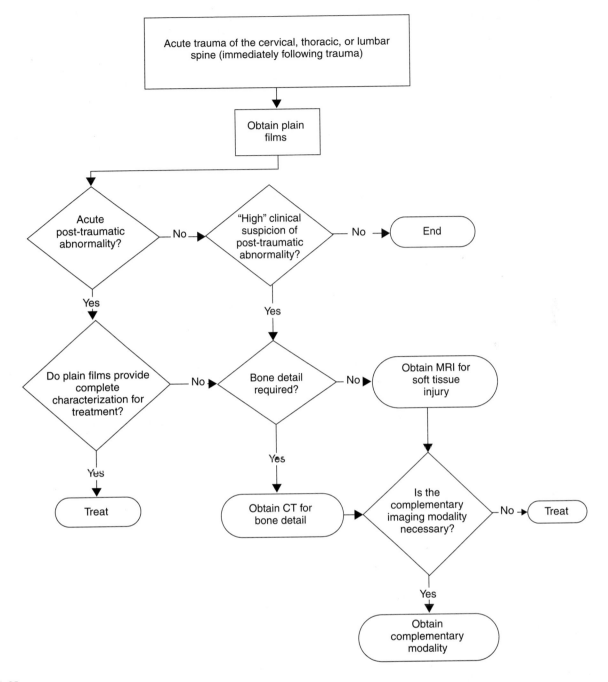

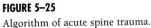

FIGURE 5–25

Algorithm of acute spine trauma.

muscle spasm. Furthermore, Matsumoto and coworkers (1998) found no correlation between nonlordotic cervical curvature or local angular kyphosis in patients with whiplash injury: in their studies, these "abnormal" curvatures were found equally frequently in patients with whiplash injury and asymptomatic subjects.

If clinical factors indicate that the likelihood of significant injury is high and if bony detail is necessary, CT should be performed (Fig. 5–1). If soft tissue evaluation (and, in particular, cord evaluation) is necessary, MRI should be performed (Fig. 5–26). Similarly, if plain films demonstrate a fracture or fractures but do not completely characterize the extent of injury, further evaluation with

either CT or MRI should be performed (Fig. 5–27). In some cases, plain films and CT or MRI alone is inadequate, and all three must be obtained for full characterization of the lesion (Fig. 5–28).

The report of radiographic studies in acute injury should state whether a fracture is present, whether there is indirect or direct evidence of soft tissue injury, and whether there is spinal canal or foraminal stenosis or neural compression. The degree of stenosis and neural compression should be graded as described in Chapter 2. Note, however, that the degree of canal stenosis has little or no correlation with neurologic recovery (or surgical results) (Atlas 1986, Shuman 1985). In many cases where fractures are present,

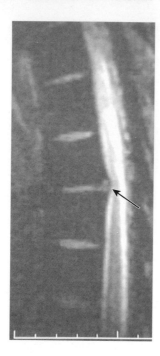

FIGURE 5-26

Trauma with negative plain films and soft tissue injury characterized by MRI. A 25-year-old man with lower extremity weakness following an MVA. Plain films of the thoracic spine (not shown) were negative. Sagittal GRE T2WI (shown here) demonstrates a cranially and caudally dissecting disc extrusion at T7–8 (arrow) with associated compression of the spinal cord. In this case, MRI was necessary to demonstrate pathology not evident on plain radiographs.

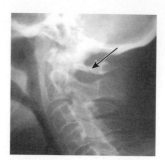

A

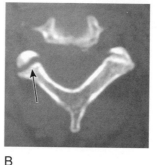

B

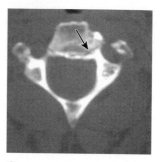

C

FIGURE 5-27

Fracture seen on plain films but more fully characterized with CT. A 41-year-old man with neck pain following an MVA. A, Lateral plain film demonstrates discontinuity of the posterior C1 ring (arrow). B, Axial CT study at the level of the C2–3 facet joints shows subluxation and widening of the left facet joint (arrow). C, Axial CT study through the base of the C2 vertebral body demonstrates a lucency along the posterior, inferior corner of the vertebral body (arrow). CT frequently detects additional injuries not visible on plain films.

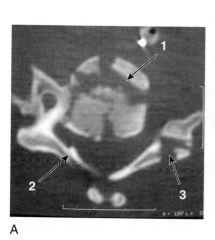

A

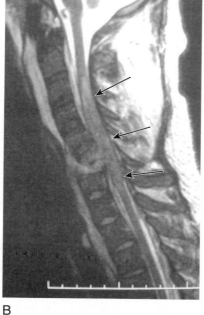

B

FIGURE 5-28

Complex trauma requiring plain films, CT, and MRI to completely characterize the injury. A 21-year-old man after diving injury. A, Axial CT study of the cervical spine shows multiple fracture lines involving the vertebral body (arrow 1), lamina (arrow 2), and lateral mass (arrow 3). B, Sagittal T2WI demonstrates extensive multilevel cord swelling and T2 prolongation (arrows). CT better characterizes the extent of bony abnormality, whereas MRI is necessary to delineate the extent of cord abnormality.

characterization by fracture mechanism (such as flexion or extension) is possible. The spine imager may wish to comment on stability, using, for example, the rules published by Daffner and associates (1990), which include a displaced vertebra, widened interlaminar or interspinous distance, perched or dislocated facets, increased interpedicular distance, and a disrupted posterior vertebral body line. However, the definition of instability is controversial and no single scheme to classify stability has been accepted (El-Khoury 1993).

FIGURE 5–29
Algorithm of subacute presentation following trauma. s/p, status post.

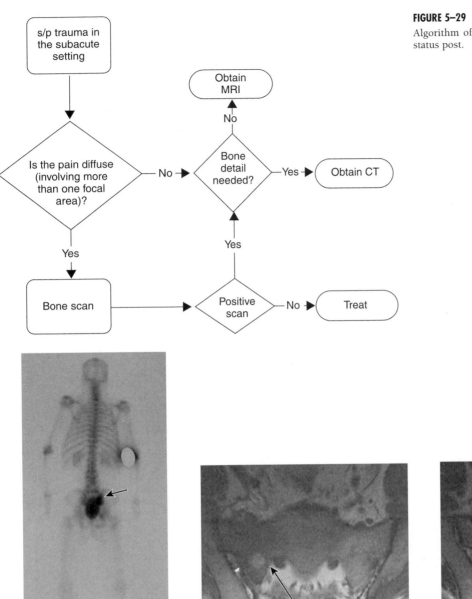

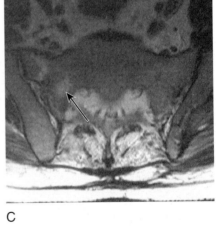

A   B   C

FIGURE 5–30

Bone scintigraphy which demonstrated a clinically unsuspected fracture. A 48-year-old man with chronic back pain after spine surgery, with a fall approximately 2 weeks prior to imaging with sacral pain. *A,* Nuclear medicine planar image demonstrates abnormal increased radiotracer localization of the right sacrum (*arrow*) (somewhat obscured by activity in the overlapping bladder). *B,* Axial T1WI through the sacrum demonstrates T1 prolongation in the right sacral ala (*arrow*). *C,* Axial T2WI through the sacrum demonstrates corresponding T2 prolongation within the right sacral ala (*arrow*). The findings are those of an acute fracture, corresponding to the patient's trauma of approximately 2 weeks before but not evident on plain films (not shown).

SUBACUTE PRESENTATION AFTER TRAUMA WITH CONTINUED PAIN

Most patients with spine trauma will have undergone plain film evaluation immediately after trauma. Plain films obtained either immediately after trauma or in the subacute period should be reviewed prior to CT or MR imaging; these may sufficiently characterize the lesion to obviate further imaging. As noted earlier, some patients undergo flexion/extension films on a delayed basis to evaluate possible soft tissue injury and "instability" (Vandemark 1990), but abnormal alignment does not necessarily indicate ligamentous injury (Ronnen 1996).

If the patient's plain films are negative and the patient's pain is intense and focal, an occult fracture should be suspected. CT examination with thin cuts through the level of symptoms should be performed (Figs. 5–1 and 5–6). If a soft tissue injury is suspected (e.g., post-traumatic disc herniation), then MRI should be performed (Fig. 5–14). Occasionally, post-traumatic pain is evaluated with MRI first but requires further characterization with CT (Fig. 5–17) or vice versa.

In patients with diffuse pain throughout the spine or body following trauma, a bone scan is frequently helpful (Fig. 5–29). Bone scintigraphy is quite sensitive to fracture and may allow discovery of a previously undiscovered fracture (Fig. 5–30). Of course, positive bone scintigraphy may also result from a wide variety of other lesions, including degenerative disease, infection, and postoperative changes. In addition, bone scans provide little information regarding soft tissue injury.

The report in subacute cases with post-traumatic abnormalities should contain the same information as the report in the acute case (see earlier). Some assessment of whether these abnormalities account for the patient's pain should be attempted as well, and occasionally recommendations for additional complementary imaging studies is warranted.

FRACTURE FOUND WITH NO HISTORY OF TRAUMA

When an imaging study performed for evaluation of spine pain reveals a fracture, it is first necessary to determine whether the fracture is acute and might account for the patient's symptoms (Fig. 5–31). Acute fractures may show "raw" margins or displaced and unincorporated flecks of bone on plain films and CT (Figs. 5–7 and 5–20), whereas MRI may demonstrate T1 and T2 prolongation (Figs. 5–14 and 5–20). Such findings should cause re-evaluation of the patient's history for possible trauma. If there is clearly no history of trauma, the possibility of a pathologic fracture, either through osteoporosis (Figs. 5–14 and 5–32) or tumor (see Chapter 4) should be considered. Fractures through osteoporosis in the lumbar spine usually resemble typical post-traumatic fractures. Sacral insufficiency fractures, however, may have a variety of appearances, depending on their age and the imaging modality used. Plain films may demonstrate little abnormality or a diffuse area of ill-defined sclerosis (in the healing stage). MRI typically demonstrates T1 and T2 prolongation. Such lesions are liable to be misdiagnosed as possible tumor; CT usually

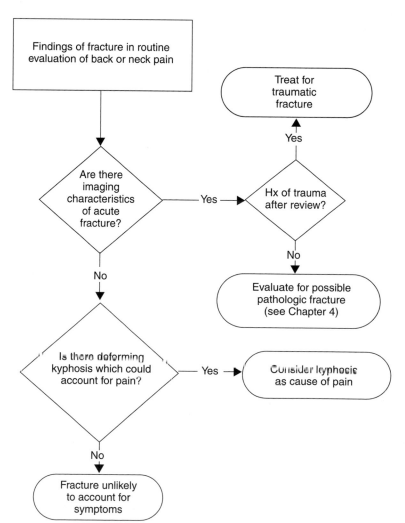

FIGURE 5–31

Algorithm of findings of fracture with no history of trauma. Hx, history.

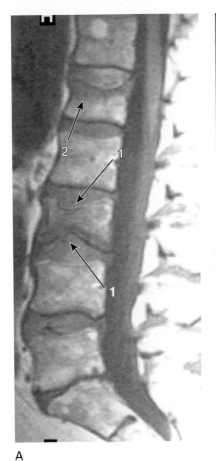

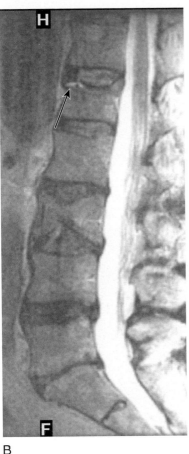

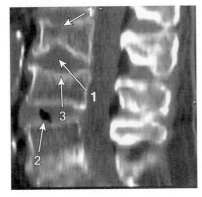

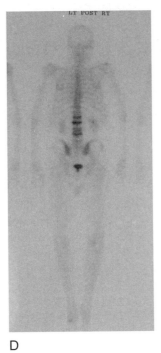

FIGURE 5–32

Acute fracture with no specific history of trauma. A 79-year-old man with both chronic and acute back pain and no history of trauma. *A,* Sagittal T1WI demonstrates biconcave deformity of L3 *(arrows 1)* with T1 prolongation of the vertebral marrow. There is also 30% loss of height at the L1 level, along with a well-defined band of T1 prolongation paralleling the superior margin of the vertebral body *(arrow 2)* consistent with a benign osteoporotic compression fracture. *B,* Sagittal T2WI demonstrates (when correlated with the T1WI) multilevel degenerative disc disease, including L2–3 moderate disc dehydration, L3–4 moderate disc dehydration, L4–5 moderate disc dehydration as well as a focus of gas and degenerative disc bulging, and L5–S1 severe loss of disc height and hydration with subchondral Modic Type II degenerative changes. There is little if any T2 prolongation corresponding to the T1 prolongation seen on the T1WI within the L1 and L3 vertebrae, although there is a slender focus of T2 prolongation along the superior margin of the L1 vertebral body *(arrow)*. Incidentally noted is a T12 hemangioma with T1 and (to a lesser degree) T2 prolongation relative to adjacent marrow. *C,* Sagittal CT reconstruction performed 2 months after the MRI study demonstrates the biconcave deformity at the L3 *(arrows 1)* level along with a vacuum phenomenon at the L4–5 level *(arrow 2)*. In addition, there is new deformity of the L4 vertebral body *(arrow 3)* consistent with development of yet another compression fracture. *D,* Nuclear medicine study done at the time of the CT examination shows abnormal increased radiotracer localization within the L1, L2, and L4 (and to a lesser extent, the L3) vertebral bodies, consistent with healing fractures.

demonstrates the lucency of the fracture line (Figs. 5–33 and 5–34) and (depending on the chronicity of the process) reactive changes of endosteal new bone along the fracture margins. Pathologic fractures may also occur through tumor. For a discussion of the differentiation of benign and malignant compression fractures, see Chapter 4.

If the imaging characteristics are those of a chronic fracture, this may or may not represent a cause of pain. Deforming kyphosis (>30 degrees) at the level of the fracture may lead to pain in some patients (Haher 2000)

(Figs. 5–18 and 5–35). In the absence of such deforming kyphosis, the presence of a chronic-appearing fracture should not necessarily be assumed to be the cause of the patient's symptoms, and evaluation for other causes of pain should be pursued. Some patients develop a syrinx following trauma (Fig. 5–36); if expansile, such a syrinx may produce associated neurologic findings.

The report on such fractures should indicate whether they are likely to be a source of symptoms and whether there are other abnormalities present on the scan that would better

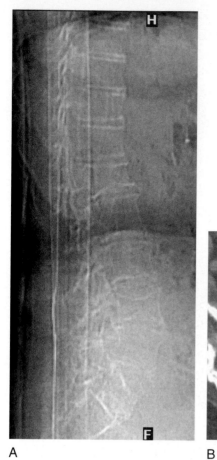

A

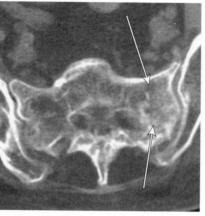

B

FIGURE 5–33

CT of a healing sacral insufficiency fracture. A 74-year-old woman with central low back pain. *A,* Sagittal scout view from the patient's CT scan shows multilevel degenerative disc disease, demineralization, and wedging of the T12 vertebral body. *B,* CT scan of the sacrum demonstrates abnormal texture of the left sacral ala *(arrows)* consistent with a healing sacral insufficiency fracture.

explain the patient's symptoms; the report should also recommend appropriate further work-up. Chronic fractures that appear healed on MRI and CT and demonstrate no severe kyphosis are unlikely to explain acute or ongoing pain. Further work-up may require obtaining additional clinical history (e.g., for suspected metastatic malignancy) or obtaining complementary imaging modalities (e.g., obtaining a bone scan to exclude an acute fracture when plain films show wedged vertebral bodies). Statistically, the most likely cause of back pain is degenerative disease (see Chapter 2).

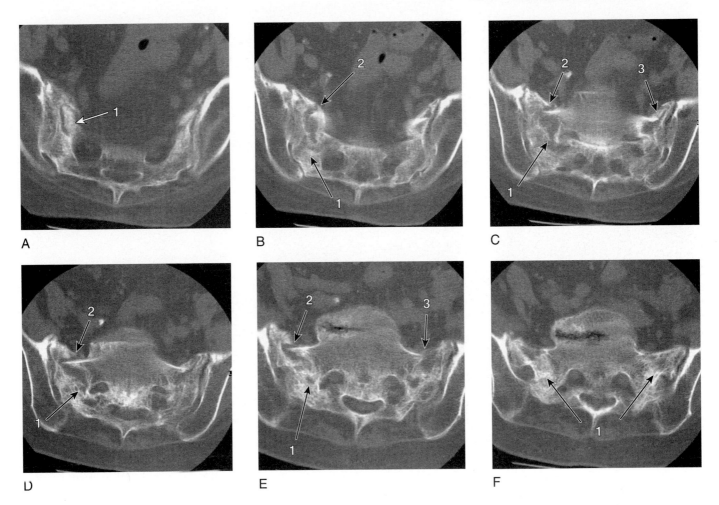

FIGURE 5–34

Sacral insufficiency fracture on CT. A 73-year-old woman with known osteoporosis and low back pain. An outside MRI (not shown) was interpreted as suspicious for tumor (the possibility of healing fracture was not mentioned) and the patient was referred for biopsy. *A–F,* Sequential 5-mm CT images demonstrate diffuse textural abnormality particularly of the right sacrum (*arrows 1*) from healing insufficiency fracture. Deformity and cortical discontinuity along the anterior margin of the right sacral ala (*arrows 2*), and, less conspicuously, the left sacral ala (*arrows 3*) are apparent. The findings are characteristic of a healing sacral insufficiency fracture.

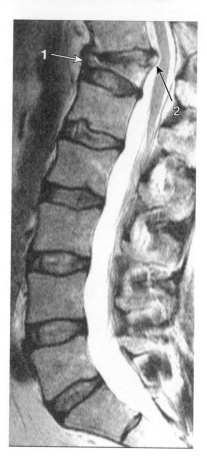

FIGURE 5–35

Chronic fracture with pain secondary to accentuated kyphosis. A 56-year-old man after fracture 1 year prior to MR examination with a known T12 fracture. The patient had pain following the fracture which gradually diminished, but had new and different pain in approximately the same location which developed about 1 year following the fracture. Sagittal T2WI demonstrates marked anterior wedging of the T12 vertebra (*arrow 1*) with loss of more than 70% of anterior vertebral body height, as well as middle column failure and retropulsion of the posterior, upper margin of the T12 vertebra (*arrow 2*) with associated central canal narrowing. The spinal cord is draped over the posterior T12 vertebral margin and mildly deformed at the level of the fracture. There is marked accentuation of kyphosis at this level. Given the clinical history and imaging findings, the patient's pain is most likely coming from accentuation of his kyphosis.

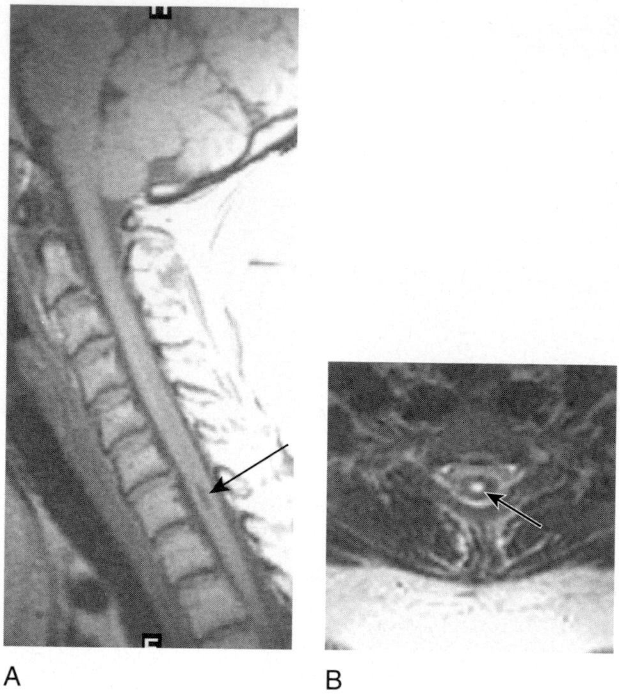

A   B

FIGURE 5–36

Post-traumatic syrinx. A 29-year-old woman who had a motor vehicle accident 5 months prior to imaging with persistent neck pain. *A,* Sagittal T1WI demonstrates a focus of T1 prolongation within the lower cervical spinal cord at the C7 level (*arrow*). *B,* Axial T2WI demonstrates a 4-mm central focus of T2 prolongation within the spinal cord (*arrow*).

References

Acheson MB, Livingston RR, Richardson ML, Stimac GK. High-resolution CT scanning in the evaluation of cervical spine fractures: comparison with plain film examinations. AJR Am J Roentgenol 1987; 148:1179–1185.

An HS, Andreshak TG, Nguyen C, Williams A, Daniels D. Can we distinguish between benign versus malignant compression fractures of the spine by magnetic resonance imaging? Spine 1995; 20:1776–1782.

Atlas SW, Regenbogen V, Rogers LF, Kim KS. The radiographic characterization of burst fractures of the spine. AJR Am J Roentgenol 1986; 147:575–582.

Berquist TH. Imaging of adult cervical spine trauma. Radiographics 1988; 8:667–694.

Bhalla S, Reinus WR. The linear intravertebral vacuum: a sign of benign vertebral collapse. AJR Am J Roentgenol 1998; 170:1563–1569.

Blacksin MF, Lee HJ. Frequency and significance of fractures of the upper cervical spine detected by CT in patients with severe neck trauma. AJR Am J Roentgenol 1995; 165:1201–1204.

Boechat MI. Spinal deformities and pseudofractures. AJR Am J Roentgenol 1987; 148:97–98.

Daffner RH. Imaging of Vertebral Trauma. Rockville, MD, Aspen, 1988.

Daffner RH, Deeb ZL, Goldberg AL, Kandabarow A, Rothfus WE. The radiologic assessment of post-traumatic vertebral stability. Skeletal Radiol 1990; 19:103–108.

Daffner RH, Deeb ZL, Rothfus WE. The posterior vertebral body line: importance in the detection of burst fractures. AJR Am J Roentgenol 1987; 148:93–96.

Edeiken-Monroe B, Wagner LK, Harris JH. Hyperextension dislocation of the cervical spine. AJR Am J Roentgenol 1986; 146:803–808.

El-Khoury GY, Kathol MH, Daniel WW. Imaging of acute injuries of the cervical spine: value of plain radiography, CT, and MR imaging. AJR Am J Roentgenol 1995; 164:43–50.

El-Khoury GY, Whitten CG. Trauma to the upper thoracic spine: anatomy, biomechanics, and unique imaging features. AJR Am J Roentgenol 1993; 160:95–102.

Eustace S, Guidone P, El-Khoury GY. Newer trends in imaging of cervical spine trauma. Contemp Spine Surg 2000; 1:27–34.

Finch PM, Taylor JR. Functional anatomy of the spine. In Waldman SD, Winnie AP (eds). Interventional Pain Management. Philadelphia, WB Saunders, 1996.

Flanders AE, Schaefer DM, Doan HT, Mishkin MM, Gonzalez CF, Northrup BE. Acute cervical spine trauma: correlation of MR imaging findings with degree of neurologic deficit. Radiology 1990; 177:25–33.

Haher TR, Merola AA, Caruso SA, Mills E. Posttraumatic spinal deformity. Contemp Spine Surg 2000; 1:47–53.

Harris JH, Edeiken-Monroe B. The Radiology of Acute Cervical Spine Trauma, 2nd ed. Baltimore, Williams & Wilkins, 1987.

Jonsson K, Niklasson J, Josefsson PO. Avulsion of the cervical spinal ring apophyses: acute and chronic appearance. Skeletal Radiol 1991; 20:207–210.

Katzberg RW, Benedetti PF, Drake CM, Ivanovic M, Levine RA, Beatty CS, Nemzek WR, McFall RA, Ontell FK, Bishop DM, Poirier VC, Chong BW. Acute cervical spine injuries: prospective MR imaging assessment at a level 1 trauma center. Radiology 1999; 213:203–212.

Keats TE. Atlas of Normal Roentgen Variants That May Simulate Disease, 5th ed. St. Louis, Mosby–Year Book, 1992.

Klein GR, Vaccaro AR, Albert TJ, Schweitzer M, Keely D, Karasick D, Colter JM. Efficacy of magnetic resonance imaging in the evaluation of posterior cervical spine fractures. Spine 1999; 24:771–774.

Kulkarni MV, Bondurant FJ, Rose SL, Narayana PA. 1.5 tesla magnetic resonance imaging of acute spinal trauma. Radiographics 1988; 8:1059–1082.

Lafforgue PF, Chagnaud CJ, Daver LMH, Daumen-Legre VMS, Peragut JC, Kasbarian MJ, Volot F, Acquaviva PC. Intervertebral disk vacuum phenomenon secondary to vertebral collapse: prevalence and significance. Radiology 1994; 193:853–858.

Le Hir PX, Sautet A, Le Gars L, Zeitouin F, Tubiana JM, Arrive L, Laredo JD. Hyperextension vertebral body fractures in diffuse idiopathic skeletal hyperostosis: a cause of intravertebral fluidlike collections on MR imaging. AJR Am J Roentgenol 1999; 173:1679–1683.

Lee C, Kim KS, Rogers LF. Sagittal fracture of the cervical vertebral body. AJR Am J Roentgenol 1982; 139:55–60.

Lee C, Woodring JH. Unstable Jefferson-variant atlas fractures: an unrecognized cervical injury. AJR Am J Roentgenol 1992; 158:113–118.

Lewis CA, Castillo M, Hudgins PA. Cervical prevertebral fat stripe: a normal variant simulating prevertebral hemorrhage. AJR Am J Roentgenol 1990; 155:559–560.

Matsumoto M, Fujimura Y, Suzuki N, Toyama Y, Shiga H. Cervical curvature in acute whiplash injuries: prospective comparative study with asymptomatic subjects. Injury 1998; 29:775–778.

Naul LG, Peet GJ, Maupin WB. Avascular necrosis of the vertebral body: MR imaging. Radiology 1989; 172:219–222.

Nunez DB, Quencer RM. The role of helical CT in the assessment of cervical spine injuries. AJR Am J Roentgenol 1998; 171:951–957.

Nunez DB, Zuluaga A, Fuentes-Bernado DA, Rivas LA, Becerra JL. Cervical spine trauma: how much more do we learn by routinely using helical CT? Radiographics 1996; 16:1307–1321.

Pech P, Kilgore DP, Pojunas KW, Haughton VM. Cervical spine fractures: CT detection. Radiology 1985; 157:117–120.

Pettersson K, Hildingsson C, Toolanen G, Fagerlund M, Bjornebrink J. Disc pathology after whiplash injury: a prospective magnetic resonance imaging and clinical investigation. Spine 1997; 22:283–288.

Ronnen HR, de Korte PJ, Brink PRG, van der Bijl HJ, Tonino AJ, Franke CL. Acute whiplash injury: is there a role for MR imaging? A prospective study of 100 patients. Radiology 1996; 201:93–96.

Ryan PJ, Fogelman I. Osteoporotic vertebral fractures: diagnosis with radiography and bone scintigraphy. Radiology 1994; 190:669–672.

Shanmuganathan K, Mirvis SE, Levine AM. Rotational injury of cervical facets: CT analysis of fracture patterns with implications for management and neurologic outcome. AJR Am J Roentgenol 1994; 163:1165–1169.

Shuman WP, Rogers JV, Sickler ME, Hanson JA, Crutcher JP, King HA, Mack LA. Thoracolumbar burst fractures: CT dimensions of the spinal canal relative to postsurgical improvement. AJR Am J Roentgenol 1985; 145:337–341.

Swischuk LE, Swischuk PN, John SD. Wedging of C3 in infants and children: usually a normal finding and not a fracture. Radiology 1993; 188:523–526.

Terk MR, Hume-Neal M, Fraipont M, Ahmadi J, Colletti PM. Injury of the posterior ligament complex in patients with acute spinal trauma: evaluation by MR imaging. AJR Am J Roentgenol 1997; 168:1481–1486.

Vandemark RM. Radiology of the cervical spine in trauma patients: practice pitfalls and recommendations for improving efficiency and communication. AJR Am J Roentgenol 1990; 155:465–472.

West OC, Anbari MM, Pilgram TK, Wilson AJ. Acute cervical spine trauma: diagnostic performance of single-view versus three-view radiographic screening. Radiology 1997; 204:819–823.

Woodring JH, Goldstein SJ. Fractures of the articular processes of the cervical spine. AJR Am J Roentgenol 1982; 139:341–344.

Yuh WTC, Zachar C, Barloon TJ, Sato Y, Sickels WJ, Hawes DR. Vertebral compression fractures: distinction between benign and malignant causes with MR imaging. Radiology 1989; 172:215–218.

Zanetti M, Bruder E, Romero J, Hodler J. Bone marrow edema pattern in osteoarthritic knees: correlation between MR imaging and histologic findings. Radiology 2000; 215:835–840.

6 Infectious Spondylitis

DONALD L. RENFREW

A patient may present with a history so characteristic of infectious spondylitis that it is obvious that he or she almost certainly has the disease. For example, an intravenous (IV) drug abuser with a new onset of severe, unremitting backache, chills and fever, and an elevated white blood cell (WBC) count is presumed to have infectious spondylitis until proven otherwise. Other patients fall into a more indeterminate category: for example, a patient with a recent discectomy who has worsening backache but a normal WBC count and no fever, or an elderly man who has undergone prostatic resection and has subsequently developed a severe, persistent backache. Since an elevated WBC count and fever

occur only in approximately half of patients with discitis (Carragee 1997b, Hadjipavlou 2000, Hitchon 1992), their absence does not exclude the diagnosis. Indeed, the only clinical feature that virtually all these patients share is backache, but since up to 80% of the general population suffers from this malady (Waddell 1998), backache is hardly a specific finding. To facilitate the work-up and diagnosis of these patients and to put imaging within a context, we present several "clinical scenarios" that fit most patients who have infectious spondylitis. We present suggested pathways for evaluation of patients along with the scenarios, incorporating both clinical findings and imaging data. Before

TABLE 6–1. Findings of Infectious Spondylitis

Finding	Differential Diagnosis
T1 prolongation in subchondral marrow *with* or *without* associated T2 prolongation	Infectious spondylitis Degenerative change (pre- or post-op) Renal osteodystrophy Neoplasm Stress injury
T2 prolongation within the intervertebral disc	Infectious spondylitis Degenerative change (pre- or post-op) Renal osteodystrophy Neoplasm
Contrast enhancement of the disc, subchondral marrow, and epidural space	Infectious spondylitis Degenerative change (pre- or post-op) Neoplasm
Erosion of vertebral endplates	Infectious spondylitis Degenerative change (pre- or post-op) Renal osteodystrophy
Epidural fluid collection	Infectious spondylitis Sarcoidosis Ankylosing spondylitis Neoplasm
Paraspinous soft tissue abnormality	Infectious spondylitis Neoplasm
Posterior element involvement	Infectious spondylitis Neoplasm Arthritis

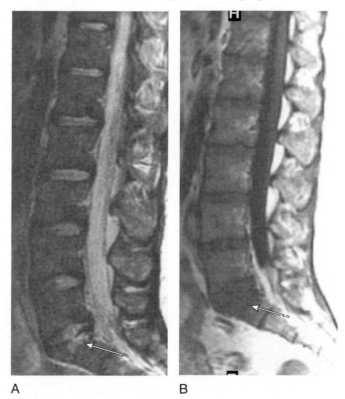

A   B

FIGURE 6–1

Infectious discitis with subchondral marrow signal intensity change. A 44-year-old woman after discography (at another institution) 5 months previously. *A*, Sagittal T2WI demonstrates abnormal subchondral T2 prolongation (*arrow*). *B*, Sagittal T1WI shows subchondral T1 prolongation (*arrow*). There is minimal disc T1 and T2 prolongation, and no epidural mass or paraspinous mass is present.

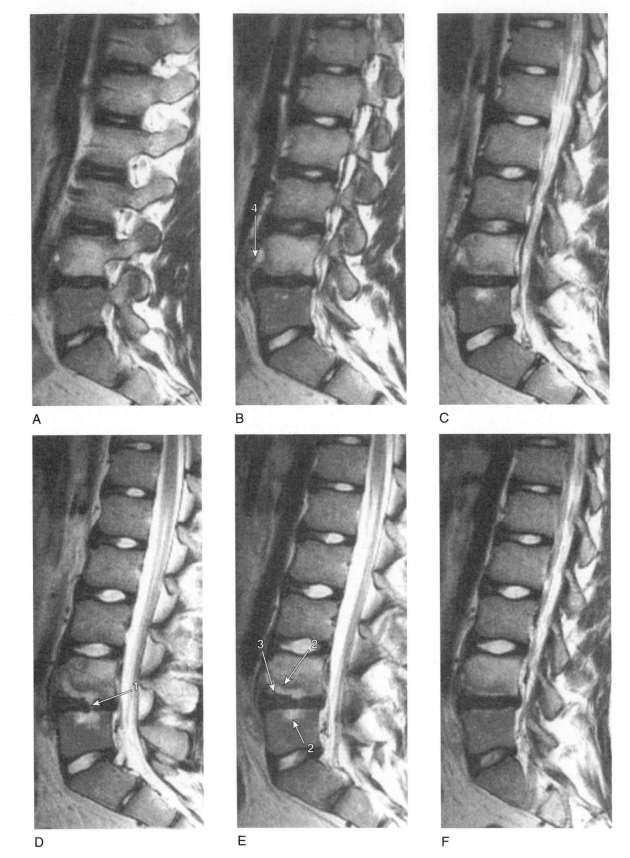

FIGURE 6–2

Infectious discitis with subchondral marrow signal intensity change more obvious on gradient-echo images. A 14-year-old boy with central low back pain. The patient had no history of fever, chills, or other constitutional symptoms. *A–F,* Sequential sagittal fast spin-echo (FSE) T2WIs demonstrate multiple abnormalities at the L4–5 level, including overall decreased signal intensity within the disc with a central focus of T2 prolongation *(arrow 1),* T2 prolongation along both sides of the L4–5 disc *(arrow 2),* erosions of the end plates *(arrow 3),* and anterior soft tissue abnormality *(arrow 4).*

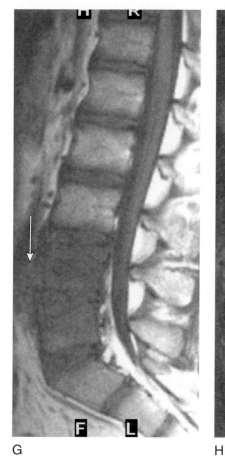

G

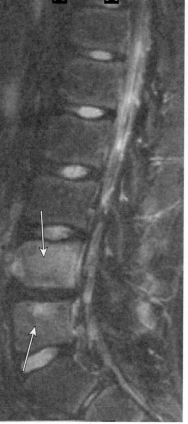

H

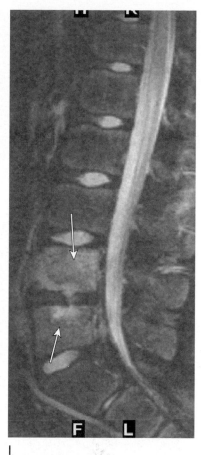

I

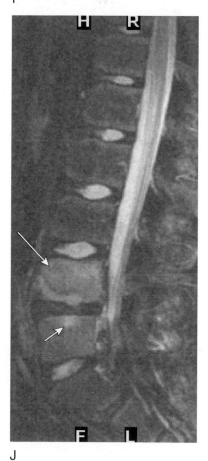

J

FIGURE 6–2   *(Continued)*

G, Sagittal T1WI demonstrates extensive T1 prolongation of the marrow within L4 and L5 vertebral bodies, as well as abnormal soft tissue anteriorly *(arrow)*. *H–J,* Sequential sagittal short tau inversion recovery (STIR) images again demonstrate T2 prolongation in the L4 and L5 vertebrae *(arrows)*. The conspicuity and extent of abnormal marrow signal are greater on the STIR image compared to the FSE images.

(Illustration continued on following page)

presenting the clinical scenarios, however, we describe and illustrate the imaging findings of infectious spondylitis (Table 6–1).

Finding 1: T1 Prolongation within Subchondral Marrow *with* or *without* T2 Prolongation

Adult spinal infection typically begins in the subchondral marrow on one side of the disc (St. Amour 1994). Abnormal signal intensity in the subchondral marrow is usually the first imaging finding (Dagirmanjian 1996, Smith 1989), although by the time imaging is performed additional findings are often present. As inflammatory tissue replaces marrow fat, both T1 and T2 are prolonged (with associated decreased signal intensity on T1-weighted image [T1WI] and increased signal intensity on T2WI) (Fig. 6–1). Standard T2WIs are relatively insensitive to early changes, and fat-suppressed or short tau inversion recovery (STIR) images show subchondral signal intensity changes earlier and with more conspicuity than T2WI (Meyers 1991, Szypryt 1988, Thrush 1990) (Fig. 6–2). Thus, normal signal intensity on T2WI certainly does not exclude discitis;

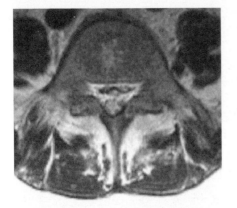

K

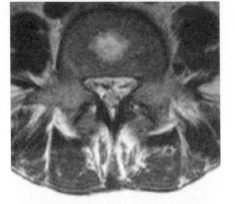

L

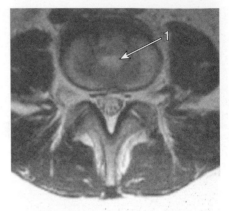

M

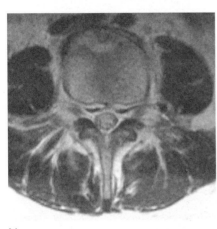

N

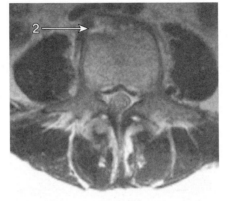

O

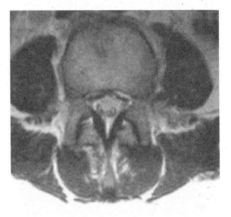

P

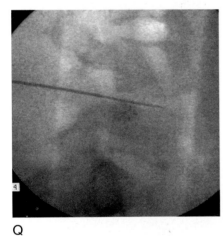

Q

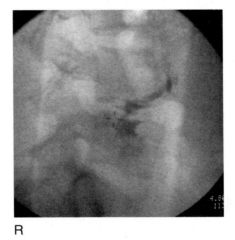

R

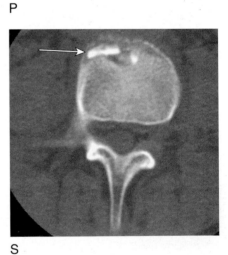

S

FIGURE 6–2 *(Continued)*

K–P, Sequential axial T2WI from just below the L5 pedicle through the L3–4 disc demonstrates punctate T2 prolongation in the central disc *(arrow 1)* with larger areas of T2 prolongation in the marrow on either side of the disc. The abnormal signal intensity within the L4 vertebral body leads to the right, anterolateral aspect of the vertebral body where there is associated abnormal soft tissue *(arrow 2). Q,* C-arm fluoroscopically directed image taken during disc biopsy/aspiration. No pus was forthcoming at the time of aspiration. *R,* Following aspiration and biopsy, contrast material was injected into the disc, with dissection into the marrow of the L4 vertebra above and the L5 vertebra below, as well as along the anterior aspect of the L4 vertebra. *S,* Axial 3-mm CT done just below the L4 pedicle level following injection of the disc with contrast agent demonstrates contrast in the anterior aspect of the vertebral body with overlying expansion and destruction of cortex *(arrow). Staphylococcus aureus* was cultured from the disc. Treatment with appropriate antibiotics followed, with patient recovery.

indeed, in Dagirmanjian and coworkers' series (1996) there was normal signal intensity on T2WI in nearly half the cases. Less frequently, patients with proven discitis may present with abnormal signal intensity on T2WI but not T1WI (Gillams 1996, Thrush 1990), with abnormal signal intensity only after contrast enhancement (Gillams 1996), or with falsely negative STIR images (Gillams 1996). Of course, other material replacing subchondral marrow,

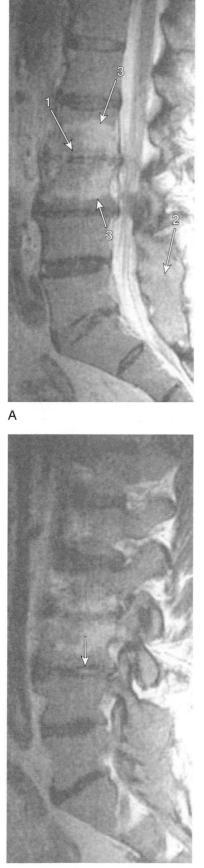

A

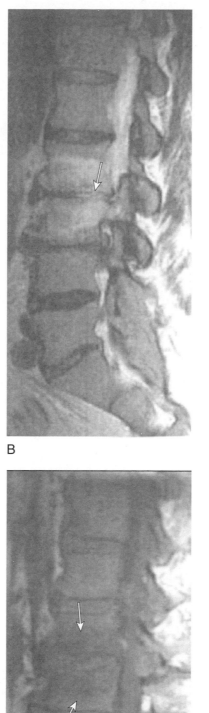

B

C

D

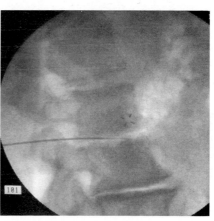

E

FIGURE 6–3

Degenerative disc disease resembling infectious spondylitis. A 78-year-old man after remote posterior spine fusion from L4 through S1, and more recent (3 months prior) transurethral resection of the prostate with persistent, severe low back pain even at rest. *A*, Sagittal T2WI demonstrates multilevel severe degenerative disc disease, including L1–2 mild loss of disc height and hydration, L2–3 severe loss of disc height with linear T2 prolongation within the disc (*arrow 1*), L3–4 severe loss of disc height and hydration, and L4–5 moderate disc dehydration. There is a solid fusion posteriorly at L4–S1 (*arrow 2*). Extensive subchondral marrow changes surround the L2–3 disc, with T2 prolongation (*arrow 3*). *B*, Left parasagittal T2WI shows T2 prolongation within the intervertebral disc (*arrow*). *C*, Right parasagittal T2WI shows similar but less dramatic T2 prolongation of the L3–4 disc (*arrow*) and again shows T2 prolongation in the subchondral marrow adjacent to the L2–3 disc. *D*, Sagittal T1WI demonstrates T1 shortening surrounding the L2–3 disc (*arrows*). Because of the history of prior prostatic surgery, unremitting pain, and extensive marrow changes (with less impressive T2 prolongation within the disc), biopsy was performed. *E*, C-arm fluoroscopy image taken during disc biopsy and aspiration. Biopsy revealed no evidence of infectious or inflammatory cells, and cultures were negative. The patient's back pain slowly diminished over the next several months, and approximately 1 year later he was doing well with no evidence of ongoing infection and no constitutional symptoms.

including but not limited to degenerative fibrovascular changes (de Roos 1987, Modic 1988, Stabler 1996) (Fig. 6–3), neoplasm (Dagirmanjian 1997), and reaction to stress injury (Siegelman 1999), may have a similar or identical imaging appearance with T1 and T2 prolongation. Postprocedural "aseptic" discitis, whether using conventional (Grane 1988) or laser (Tonami 1989) surgery or following chymopapain injection, may share the imaging characteristics of Modic Type I (Modic 1988) degenerative change, with T1 and T2 prolongation (see Chapter 2).

Infection may spread to both sides of the intervertebral disc via metaphyseal anastomosing arteries without involvement of the intervening disc itself (Smith 1989). Granulomatous infectious spondylitis more frequently presents in this fashion than does pyogenic infectious spondylitis, perhaps because of higher oxygen requirements or lack of lytic enzymes (Sharif 1995, Smith 1989).

Finding 2: Increased Signal Intensity of the Intervertebral Disc on T2WI

As noted earlier, although adult infectious spondylitis typically begins in the subchondral marrow, by the time the patient undergoes imaging, the infection has usually penetrated the disc itself. Thus, although it is possible (as noted in the Finding 1 section) to have abnormal marrow signal on one or both sides of an apparently normal disc (McHenry 1988), more frequently some T2 prolongation within the disc will be present (Dagirmanjian 1996, Keenan 1997, Meyers 1991, Modic 1985, Sharif 1992, St. Amour 1994, Szypryt 1988, Thrush 1990) (Figs. 6–2 and 6–4). T2 shortening has also been reported in a few patients (Modic 1985, Meyers 1991, Thrush 1990) (Fig. 6–5). Disruption of the "nuclear cleft" on T2WI has also been reported as a sign of infectious spondylitis (Dagirmanjian 1997), but moderate or severe degenerative change may demonstrate the same imaging finding. Indeed, not only does loss of the nuclear cleft accompany degenerative change of the disc but degenerative change without infection may cause T2 prolongation as well (Grane 1998, Stabler 1996) (Fig. 6–3). Because degenerative disc disease is so common, the cause of minimal T2 prolongation within the disc in a given patient is more likely degenerative than infectious in most practices. Renal osteodystrophy may demonstrate striking T2 prolongation of the intervertebral disc (Kaplan 1987), although extensive erosions do not occur until the patient has been on dialysis for at least 3 years (Sundaram 1987). Although renal osteodystrophy may be suspected as the cause of T2 prolongation of the disc, these patients are immunocompromised and susceptible to infection, so those with such abnormal discs and back pain routinely require biopsy to exclude infectious spondylitis (Kaplan 1987); analysis of the biopsied material should include evaluation for crystals.

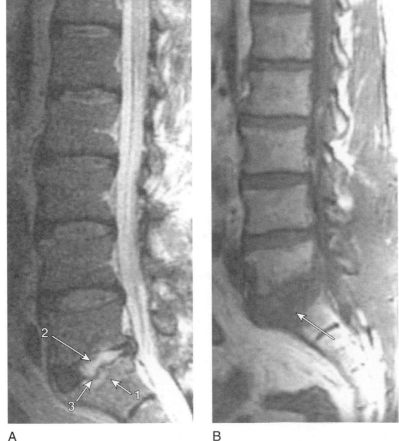

A   B

FIGURE 6–4

Infectious discitis with T2 prolongation within the intervertebral disc. A 73-year-old man after L5–S1 discectomy. *A,* Sagittal T2WI shows T2 prolongation within the subchondral marrow (particularly on the S1 side) (*arrow 1*) as well as within the intervertebral disc (*arrow 2*). There is erosion along the superior margin of the S1 vertebra (*arrow 3*). There is also extension of abnormal soft tissue posteriorly into the anterior aspect of the spinal canal. *B,* Sagittal T1WI demonstrates dramatic T1 prolongation in the upper half of the S1 vertebra (*arrow*).

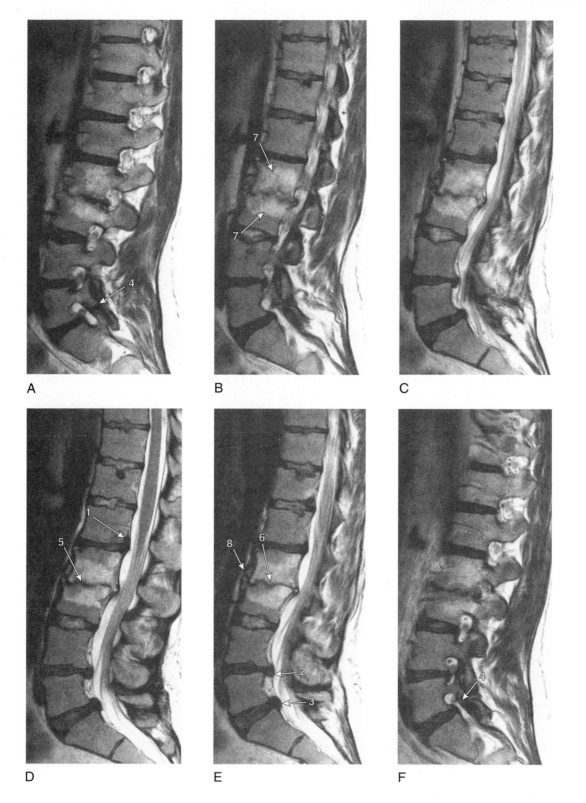

A   B   C

D   E   F

FIGURE 6–5

Infectious discitis with T2 shortening within the intervertebral disc. A 27-year-old woman with chronic, active hepatitis on large doses of oral steroids, with a 2-month history of worsening, central low back pain. *A–F,* Sequential sagittal T2WIs demonstrate multilevel degenerative disc disease, with T10–11, T11–12, and T12–L1 disc dehydration, degenerative disc bulging, and extensive vertebral marginal irregularities and Schmorl's nodes, L1–2 severe loss of disc height and hydration, and a 4.4-mm cranially dissecting disc extrusion *(arrow 1),* L3/L4 Schmorl's node formation, L4–5 moderate loss of disc height and hydration with a 6.6-mm disc extrusion *(arrow 2)* and Schmorl's node formation, and L5–S1 moderate disc dehydration with a 6.8-mm disc protrusion *(arrow 3)* as well as 10% lytic spondylolisthesis with bilateral pars defects *(arrow 4).* Despite the multilevel vertebral marginal irregularities and lower lumbar disc degenerative changes and spondylolysis, the patient denied any pain prior to 2 months previous to the scan. The L2–3 level demonstrates severe loss of disc height and hydration with no substantial area of T2 prolongation within the disc *(arrow 5).* There are, however, erosions along the disc margin *(arrow 6)* and extensive T2 prolongation within the subchondral marrow paralleling the disc margin *(arrow 7).* There is also a 6 × 14-mm soft tissue lesion along the anterior aspect of the L2 vertebrae *(arrow 8).* *(Illustration continued on following page)*

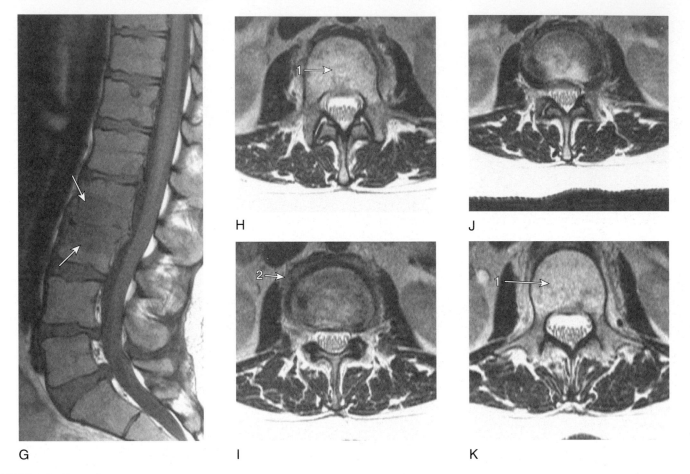

FIGURE 6–5 *(Continued)*

G, Sagittal T1WI shows T1 prolongation of L2 and L3 *(arrows)* corresponding to the T2 prolongation seen on the T2WIs. *H–K,* Sequential axial T2WIs from the L3 to the L2 pedicle demonstrate T2 prolongation within the marrow *(arrow 1)* and abnormal soft tissue anterior to the L2 vertebral body *(arrow 2).*

Finding 3: Contrast Enhancement of the Subchondral Marrow, Disc, and Epidural Space

Both the abnormal subchondral marrow and the abnormal intervertebral disc may demonstrate increased contrast enhancement in infectious spondylitis (Boden 1992, Dagirmanjian 1996, Post 1990, Thrush 1990) (Fig. 6–6). Degenerative change (Grane 1998), neoplasm, and even postoperative changes (Fig. 6–7) may also demonstrate marrow enhancement, however, so contrast enhancement will not allow differentiation of these entities. With respect to marrow changes, administration of contrast material may actually mask subchondral marrow abnormality and make the disease less conspicuous (Thrush 1990) (Fig. 6–8). In rare instances, marrow abnormality may be seen only following contrast enhancement (Gillams 1996). Disc enhancement, being seen in both degenerative (Grane 1998, Stabler 1996) and postoperative change (Post 1990, Sharif 1992), provides no differentiating power between infection and other disease entities. Although Ross and associates (1996) noted that asymptomatic postoperative patients have a different pattern of contrast enhancement of the disc (with two bands of enhancement paralleling the end plates) (Fig. 6–7) than do those with disc space infection (with amor-

phous enhancement), Post and colleagues (1990) reported several different patterns of contrast enhancement of the abnormal disc in infectious spondylitis, one of which was thin, linear areas of enhancement along the disc periphery.

With respect to epidural and paraspinal abscesses and phlegmonous tissue, however, the contrast-enhanced study provides great benefit. Epidural abscesses can be difficult to identify on precontrast studies. Epidural abscesses, however, become obvious after administration of contrast material as areas of intense contrast enhancement within the spinal canal (Dagirmanjian 1996, Kuker 1997, Post 1990, Sharif 1992). The contrast enhancement pattern may provide benefit in the selection of an area of biopsy (Post 1992). Dagirmanjian and associates (1996) found that solidly enhancing lesions corresponded to areas of phlegmon (not amenable to drainage), whereas lesions with peripheral enhancement corresponded to abscesses (likely requiring drainage).

Finding 4: Erosion of Vertebral End Plates

As infection progresses, the vertebral margins adjacent to the disc may be destroyed with loss of the usual pristine thin line of signal absence corresponding to immobile protons in the

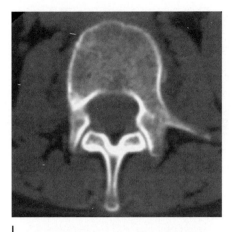

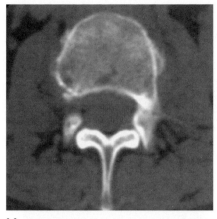

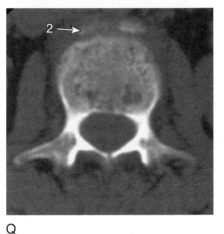

L

M

N

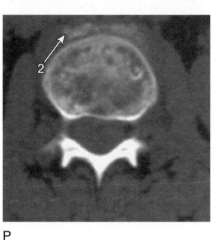

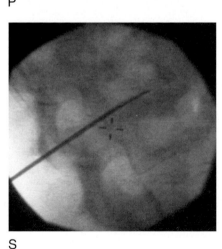

O

P

Q

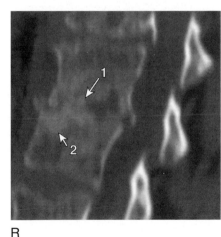

R

S

FIGURE 6–5 *(Continued)*

L–Q, Selected (every other) sequential 3-mm CT examinations from the L3 through the L2 pedicle demonstrate destructive and erosive changes along the disc margin *(arrow 1)* and abnormal calcification along the ventral aspect of L2 *(arrow 2). R,* Sagittal reconstruction CT examination demonstrates L2–3 erosions, collapse of the L2–3 disc *(arrow 1),* and increased density within the anterior, superior aspect of the L3 vertebral body *(arrow 2). S,* C-arm fluoroscopically directed view of biopsy/aspiration. No pus was aspirated, but the culture grew gram-positive cocci. The patient was treated with antibiotics with an uneventful recovery.

cortical bone (Dagirmanjian 1996, Dagirmanjian 1997, Modic 1985, Smith 1989, Thrush 1990) (Figs. 6–2 and 6–4 to 6–6). Chemical shift artifact may normally cause the end plate on the side of the disc toward the lower end of the gradient field to appear thin while the side of the disc at the higher end of the gradient field appears thick (Wolansky 1999). This may result in "pseudosparing" of the end plate adjacent to an abnormal disc, with the end plate being more conspicuous at the diseased level than at other, normal levels. Pseudosparing is conspicuous on T1WI but minimal on proton density or T2WI.

As with the other findings of infection, erosion is a finding that may be seen in other processes, including degenerative disc disease (Fig. 6–3) (either without [Grenier 1987, Stabler 1996] or with [Grane 1998] associated surgery), spondyloarthropathy in hemodialysis patients (Kaplan 1987, Naidich 1988, Sundaram 1987), gout (Duprez 1996, Fenton 1995), and rheumatoid arthritis. In addition to this lack of specificity, the cortical end plates are not invariably eroded in infectious spondylitis but may appear intact, even on proton density and T2WI (Sharif 1992).

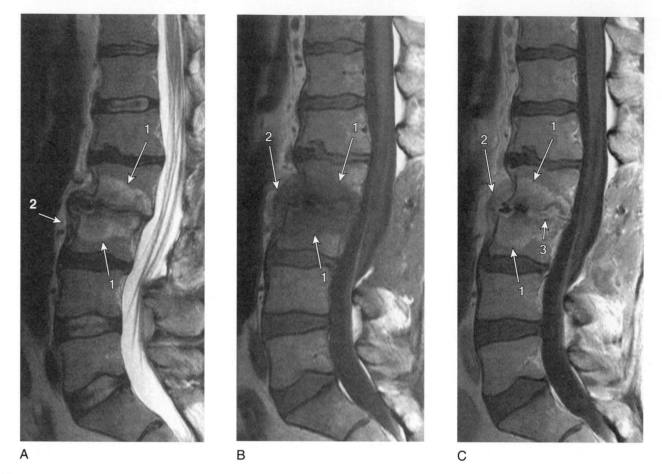

FIGURE 6–6

Infectious discitis with contrast enhancement of the subchondral marrow and intervertebral disc. A 53-year-old man after posterior decompression at the L2 and L3 levels with biopsy-proven *Pseudomonas* discitis. *A,* Sagittal T2WI demonstrates multilevel abnormality, including T11–12 mild loss of disc height and hydration with irregularity along the vertebral body margins, L1–2 severe loss of disc height and hydration with reversal of lordosis and irregularity along the vertebral body margins, and L3–4 mild loss of disc height with moderate disc dehydration. At L2–3, there is severe loss of disc height and hydration, along with erosion of the vertebral body margins and retrolisthesis. Extensive areas of T2 prolongation surround the intervertebral disc *(arrow 1).* There is soft tissue along the anterior aspect of the disc and upper L3 and lower L2 vertebral bodies *(arrow 2). B,* Sagittal T1WI demonstrates L2–3 narrowing, T1 prolongation paralleling the disc *(arrow 1),* and abnormal anterior soft tissue *(arrow 2). C,* Sagittal postcontrast T1WI demonstrates extensive contrast enhancement of the abnormal marrow adjacent to the L2–3 disc *(arrow 1),* as well as the anterior soft tissue lesion *(arrow 2).* Note the disc itself demonstrates marked contrast enhancement *(arrow 3),* despite the relative lack of T2 prolongation.

Finding 5: Epidural Fluid Collection (Epidural Abscess)

Epidural abscess usually has accompanying findings of infection in the subchondral marrow and disc (Friedman 1994, Kuker 1997) (Fig. 6–9). Epidural abscess may have potentially disastrous consequences with spinal cord compression (Friedman 1994, Kuker 1997). Several other processes may result in epidural fluid collection or soft tissue masses resembling fluid, including sarcoidosis, ankylosing spondylitis, and tumors such as lymphoma (Kuker 1997), but these processes usually do not demonstrate the other findings of infectious spondylitis noted earlier. Contrast-enhanced scans improve detection and delineation of epidural abscess (Kuker 1997, Post 1990), particularly if no proton density images have been obtained (Sharif 1992).

Finding 6: Paraspinal Soft Tissue Abnormality

Although epidural abscesses *usually* present with other findings of infectious spondylitis, paraspinal soft tissue masses of infectious spondylitis virtually *always* are accompanied by imaging abnormalities of the subchondral marrow and disc (Figs. 6–2, 6–5, 6–6, and 6–8). The differential diagnosis of paraspinous masses includes tumors. Such tumors, including plasmacytoma, eosinophilic granuloma, aneurysmal bone cyst, giant cell tumors, and chordoma, may have accompanying marrow and even disc changes mimicking infectious spondylitis (Dagirmanjian 1996). Paraspinal soft tissue abnormalities may offer a good site for biopsy (Post 1990). Large paraspinal masses, particularly if calcified, favor granulomatous infection (Sharif 1995, Smith 1989). As noted earlier in Finding 3, solidly enhanc-

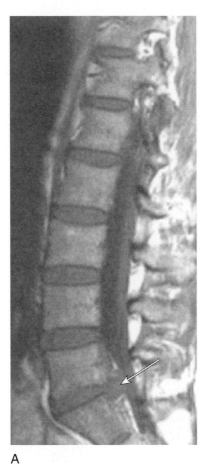

A

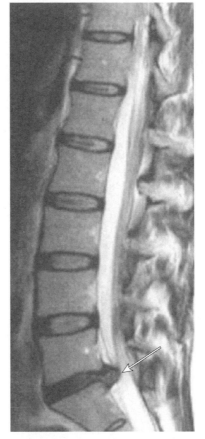

B

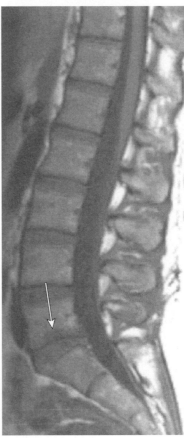

C

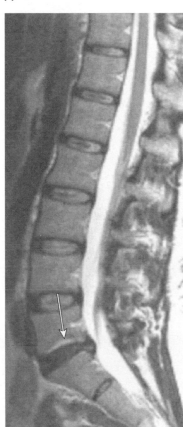

D

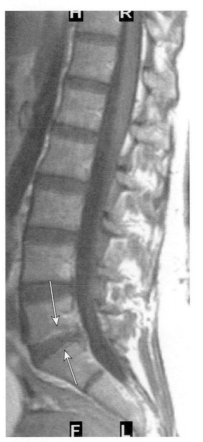

E

FIGURE 6–7

Postoperative changes resembling infectious spondylitis. A 44-year-old woman with low back and left leg pain who underwent discectomy with complete pain relief and was imaged postoperatively as part of a research study. *A*, Preoperative sagittal T1WI shows a 10.9-mm disc extrusion at L5–S1 *(arrow)*. Note normal subchondral marrow signal intensity. *B*, Preoperative sagittal T2WI also demonstrates the disc extrusion *(arrow)*, again with normal subchondral marrow. *C*, Postoperative precontrast sagittal T1WI shows resection of the disc extrusion. There is T1 prolongation, particularly along the L5 end plate *(arrow)*. *D*, Postoperative sagittal T2WI demonstrates T2 prolongation along the L5 end plate *(arrow)*. *E*, Postoperative postcontrast sagittal T1WI shows contrast enhancement of the subchondral marrow *(arrows)*. Such subchondral contrast enhancement may be normal in the postoperative period and does not necessarily indicate infection or any complication of surgery.

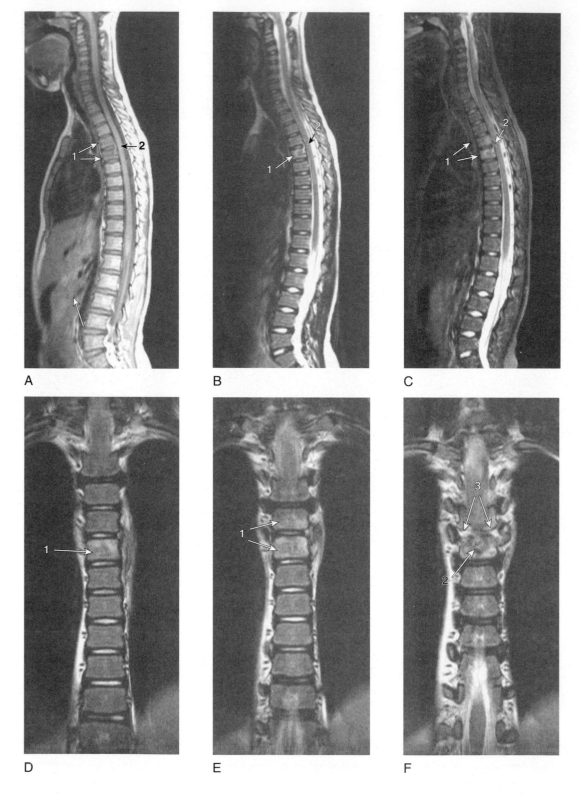

FIGURE 6–8

Infectious discitis with subchondral marrow changes becoming less conspicuous on contrast-enhanced examination. A 7-year-old girl referred for evaluation of "painful scoliosis." During scanning, the patient's mother (a pediatric intensive care unit nurse) also related that the patient had been increasingly lethargic and less active over the prior 2 months. The first three imaging sequences were done with a large field of view to image the entire spine because of the clinical history given. *A,* Sagittal T1WI demonstrates T1 prolongation within the T5 and T6 vertebral bodies *(arrow 1)* with an abnormal focus of intermediate signal intensity crossing the posterior aspect of the vertebral body *(arrow 2). B,* Sagittal fast spin-echo T2WI demonstrates T2 prolongation within the T6 vertebral body *(arrow 1)* and also along the dorsal aspect of the T5–6 intervertebral disc *(arrow 2). C,* Sagittal gradient-recalled echo T2WI demonstrates T2 prolongation not only of T6 but also T5 *(arrow 1)* and again demonstrates abnormal signal intensity along the posterior aspect of the T5–6 intervertebral disc *(arrow 2). D–F,* Sequential anterior-to-posterior coronal T2WIs demonstrate T2 prolongation of the T5 and T6 vertebral bodies *(arrow 1),* inhomogeneous signal intensity along the posterior aspect of the T6 vertebral body *(arrow 2),* and T2 prolongation along the posterior disc margin leading to abnormal signal intensity within the costovertebral joints bilaterally *(arrow 3).*

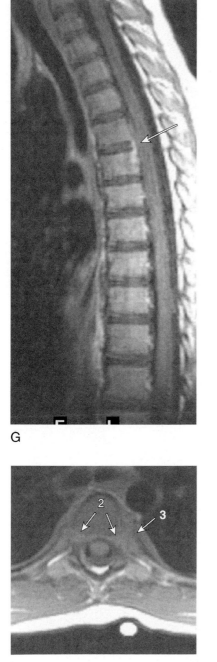

G

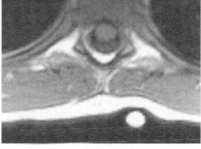

H

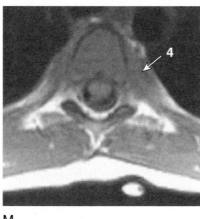

I

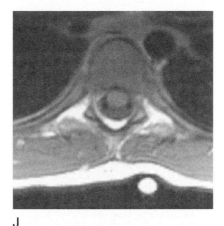

J

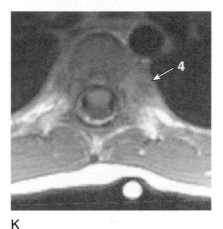

K

L

M

FIGURE 6–8 *(Continued)*

G, Sagittal postcontrast T1WI with a smaller field of view than *A* demonstrates contrast enhancement along the posterior margin of the disc *(arrow).* Note that there is contrast enhancement of the marrow, reducing T1 prolongation and making the marrow signal abnormality *less* conspicuous on postcontrast injection images. *H–M,* Sequential axial precontrast T1WIs from the T7 pedicle through the T5 pedicle demonstrate a normal appearance along the neurocentral synchondrosis at T7 *(arrow 1)* but abnormal widening of this structure at T6 *(arrow 2).* In addition, there is abnormal signal intensity along the interface between the left 6th rib and adjacent T5 and T6 vertebrae *(arrow 3)* with excessive soft tissue and poor definition of the rib head *(arrow 4).* *(continued)*

ing lesions usually represent phlegmonous infection, whereas lesions with peripheral enhancement corresponded to abscesses (Dagirmanjian 1996).

Finding 7: Posterior Element Abnormality

Less than 5% of the time, infectious spondylitis presents with posterior element involvement (particularly of the facet joints) (Ehara 1989, Hadjipavlou 2000, Rombauts 2000). Such involvement often is accompanied by a posterior paraspinous mass representing either phlegmon or abscess (Ehara 1989, Rombauts 2000). The differential diagnosis of such abnormalities includes neoplasm and inflammatory arthritis.

Clinical Scenarios

Although great variability exists in the presentation of patients with infectious spondylitis (as noted by Keenan and Benson [1997]), many patients fall into one of four categories, characterized here as "clinical scenarios." These include the following:

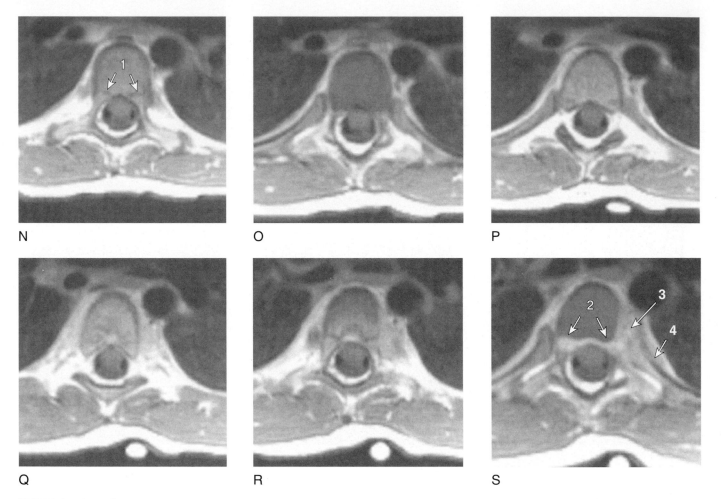

FIGURE 6–8   *(Continued)*

N–S, Sequential axial postcontrast T1WIs from the T7 through the T5 pedicle (compare with precontrast studies) again demonstrate a normal-appearing neurocentral synchondrosis at T7 *(arrow 1)* but abnormal contrast enhancement along the neurocentral synchondrosis at T6 *(arrows 2)* extending into the left costovertebral joint *(arrow 3),* with abnormal contrast enhancement of the rib head *(arrow 4).* The patient was admitted to the hospital and found to have an elevated C-reactive protein and erythrocyte sedimentation rate as well as a positive *Streptococcus* titer. Antibiotics were administered, with relief of patient pain.

1. There is a strong clinical suspicion of infectious spondylitis.
2. There are imaging features (ranging from equivocal to strongly suggestive) of infectious spondylitis with no constitutional symptoms.
3. The patient has had manipulation of the disc.
4. A known disc infection is being followed.

The evaluation of the patient may vary in these circumstances, as noted in the following sections.

CLINICAL SCENARIO 1: THERE IS A STRONG CLINICAL SUSPICION OF INFECTIOUS SPONDYLITIS (Fig. 6–10)

The physician should suspect that a patient with severe, unremitting, nonmechanical back pain may have infectious spondylitis. Approximately half of patients with infectious spondylitis have an elevated WBC count and are febrile. The presence of one or more of the risk factors listed in Table 6–2 increases the likelihood of infectious spondylitis. As St. Amour and colleagues (1994) and, more recently, Carragee (1997b) have emphasized, the epidemiology of

TABLE 6–2. Risk Factors for Infectious Spondylitis

Diabetes (St. Amour 1994, Hitchon 1992, Carragee 1997b, Joughin 1997, Kapellar 1997, Wong 1999)

IV drug abuse (St. Amour 1994, Friedman 1994, Wong 1999)

Immunosuppression (alcoholism, steroid therapy, radiation therapy, AIDS) (St. Amour 1994, Carragee 1997b, Wong 1999, Joughin 1991)

Prior disc surgery or other instrumentation (St. Amour 1994, Wong 1999)

Urinary tract instrumentation, including TURP (transurethral resection of the prostate) (St. Amour 1994, Carragee 1997, Joughin 1991, Kapellar 1997)

Infection elsewhere (Friedman 1994, Carragee 1997, Wong 1999)

the "typical" patient with infectious spondylitis has changed through time. Patients with discitis now tend to be older and are more likely to be immunocompromised than in prior eras.

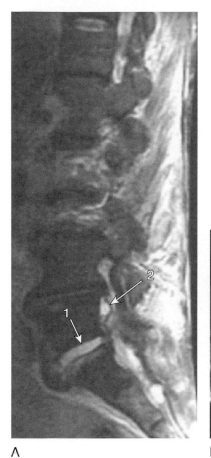

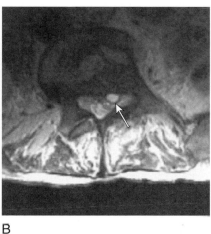

Λ   B

FIGURE 6–9

Infectious discitis with epidural abscess. An 81-year-old woman with back pain. *A,* Sagittal T2WI demonstrates multilevel degenerative changes and scoliosis. L5–S1 shows T2 prolongation and greater height compared to other levels *(arrow 1).* There is also a pocket of T2 prolongation along the dorsal surface of the L5 *(arrow 2). B,* Axial T2WI at the mid L5 vertebral body level demonstrates the focal area of T2 prolongation along the left subarticular aspect of the disc margin *(arrow)* representing a small epidural abscess.

In patients for whom there is a strong clinical suspicion of infectious spondylitis, magnetic resonance imaging (MRI) is the imaging method of choice (Fig. 6–10). A normal MRI examination virtually excludes discitis. In those cases where there is a strong clinical suspicion of infection, IV contrast agent should be given for several reasons: (1) two different studies (Dagirmanjian 1996, Gillams 1996) have included cases in which the noncontrast images were normal and the infection was only evident on postcontrast enhanced views; (2) in those cases of epidural abscess, contrast examinations make the abnormality much more conspicuous (Post 1990); and (3) in those cases with a paraspinous soft tissue abnormality, contrast differentiates between phlegmon and abscess (Dagirmanjian 1996). If the only level of abnormality demonstrates a vacuum phenomenon of the disc (which may be difficult to determine on MRI and is easier to recognize on plain films or computed tomography [CT]), this also virtually excludes discitis, because such gas collections are nearly always secondary to degeneration rather than infection (Bielecki 1986, Grenier 1987, Rothman 1996). Note, however, that a gas collection *outside* the disc in a paravertebral soft tissue mass, far from excluding infection, actually strongly *favors* it. Isolated disc dehydration (with T1 and T2 shortening) without associated subchondral marrow signal intensity changes or end plate erosions is virtually never seen in infection.

If there is a strong clinical suspicion of infection and the MRI examination is abnormal but not strongly suggestive of an infection (having features that favor simple degenerative disc disease), two laboratory tests may be helpful: the erythrocyte sedimentation rate (ESR) and C-reactive protein. The ESR is virtually always elevated in immunocompetent patients with bacterial infectious spondylitis (Hitchon 1992, Carragee 1997b, Sharif 1992). Since the ESR is also elevated in several other disease processes, and since many of these patients are not immunocompetent, C-reactive protein may be more sensitive and specific (Fouquet 1992, Grane 1998). If these tests are negative, then infectious spondylitis is highly unlikely.

The MR findings of infectious spondylitis are multiple and nonspecific, and many patients either have an elevated ESR or are immunocompromised (invalidating the results of the ESR). At this point in the algorithm (Fig. 6–10), it is necessary to evaluate the MRI for a lesion amenable to biopsy. Any disc with markedly increased signal intensity or any fluid pocket (identified as an area of T1 and T2 prolongation without contrast enhancement) is an excellent candidate. Discs of uniformly decreased SI on both T1 and T2WI are less likely to be productive sites for biopsy but have been reported as infected (Meyers 1991, Modic 1985, Thrush 1990). If no lesion seems to be a good candidate for biopsy on the basis of the lumbar MRI, it may be reasonable to perform an abdominal and pelvic CT scan to see if there is a retroperitoneal site of possible infection to biopsy.

When biopsy is performed, samples should be sent not only for Gram stain and culture and sensitivity of any aspirated material, but cores of tissue should also be obtained for culture and histopathology. Unless gross pus is aspirated

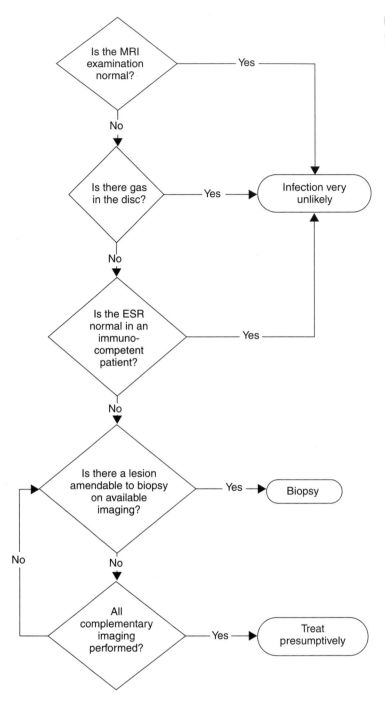

FIGURE 6–10
Clinical Scenario 1. Strong clinical suspicion of infectious spondylitis. ESR, erythrocyte sedimentation rate.

during the procedure, the differential diagnosis often includes tumor, and the histopathologic analysis is helpful in excluding malignancy. In addition, cultures of infectious spondylitis (even when gross pus is aspirated and the patient is not on antibiotics) are frequently negative, and histologic analysis confirming inflammatory tissue at the site of biopsy is helpful.

Ultimately, some of these patients need to be treated presumptively for infection, without culture proof of bacterial infection, on the basis of a typical clinical history and characteristic MRI features (Honan 1996, Joughin 1991). Positive blood cultures obtained during a fever spike along with typical imaging features are considered sufficient to

guide appropriate therapy in those cases when material from biopsy does not provide a specific organism (Honan 1996).

CLINICAL SCENARIO 2: THERE ARE IMAGING FEATURES OF INFECTIOUS SPONDYLITIS WITH NO CONSTITUTIONAL SYMPTOMS (Fig. 6–11)

Occasionally, patients without fever, chills, malaise, or other constitutional symptoms of infection have imaging features that suggest infectious spondylitis. Such imaging features may include apparent destruction of the vertebral end plates, increased signal intensity of the disc on T2WI, or a paraspinal mass with a central area of fluid signal

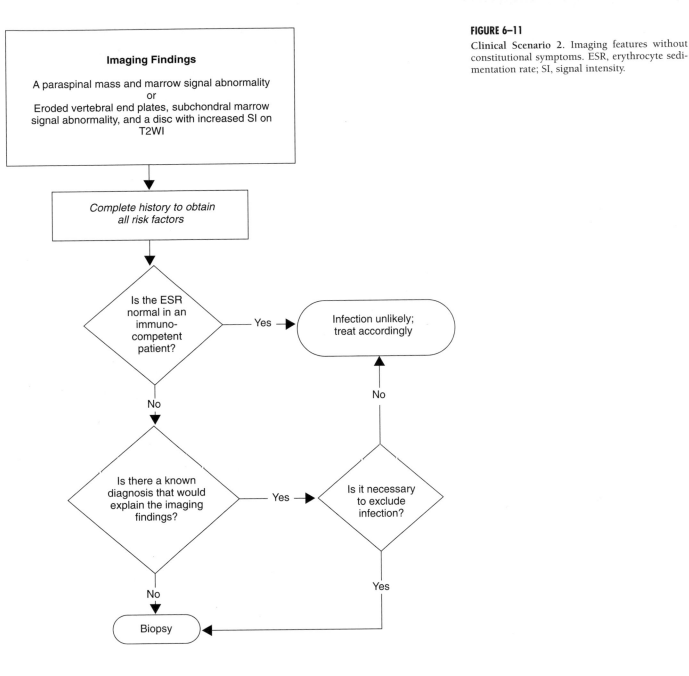

FIGURE 6–11
Clinical Scenario 2. Imaging features without constitutional symptoms. ESR, erythrocyte sedimentation rate; SI, signal intensity.

(Figs. 6–2, 6–8, and 6–12). Review of the patient's history with attention to the risk factors in Table 6–2 may reveal one or more risk factors. This may indicate that use of the algorithm presented in Clinical Scenario 1 (Fig. 6–10) is in order. Whether the patient has risk factors or not, the best first step is probably to obtain an ESR and/or C-reactive protein test. If these laboratory tests are negative in the setting of mechanical back pain and imaging findings of mildly eroded vertebral end plates, subchondral marrow changes, and increased signal intensity in the disc, it is highly likely that the patient has degenerative disc disease rather than infectious spondylitis.

Some patients may have a diagnosis that would explain the imaging findings without the necessity of biopsy. Patients with neuropathic arthropathy, which may be considered an extremely advanced form of degenerative disc disease, may share many of the findings of infectious spondylitis, including subchondral marrow changes and increased signal intensity of the disc on T2WI (Wagner 2000). If a patient has paraplegia or some other cause of neuropathic arthropathy and joint disorganization and debris, biopsy may not be necessary to establish the diagnosis. Similarly, a patient with known multiple myeloma, marrow abnormality, and a paraspinal soft tissue mass with involvement of the intervertebral disc (Dagirmanjian 1996) probably does not require biopsy.

Patients with tuberculous spondylitis may present with fewer (and later-onset) constitutional symptoms than those with bacterial spondylitis (Sharif 1995). These patients may present with large, multilocular paraspinous abscesses or dramatic, multilevel spine changes suggestive of neoplasm (Sharif 1995, Smith 1989).

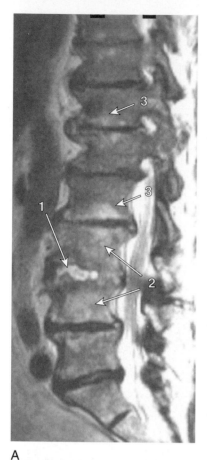

A

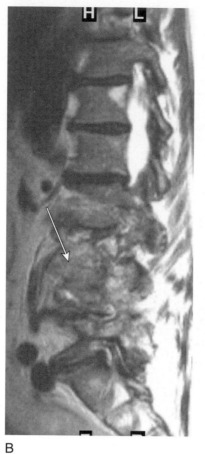

B

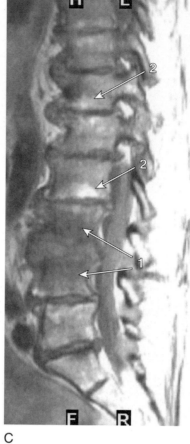

C

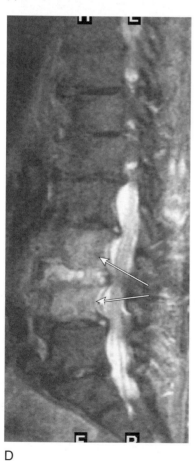

D

FIGURE 6–12

Infectious spondylitis in a patient with no constitutional symptoms but with imaging findings of infection. An 85-year-old woman with low back and left leg pain. The patient had no fever, chills, or weight loss. *A,* Sagittal T2WI demonstrates multilevel degenerative changes of the lumbar spine. At the L3–4 level, there is widening of the disc compared to the other (degenerated) lumbar discs, and there is marked T2 prolongation (*arrow 1*). Note relatively subtle T2 prolongation in the L3 and L4 vertebral bodies (*arrow 2*), compared to the much more striking subchondral T2 prolongation at T12–L1 and L2–3 from Modic Type II changes (*arrows 3*). *B,* Left parasagittal T2WI lateral to the vertebral bodies demonstrates a disorganized appearance of soft tissues in the left paravertebral area (*arrow*). *C,* Sagittal T1WI shows T1 prolongation of the L3 and L4 vertebral marrow (*arrow 1*). The T12–L1 and L2–3 subchondral Modic Type II changes demonstrate T1 shortening (*arrows 2*). *D,* Sagittal gradient-recalled echo T2WI demonstrates much more conspicuous marrow abnormality of the L3 and L4 marrow than does the fast spin-echo T2WI (*arrows*) (compare with *A*). Again demonstrated is disc expansion and T2 prolongation.

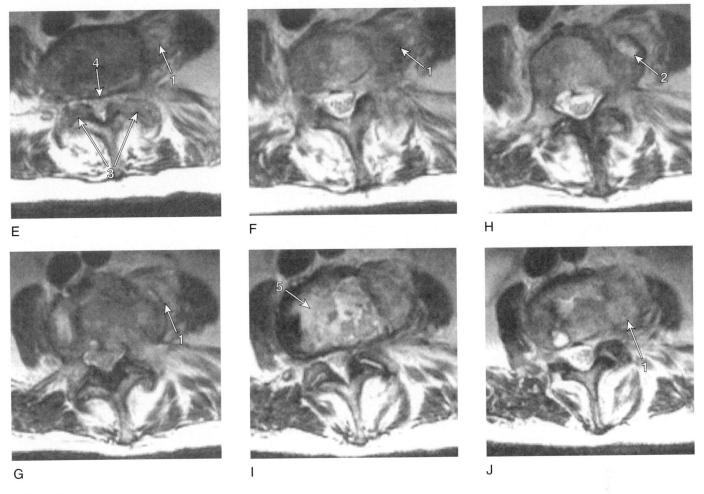

FIGURE 6–12 *(continued)*

E–J, Sequential axial T2WIs from the level of the L4–5 disc to just above the L3–4 disc demonstrate abnormal soft tissue separating the right psoas muscle from the vertebral body *(arrow 1)* (compare to the left side, where the psoas muscle is in a more normal position). There is a focus of T2 prolongation within the central portion of the soft tissue lesion consistent with pus or necrotic debris *(arrow 2)*. Incidentally noted at the L4–5 level is severe facet arthropathy *(arrow 3)* and moderate spinal canal stenosis *(arrow 4)* from a combination of facet arthropathy and degenerative disc bulging. The L3–4 intervertebral disc demonstrates extensive abnormal signal intensity with T2 prolongation *(arrow 5)*. The patient had blood cultures done and also cultures of biopsy material from the L3–4 disc; both of these were positive for *Streptococcus bovis*. She was treated with intravenous antibiotics.

CLINICAL SCENARIO 3: THE PATIENT HAS HAD MANIPULATION OF A DISC (Fig. 6–13)

Patients who do not have infectious spondylitis but who have undergone manipulation of the disc, particularly discectomy, may have many imaging features that suggest infection (Fig. 6–7). Indeed, many have pointed out the overlap in imaging findings in those patients who have undergone discectomy without and with infection, and note that imaging is of limited use in this scenario (Bircher 1988, Fouquet 1992, Grane 1998, Post 1990, Sharif 1992). Laboratory tests, however, are quite helpful. Although the postoperative ESR is routinely elevated in the first few days after surgery, it should begin to drop about 4 days after surgery and show a steady decrease for the next 6 weeks, with an ESR of less than 50 at 2 weeks and less than 15 at 6 weeks (Bircher 1988, Jonsson 1991). Grane and coworkers (1998) report an even more dramatic response with C-reactive protein, which should return to normal by 6 days after surgery.

If the patient demonstrates abnormal laboratory values but has no neurologic findings, many authors would forego imaging and treat medically (Bircher 1988, Fouquet 1992, Grane 1998). If MR imaging is performed, perhaps the most important features to be searched for are epidural abscess and paraspinal abscess, for these may require surgical intervention. Boden and associates (1992) thought that the triad of abnormal contrast enhancement of the subchondral marrow, disc space, and posterior annulus was unlikely in an uninfected patient. Ross and colleagues (1996) noted that linear enhancement of the end plates is seen in asymptomatic postoperative patients, but Post (1990) and Grane (1998) and their coworkers have reported the same pattern of contrast enhancement in patients with infectious spondylitis. Although MRI may be helpful in excluding catastrophic complications of infection such as extensive epidural abscess or large paraspinal abscess, MRI alone is unlikely to definitely exclude or establish the diagnosis of infectious spondylitis in the postoperative patient.

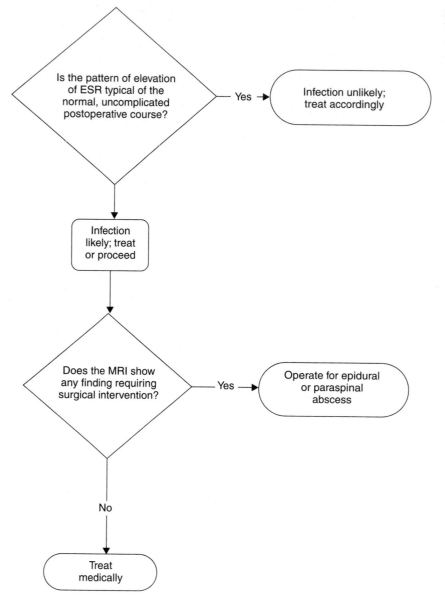

FIGURE 6–13
Clinical Scenario 3. Status after disc manipulation. ESR, erythrocyte sedimentation rate.

CLINICAL SCENARIO 4: A KNOWN DISC INFECTION IS BEING FOLLOWED

Two studies have shown that MRI in a patient with known discitis may be misleading. Gillams and associates (1996) noted that the soft tissue component of the infection typically decreased and the marrow inflammatory changes usually converted to fat. However, lack of these changes and progression of cortical and subchondral bony changes as well as disc abnormalities did not indicate failed treatment. Similarly, Carragee (1997a) noted several cases where the MRI findings indicated little change or even deterioration despite clinical improvement.

Organisms

From an imaging standpoint, perhaps the most pragmatic thing to know about the organisms producing pyogenic infectious spondylitis is that there is no way to distinguish between the various species of organisms on the basis of imaging. All pyogenic infections, whether caused by *Staphylococcus aureus* (the most frequent offender) (Carragee 1997b, Joughin 1991, Hadjipavlou 2000), *Escherichia coli*, *Streptococcus viridans*, or some other species, produce similar imaging features. Organisms that may be considered contaminants and/or of low virulence may actually prove to be the offending agent. For example, Carragee (1997b) found that *Staphylococcus epidermidis*, *Propionibacterium acnes*, and diphtheroid species were responsible for infections in 37% of his series. Therefore, a typical "contaminant" obtained via a biopsy using appropriate technique should be considered a possible pathogen and treated accordingly.

Granulomatous infectious spondylitis may have the same imaging features as pyogenic infectious spondylitis. In some patients, however, granulomatous infectious spondylitis may produce changes more typical of neoplastic involvement, including multilevel involvement, posterior element involvement, relative sparing of the intervertebral disc, and large paraspinal soft tissue masses (Dagirmanjian 1997, Smith 1989, Thrush 1990). Olson and colleagues (1998) reported that the imaging findings in coccidioidomycosis infections are nonspecific, with abnormal discs, subchondral marrow, and adjacent epidural and soft tissue masses seen as in other cases of infectious spondylitis.

Reporting in Infectious Spondylitis

Infectious spondylitis is an unusual and sometimes unsuspected diagnosis, and it is imperative that any radiologist considering this diagnosis should alert the referring clinician. The MRI report of infectious spondylitis, like other radiology reports, should be broken into two components: the body and the conclusion. The body includes a description of findings, whereas diagnosis(es) and recommendations are placed in the conclusion. The recommendations of the algorithms should be used in generating the conclusion of an MRI report of the patient either known or suspected to have infectious spondylitis. In Clinical Scenario 1 (Fig. 6–10), note should be made of any "classic" findings of infectious spondylitis such as marked T2 prolongation within the disc, epidural or paraspinous soft tissue abnormalities, and, to a lesser degree, subchondral marrow signal abnormality. As noted by Dagirmanjian and coworkers (1996, 1997), however, the *absence* of T2 prolongation should not dissuade the radiologist from suggesting the diagnosis in the appropriate setting; indeed, as noted earlier in the Findings sections, infectious spondylitis may be accompanied by nearly any combination of imaging features, and it is hard to exclude infectious spondylitis by MRI examination unless the study is completely normal. In the case of a vacuum phenomenon of the disc, however or where there is isolated disc dehydration with no accompanying subchondral marrow abnormality or end plate erosion, the diagnosis needs to be regarded as extremely unlikely.

The radiologist should offer the suggestion that infection is possible in Clinical Scenario 2 (Fig. 6–11) and try to obtain correlation with serum chemistry abnormalities (since this is the most cost-effective way to exclude the diagnosis). The clinician may object that there are "no clinical findings of infection." In fact, constitutional symptoms are frequently lacking in patients with infectious spondylitis and the only clinical finding universally present in these patients is backache, which the patient almost certainly has (otherwise, he or she would not be undergoing imaging in the first place).

The report for Clinical Scenarios 3 (status following disc manipulation) (Fig. 6–11) and 4 (following a known disc infection) should usually not venture much beyond description unless there are dramatic findings such as a large epidural or paraspinal abscess. The overlap of septic and aseptic findings in the patient after discectomy is simply too great to allow firm conclusions on the basis of imaging without dramatic imaging findings, and the clinician should be made aware of this. Similarly, we emphasize that pronouncements of "worsening" based on imaging findings on serial studies alone may be misleading and not correlate with the clinical picture.

Conclusion

Infectious spondylitis has multiple imaging features, many of which overlap with several other diseases, particularly degenerative disc disease. Given the relative prevalence of degenerative change (nearly universal) and infection (quite rare), a given patient with subchondral marrow changes, erosions along the vertebral end plates, and T2 prolongation within the intervertebral disc is more likely to have degenerative disc disease than infectious spondylitis, unless the disc is frankly distended with fluid or there is an accompanying epidural or paraspinous abscess. Because of the nonspecificity of the imaging findings, these patients frequently come to biopsy. Such a biopsy should be readily accomplished with either C-arm fluoroscopic or CT guidance and should provide enough information for reasonable treatment to follow. In cases of prior disc surgery, imaging for the most part should play a secondary role to laboratory evaluation. In following infection, imaging findings and clinical course may vary dramatically, also limiting the role of imaging.

References

Bielecki DK, Sartoris D, Resnick D, Van Lom K, Fierer J, Hadhighi P. Intraossseous and intradiscal gas in association with spinal infection: report of three cases. AJR Am J Roentgenol 1986; 147:83–86.

Bircher MD, Tasker T, Crawshaw C, Mulholland RC. Discitis following lumbar surgery. Spine 1988; 13:98–102.

Boden SD, Davis DO, Dina TS, Sunner JL, Wiesel SW. Postoperative diskitis: distinguishing early MR imaging findings from normal postoperative disk space changes. Radiology 1992; 184:765–771.

Carragee EJ. The clinical use of magnetic resonance imaging in pyogenic vertebral osteomyelitis. Spine 1997a; 22:780–785.

Carragee EJ. Pyogenic vertebral osteomyelitis. J Bone Joint Surg Am 1997b; 79:874–880.

Dagirmanjian A, Schils J, McHenry M, Modic MT. MR imaging of vertebral osteomyelitis revisited. AJR Am J Roentgenol 1996; 167:1539–1543.

Dagirmanjian A, Schils J, McHenry M, Modic MT. Spinal osteomyelitis. Semin Spine Surg 1997; 9:38–50.

de Roos A, Kressel H, Spritzer C, Dalinka M. MR imaging of marrow changes adjacent to end plates in degenerative lumbar disk disease. AJR Am J Roentgenol 1987; 149:531–534.

Duprez TP, Malghem J, VandeBerg BC, Noel EA, Munting EA, Maldague BE. Gout in the cervical spine: MR pattern mimicking diskovertebral infection. AJNR Am J Neuroradiol 1996; 17:151–153.

Ehara S, Khurana JS, Kattapuram SV. Pyogenic vertebral osteomyelitis of the posterior elements. Skeletal Radiol 1989; 18:175–178.

Fenton P, Young S, Prutis K. Gout of the spine: two case reports and review of the literature. J Bone Joint Surg1995; 77A:767–771.

Fouquet B, Goupile P, Jattiot F, Cotty P, Lapierre F, Valat JP, Amouroux J, Benatre A. Discitis after lumbar disc surgery: features of "aseptic" and "septic" forms. Spine 1992; 17:356–358.

Friedman DP, Hills JR. Cervical epidural spinal infection: MR imaging characteristics. AJR 1994; 163:699–704.

Gillams AR, Chaddha B, Carter AP: MR appearances of the temporal evolution and resolution of infectious spondylitis. AJR Am J Roentgenol 1996; 166:903–907.

Grane P, Josephsson A, Seferlis A, Tullberg T. Septic and aseptic postoperative discitis in the lumbar spine: evaluation by MR imaging. Acta Radiol 1998; 39:108–115.

Grenier N, Grossman RI, Schiebler ML, Yeager BA, Goldberg HI, Kressel HY. Degenerative lumbar disk disease: pitfalls and usefulness of MR imaging in detection of the vacuum phenomenon. Radiology 1987; 164:861–865.

Hadjipavlou AG, Mader JT, Necessary JT, Muffoletto AJ. Hematogenous pyogenic spinal infections and their surgical management. Spine 2000; 25:1668–1679.

Hitchon PW, Osenbach RK, Yuh WTC, Menezes AH. Spinal infections. Clin Neurosurg 1992; 38:373–387.

Honan M, White GW, Eisenberg GM. Spontaneous infectious discitis in adults. Am J Med 1996; 100:85–89.

Jonsson B, Soderholm R, Stromqvist B. Erythrocyte sedimentation rate after lumbar spine surgery. Spine 1991; 16:1049–1050.

Joughin E, McDougall C, Parfitt C, Yong-Hing K, Kirkaldy-Willis WH. Causes and clinical management of vertebral osteomyelitis in Saskatchewan. Spine 1991; 16:261–264.

Kapeller P, Fazekas F, Krametter D, Koch M, Roob G, Schmid R, Offenbacher H. Pyogenic infectious spondylitis: clinical, laboratory, and MRI features. Eur Neurol 1997; 38:94–98.

Kaplan P, Resnick D, Murphey M, Heck L, Phalen J, Egan D, Rutsky E. Destructive noninfectious spondyloarthropathy in hemodialysis patients: a report of four cases. Radiology 1987; 162:241–244.

Keenan TL, Benson DR. Differential diagnosis and conservative treatment of infectious diseases. In Frymoyer JW (ed). The Adult Spine: Principles and Practice, 2nd ed. Philadelphia, Lippincott-Raven, 1997.

Kuker W, Mull M, Mayfrank L, Topper R, Thron A. Epidural spinal infection: variability of clinical and magnetic resonance imaging findings. Spine 1997; 22:544–550; discussion 551.

McHenry MC, Duchesneau PM, Keys TF, Rehm SJ, Boumphrey RS. Vertebral osteomyelitis presenting as spinal compression fracture: six patients with underlying osteoporosis. Arch Intern Med 1988; 148:417–423.

Meyers SP, Wiener SN. Diagnosis of hematogenous pyogenic vertebral osteomyelitis by magnetic resonance imaging. Arch Intern Med 1991; 151:683–687.

Modic MT, Feiglin DH, Piraino DW, Boumphrey F, Weinstein MA, Duchesnaue PM, Rehm S. Vertebral osteomyelitis: assessment using MR. Radiology 1985; 157:157–166.

Modic MT, Steinberg PM, Ross JS, Masaryk TJ, Carter JR. Degenerative disk disease: assessment of changes in vertebral body marrow with MR imaging. Radiology 1988; 166:193–199.

Naidich JB, Mossey RT, McHeffrey-Atkinson B, Karmel MI, Bluestone PA, Mailloux LU, Stein HL. Spondyloarthopathy from long-term hemodialysis. Radiology 1988; 167:761–764.

Olson EM, Duberg AC, Herron LD, Kissel P, Smilovitz D. Coccidioidal spondylitis: MR findings in 15 patients. AJR 1998; 171:785–789.

Palestro CJ, Kim CK, Swyer AJ, Vallabhajosula S, Goldsmith SJ. Radionuclide diagnosis of vertebral osteomyelitis: Indium-111 leukocyte and technetium 99m–MDP bone scintigraphy. J Nucl Med 1991; 32:1861–1865.

Post MJD, Sze G, Quencer RM, Eismont FJ, Green BA, Gahbauer H. Gadolinium-enhanced MR in spine infection. J Comput Assist Tomogr 1990; 14:721–729.

Rombauts PA, Linden PM, Buyse AJ, Snoecx MP, Lysens RJ, Gryspeerdt SS. Septic arthritis of a lumbar facet joint caused by *Staphylococcus aureus*. Spine 2000; 25:1736–1738.

Rothman SLG. The diagnosis of infections of the spine by modern imaging techniques. Orthop Clin North Am 1996; 27:15–31.

Ross JS, Zepp R, Modic MT. The postoperative lumbar spine: enhanced MR evaluation of the intervertebral disc. AJNR Am J Neuroradiol 1996; 17:323–331.

Sharif HS. Role of MR imaging in the management of spinal infections. AJR 1992; 158:1333–1345.

Sharif HS, Morgan JL, Al Shahed MS, Aabed Al Thagafi MY. Role of CT and MR imaging in the management of tuberculous spondylitis. Radiol Clin North Am 1995; 33:787–804.

Siegelman ES. Imaging corner. Spine 1999; 24:2175–2176.

Smith AS, Weinstein MA, Mizushima A, Coughlin B, Hayden SP, Lakin MM, Lanzier CF. MR imaging characteristics of tuberculous spondylitis versus vertebral osteomyelitis. AJNR Am J Neuroradiol 1989; 10:619–625.

St. Amour TE, Hodges SC, Laakman RW, Tarnas DE. Osteomyelitis of the spine. In St. Amour TE, Hodges SC, Laakman RW, Tarnas DE (eds). MRI of the Spine. New York, Raven Press, 1994.

Stabler A, Doma AB, Baur A, Kruger A, Reiser MF. Reactive bone marrow changes in infectious spondylitis: quantitative assessment with MR imaging. Radiology 2000; 217:863–868.

Sundaram M, Seelig R, Pohl D. Vertebral erosions in patients undergoing maintenance hemodialysis for chronic renal failure. AJR Am J Roentgenol 1987; 149:323–327.

Szypryt E, Hardy JG, Hinton CE, Worthington BS, Mulholland RC. A comparison between magnetic resonance imaging and scintigraphic bone imaging in the diagnosis of disc space infection in an animal model. Spine 1988; 13:1042–1048.

Thrush A, Enzmann D. MR imaging of infectious spondylitis. AJNR Am J Neuroradiol 1990; 11:1171–1180.

Tonami H, Kuginuki M, Kuginuki Y, Matoba M, Yokota H, Higashi K, Yamamoto I, Nishijima Y. MR imaging of subchondral osteonecrosis of the vertebral body after percutaneous laser diskectomy. AJR 1999; 173:1383–1386.

Waddell G. The Back Pain Revolution. New York, Churchill Livingstone, 1998.

Wagner SC, Schweitzer ME, Morrison WB, Przybylski GJ, Parker L. Can imaging findings help differentiate spinal neuropathic arthropathy from disk space infection? Initial experience. Radiology 2000; 214:693–699.

Wolansky LJ, Heary RF, Patterson T. Friedenberg JS, Tholany J, Chen JK, Patel N, Doddakashi S. Pseudosparing of the endplate: a potential pitfall in using MR imaging to diagnose infectious spondylitis. AJR 1999; 172:777–780.

7

Congenital and Developmental Anomalies

DONALD L. RENFREW • SANJAY SALUJA • MICHAEL W. HAYT

Some patients with congenital anomalies may undergo imaging shortly after birth, either before or after surgery. These same patients may undergo additional imaging years later when a complication is suspected. Other patients undergo initial imaging in later childhood or even adulthood, sometimes because of symptoms secondary to an anomaly, but often because of unrelated symptoms with the incidental discovery of an anomaly. This chapter provides definitions and illustrates the imaging features of the more commonly encountered congenital anomalies and reviews some common clinical scenarios. The imaging of congenital anomalies is briefly reviewed.

Although most sources discussing congenital anomalies review embryology, we will not. We note that there are more than three dozen terms to learn in describing congenital anomalies, even without introduction of such concepts as neurulation, canalization, and retrogressive differentiation. Furthermore, controversy exists with regard to the embryology of many these entities (Barkovich 2000, Goske 1994, Osborn 1994, St. Amour 1994). In many patients multiple anomalies coexist, calling into question the rationale of memorizing a specific, single-hit embryologic insult with resultant abnormality when the imaging issue is cataloging and describing all defects present in a given individual.

Imaging of Congenital Anomalies

Multiple anomalies at separate locations in the spine frequently coexist. In symptomatic congenital anomalies, it is usually necessary to image the entire spinal cord and, often, the brain as well.

PLAIN FILMS

Plain films are of value in obtaining an overview of the spine, measuring scoliosis and kyphosis, and to a certain extent evaluating segmentation anomalies. They are of little benefit in evaluation of the soft tissues, of course, and

usually need to be complemented by additional imaging methods (particularly magnetic resonance imaging [MRI]).

ULTRASOUND

Ultrasound may detect congenital anomalies of the spine in utero and result in prenatal MRI and even surgical repair (Adzick 1998). After delivery, ultrasound may also be of benefit to visualize the spinal cord, canal, and soft tissue masses, either through unossified portions of the canal or at surgery. Definitive imaging usually requires MRI, however.

COMPUTED TOMOGRAPHY

For the most part, MRI has supplanted computed tomography (CT) as the method of choice for imaging congenital spine anomalies (Tortori-Donati 1990). In some cases the two techniques may be complementary. For example, in evaluating a possible osseous component in diastematomyelia, CT can be helpful.

MAGNETIC RESONANCE IMAGING

MRI is, generally speaking, the imaging method of choice for evaluation of congenital anomalies. It allows characterization of soft tissues and evaluation of bony anomalies. Axial and sagittal T1 and T2WI should be obtained of the spine, supplemented by coronal images in cases of scoliosis or complex congenital anomalies. Fluid-attenuated inversion recovery (FLAIR) images are helpful in evaluation of dermoids and epidermoids, which can otherwise mimic cerebrospinal fluid (CSF) on all imaging sequences (Barkovich 2000).

Findings of Congenital Spine Abnormalities

The commonly encountered imaging findings of congenital spinal abnormalities are listed in Table 7–1, along with the anomalies that cause the findings. These terms may be confusing, because authorities use different terms for the same

TABLE 7–1. Common Imaging Findings of Congenital Spine Abnormalities

Imaging Finding	Anomalies, Terminology, Differential Diagnosis, and Comments
Abnormal posterior opening of the spinal canal	**Dysraphism**, from Gr. *dys* + *raphe* (seam). An abnormal posterior opening of the spinal canal. Also called **spina bifida** and **rachischisis**. Dysraphism may accompany any of several congenital anomalies (e.g. myelocele, myelomeningocele). The small vertical clefts sometimes seen in the spinous process of L5 and S1 are *not* examples of dysraphism (Byrd 1991).
CSF in herniated meninges, outside the normal spinal canal	This finding is also seen in any of several congenital anomalies, namely those with the suffix "cele" (Gr. *kele* or hernia), which refers to herniation of CSF outside of the spinal canal. In **simple meningocele**, there is herniation of the meninges and CSF through a dysraphic defect into the posterior soft tissues.
CSF and neural elements outside the normal spinal canal	This finding is seen in **myelocele** (Gr. *myelo* denoting the spinal cord), which is herniation of meninges and neural tissue not covered by skin and flush with the plane of the back, and **myelomeningocele**, which is herniation of meninges and neural tissue not covered by skin and associated with an elevated back mass.
Partial or complete duplication of the spinal cord	**Diastematomyelia** (Gr. *diastema* an interval + *myelos* spinal cord), in which there is partial or complete splitting of the spinal cord into two parts, each of which has one set of dorsal and one set of ventral roots; and **Diplomyelia** with two distinct cords, each with its own dual set of ventral and dorsal roots.
Septation of the spinal canal	This finding accompanies approximately 50% of cases of diastematomyelia. The septation may be cartilaginous, osseous, or a combination of the two and results in tethering of the cord with associated symptoms.
CSF intensity lesion within the spinal cord and paralleling the long axis of the cord	**Hydromyelia** refers to dilation of the central canal of the spinal cord and has an ependymal lining. **Syringomyelia** refers to a CSF fluid collection that has dissected out of the central canal and is hence not lined with ependyma. **Syringohydromyelia** (also called **hydrosyringomyelia** and **syrinx**) denotes either one or both hydromyelia/syringomyelia, since the imaging (and even histologic) distinction between these two entities may not be possible in a given case (Barkovich 2000, Osborn 1994, Sherman 1986).
Abnormal position of the conus medullaris.	In infants ≤ 3 months of age, the conus may be at the body of L3 (Byrd 1991). In 99% of normal adults, the conus medullaris ends above the L2–3 disc level (Saifuddin 1998). An abnormally low conus is a sign of a tethered spinal cord. There are multiple associated anomalies, including fibrolipoma of the filum terminale, diastematomyelia, myelocele, and myelomeningocele. Axial images may be necessary to distinguish the distal conus medullaris and the cauda equina, since these structures may blend together on sagittal studies (Gundry 1994, Osborn 1994). Occasionally even on axial images it is not clear where the conus ends and the filum begins in which case Tortori-Donant and associates (1990) have proposed the term *neurofibrous structure*.
Abnormal tapering of the conus medullaris	The distal conus medullaris should be slightly bulbous above a smoothly tapered point. An abnormally thinned and "stretched" conus is a sign of a tethered cord. A blunted appearance of the cord may be seen in caudal regression syndrome, especially when there is an accompanying tethered cord (Barkovich 2000).
Abnormality of the filum terminale	The filum terminale is normally 2 mm in maximum diameter at the L5–S1 level. A small amount of fat is often seen within the filum, but filum terminale demensions > 2 mm or extensive fat within the filum (lipomas and fibrolipomas of the filum) are not normal.
Intramedullary, intradural-extramedullary, and extradural masses	Congenital anomalies presenting as masses are occasionally difficult to distinguish from other masses of the spine, but the presence of segmentation anomalies or dysraphism accompanying a mass is a strong indication that the mass is congenital. **Lipomas:** These may be applied to the posterior surface or split the spinal cord. Lipomas may be seen within the canal with associated dysraphism. Lipomas may also be seen posterior to dysraphism with posterior herniation of the meninges and neural tissue (**lipomyelomeningocele**). **Dermoids:** These are cystic or complex lesions lined by a squamous epithelium containing skin appendages. **Epidermoids:** These are cystic or complex lesions composed of the superficial (epidermal) elements of the skin. **Teratomas:** Sacrococcygeal types may occur in the presacral or postsacral space. These tumors generally demonstrate inhomogeneous signal intensity. **Neurenteric cysts:** These are fluid-containing cysts lined by epithelial and goblet cells. These cysts may lie anterior or posterior to the spinal cord within the canal; approximately 50% have associated segmentation anomalies (Barkovich 2000).
Axially oriented tracts of abnormal signal intensity within the posterior soft tissues	The congenital anomaly associated with this finding is the **dorsal dermal sinus**: a tube lined with epithelium that extends from the skin for a variable distance and that may reach the spinal canal. Dorsal dermal sinuses are frequently associated with dermoids or epidermoids (Barkovich 1991).

TABLE 7–1. (*continued*)

Imaging Finding	Anomalies, Terminology, Differential Diagnosis, and Comments
Absent or diminutive appearance of the caudal spine	**Caudal regression** refers to nondevelopment of the caudal aspect of the inferior spine. Only the coccyx may be involved with no clinical consequence, or the abnormality may extend more superiorly (even into the lower thoracic spine). A wedge-shaped or blunted conus may accompany caudal regression.
Abnormally low position of the cerebellar tonsils	The cerebellar tonsils normally end above the foramen magnum; tonsils between 1 and 5 mm below the tonsils are "low lying" but not necessarily associated with symptoms. **Chiari I malformation:** The tonsils are > 5 mm below the foramen magnum, the fourth ventricle is in normal position, and there is a small posterior fossa. **Chiari II malformation:** The tonsils are > 5 mm below the foramen magnum and the fourth ventricle is in an abnormally low position. Almost all patients with Chiari II malformation present at birth with a myelomeningocele, and there are multiple additional abnormalities including beaking of the tectum, a cervicomedullary kink, hypogenesis of the corpus callosum, and hydrocephalus.
Segmentation anomalies	Abnormal segmentation of the spine takes several forms, ranging from a partially absent disc or fusion of a facet joint to a multisegmental anomaly with the elements of the spine forming a confusing jumble. **Wedge vertebrae:** may occur with decreased height of the anterior or lateral aspect of the vertebra. Wedge vertebra may be associated with scoliosis or abnormal kyphosis or lordosis. **Butterfly vertebrae:** may occur with hypoplasia of the central portion of the vertebral body. **Block vertebrae:** occur when the vertebrae fail to segment appropriately.

entity or the same term for different entities. We present what we think is the simplest set of terms that will allow the spine imager to diagnose and describe most congenital anomalies (Barkovich 2000, Byrd 1991, Goske 1994, Osborn 1994). These are presented in Table 7–2 for easy reference when reading the Common Clinical Scenarios section (see later). To help the reader digest the large number of terms and relative complexity of this area, some of the points made in Table 7–2 are repeated in the text.

Common Clinical Scenarios in Congenital and Developmental Anomalies

A patient with a congenital anomaly of the spine may present with any one of several different clinical scenarios (see Table 7–2).

PRESENTATION AT BIRTH

Spinal Dysraphism Associated with a Non–Skin-Covered Back (Dorsal) Mass. Infants born with an obvious back mass usually undergo immediate surgery, although occasionally such infants are imaged either in utero via ultrasound or immediately after delivery but before surgery. If the dysraphism is associated with a flat plate of neural tissue (the *placode*) flush with the dorsal body surface, this is a *myelocele*; if there is an associated lipoma causing a back mass, this is a called a *lipomyelocele* (Fig. 7–1); if there is a dilated meningeal-lined CSF-filled sac causing a back mass, this is a *myelomeningocele*. If imaging is performed either prior to surgery or shortly after surgery, every attempt should be made to image the entire neuraxis and document all associated abnormalities, including tethering of the cord and position of the conus, segmentation anomalies of the spine, Chiari II malformation, diastematomyelia, lipomas,

TABLE 7–2. Clinical Scenarios of Congenital Anomalies

Clinical Scenario	Lesions
Presentation at birth	
Spinal dysraphism associated with a non–skin-covered back mass	Myelocele Myelomeningocele
Spinal dysraphism with a skin-covered back mass	Lipomyelomeningocele Myelocystocele Posterior meningocele
Obvious genitourinary abnormalities or other findings of caudal dysplasia	Caudal regression syndrome
Sacral dimple or other worrisome midline skin lesion	Dorsal dermal sinus Any of several additional lesions
Presentation later in life	

Any of several nonspecific symptoms (including lower extremity weakness, painful scoliosis, bowel and bladder control problems) or incidentally discovered abnormality found during imaging for an unrelated, symptom-producing lesion	Meningocele
	  Simple posterior
	  Lateral thoracic
	  Anterior sacral
	Diastematomyelia
	Dorsal dermal sinus
	Syringohydromyelia
	Spinal lipoma
	Tight filum terminale
	Neurenteric cyst
	Occult caudal regression syndrome
	Segmentation anomalies

Data From Byrd 1991, Goske 1994, Schut 1997.

neurenteric cysts, dermoids, and epidermoids. The report should include the levels of dysraphism, the size of the herniated CSF collection, the level of the conus, and a description of all associated anomalies.

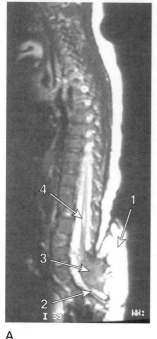
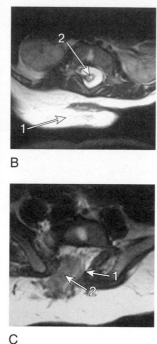

FIGURE 7–1

Lipomyelocele. A 3-month-old infant with a back mass. *A,* Sagittal T2WI demonstrates a dorsal lipoma *(arrow 1)*, dysraphism of the lower spine *(arrow 2)*, and a low-lying spinal cord with syrinx *(arrow 4)* extending directly into a neural placode *(arrow 3)*. *B,* Axial T2WI demonstrates the dorsal lipoma *(arrow 1)* and syrinx *(arrow 2)*. *C,* Axial T2WI at a slightly lower level demonstrates the dorsal dysraphism *(arrow 1)* and neural placode *(arrow 2)*.

After surgical repair of a myelocele or myelomeningocele, imaging will be performed again if neurologic symptoms develop (Fig. 7–2). These include changes in bowel or bladder control, lower extremity weakness, and increasing scoliosis. In the event of development of these symptoms, the entire neuraxis should again be imaged. A significant undiagnosed anomaly such as a Chiari II malformation with hydrocephalus malformation may be found. Syringomyelia should be sought (Fig. 7–3), particularly in those cases of increasing or painful scoliosis. A constricting dural ring at the site of prior surgery may be identified (usually more easily seen on CT-myelogram than on MRI). Ischemia from vascular compromise may be suggested by a sudden change in caliber of the spinal cord. In a patient with none of these findings, the presumptive diagnosis is retethering of the spinal cord (Fig. 7–4). Retethering of the cord is generally a diagnosis of exclusion, although phase-contrast MRI shows promise as a method of demonstrating decreased cord motion in cases of both tethered and re-tethered cord (Barkovich 2000).

Spinal Dysraphism Associated with a Skin-Covered Back Mass. These infants also usually undergo immediate surgery. If the skin covers a lipoma to which the distal cord is attached through the dysraphic spine, this is a *lipomyelocele* (without associated herniation of meninges) or *lipomyelomeningocele* (with associated herniation of meninges). If the skin covers a cystic lesion that leads directly to the central cavity in a spinal cord with syringohydromyelia, then the diagnosis is *myelocystocele*. If the

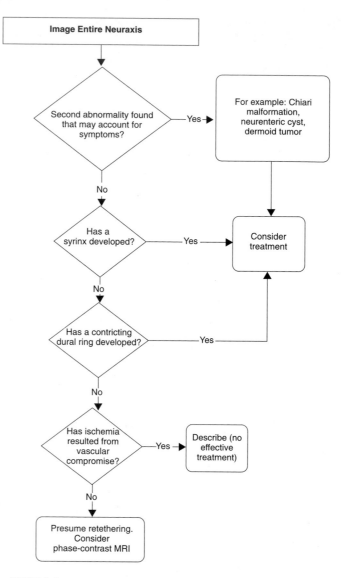

FIGURE 7–2

Algorithm for symptoms following surgical repair of a congenital anomaly.

skin covers CSF-distended meninges without neural elements, this is a *meningocele* (Fig. 7–5). As in the prior clinical scenario, every attempt should be made to image the entire neuraxis and document all associated anomalies. Reporting and later development of symptoms in the postoperative patient are also handled as in the prior scenario (Fig. 7–6).

Obvious Genitourinary Abnormalities or Other Findings of Caudal Dysplasia. Patients with suspected or obvious findings of caudal regression syndrome also should undergo imaging of the entire neuraxis, again searching for additional pathology. The distal spinal cord should be scrutinized for an abnormal appearance, since a blunted or attenuated conus is a sign of cord tethering in caudal regression (Fig. 7–7) (Barkovich 2000). The report in these cases needs to include a description of the level of abnormality, location of the conus (and description of its appearance), and any associated anomalies of the spine. CT of the abdomen and pelvis may complement MRI of the spine, allowing diagnosis of associated genitourinary and bowel abnormalities.

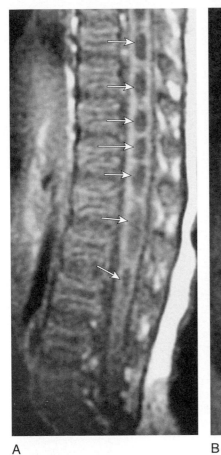

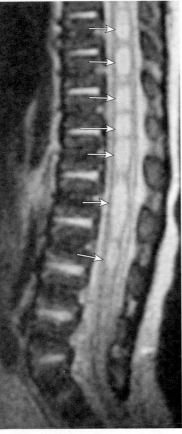

A   B

FIGURE 7–3

Syringomyelia accompanying repaired meningocele. A 1-year-old child with myelomeningocele repair at birth and now with new onset of calf weakness. *A,* Sagittal T1WI demonstrates extensive syringomyelia *(arrows).* Note low-lying conus. *B,* Sagittal T2WI demonstrates extensive syringomyelia *(arrows)* with multiple areas of T2 prolongation expanding the cord, which ends abnormally low. The syrinx was new from prior studies (not shown).

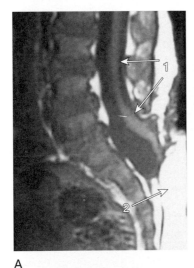

A

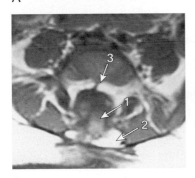

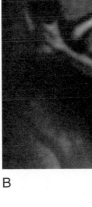

C   B

FIGURE 7–4

Retethering of the cord following myelomeningocele repair. The patient underwent surgical correction of a lumbosacral meningocele 3 years before this examination. The patient presented with increasing deformity of the left foot. *A,* Sagittal T1WI demonstrates a tethered cord *(arrow 1)* and dorsal spinal dysraphism *(arrow 2). B,* Sagittal T2WI demonstrates the tethered cord *(arrow 1)* along with dorsal dysraphism *(arrow 2).* Note expansion of spinal canal *(arrow 3). C,* Axial T1WI demonstrates the posteriorly located, tethered spinal cord *(arrow 1),* dorsal dysraphism *(arrow 2),* and a prominent central septum *(arrow 3).*

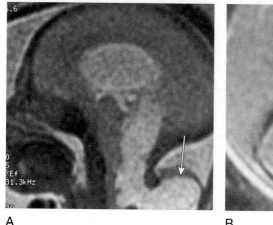

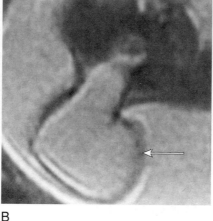

A   B

FIGURE 7–5

Meningocele. A woman with 31-week pregnancy referred for MRI because of abnormal ultrasonographic examination (not shown). *A*, Sagittal fast spin-echo (FSE) T2W1 demonstrates a posterior cervical meningocele (*arrow*). *B*, Axial FSE T2W1 demonstrates the posterior meningocele (*arrow*). There is dysraphism of the posterior elements and cerebrospinal fluid in herniated meninges, outside the normal spinal canal.

Sacral Dimple or Other Worrisome Midline Skin Lesion. The location of the sacral dimple should be marked and all images carefully windowed to make the relatively low signal intensity tract of a dorsal dermal sinus tract stand out. Every effort should be made to document the interior terminus of a dorsal dermal sinus, which may be several levels removed from the cutaneous lesion.

Other cutaneous lesions (e.g., a skin tag, hairy patch, or midline nevus) may also be seen with any of several congenital anomalies, but the type and location of the cutaneous lesion are not predictive of the type and location of anomaly (Schut 1997). The decision whether to image these individuals is made on the basis of other clinical findings, some of which are obvious at birth (e.g., clubfoot) and others of which may become apparent only later (e.g., lower extremity weakness, bowel or bladder functional abnormalities). If imaging is undertaken, the entire neuraxis should be screened since the spinal anomaly may be at different levels than the cutaneous abnormality.

PRESENTATION LATER IN LIFE

Patients who do not present as neonates and who have congenital spinal anomalies may present with symptoms related to their anomaly or have their anomaly discovered incidentally when undergoing imaging for an unrelated complaint (e.g., radicular pain from a herniated disc). The clinical symptoms manifested by patients with congenital anomalies are nonspecific (Schut 1997) and include backache, radicular pain, changes in bowel and bladder function, lower extremity weakness, and painful scoliosis. Any of several congenital anomalies (and any of several other abnormalities) may cause such symptoms. We briefly review the lesions that may be found in such patients. To reiterate, many patients with congenital anomalies have multiple lesions; therefore, discovery of one congenital anomaly should cause the spine imager to search diligently for additional lesions.

Meningoceles. Meningoceles occur in three basic varieties: (1) simple (posterior) meningoceles, (2) lateral thoracic meningoceles, and (3) anterior sacral meningoceles.

First, when the CSF-containing meninges herniate through the dysraphic defect posteriorly without associated neural tissue, this is called *meningocele* (or *posterior meningocele* or *simple meningocele*) (Fig. 7–5). When ana-

lyzing and reporting meningoceles, it is important to scrutinize the neural elements. Although, technically, no neural elements should be contained in meningoceles (otherwise they should be called *myelo*meningoceles), a single nerve root does not disqualify a lesion as a meningocele. The presence of a nerve root is important to the surgeon, because if the meningocele is resected the surgeon will attempt to avoid resecting the nerve root. In addition to evaluation of all nervous tissue, the position of the conus and the appearance of the filum should be specifically evaluated and reported, because tethered cord is an important collateral abnormality in simple meningocele.

The second type is a *lateral thoracic meningocele*. Meningoceles may also occur without dysraphism. Outpouchings of CSF-filled dura may extend through a neural foramina with associated remodeling of the adjacent bone. Most patients with lateral thoracic meningoceles have neurofibromatosis. The report regarding a lateral thoracic meningocele should include the level and size of the meningocele, mention any associated kyphosis (which often accompanies the meningocele), and describe whether any neural elements (cord or nerve roots) are included in the meningocele. Description of the effect on adjacent organs (e.g., compression of lung tissue) and accompanying hydrocephalus should also be part of the report. If (as is usually the case) the patient has neurofibromatosis, a description of all associated soft tissue masses should be included.

The third type is an anterior sacral meningocele. These lesions consist of outpouching of the dura anteriorly with an associated scimitar-shaped sacrum and/or a defect within the sacrum communicating with a CSF-filled cyst within the pelvis (Fig. 7–8). The cyst may be complex and multiloculated. Continuity between the cyst and the sacral canal may be demonstrated directly on sagittal and axial MRI studies or with CT performed after intrathecal contrast (Barkovich 2000). The report should include the size and position of the meningocele and where communication with the spinal canal has been identified. Specific mention of possible cord tethering and associated (dorsal) lipomas should be made. It is imperative to make every attempt to identify the sacral nerve roots and whether these are included within the meningocele: the presence of nerve roots within the meningocele alters the surgical approach (Barkovich 2000).

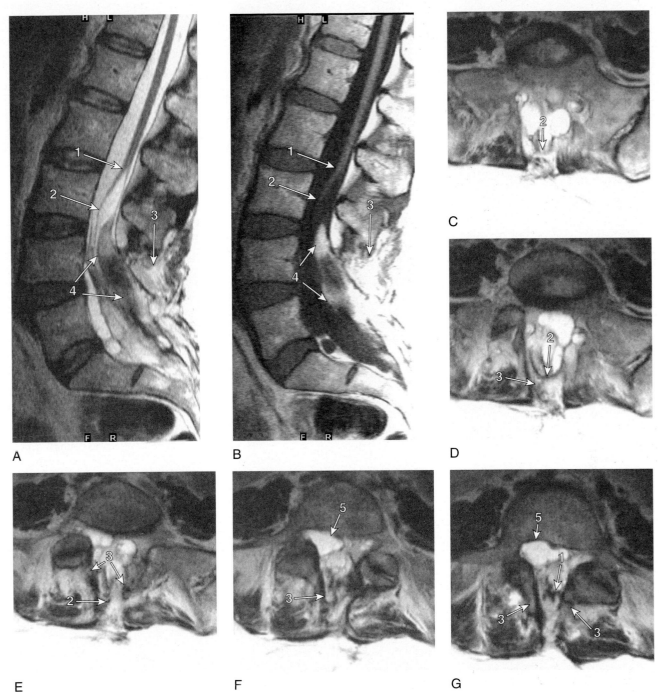

FIGURE 7–6

Repaired lipomyelomeningocele with superimposed degenerative changes. A 53-year-old woman with a history of surgery performed just after birth and at 2 years of age. The patient had a fall approximately 3 weeks prior to the MRI study, with low back pain. *A,* Sagittal T2WI demonstrates a tethered cord with the conus at the L2–3 intervertebral disc level (*arrow 1*), an abnormal course of the nerve roots within the spinal canal (*arrow 2*), dorsal dysraphism (*arrow 3*), and a spinal canal lesion at the L4 level (*arrow 4*). *B,* Sagittal T1WI demonstrates the tethered cord (*arrow 1*), distorted cauda equina (*arrow 2*) (although not as well as the T2WI), dorsal dysraphism (*arrow 3*), and central lesion at the L4 level (*arrow 4*). The lesion at the L4 level demonstrates intermediate signal intensity on T2WI with T1 shortening, consistent with fat and indicative of a lipomeningocele (in this case, repaired). *C–N,* Sequential axial T2WI from the sacrum through the L3–4 disc demonstrates the lipoma (*arrows 1*) extending through the dorsal dysraphic defect (*arrows 2*) into the dorsal soft tissues. There is an elongated and dysplastic appearance of the laminae and posterior elements (*arrows 3*). The nerve roots within the lower thecal sac have a clumped appearance (*arrows 4*). There is cyst formation along the right ventral aspect of the distal spinal canal (*arrow 5*). *O–Z,* Sequential axial T1WI matching images. *C–N* also demonstrate the lipoma (*arrow 1*), dorsal dysraphic defect (*arrows 2*), and dysplastic posterior elements (*arrows 3*). Although there are many findings of repaired lipomyelomeningocele, the cause of the patient's low back pain may be the degenerative changes rather than her residual congenital spinal abnormalities. No acute fracture is identified.

(continued)

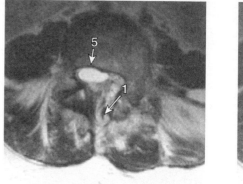

H

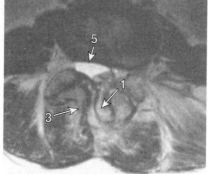

I

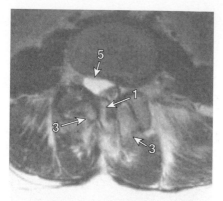

J

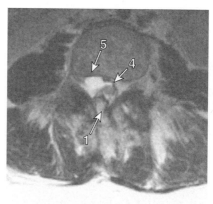

K

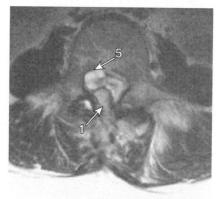

L

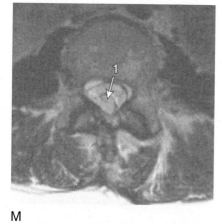

M

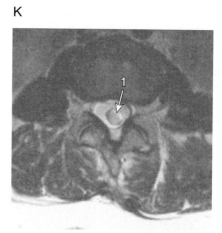

N

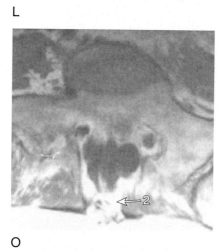

O

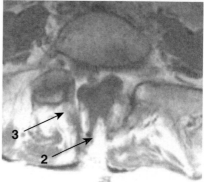

P

FIGURE 7–6 (*continued*)

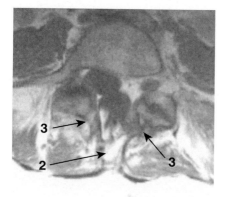

Q

R

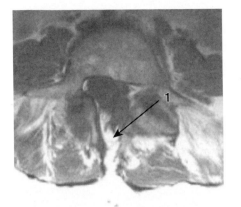

S

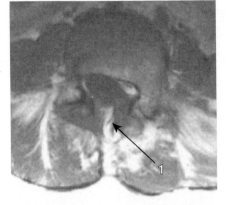

T

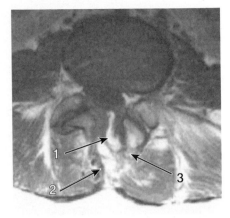

U

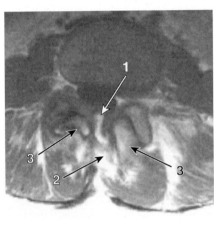

V

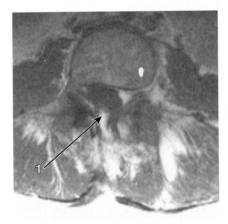

W

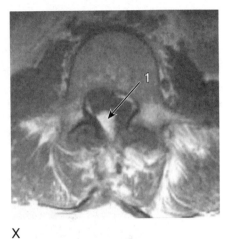

X

FIGURE 7–6 (continued)

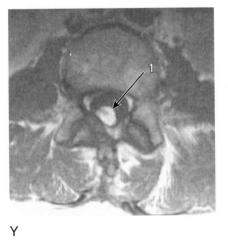

Y

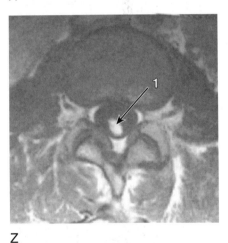

Z

Diastematomyelia. When there is incomplete or complete splitting of the spinal cord, with each of the two parts of the cord containing ventral and dorsal roots, this is called *diastematomyelia* (Fig. 7–9). Given the dramatic imaging findings, many cases of diastematomyelia are surprisingly asymptomatic. Those patients that do manifest symptoms have other collateral pathology or a bony or fibrous septum separating and tethering the two portions of the spinal cord. This tethering leads to symptoms. Important points to keep in mind in reporting cases of diastematomyelia are that the specific location of all parts of the septum must be

designated and that there may be discontinuity in the septum (with one portion of the septum lying more inferior and another more superior). Full characterization of the septum, which may contain fibrous, cartilaginous, and bony elements, often requires the use of both MR and CT scanning.

Dorsal Dermal Sinus. When there is a sinus tract leading from the posterior skin surface into the patient, this is a dorsal dermal sinus (Fig. 7–10). Since the tract may lead all the way to the spinal canal, patients may present with intermittent meningitis. The tract may also extend several levels

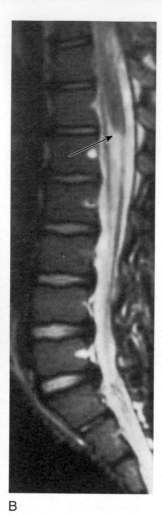

FIGURE 7–7

Blunted conus in caudal regression syndrome. A 6-year-old boy with urinary incontinence and unilateral leg weakness. *A,* Lateral plain film demonstrates absence of the lowest sacral segment *(arrow). B,* Sagittal T2WI demonstrates an abnormal, wedge-shaped conus typical of caudal regression syndrome *(arrow).* The conus is normally located at the T12–L1 level, however, without evidence of a low-lying cord.

cephalad or caudad from the skin site. The report should include, if at all possible, the exact location of both the skin entrance site and internal terminus of the tract as well as specific mention of any additional congenital anomalies. With respect to additional abnormalities, dorsal dermal sinus tracts may be associated with dermoids, epidermoids, or lipomas anywhere along the course of the tract, including within the spinal canal (Barkovich 1991).

Syringohydromyelia. *Hydromyelia* refers to expansion of the central canal (which is lined by ependyma); *syringomyelia* refers to fluid within the spinal cord (distributed parallel to the long axis of the cord) that is not within the central canal and hence not lined with ependyma. Since these two entities are difficult to separate (not only on imaging, but histologically as well), the term *syringohydromyelia* (or *hydrosyringomyelia,* or *syrinx*) has been used to denote longitudinal fluid collections of either variety (Barkovich 2000, Osborn 1994, Sherman 1986) (Fig. 7–11). A syrinx may be associated with additional congenital anomalies (Fig. 7–9) or a cord tumor, and patients with a small syrinx should routinely be evaluated with contrast agent to evaluate whether the syrinx enhances or if spinal cord adjacent to the syrinx enhances (indicating a possible neoplasm). A small, benign syrinx is usually asymptomatic and is generally of no clinical consequence, but it is not possible to reliably predict whether a syrinx will expand, and an expanding syrinx may result in neurologic damage (Osborn 1994). Therefore, it is usually recommended that an asymptomatic syrinx be followed to ensure that there is no progression of size. The report should indicate the size (length and diameter) and position (relative to the vertebral bodies), the contrast enhancement pattern, and any associated additional congenital anomalies.

Lipoma. Lipomas of the cord may occur at the posterior margin of myeloceles or myelomeningoceles (which are termed *lipomyeloceles* [Fig. 7–1] or *lipomyelomeningoceles* [Figs. 7–9 and 7–12]), within the filum terminale (Fig. 7–13), or within the dura. Congenital intradural spinal lipomas occur in the posterior aspect of the spinal canal and lie either along the posterior margin of the cord (Fig. 7–14) or within a groove within the posterior aspect of the cord (Fig. 7–15). Unlike almost all other tumors, it is possible to

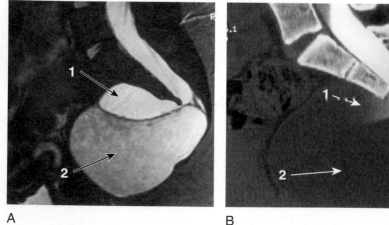

FIGURE 7–8

Sacral meningocele. An 11-year-old child with hypertension, enuresis, and a pelvic mass. *A,* Sagittal T2WI demonstrates a defect in the lower sacrum, with apparent communication between the thecal sac and an anterior meningocele *(arrow 1),* along with a larger and more inferior cyst *(arrow 2). B,* Sagittal reconstruction CT-myelogram demonstrating communication between the thecal sac and anterior meningocele *(arrow 1)* and lack of communication with the lower cyst *(arrow 2).* Note the portion of distal sacrum inferior to the cyst *(arrow 3).*

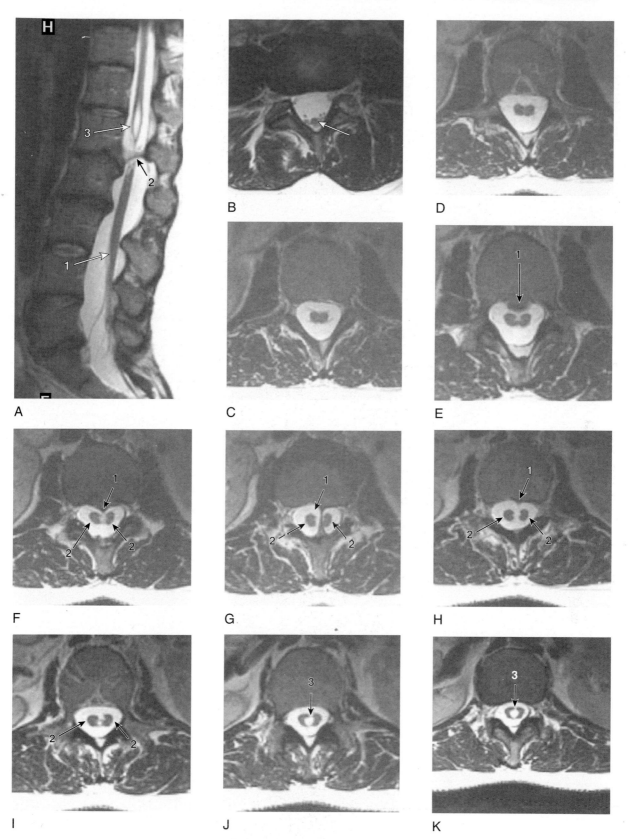

FIGURE 7–9

Diastematomyelia. A 36-year-old woman with chronic low back pain. *A,* Sagittal T2WI demonstrates a low-lying neurofibrous structure *(arrow 1),* a septum of tissue cleaving the spinal cord emanating from the posterior surface of L1 *(arrow 2),* and a syrinx *(arrow 3)* above the level of the septum. There are degenerative changes of the L2–3 and L5–S1 intervertebral discs. *B,* Axial T2WI at the L4–5 level demonstrates thickening of neurofibrous structures, representing either the stretched and tethered conus or thickened filum terminale *(arrow),* along with a capacious spinal canal. *C–K,* Sequential inferior-to-superior axial T2WIs demonstrate a septum *(arrows 1)* separating the cord into distinct halves *(arrows 2)* (diastematomyelia). There is a 5.5-mm syrinx *(arrow 3)* above the level of the septum.

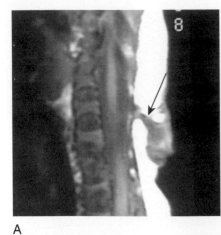

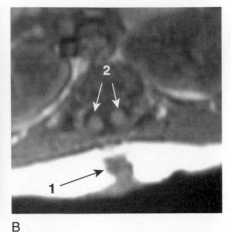

A

B

FIGURE 7–10

Dorsal dermal sinus. A 1-day-old infant girl with a skin-covered back mass. *A,* Sagittal T1WI demonstrates a dorsal dermal sinus connecting the spinal canal to the posterior skin surface *(arrow).* *B,* Axial T1WI demonstrates the dorsal dermal sinus *(arrow 1)* as well as diastematomyelia *(arrow 2).*

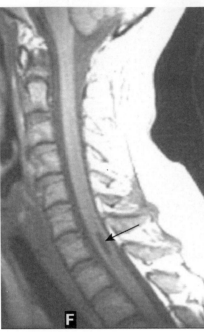

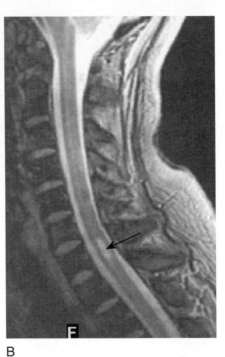

A

B

FIGURE 7–11

Syrinx. A 36-year-old woman with neck and shoulder pain. *A,* Sagittal T1WI demonstrates a 15 × 4-mm focus of T1 prolongation *(arrow)* at the C7 level. *B,* Sagittal T2WI demonstrates corresponding T2 prolongation *(arrow).* No contrast enhancement of the lesion or associated Chiari malformation was identified. *C,* Sagittal T1WI, and *D,* Sagittal T2W1, obtained 12 months after *A,* documenting stability of the lesion. Although typically stable, such lesions are usually followed because expansion (and associated irreversible neurologic damage) may be accompanied by minimal symptoms, and patients with expanding syringes are considered to be surgical candidates for shunting.

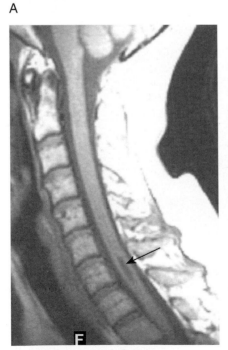

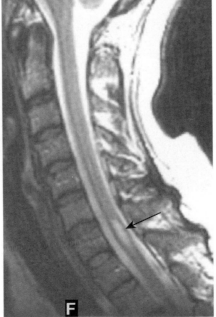

C

D

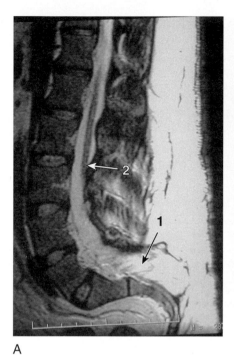

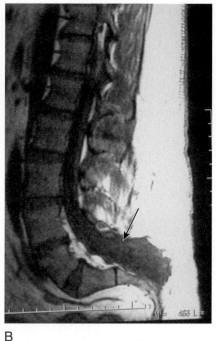

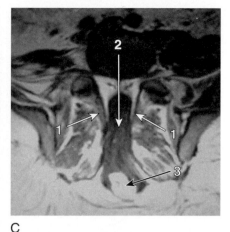

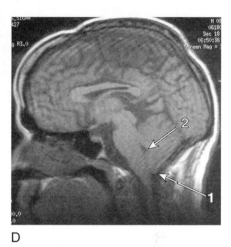

FIGURE 7–12

Repaired lipomyelomeningocele. A 34-year-old man with low back pain and urinary dysfunction. *A*, Sagittal T2WI demonstrates a large lipomyelomeningocele. there was a skin covering, but the distal cord was attached to a lipoma through a dysraphic spine. Cerebrospinal fluid (CSF) projects through a dorsal dysraphic defect (*arrow 1*). Note the low-lying conus (*arrow 2*) from an associated tethered cord. *B*, Sagittal T1WI also shows CSF projecting through the dorsal dysraphic defect (*arrow*). *C*, Axial T2WI demonstrates the elongated appearance of the posterior elements (*arrows 1*) associated with spinal dysraphism (*arrow 2*). The cord was connected to a dorsal lipoma (*arrow 3*). *D*, Sagittal T1WI of the brain shows Chiari II malformation. The cerebellar tonsils are low and pointed (*arrow 1*), and the fourth ventricle is also low (*arrow 2*).

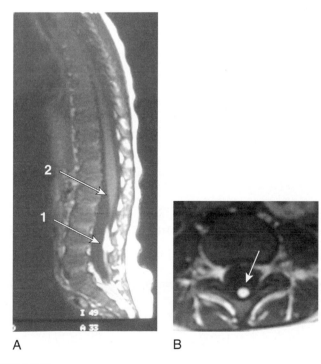

FIGURE 7–13

Lipoma of the filum terminale. A 16-month-old boy. *A*, Sagittal T1WI demonstrates a lipoma of the filum terminale (*arrow 1*) with an associated low-lying conus (*arrow 2*). *B*, Axial T1WI demonstrates the lipoma of the filum terminale (*arrow*).

histologically characterize lipomas because of the unique imaging characteristics of fat: lipid will demonstrate high signal intensity on T1-weighted image (T1WI) (T1 shortening) with fading (but still relatively bright) signal intensity on T2WI, and signal will diminish greatly on fat-suppression sequences. The report of a lipoma should include the size and position of the lipoma and a description of the imaging characteristics that establish its histologic characterization. A description of the spinal cord appearance (such as narrowing or tethering) should be provided. As with all congenital anomalies, the presence of a lipoma should alert the interpreting radiologist to search for additional congenital lesions.

Tight Filum Terminale. The normal filum terminale leads from the conus medullaris through the lumbar and sacral subarachnoid space to end at the posterior margin of the coccyx. In the normal individual, the conus medullaris terminates at or above the L2–3 level (Saifuddin 1998) and the filum is at most 2 mm in diameter at the L5/S1 level.

The thickened filum terminale causes fixation of the spinal cord and may become symptomatic in childhood or adolescence secondary to the relatively greater growth of the vertebra compared to the spinal cord, causing increased tension on the cord. In the adult, symptoms follow from tension on the cord from repeated neck flexion, trauma, or spondylotic canal stenosis (Pang 1982). Nondermatomal pain referred to the anorectal region, progressive sensorimotor deficits of the lower extremities, and bladder and

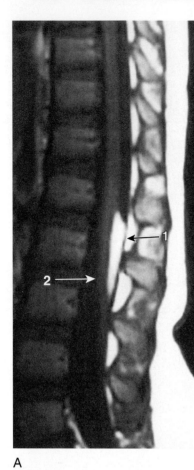

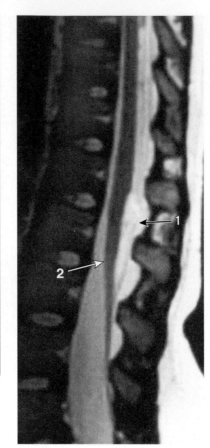

A

B

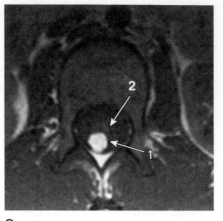

C

FIGURE 7–14

Congenital lipoma with associated tethered cord. *A*, Sagittal T1WI demonstrates an oblong lipoma (*arrow 1*) posterior to a tethered spinal cord (*arrow 2*); the tip of the conus and lipoma are at L3. *B*, Sagittal T2WI again demonstrates the lipoma (*arrow 1*) posterior to a tethered spinal cord (*arrow 2*). *C*, Axial T1WI demonstrates the lipoma (*arrow 1*) posterior to the distal spinal cord (*arrow 2*).

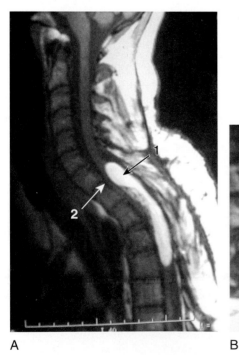

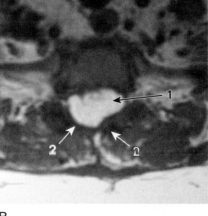

A

B

FIGURE 7–15

Congenital lipoma (postoperative). A 30-year-old woman after surgery for congenital lipoma with incontinence and difficulty with ambulation. *A*, Sagittal T2WI demonstrates large intradural lipoma (*arrow 1*) extending from C7 to T4. The spinal cord (*arrow 2*) is attenuated at the level of the lesion, with the lipoma dorsal to the flattened cord. *B*, Axial T2WI through the lipoma (*arrow 1*) (which fills the spinal canal) demonstrates a combination of postoperative and dysraphic change posteriorly (*arrow 2*).

bowel dysfunction may be present in both adults and children; progressive foot and spine deformities are more frequently seen in children (Pang 1982). Patients with a thickened filum with a cord in a fixed, abnormally low position and such symptoms are said to have "tight filum terminale syndrome" (Byrd 1991) or "tethered cord syndrome" (Pang 1982).

Frequently, there may be a small amount of fat within the proximal (Fig. 7–16) or distal filum, and patients with proximal filum measurements of up to 3 mm *without* cord

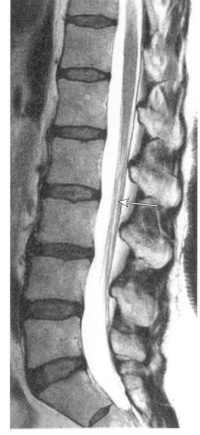

A

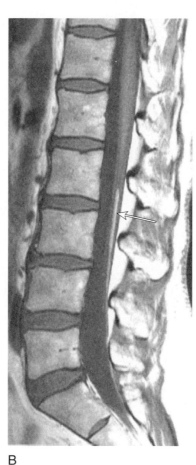

B

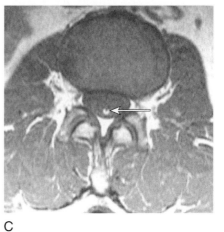

C

FIGURE 7–16

Fatty filum. A 57-year-old woman with recent onset of low back and bilateral leg pain. *A*, Sagittal T2WI demonstrates mild disc dehydration throughout the lumbar spine with Schmorl's node formation, along with L3–4 disc narrowing. Note that the fatty filum terminale is inconspicuous on this imaging sequence, since it is adjacent to cerebrospinal fluid (CSF) *(arrow)*. *B*, Sagittal T1WI demonstrates the fatty filum *(arrows)*; T1 shortening within the fat renders the lesion much more conspicuous than adjacent CSF. *C*, Axial T1WI at the L2–3 disc level demonstrates the fatty filum *(arrow)* in the posterior canal.

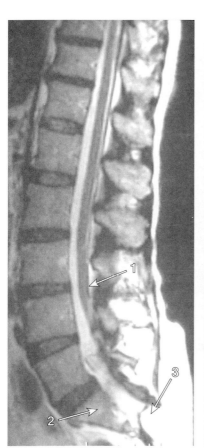

A

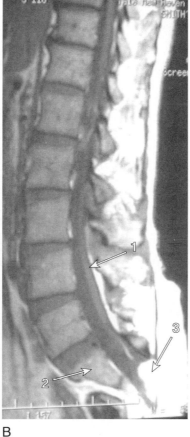

B

FIGURE 7–17

Tethered cord with accompanying caudal regression and lipomyelomeningocele. A 51-year-old woman with back pain and urinary incontinence. *A*, Sagittal T2WI demonstrates a tethered cord with an abnormally elongated and tapered conus *(arrow 1)*, caudal regression with an atretic sacrum *(arrow 2)*, and dysraphism with a dorsal lipoma *(arrow 3)*. *B*, Sagittal T1WI also demonstrates the low-lying neurofibrous structure *(arrow 1)*, atretic sacrum *(arrow 2)*, and dysraphism with a dorsal lipoma *(arrow 3)* with T1 shortening diagnostic of fat.

tethering or symptoms have been reported (Uchino 1991). Therefore, discovery of fat within the filum does not necessarily lead to a diagnosis of tethered cord syndrome. Imaging of the distal conus with motion-sensitive imaging sequences holds promise in making the diagnosis (Barkovich 2000), but at present the main imaging clues are the position of the conus and the diameter of the filum terminale. Reporting of this entity should include the position of the conus and diameter of the filum, and an attempt should be made to correlate with any symptoms that might be related to low-lying conus. The lower posterior canal should be scrutinized for associated dysraphic changes.

Although a thickened filum terminale and low-lying cord may be a relatively isolated (yet symptom-producing) lesion, a low-lying, tethered cord may also accompany many of the more complex congenital anomalies (e.g., myelomeningocele, diastematomyelia). For this reason, discovery of a thickened filum terminale and low-lying cord should prompt a search for additional anomalies (Fig. 7–17). Conversely, the report of all complex congenital anomalies needs to include a description of the end of the spinal cord and filum terminale regarding appearance and location.

It may be difficult to distinguish between the conus and a thickened filum terminale, particularly on sagittal studies (Barkovich 2000, Gundry 1994, Osborn 1994); Tortori-

Donant and associates (1990) have proposed the term *neurofibrous structure* to delineate the conus/filum terminale complex in difficult cases.

Neurenteric Cyst. Neurenteric cysts are fluid-filled pockets lined with epithelium (Gleeson 1961) that may occur in the spinal canal and thus mimic arachnoid cysts (St. Amour 1994). The clue to differentiating neurenteric cysts from arachnoid cysts or cystic tumors within the spinal canal is the frequent coexistence of spinal segmentation anomalies (Barkovich 2000, St. Amour 1994) (Fig. 7–18). The report of these abnormalities should include the size and location of the cyst, grade of associated neural compression, and mention of any additional congenital anomalies, including, in particular, segmentation anomalies at or near the level of the lesion. It may not always be possible to distinguish a neurenteric cyst from an arachnoid cyst (Geremia 1988).

Occult Caudal Regression Syndrome. Although gross caudal regression is obvious at birth, lesser forms of the abnormality may present only later in life; as with other congenital anomalies, the symptoms produced by caudal regression syndrome are nonspecific (Schut 1997). Limited forms of caudal regression syndrome (e.g., isolated absence of the coccyx) may be an incidental finding without clinical consequence (Osborn 1994). The report in caudal regres-

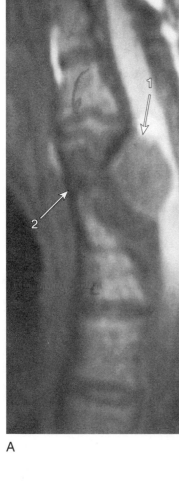
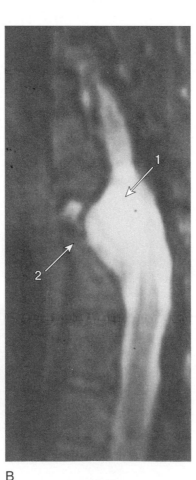

A   B

FIGURE 7–18

Neurenteric cyst with associated segmentation anomaly. A 31-year-old woman with long-standing paraplegia. *A,* Sagittal T1WI demonstrates a cervicothoracic junction mass with both an extradural and intradural component. Note associated segmentation of the vertebrae anterior to the lesion *(arrow 2). B,* Sagittal T2WI demonstrates the neurenteric cyst *(arrow 1)* and associated spinal segmentation anomaly *(arrow 2).*

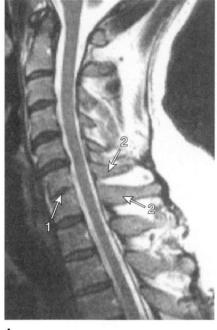
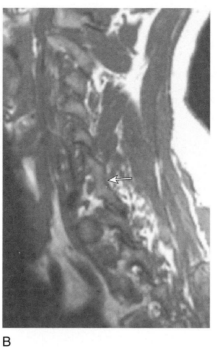

A

B

FIGURE 7-19

Segmentation anomaly of the cervical spine. A 34-year-old man with neck and shoulder pain following a motor vehicle accident. *A,* Sagittal T2WI demonstrates multilevel degenerative changes, including C5–6 degenerative disc bulging. At the C6–7 level, there is a rudimentary disc with apparent fusion along the posterior disc margin *(arrow 1)*. The spinous processes appear separated posteriorly, however *(arrow 2)*. *B,* Right parasagittal T1WI demonstrates nonsegmentation of the left C6–7 facet joint, with bone marrow crossing the joint *(arrow)*.

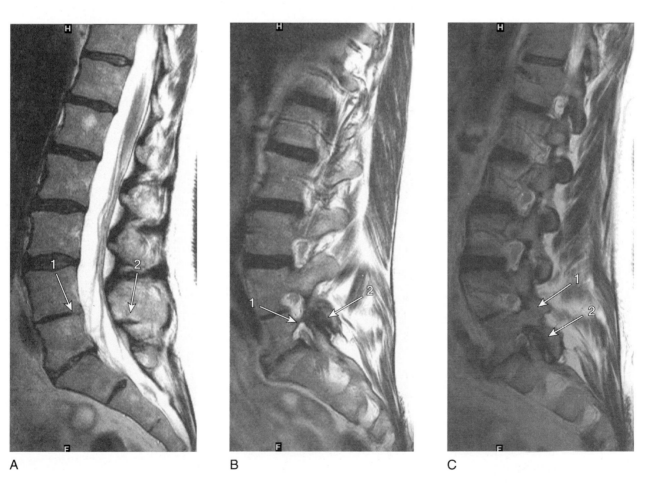

A

B

C

FIGURE 7-20

Segmentation anomaly of the lumbar spine. A 54-year-old woman with low back pain. *A,* Sagittal T2WI demonstrates multilevel degenerative disc disease with disc narrowing and dehydration, most pronounced at the L5–S1 level. There is an incomplete L4–5 intervertebral disc, with marrow crossing the posterior disc space *(arrow 1)*. Posteriorly, there is a single fused spinous process with an anterior cleft *(arrow 2)*. *B,* Right parasagittal T2WI demonstrates an abnormal right L5 pedicle *(arrow 1)* and a malformed and degenerated L5–S1 facet joint *(arrow 2)*. *C,* Left parasagittal T2WI demonstrates fusion across the L4–5 facet joint *(arrow 1)* and degenerative changes of the L5–S1 facet joint *(arrow 2)*. *(continued)*

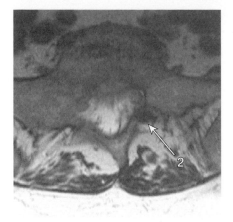

D

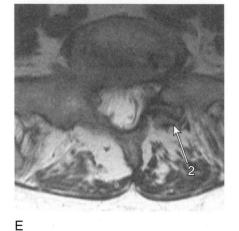

E

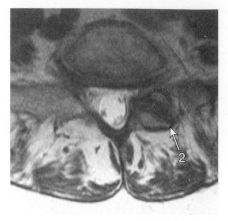

F

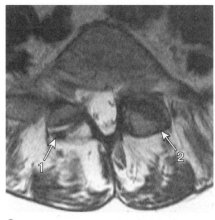

G

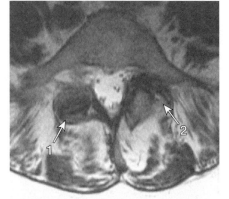

H

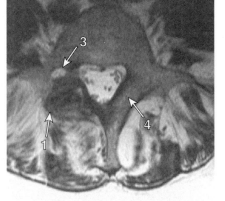

I

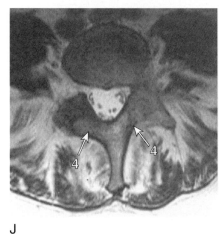

J

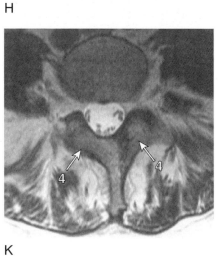

K

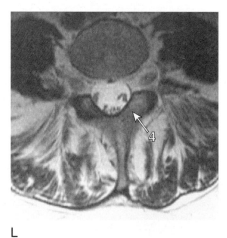

L

FIGURE 7–20 (continued)

D–L, Sequential axial T2WIs from the S1 pedicle through the lower L4 vertebra demonstrates a markedly asymmetric appearance of the L5–S1 facet joints, with the right (arrow 1) having a more coronal orientation and being hypoplastic relative to the left (arrow 2). The right pedicle is discontinuous through its mid portion (arrow 3), and the L5 laminae (arrows 4) are short, thick, and dysplastic.

sion syndrome presenting later in life should include the levels of anomaly and any additional anomalies, particularly tethered cord. As noted earlier, the conus in a patient with caudal regression syndrome may be blunted, wedge-shaped, or tethered (Fig. 7–7).

Segmentation Anomalies. Incomplete discs or fusion across facet joints are examples of relatively frequently encountered segmentation anomalies. These anomalies may occasionally resemble the findings seen in patients who have undergone interbody fusion. Usually congenital anomalies may be distinguished from postoperative findings because of an "hourglass" configuration at the level of the disc and accompanying abnormalities of the facets (Figs. 7–19 and 7–20). In some cases, segmentation

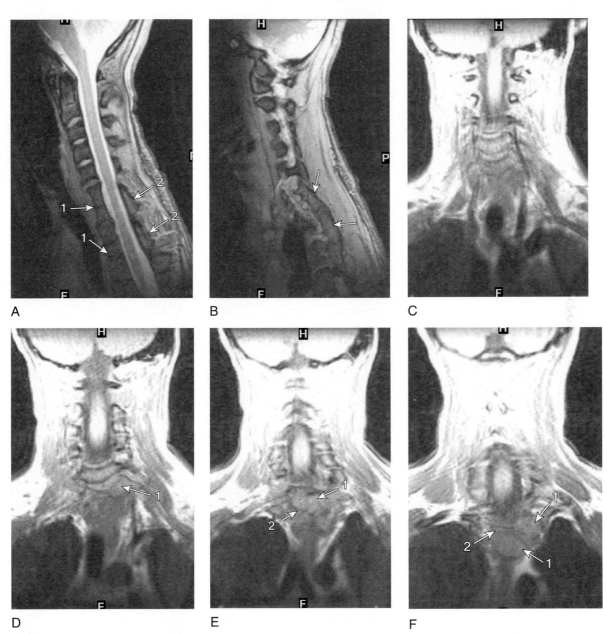

FIGURE 7–21

Complex cervical segmentation anomaly with scoliosis. A 14-year-old girl with scoliosis. *A*, Sagittal T2WI of the cervical spine demonstrates multilevel segmentation anomalies beginning at C6–7 and involving several segments of the upper thoracic spine (*arrows 1*). Posteriorly, there is fusion of segments (*arrows 2*). *B*, Right parasagittal T2WI demonstrates abnormal formation of the right lateral masses with fusion from C6 through T4 (*arrows*). *C–G*, Sequential anterior-to-posterior coronal T1WIs demonstrates multiple abnormalities, with wedge vertebral bodies (*arrows 1*) as well as incompletely formed and dystrophic intervertebral discs (*arrows 2*). There is scoliosis apex to the left.

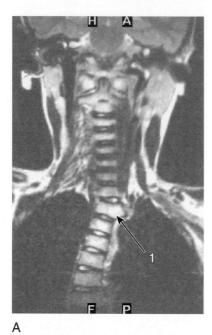

A

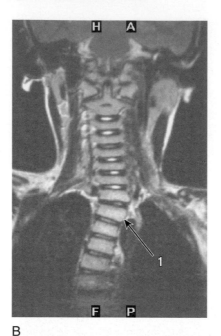

B

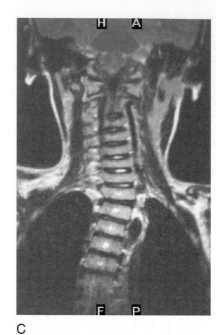

C

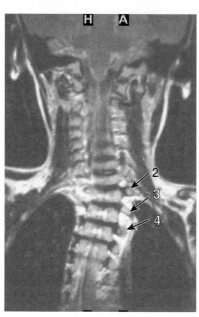

D

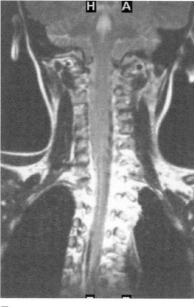

E

FIGURE 7–22

Segmentation anomaly with scoliosis. A 9-year-old child with scoliosis. *A–E,* Sequential anterior-to-posterior coronal T2WIs demonstrate abnormal widening of the T2 vertebral body on the left side (*arrow 1*). Posteriorly, the 1st (*arrow 2*), 2nd (*arrow 3*), and 3rd (*arrow 4*) ribs appear normally formed.

anomalies involve multiple vertebrae in a confused jumble of parts (Fig. 7–21). Although simple segmentation anomalies tend to be asymptomatic, more complex or severe anomalies may be associated with symptoms. Wedge vertebrae may be associated with scoliosis (Figs. 7–21 and 7–22) or loss, accentuation, or reversal of kyphosis or lordosis (Fig. 7–23). Butterfly vertebra may also be associated with abnormalities of alignment (Figs. 7–24 and 7–25). Segmentation abnormalities of the craniovertebral junction are relatively frequent and may be

associated with limitations of motion and abnormal alignment (Fig. 7–26). The classic clinical triad of a short neck, a low posterior hairline, and restriction of motion may be present in the multisegmental cervical anomaly known as *Klippel-Feil syndrome* (Brinker 1997). Patients with this syndrome may demonstrate any of several additional anomalies, including Sprengel's deformity (elevation of the scapula with or without an associated omovertebral bone) (Fig. 7–27). As noted earlier, the presence of segmentation anomalies may assist in differentiating

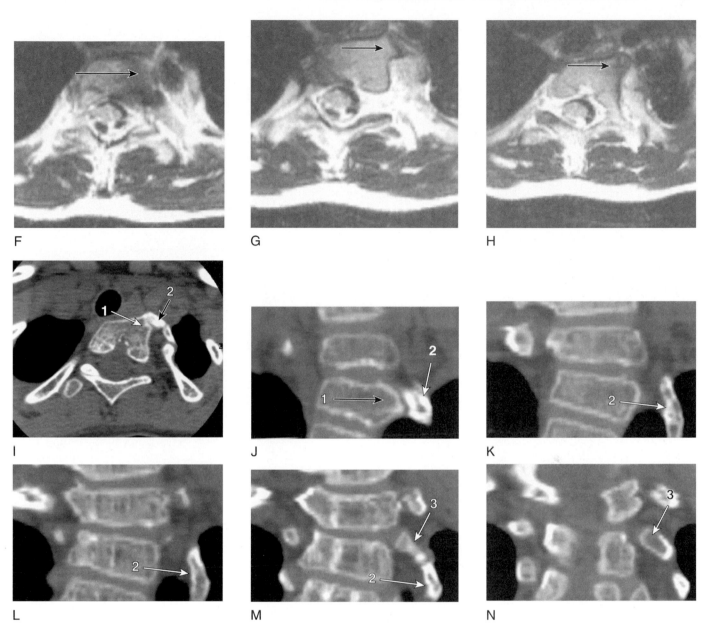

FIGURE 7–22 *(continued)*

F–H, Sequential inferior-to-superior T2WIs through the T2 vertebra demonstrates abnormal overgrowth along the anterolateral, left side of the vertebra *(arrows).* *I,* Axial CT at the level of the T2 vertebral body (compare with *G*) demonstrates overgrowth of the left side of the vertebral body *(arrow 1)* as well as an apparent accessory rib *(arrow 2).* *J–N,* Sequential anterior-to-posterior curved coronal CT reconstructions demonstrate the overgrowth of the left side of the T2 vertebral body *(arrow 1)*and the abnormal bone *(arrows 2)* arcing back to contact the 2nd rib *(arrow 3).* In such complicated cases, MRI and CT may be complementary in demonstrating the abnormality.

neurenteric cysts from other cystic lesions of the canal, since neurenteric cysts may have an associated segmentation anomaly and arachnoid cysts do not. Congenital anomalies may also cause confusion by mimicking fractures or tumors (Gehweiler 1983, Lederman 1986, Wiener 1990).

Conclusion

Scanning and reporting congenital anomalies present several challenges. By taking into account the patient's presenting complaint, performing the appropriate imaging examination, and using appropriate terminology, the radiologist should make a significant contribution to the

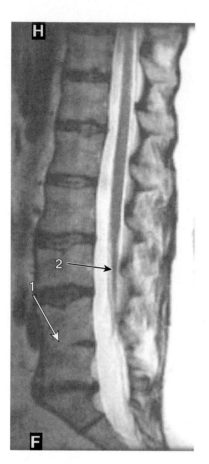

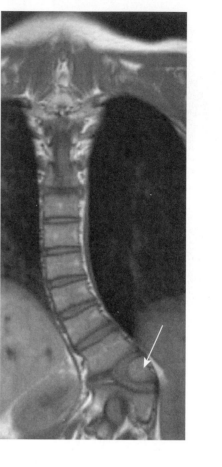

FIGURE 7–23

Segmentation anomaly with loss of lordosis. A 52-year-old woman with low back and right hip pain, along with foot numbness when walking. Sagittal T2WI demonstrates multilevel degenerative changes with Schmorl's node formation and disc dehydration, as well as L5–S1 degenerative disc bulging. A segmentation anomaly of L4-5 (*arrow 1*) is associated with reversal of normal lumbar lordosis at this level; in addition, note the tethered cord with the neurofibrous structure located at L3 or below (*arrow 2*).

FIGURE 7–25

Segmentation anomaly with scoliosis. A 13-year-old child with painful scoliosis. Coronal T1WI demonstrates a wedge vertebral body (*arrow*) at the thoracolumbar junction with associated scoliosis.

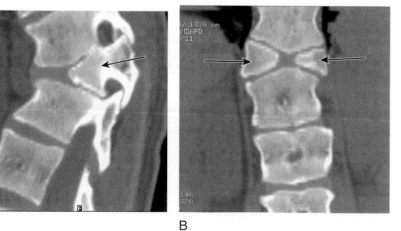

A   B

FIGURE 7–24

Segmentation anomaly associated with painful kyphosis. A 17-year-old patient with painful kyphosis. *A,* Sagittal reconstruction lateral view demonstrates a wedge vertebral body (*arrow*) posteriorly with focal kyphosis. *B,* Coronal reconstruction demonstrates a butterfly segment, with lateral wedges (*arrows*).

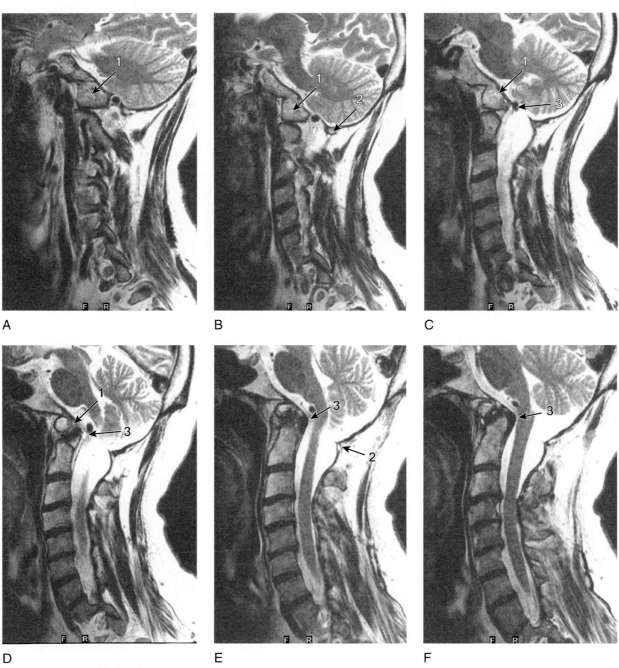

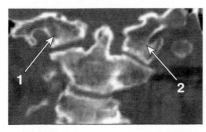

FIGURE 7–26

Segmentation anomaly of the skull base. A 49-year-old man with neck and right shoulder pain. *A–F,* Sequential right-to-left sagittal T2WIs demonstrate incorporation of the lateral mass of C1 with the occiput *(arrows 1),* a rudimentary posterior arch of C1 *(arrows 2),* and abnormal angulation at the craniocervical junction *(arrow 3). G,* Curved coronal reconstruction CT through the skull base demonstrates incorporation of the lateral masses of C1 and the occipital condyles. On the left side *(arrow 1),* the overall height of the occiput-C1 fused mass is considerably shorter than it is on the left *(arrow 2),* tilting the head on the spine.

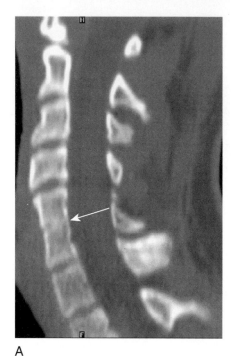

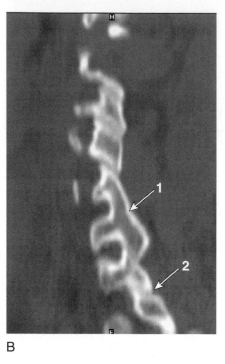

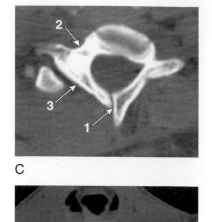

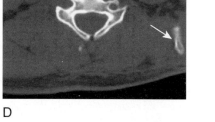

A   B   C   D

FIGURE 7–27

Klippel-Feil syndrome. A 19-year-old patient with known deformity. *A,* Sagittal CT reconstructions demonstrates C5–6 segmentation anomaly with fusion of the disc *(arrow).* *B,* Left parasagittal CT reconstruction demonstrates fusion of the C5–6 facet joint *(arrow 1)* and C6–7 facet joint *(arrow 2).* *C,* Axial CT at the C7 pedicle level demonstrates a cleft arch posteriorly *(arrow 1),* a thickened right pedicle *(arrow 2),* and lamina *(arrow 3)* with resultant rotation of the vertebral because of hypertrophy of the right side. *D,* Axial CT at the C5 level demonstrates a left omovertebral bone *(arrow).*

care of these patients. An important caveat during imaging is the coexistence of lesions both at the same and at different ends of the neuraxis. For example, careful scrutiny of a dermal sinus may demonstrate an associated epidermoid, whereas a patient with a lumbar myelomeningocele may also have a Chiari II malformation at the base of the skull.

References

Adzick NS, Sutton LN, Cromblehome TM, Flake AW. Successful fetal surgery for spina bifida. Lancet 1998; 352:1675–1676.

Barkovich AJ. Congenital anomalies of the spine. In Barkovich AJ. Pediatric Neuroimaging, 3rd ed. Philadelphia, Lippincott Williams & Wilkins, 2000.

Barkovich AJ, Edwards MSB, Cogen PH. MR evaluation of spinal dermal sinus tracts in children. AJNR Am J Neuroradiol 1991; 12:123–129.

Brinker MR, Weeden SH, Whitecloud TS. Congenital anomalies of the cervical spine. In Frymoyer JW (ed). The Adult Spine: Principles and Practice, 2nd ed. Philadelphia, Lippincott-Raven, 1997.

Byrd SE, Darling CF, McLone DG. Developmental disorders of the pediatric spine. Radiol Clin North Am 1991; 29:711–752.

Gehweiler JA, Daffner RH, Roberts L. Malformations of the atlas vertebra simulating the Jefferson fracture. AJR Am J Roentgenol 1983; 140:1083–1086.

Geremia GK, Russell EJ, Clasen RA. MR imaging characteristics of a neurenteric cyst. AJNR Am J Neuroradiol 1988; 9:978–980.

Gleeson JA, Stovin PGI. Mediastinal enterogenous cysts associated with vertebral anomalies. Clin Radiol 1961; 12:41–48.

Goske MJ, Modic MT, Yu S. Pediatric spine: normal anatomy and spinal dysraphism. In Modic MT, Masaryk TJ, Ross JS (ed). Magnetic Resonance Imaging of the Spine, 2nd ed. St. Louis, Mosby–Year Book, 1994.

Gundry CR, Heithoff KB. Imaging evaluation of patients with spinal deformity. Orthop Clin North Am 1994; 25:247–264.

Lederman HM, Kaufman RA. Congenital absence and hypoplasia of pedicles in the thoracic spine. Skeletal Radiol 1986; 5:219–223.

Osborn AG. Normal anatomy and congenital anomalies of the spine and spinal cord. In Osborne AG. Diagnostic Neuroradiology. St. Louis, Mosby, 1994.

Pang D, Wilberger JE Jr. Tethered cord syndrome in adults. J Neurosurg 1982; 57:32–47.

Saifuddin A, Burnett SJD, White J. The variation of position of the conus medullaris in an adult population: a magnetic resonance imaging study. Spine 1998; 23:1452–1456.

Schut L, Sutton LN, Duhaime AC. Congenital neurologic disorders of the lumbar spine presenting in the adult. In Frymoyer JW (ed). The Adult Spine: Principles and Practice, 2nd ed. Philadelphia, Lippincott-Raven, 1997.

Sherman JL, Barkovich AJ, Citrin CM. The MR appearance of syringomyelia: new observations. AJNR Am J Neuroradiol 1986; 7:985–995.

St Amour TE, Hodges SC, Laakman RW, Tamas DE. MRI of the Spine. New York, Raven Press, 1994.

Tortori-Donati P, Cama A, Rosa ML, Andreussi L, Taccone A. Occult spinal dysraphism: neuroradiological study. Neuroradiology 1990; 31:512–522.

Uchino A, Mori T, Ohno M. Thickened fatty filum terminale: MR imaging. Neuroradiology 1991; 33:331–333.

Wiener MD, Martinez S, Forsberg DA. Congenital absence of a cervical spine pedicle: clinical and radiologic findings. AJR Am J Roentgenol 1990; 155:1037–1041.

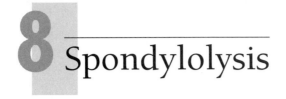

8 Spondylolysis

DONALD L. RENFREW

Any discussion of *spondylolysis* (defects within the pars interarticularis) must also address *spondylolisthesis* (forward slippage of a superior on an inferior vertebrae). Spondylolysis is a specific diagnosis, whereas spondylolisthesis is a finding that a number of different disease processes share. Wiltse's classification scheme of spondylolisthesis (Grobler 1997, Wiltse 1976) offers five types (Table 8–1). Because this book is divided into chapters by disease (rather than finding), this chapter covers Types I (dysplastic) and II (isthmic) spondylolisthesis, whereas Chapter 2 covers Type III (degenerative). This chapter addresses both Types I and II because, although some cases of spondylolisthesis clearly fall into one or the other type, many cases have features of both (Grobler 1997, Wiltse 1976). The chapter also deals with spondylolysis without spondylolisthesis.

Spondylolysis is generally held to be a fatigue fracture of the pars interarticularis (Wiltse 1975) and is distinctly unusual in infants and those who have never ambulated. It may be the result of uneven ossification of the maturing isthmus, leading to a stress riser with resultant fracture (Sagi 1998). As noted by Wiltse and associates (1975) in the original article promoting the fatigue fracture hypothesis, however, spondylolysis defects display several differences from fatigue fractures elsewhere, including an earlier age of onset, an (at least partially) hereditary basis, lack of fluffy periosteal reaction, and persistence of the defect through time. Spondylolysis generally affects about 5% of the population, although its incidence is higher in some groups, including some identifiable genetic cohorts (e.g., Inuits) and individuals with Scheuermann's disease (see Chapter 2) (Rossi 1978). Many athletic activities increase the risk of developing spondylolysis, including not only lifting weights but also playing American football (particularly as a lineman),

gymnastics, javelin throwing, and pole vaulting (Grobler 1997, Rossi 1978). Indeed, any activity producing prolonged or forced extension of the lower back may place an adolescent at risk for the development of spondylolysis, although the process need not necessarily be painful. Most defects occur in the L5 (approximately 80%) or the L4 (approximately 10%) pars, but locations throughout the lumbar spine may be seen. Spondylolysis has also been reported in the cervical spine, although this is almost always associated with dysplastic changes of the posterior elements and may occur via a different mechanism than lumbar spondylolysis (Redla 1999).

Imaging

Spondylolysis may be evaluated with plain films, nuclear medicine, computed tomography (CT), or magnetic resonance imaging (MRI) (Table 8–2). Fluoroscopically directed injections of pars defects and/or the adjacent facet joints may also be performed. Plain film tomography, although of historic interest, is inferior in many ways to thin-cut CT with reconstructions and also results in much higher radiation exposure. The choice of imaging modality depends on the clinical scenario (see later).

PLAIN FILMS

When performing plain films for evaluation of pars defects, either oblique films or flexion/extension laterals or both should be included as part of the examination. Some pars defects may be difficult to see, even on oblique radiographs, and plain films will not be able to assess important collateral pathology such as foraminal stenosis and disc herniation. Plain films are the method of choice if serial follow-up studies of a known spondylolisthesis are necessary: a standard technique is generally reproducible and assessment of progression of spondylolisthesis may be made relatively inexpensively.

NUCLEAR MEDICINE

Nuclear medicine is widely used for both detecting spondylolysis and in assessing its "activity." It is generally held that a positive bone scan with negative plain films indicates a "subradiologic" stage of disease that may progress unless

TABLE 8-1. Types of Spondylolisthesis

Type	Description
I	Congenital or dysplastic
II	Isthmic
III	Degenerative
IV	Post-traumatic
V	Pathologic
VI	Postsurgical

Grobler 1997.

TABLE 8-2. Imaging Findings of Spondylolysis

Finding	Differential Diagnosis
CT	
Interruption of the pars cortex	Spondylolysis Volume averaging Facet joint, especially on axial studies Facet arthropathy
MRI	
Interruption of the pars cortex	Spondylolysis Volume averaging Facet joint, especially on axial studies Facet arthropathy
Abnormal signal intensity of the pedicle or pars	Spondylolysis Volume averaging Normal variant with fat-containing marrow
Increased AP diameter of the central canal	Spondylolysis Hypoplasia of posterior elements Segmentation anomaly
Bone scan	

Increased uptake in the region of the pars	Bilateral:
	  Spondylolysis
	  Facet arthropathy
	Unilateral
	  Spondylolysis
	  Facet fracture
	  Osteoid osteoma

AP, anteroposterior.

treated, whereas a negative bone scan with an obvious pars defect on plain films indicates an old (and presumably asymptomatic) lesion (Elliott 1988, Lowe 1984). Planar images may be falsely negative, and single photon emission CT (SPECT) images are routinely employed in those cases where spondylolysis is suspected (Harvey 1998). Raby and Mathews (1993) found that having a positive SPECT study predicted a successful surgical outcome and that, conversely, those patients who did not have a positive SPECT study did not fare as well.

COMPUTED TOMOGRAPHY

In many published studies, computed tomography forms the reference standard for the diagnosis of spondylolysis. In addition, before the advent of MRI, CT was in a unique position to diagnose collateral pathology associated with spondylolysis (Grogan 1982, McAfee 1982). Newer, faster scanners with increased tube heat capacity may obtain thin (1-mm) cuts through the area of the pars in the lumbar spine. This technique allows high-quality sagittal and coronal reconstructions, which may be useful in optimal visualization of the spondylolysis: the pars, at least in some patients, is oblique to all three standard anatomic planes (Johnson 1989, Harvey 1998). Whether 1-mm cuts or 3-mm cuts at 2-mm intervals are used for evaluation, all images should be obtained in a contiguous fashion, because "gaps" in the scan may miss the pathology (Major 1999, Ulmer 1997). We perform all scans with contiguous, nonangled slices that allow for optimal reconstructions and easier interpretation of collateral pathology.

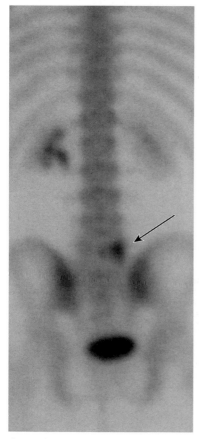
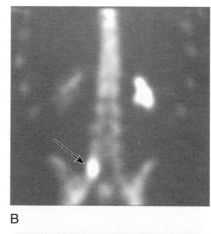
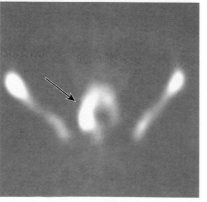

FIGURE 8–1

Nuclear medicine and CT study of pars defects. A 17-year-old patient with low back and left leg pain. *A,* Posterior bone scan with increased radiotracer localization on the right at the L5 pars level (*arrow*). *B,* Coronal SPECT image demonstrates increased radiotracer localization along the right pars defect (*arrow*). No abnormal activity is seen on the left side. *C,* Axial SPECT image also demonstrates increased radiotracer localization along the right pars (*arrow*), again without corresponding abnormality on the left side.

A

B

C

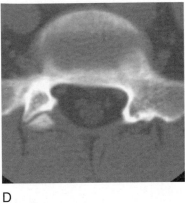

D

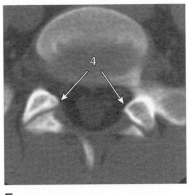

E

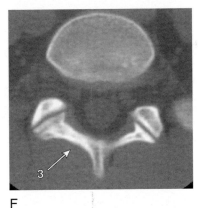

F

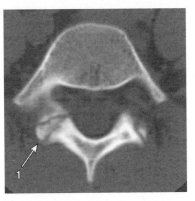

G

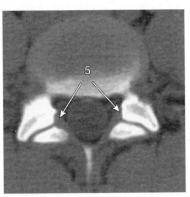

H

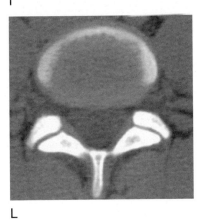

I

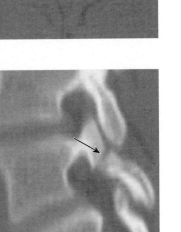

J

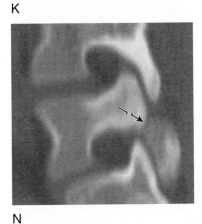

K

L

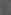

M

N

FIGURE 8–1 (*continued*)

D–L, Selected (every other) sequential 3-mm CT scans from the S1 pedicle through the L4–5 disc demonstrate bilateral pars defects (*arrow 1*). The left-sided defect demonstrates no definite osseous union. The right-sided defect demonstrates fragmentation. Note the marked sclerosis of the right pedicle and pars (*arrow 2*), corresponding to increased activity on the bone scan. Also note the asymmetry of the laminae of L5 below the level of the defect, with a thicker right (*arrow 3*) than left lamina. The pars defects are in a more coronal plane than the L5–S1 facet joints (*arrow 4*) but in approximately the same plane as the L4–5 facet joints (*arrow 5*). The pars demonstrate an undulate margin without cortication, whereas the facet joint margins are smoother and corticated. The pars defects are in the same plane as the transverse processes (*6*), whereas the facet joints lie superior and inferior to these structures. *M* and *N*, Sagittal reconstructions through the right and left pars demonstrate bilateral pars defects seen in the sagittal plane (*arrows*).

MAGNETIC RESONANCE IMAGING

A routine MR examination of the lumbar spine with 3- to 4-mm axial and sagittal T1-weighted images (T1WIs) and T2WIs provides sufficient information for the diagnosis of spondylolysis in most instances (Udeshi 1999). Note that if slice thickness is set at 5 mm, the likelihood of correct diagnosis diminishes (Campbell 1999). The increased spatial resolution available with 512 × 512-image matrix size improves visualization of subtle pars defects. As with CT examination, gaps in the MR scan are unacceptable: angling the axial cuts to the level of the disc and excluding the plane through the mid vertebral body (and pars) from imaging results in false-negative studies. As noted earlier, the pars interarticularis is often oblique to all three standard anatomic planes, and having both axial and sagittal images is critical for diagnosis (Campbell 1999). Jinkins and Rauch (1994) have noted that MRI can directly show neural impingement in spondylolysis, providing an advantage over other imaging modalities. Supporting the role of MR in the evaluation of spondylolysis, Duprez and colleagues (1999) noted that in one complex case with a retrodural cyst, all the information from plain film radiography, myelography, and facet arthrography was obtained on a routine, unenhanced MR examination.

Findings

COMPUTED TOMOGRAPHIC FINDING: INTERRUPTION OF THE PARS CORTEX

Since spondylolysis is, by definition, interruption of the pars interarticularis, direct imaging of the interruption of the cortical margins of the pars is the sine qua non of spondylolysis (Grenier 1989) (Figs. 8–1 to 8–5). Imaging features allowing differentiation between pars defects, and the zygapophyseal (facet) joints may be more easily appreciated on CT than on MRI (St. Amour 1994). In many cases, the defects are obvious and unequivocal, with little debate possible about the diagnosis. However, some pars defects may demonstrate equivocal imaging findings and may be difficult to identify. In the axial plane, it may be difficult to differentiate pars defects from normal or abnormal facet joints. Useful differentiating features include the following (Figs. 8–1, 8–2, 8–4, and 8–6) (Grogan 1982):

1. The transverse processes usually lies in the same plane as the pars defects, whereas the facets will be located either above or below the level of the transverse processes.
2. Pars defects often lie in the coronal plane, whereas facet joints are usually oblique.
3. Pars defects are generally straighter whereas facet joints curve at the margins.
4. Pars defects have irregular, jagged edges, often without a well-defined cortical margin, whereas facet joints have smooth margins with a generally well-defined cortical edge.

In addition, the facet joints are usually seen on several adjacent 3-mm images, and any pars defect large enough to be seen on several adjacent images is usually easy to identify on sagittal reconstruction images. Note, however, that volume averaging on sagittal reconstructions may give the appearance of a gap in the pars interarticularis when there is none.

Some patients may have unilateral spondylolysis with an abnormal contralateral pars that may be thickened and sclerotic (Fig. 8–7). These changes presumably result from a prior bony defect that has undergone healing (Grogan 1982, Guillodo 2000). In addition, a pars defect on one side may be accompanied by any of several defects on the contralateral side involving the pedicle, pars, or lamina (Rothman 1984, Akari 1992, Garber 1996) (Fig. 8–8).

MAGNETIC RESONANCE FINDINGS

INTERRUPTION OF THE PARS CORTEX

Visualization of the pars defect on MRI may be considerably more difficult than on CT examination: both the small size of the cortical interruption of some pars defects and the signal characteristics of cortical bone may make it difficult to appreciate cortical interruption (Figs. 8–3 and 8–8). In addition, the pars may not lie entirely in one sagittal slice, and volume averaging through adjacent fat in the sagittal plane leads to apparent discontinuity of the pars cortex, even when there is none (Fig. 8–3). In most normal pars, careful evaluation of all sagittal images will reveal that at least one sagittal image with an intact lower cortical margin is continuous from the undersurface of the pedicle to the articular margin of the inferior articular process.

ABNORMAL SIGNAL INTENSITY OF THE PEDICLE OR PARS

St. Amour (1994), Yamane (1993), and Ulmer (1997) and their coworkers all have noted reactive marrow not only in the pars interarticularis but also within the adjacent pedicle in patients with spondylolysis (Figs. 8–4 and 8–5). Such abnormal marrow may be present *prior* to frank cortical interruption of the pars as seen on CT scans (Yamane 1993) and thus represent a "stress reaction" rather than a full-blown "stress fracture." Ulmer and associates (1997) liken the abnormal signal intensity to the subchondral marrow changes Modic and colleagues (1988) described in degenerative disc disease. They note that the marrow of the pars and adjacent pedicles may demonstrate imaging characteristics of fibrovascular tissue or "Type I" change (T1 and T2 prolongation) (Figs. 8–4 and 8–5), fat or "Type II" change (T1 shortening and T2 prolongation) (Fig. 8–9), or sclerotic bone or "Type III" change (T1 prolongation and T2 shortening) (Fig. 8–10). As with visualization of cortical interruption of the pars interarticularis, volume averaging may give the false impression of abnormal signal intensity within the pars or pedicle: in one study, almost 25% of patients *without* spondylolisthesis did *not* demonstrate continuous marrow through the L4/5 level (Campbell 1999), although it should be noted that this study was performed with 5-mm-slice thickness, and thinner slices result in more consistent visualization of intact marrow fat (Udeshi 1999).

Ulmer and coworkers (1995a) found fatty change within the pars and pedicle the most common finding in patients with known spondylolysis. Some patients, however, appear to have fatty change at one or more levels as a

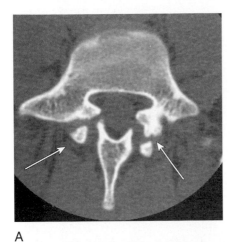

A

FIGURE 8–2

CT with interruption of the pars cortex. A 26-year-old man with central low back pain. *A,* CT 1-mm slice at the L5 pedicle level shows bilateral pars defects with fragmentation along the pars margins *(arrows)*. *B–G,* Sequential curved coronal CT reconstruction images from anterior (pedicle) *(1)* to posterior (lamina) *(arrows 2)* demonstrate the bilateral L5 pars defects *(arrow 3)* between the inferior and superior L5 articular processes.

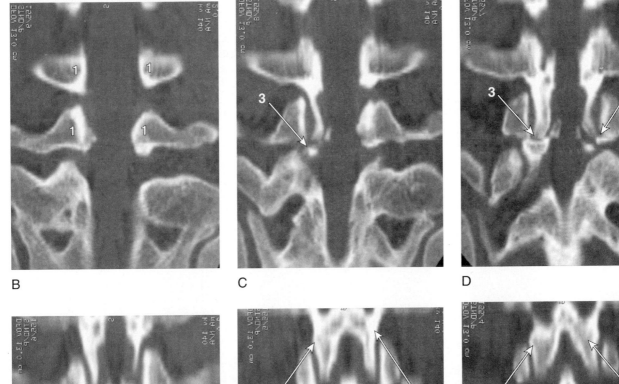

B

C

D

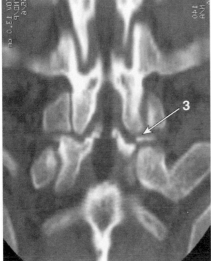

E

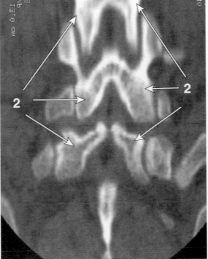

F

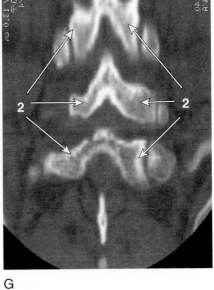

G

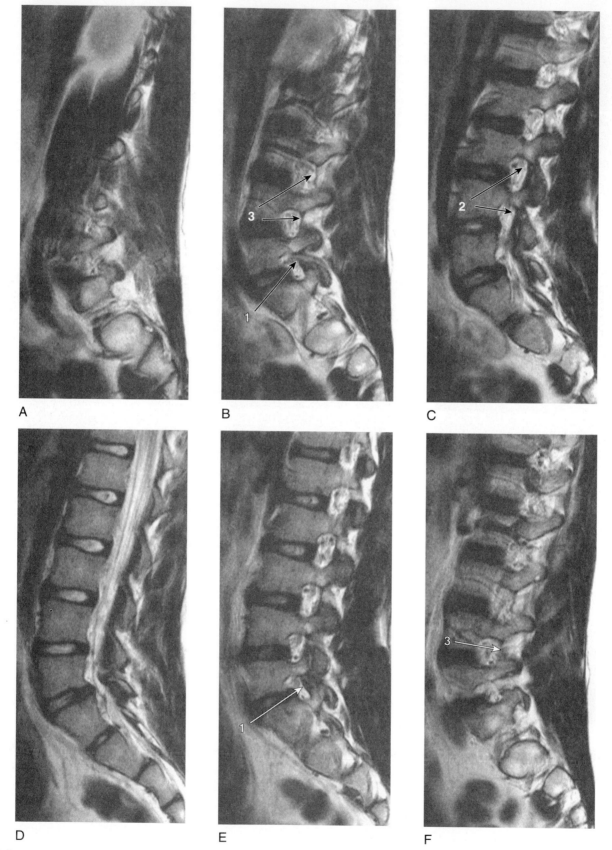

FIGURE 8–3

CT and MRI with interruption of the pars cortex. A 10-year-old girl with 9 months of central low back pain. *A–C (right)* and *D–F (left)*, Sequential sagittal T2WIs from the right to the left side fail to show any definite continuous marrow through the L5 pars *(arrow 1)*, despite the fact that continuous marrow is visualized through the L4 and L3 pars *(arrow 2)*. Note that cuts just lateral to the level of the pars may give the appearance of pars discontinuity *(arrow 3)*, even at those levels where the pars are intact. There is no dramatic spondylolisthesis or pedicle marrow signal intensity abnormality.

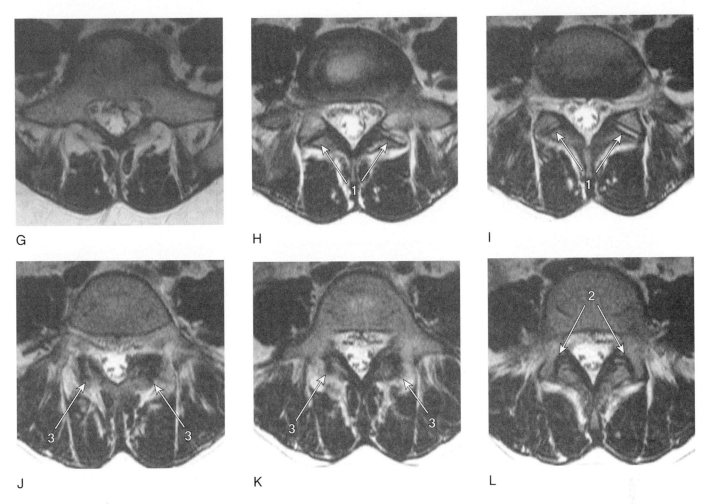

FIGURE 8–3 (*continued*)

G–L, Sequential axial T2WI from the S1 through the L5 pedicle shows the L5–S1 facet joints below (*arrow 1*), and the L4–5 facet joints above (*arrow 2*), the bilateral pars defects (*arrow 3*). More fibroproliferative change accompanies the left defect compared to the right. (*continued*)

normal variant, and isolated fatty change within the pedicle or pars may not indicate spondylolysis if no other imaging features are evident (Fig. 8–11). Clinically, the most important finding is probably fibrovascular or Modic Type I change, which is consistent with early injury and an active, reparative process (Ulmer 1995a).

INCREASED ANTEROPOSTERIOR DIAMETER OF THE CENTRAL CANAL

Sener and colleagues (1991) first noted that patients with spondylolysis may have an abnormally wide central spinal canal at the level of the pars defect, even without associated spondylolisthesis. Using the ratio of the central spinal canal dimension at the level of the slip (usually L5) and L1 with a cutoff value of 1.25, Ulmer and coworkers (1994) were able to differentiate between isthmic and degenerative spondylolisthesis with 100% accuracy. This finding is positive in a surprisingly large number of patients with little or no spondylolisthesis, being seen in more than 75% of such patients (Ulmer 1995b). The increased diameter of the central spinal canal without spondylolisthesis apparently results from posterior displacement of the posterior ele-

ments preceding anterior displacement of the anterior elements. In equivocal cases, this ancillary finding may be helpful in drawing attention to the possibility of an abnormal pars and in lending certainty to the diagnosis of pars defects (Figs. 8–3, 8–10, and 8–12).

BONE SCAN FINDING: ABNORMAL INCREASED UPTAKE IN THE PARS REGION

Increased uptake in the pars region of a bone scan is consistent with spondylolysis (Figs. 8–1 and 8–5). SPECT studies are more sensitive to imaging of early and subtle abnormalities than is planar imaging (Fig. 8–13), allowing early identification of cases with prevention of progression (Harvey 1998). The finding of a positive bone scan is probably the equivalent of seeing fibrovascular change (T1 and T2 prolongation) within the pedicles and pars on MRI. Nuclear medicine in spondylolysis (as with other lesions) is nonspecific, and anything resulting in increased turnover of bone in the posterior elements or facets may result in similar bone scan findings, including facet arthropathy, osteoid osteoma, infection, and fracture.

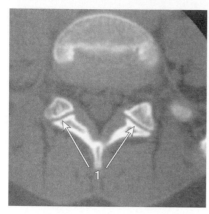

M

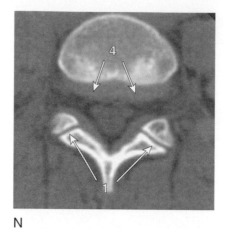

N

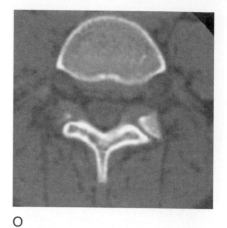

O

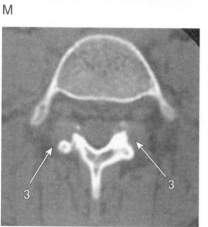

P

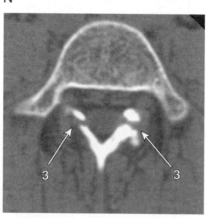

Q

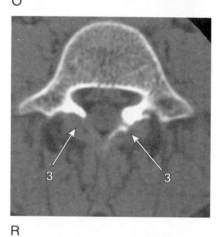

R

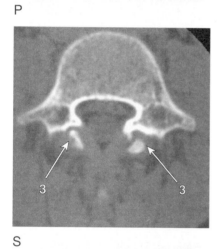

S

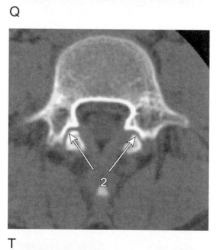

T

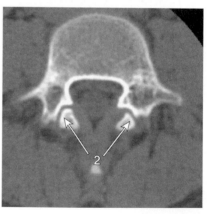

U

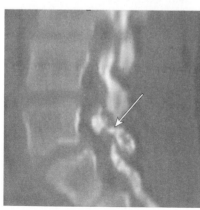

V

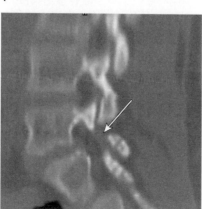

W

FIGURE 8–3 (continued)

M–U, Sequential selected (every third) 1-mm slices from the L5–S1 through the L4–5 facet joints demonstrates the L5–S1 facets below (arrow 1) and the L4–5 facets above (arrow 2) the bilateral pars defects (arrow 3) with a paucity of bony reactive change. Note the pseudodisc appearance secondary to volume averaging (arrow 4). V, Parasagittal right CT reconstruction again demonstrates the pars defect at the L5 level with a paucity of bone formation (arrow). W, Parasagittal left CT reconstruction demonstrates a defect on the left side as well (arrow).

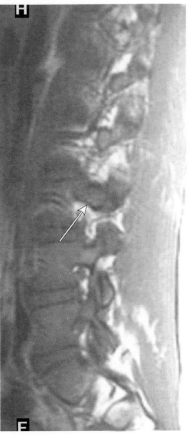

A

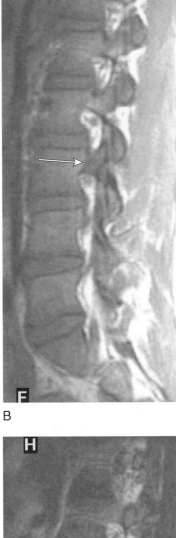

B

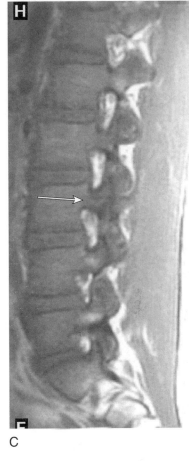

C

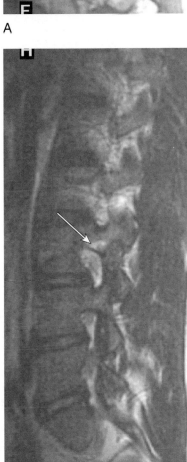

D

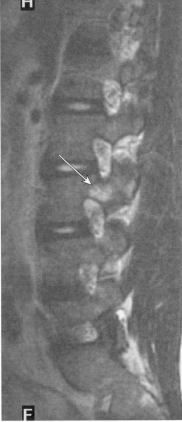

E

FIGURE 8–4

CT and MRI with interruption of the pars cortex. A 13-year-old girl with low back and bilateral thigh pain. *A* and *B*, Sequential right parasagittal T1WI show T1 prolongation at the L3 pedicle level *(arrow)*. *C*, Left parasagittal T1WI shows similar T1 prolongation at the L3 pedicle level *(arrow)*. Compare with more normal appearing marrow above and below the L3 level. *D*, Right parasagittal T2WI shows T2 prolongation in the left L3 pedicle. *E*, Left parasagittal T2WI shows T2 prolongation within the left L3 pedicle.

(continued)

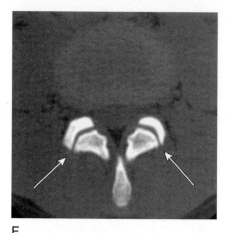

F

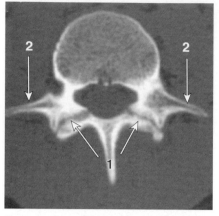

G

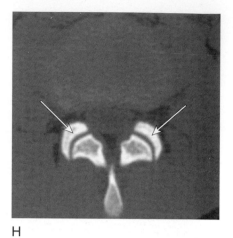

H

I

J

FIGURE 8–4 (continued)

F, Axial 1-mm CT slice through the L3–4 facet joints demonstrates a normal appearance (arrows). G, Axial 1-mm CT slice at the level of the L3 pars demonstrates bilateral pars defects (arrow 1). Note that the pars defects are at the level of the transverse processes (arrow 2). H, Axial 1-mm CT slice above the level of the pars at the L2–3 facet joints demonstrates a normal appearance (arrows). I, Right parasagittal reconstruction CT demonstrates the right L3 pars defect (arrow). J, Left parasagittal reconstruction CT demonstrates the left L3 pars defect (arrow).

Collateral Findings and Pathology

Many patients with spondylolysis have pain not only from spondylolysis but also (or exclusively) from accompanying collateral pathology (Grenier 1989, Grobler 1997, Szypryt 1989) (Table 8–3). This pathology more often manifests later in life: painful spondylolysis is usually seen in adolescents or young adults, whereas the collateral pathology frequently becomes symptomatic only during the middle or later years of life. The following sections are a brief discussion of entities that may be associated with spondylolysis, many of which we discuss at greater length elsewhere in the text.

POSTERIOR BONE AND JOINT ABNORMALITIES

The posterior elements below the level of the pars defects may show hypoplasia of the facet joints or laminae, asymmetry of the laminae, an off-center position of the spinous process, or a cleft within the posterior bony arch (Rothman 1984) (Figs. 8–1, 8–6 to 8–8, 8–12, and 8–14). Although some of these findings are clearly dysplastic (Figs. 8–7 and 8–14) and would place associated spondylolisthesis in the Wiltse Type I (dysplastic) category, others (including hypoplasia of the facets) may be cause or effect. It is not clear whether small facets result in abnormal stress, which

TABLE 8-3. Collateral Findings/Pathology with Spondylolysis

Posterior bone and joint abnormalities
Proliferative changes along the pars
Retrodural cysts
Spondylolisthesis
Foraminal stenosis
Disc herniation
Internal disc disruption

in turn causes spondylolysis, or if spondylolysis "unloads" facet joints inferior to the level of the spondylolysis and results in hypoplasia (Grobler 1993, Grobler 1997).

PROLIFERATIVE CHANGES ALONG THE PARS DEFECTS

Many times the reparative process along the pars defects is more conspicuous than the lytic defect itself, making the diagnosis (particularly on axial MR examinations) much more obvious (Figs. 8–3 and 8–10). Extensive fibroproliferative changes may lead to significant nerve root displacement, impingement, and radicular symptoms (Major 1999), even without accompanying foraminal stenosis from spondylolisthesis (see later). On axial CT images, a bony fragment or "spur" may appear to project off the antero-

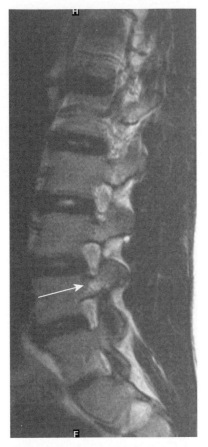

A

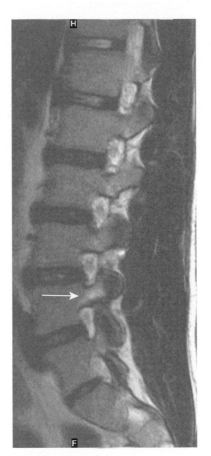

B

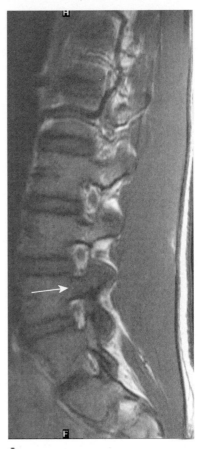

C

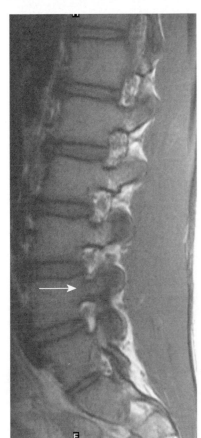

D

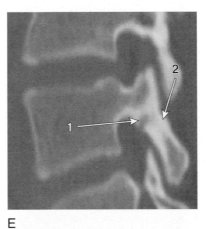

E

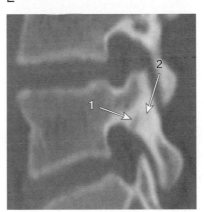

F

FIGURE 8–5

CT with incomplete interruption of the pars. A 16-year-old boy with central low back pain. Parasagittal T2WI at the level of the right (A) and left (B) pedicles shows T2 prolongation within the L4 pedicles (*arrows*). Parasagittal T1WI at the level of the right (C) and left (D) shows T1 prolongation in the same pedicles. E, Right parasagittal CT reconstruction also shows a lucency along the undersurface of the pars (*arrow 1*) with accompanying sclerosis (*arrow 2*). F, Left parasagittal CT reconstruction shows similar findings on the left side (*arrows 1 and 2*). In this patient, there were bilateral Type I pedicle signal intensity changes, with a history of recent onset of pain. The CT findings are more consistent with a chronic (and healing process). A bone scan (not shown) demonstrated unilateral uptake on the left side only.

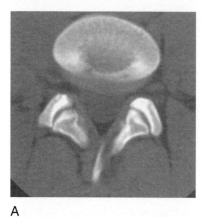

A

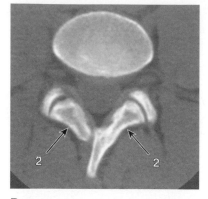

B

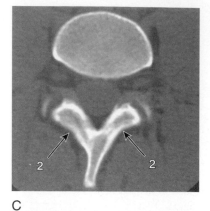

C

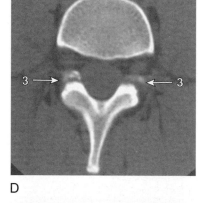

D

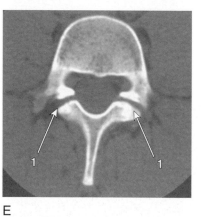

E

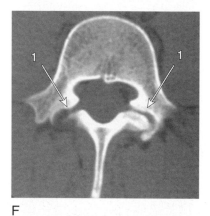

F

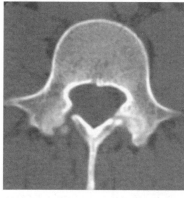

G

H

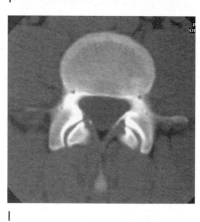

I

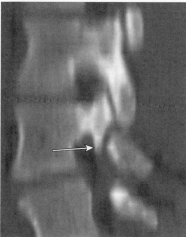

J

FIGURE 8–6

CT showing pars defects mimicking facet joints. A 22-year-old patient with central low back pain. *A–I,* Sequential 3-mm axial CT images from the L4–5 to the L3–4 facet joints demonstrate bilateral L4 pars defects *(arrow 1).* The pars defects in this case show curvature that resembles the typical appearance of facet joints, but the pars defects are slightly wider and in a somewhat more coronal plane than the facet joints above and below. Note the mild asymmetry of the posterior elements below the pars defects *(arrow 2),* and a "spur" projecting off of the inferior aspect of the pars defects *(arrow 3). J,* Left parasagittal CT reconstruction demonstrates the spur projecting from the inferior aspect of the superior portion of the pars *(arrow).*

inferior aspect of the pars defect into the spinal canal (Teplick 1986) (Fig. 8–6). MR examinations usually demonstrate the full extent of the soft tissue abnormality along the pars defects better than CT.

RETRODURAL CYSTS

One of the curious features of spondylolysis defects is their tendency to communicate with adjacent facet joints (Ghelman 1978). On occasion, injection into one of bilateral defects results in not only opacification of ipsilateral facet joints but communication across the midline posteriorly into the contralateral defect and/or facet joints (Maldague 1981). This space must lie posterior to not only the dura but also the peridural membrane described by Wiltse and associates (1993), because a needle passed from posterior enters this space prior to entering the epidural space. If this space becomes expanded with fluid, the resulting retrodural cysts may cause spinal canal stenosis and nerve root impingement (Duprez 1999) (Fig. 8–15).

SPONDYLOLISTHESIS

Wiltse's classification system (Table 8–1) provides a relatively extensive list of the causes of spondylolisthesis. In practice, most cases of spondylolisthesis are either dysplastic/lytic (often difficult to distinguish, as noted earlier) or degenerative. Minor degrees (<25%, or Grade I) of spondylolisthesis may be present in either dysplastic/lytic or degenerative spondylolisthesis. Helpful differentiating features include the following:

1. Most lytic spondylolisthesis occurs at L5/S1, whereas most degenerative spondylolisthesis occurs at L4/5.
2. Lytic spondylolisthesis is more likely to be evaluated in adolescence, whereas degenerative spondylolisthesis is a disease of predominantly the elderly.
3. Lytic spondylolisthesis has a wide central spinal canal, whereas degenerative spondylolisthesis has a narrowed central spinal canal (Ulmer 1994).
4. Lytic spondylolisthesis frequently shows hypoplasia of the facets below the level of the slip, whereas degenera-

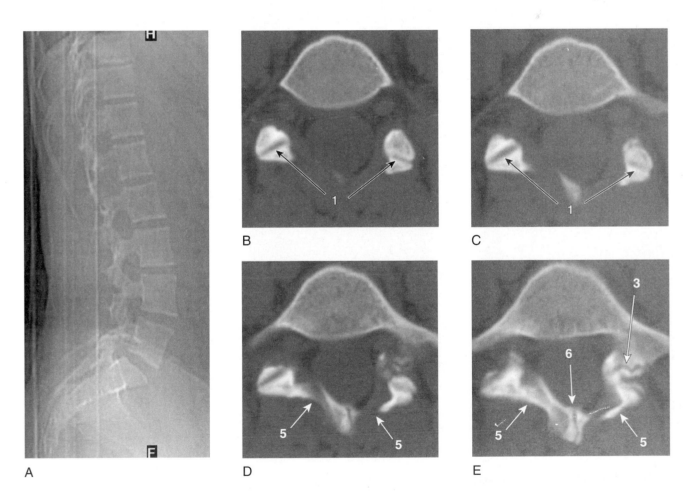

FIGURE 8–7

Pars defect on one side with a contralateral thickened and sclerotic pars. A 19-year-old woman with central low back pain. *A,* Sagittal scout radiograph from CT study demonstrates no spondylolisthesis. *B–M,* Sequential axial 3-mm CT slices from the L5–S1 facet joints (*arrow 1*) to the L4–5 (*arrow 2*) facet joints show a left pars defect with sclerosis along the margins (*arrow 3*) consistent with a chronic process. There is also sclerosis and thickening of the right pars (*arrow 4*), consistent with a possible healed defect on the right side. Note the more coronal orientation of the pars defect compared to the facet joints above and below the level of the defect. There is considerable asymmetry of the laminae below the level of the pars defect (*arrow 5*), along with failure of complete ossification of the posterior ring with a central lucency in the spinous process (*arrow 6*). The L5–S1 facet joints (*arrow 1*) are rudimentary.

(continued)

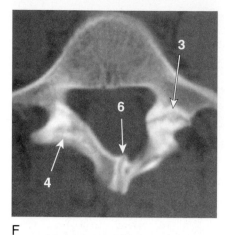

F

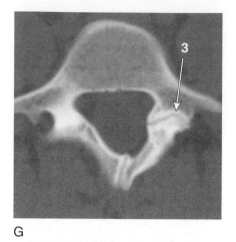

G

H

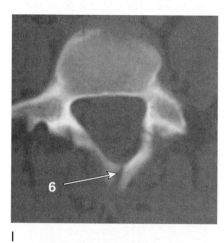

I

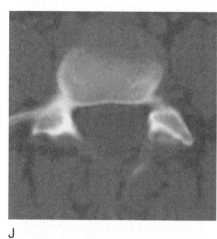

J

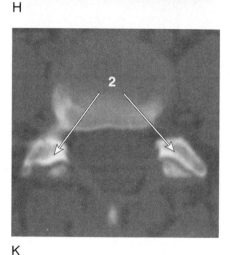

K

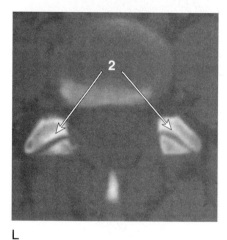

L

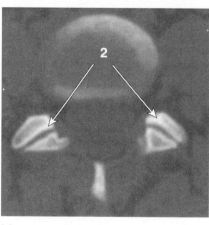

M

FIGURE 8–7   (continued)

tive spondylolisthesis is in large part secondary to facet arthropathy and is almost invariably associated with extensive productive changes along the facet joint margins.

Although these causes of spondylolisthesis are usually easily separated, there are occasions when it is difficult to differentiate the two or when both diseases coexist (Fig. 8–16).

When forward displacement of one vertebra on another exceeds 25%, there is almost always spondylolysis. Eventually, *spondyloptosis,* or complete displacement of

the superior on the inferior vertebral body, may result. At this extreme, there is rounding of the superior aspect of the lower vertebral anterosuperior border from subchondral bony and cartilaginous injury (Ikata 1996) (Fig. 8–17).

Although progression of spondylolisthesis was once thought to cease at skeletal maturity, Floman (2000) published a recent study documenting the progression of slip at L5/S1 because of disc deterioration in skeletally mature adults. This progression may result in the new onset of symptoms because of internal disc disruption or foraminal stenosis.

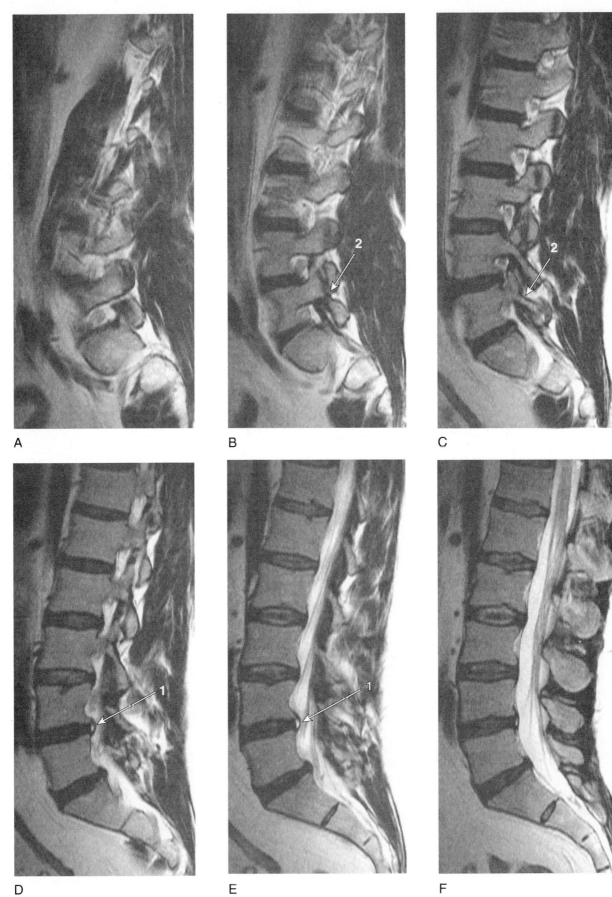

A

B

C

D

E

F

FIGURE 8–8   *See legend on page 321 (continued)*

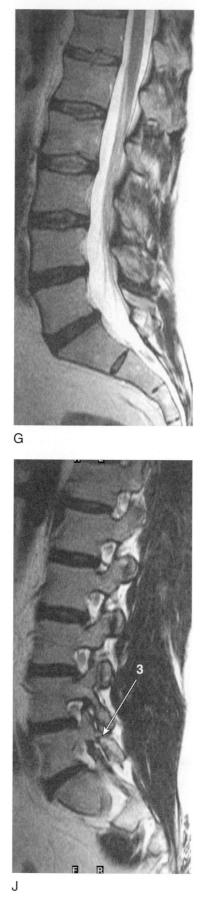

G

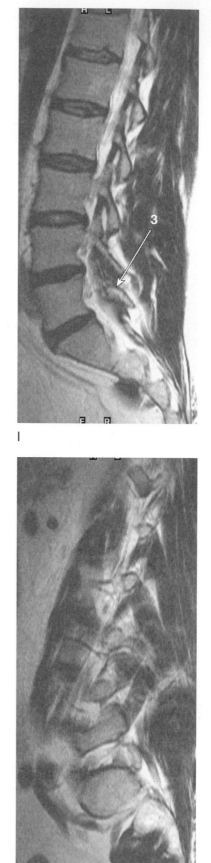

H

I

J

K

L

FIGURE 8–8 *(continued)*

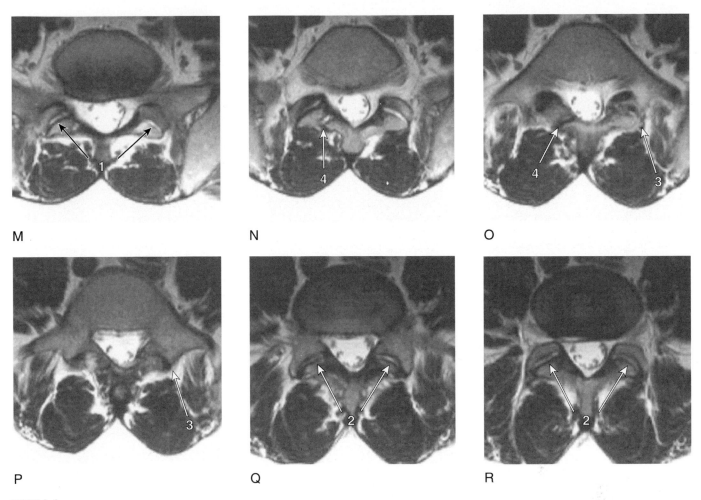

FIGURE 8–8

Pars defect with contralateral laminar defect (and additional degenerative disease). A 44-year-old patient with chronic central low back pain. *A–L,* Sequential right-to-left sagittal T2WIs demonstrate changes of Scheuermann's disease, including T12–L1 mild loss of disc height and hydration with Schmorl's node formation and vertebral marginal irregularity, L1–2 mild disc dehydration with vertebral marginal irregularity, L2–3 vertebral marginal irregularity, L3–4 mild loss of disc height and hydration with vertebral marginal irregularity, L4–5 mild loss of disc height and moderate disc dehydration with a 3-mm right central and subarticular disc protrusion (with associated T2 prolongation along the disc margin) *(arrow 1),* and L5–S1 mild loss of disc height with moderate disc dehydration and disc bulging. On the right side, the pars is intact *(arrow 2),* whereas on the left side there is discontinuity of marrow within the pars and no smooth cortical margin along the pars undersurface *(arrow 3).* No anteroposterior widening of the central canal at L5, spondylolisthesis, or abnormal signal intensity within the pedicle is identified. *M–R,* Sequential axial T2WIs from the L5–S1 facet joints *(arrow 1)* through the L4–5 facet joints *(arrow 2)* demonstrate a left pars defect *(arrow 3)* and a right laminar defect *(arrow 4). S–AA,* Selected (every third) sequential 1-mm CT slices from the L5–S1 facet joints *(arrow 1)* through the L4–5 facet joints *(arrow 2)* again show the left pars defect *(arrow 3)* and right laminar defect *(arrow 4).* There is also a pseudodisc from volume averaging through the L5–S1 disc *(arrow 5). BB–CC,* Right *(BB)* and left *(CC)* parasagittal CT reconstruction views demonstrate a right pars defect *(arrow 1)* but an intact left pars *(arrow 2).*

FORAMINAL STENOSIS

Foraminal stenosis with or without associated nerve root compression in spondylolysis may result from spondylolisthesis and direct bony encroachment between the posterosuperior corner of the lower vertebra and the pedicle of the upper vertebra (Jinkins 1994) (Fig. 8–18), abnormal soft tissue within the neural foramen that may result from annular redundancy on the side of the disc or callus on the side of the pars defect (Jinkins 1994, Major 1999), or disc herniation into the foramen (see later). Sagittal images (either direct with MR or reconstructed with CT) are of great benefit in evaluation of foraminal stenosis, because axial images may provide a misleading appearance when the foramina are "bilobed": the posterior component of the

foramen, containing only fat, may appear widely patent on axial images, whereas the anterior component that houses the stretched and compressed ganglion is quite narrow (Jinkins 1992, Jinkins 1994).

DISC HERNIATION

Disc herniation occurs more frequently above the level of the spondylolysis than below the level of the lysis (Figs. 8–10 and 8–12) and may be seen with surprising frequency: 6 of the 13 patients reported on by Grenier and coworkers (1989) in their early MRI study of spondylolysis had an accompanying disc herniation. The anteroposterior (AP) elongation of the central canal may result in less

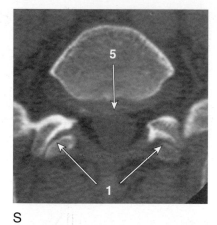

S

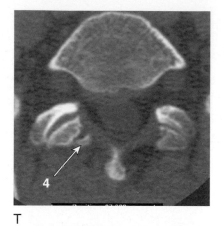

T

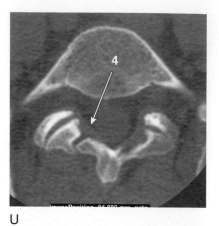

U

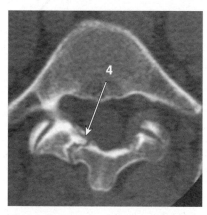

V

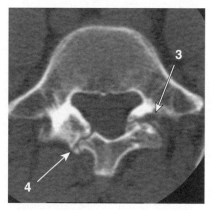

W

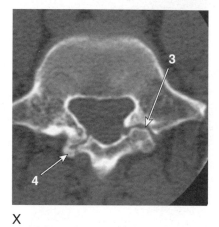

X

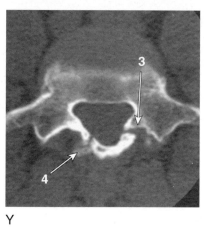

Y

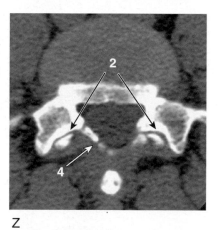

Z

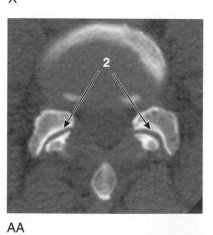

AA

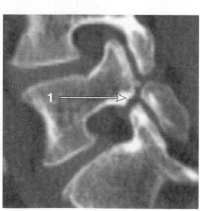

BB

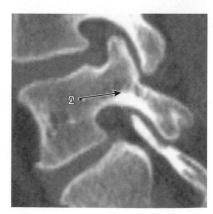

CC

FIGURE 8–8   (*continued*)

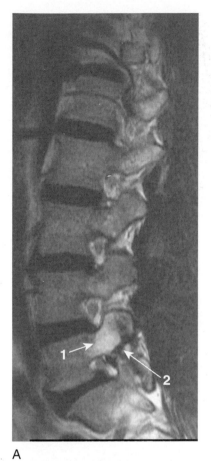

A

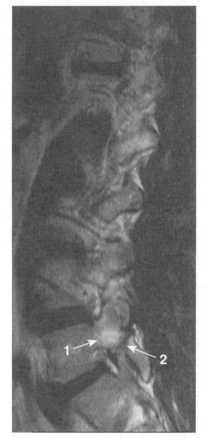

B

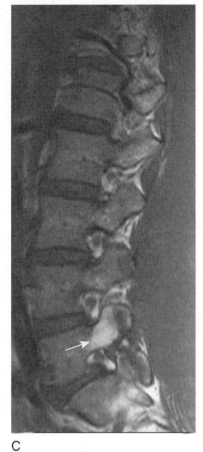

C

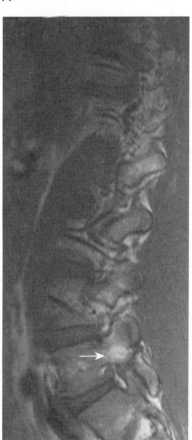

D

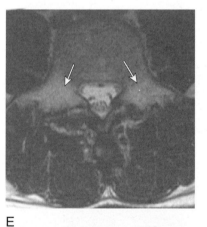

E

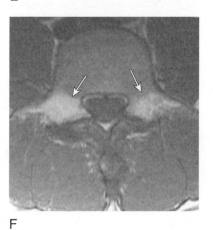

F

FIGURE 8–9

Pars defect with adjacent fatty marrow (Ulmer Type II). A 48-year-old man with low back and left leg pain. Sagittal T2WIs through the right (*A*) and left (*B*) pars demonstrates T2 prolongation within the pedicle (*arrow 1*). There are obvious pars defects (*arrow 2*) with T1 shortening along the margins consistent with sclerotic bone. Sagittal T1WIs through the right (*C*) and left (*D*) pars demonstrates T1 shortening within the pedicles (*arrows*). *E*, Axial T2WI demonstrates T2 prolongation of the pedicles and transverse processes at the L5 level (*arrows*). *F*, Axial T1WI demonstrates T1 shortening of the pedicles and transverse processes (*arrows*). The findings are those of fatty change of the pedicles bilaterally, consistent with a long-standing process.

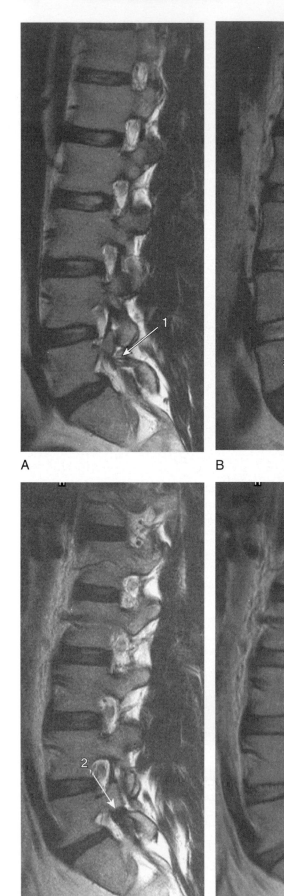

A

B

C

D

FIGURE 8–10

Pars defect with adjacent sclerosis (Ulmer Type III), with an increased central canal ratio. A 38-year-old man with central low back pain. Sagittal T2WIs through the right pars (A), central, spinal canal (B), and left pars (C) demonstrate bilateral L5 pars defects (arrow 1) with T2 shortening along the pars margins (arrow 2) (particularly on the left). There is also moderate L5–S1 disc dehydration and a 6-mm cranially dissecting disc extrusion (arrow 3). The L5:L1 central canal ratio on the midline image is 1.39 (exceeding the cutoff of 1.25 for diagnosing lytic spondylolisthesis). This ratio is calculated by dividing the anteroposterior (AP) canal diameter at L5 (double-headed arrow 4) by the diameter at L1 (double-headed arrow 5). Although somewhat easy to pass by because of the disc extrusion, there is minimal (approximately 5%) lytic spondylolisthesis of L5 on S1. D, Right parasagittal T1WI demonstrating T1 prolongation along the pars margins (arrow 1) (Ulmer Type III; see text).

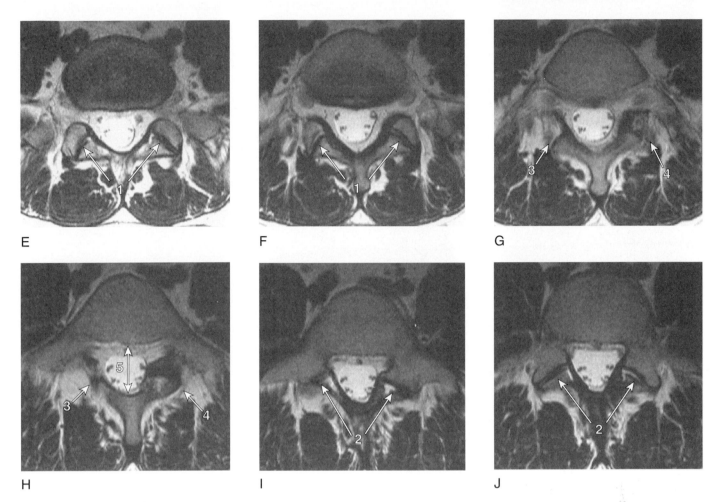

FIGURE 8–10 (*continued*)

E–J, Sequential axial T2WIs from the L5–S1 facet joints (*arrow 1*) through the L4–5 facet joints (*arrow 2*) demonstrate attenuation of the right pars (*arrow 3*) with slight bulbous thickening of the left pars (*arrow 4*), and AP elongation of the central canal (*double-headed arrow 5*).

neural compression than would otherwise be present in cases of central disc herniation below the level of a lytic defect (Figs. 8–12 and 8–19). Even without frank herniation, the disc margin at the level of spondylolisthesis may have a peculiar "squared-off" appearance along its posterior border. Part of this appearance may be secondary to volume averaging through the level of the slip, but the disc is occasionally unusually prominent through the vertebral foramina, which may represent annular redundancy and may be a cause of neural compression (see section, "Foraminal Stenosis") (Teplick 1986). When disc herniation occurs within the foramen below the level of the pars defect (at a level of spondylolisthesis), the herniation may exacerbate already existing stenosis of the foramen and lead to radicular pain (Fig. 8–20).

INTERNAL DISC DISRUPTION AND DISC DEGENERATION WITHOUT HERNIATION

Disc degeneration, as noted earlier, probably accounts for the progression of spondylolisthesis in the skeletally mature patient (Floman 2000). Disc degeneration is seen more frequently below the level of the spondylolysis (Dai 2000)

(Fig. 8–10) but may also be encountered above the level of the spondylolysis (Szypryt 1989) (Figs. 8–6 and 8–21). Indeed, some authorities advocate routine evaluation of the L4–5 disc by discography prior to surgery on adults with L5 spondylolysis because of the frequent coexistence of internal disruption at this level and the necessity of including this level in the fusion for successful results (Grobler 1997).

Clinical Scenarios

Most patients with lytic/dysplastic spondylolisthesis fall into one of two categories:

1. The patient is young, presents with low back pain (with or without radicular pain), and is suspected (on clinical grounds, including tight hamstring muscles) to have spondylolysis.
2. The patient is middle-aged or older, presents with low back pain (with or without radicular pain), and has spondylolysis on imaging.

In the former instance, the issue is usually to document the presence of spondylolysis and grade of spondylolisthesis,

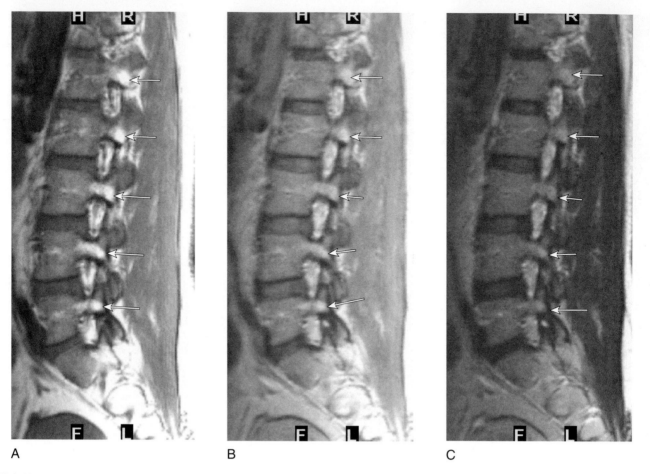

FIGURE 8–11

Fatty change within the pedicles as a normal variant. A 42-year-old woman with neck and back pain (an unremarkable cervical spine MRI was also obtained). *A,* Left parasagittal T1WI through the pedicles demonstrates multilevel T1 shortening (*arrows*). *B,* Left parasagittal proton density images through the pedicles demonstrates intermediate signal intensity within the pedicles (*arrows*). *C,* Left parasagittal T2WI through the pedicles demonstrates less signal intensity than on *A* and *B* (*arrows*). The patient had fat within the pedicles at multiple levels as a normal variant.

whereas in the latter it is to diagnose the actual cause of the patient's symptoms (which is usually *not* the patient's spondylolysis) (Grenier 1989, Grobler 1997, Szypryt 1989).

CLINICAL SCENARIO 1: THE PATIENT IS YOUNG, PRESENTS WITH LOW BACK PAIN, AND IS SUSPECTED TO HAVE SPONDYLOLYSIS

The pain diagrams offered by young patients with symptomatic spondylolysis demonstrate striking similarity (Fig. 8–22). Any young patient with pain in this pattern, particularly with a history of any of the known associated athletic risk factors (including, as noted earlier, weight lifting, gymnastics, javelin throwing, and pole vaulting) should be suspected of having spondylolysis. The absence of "red flags" in the clinical history (such as fever, weight loss, and night pain relieved by salicylates*) decreases the

likelihood of tumor and infection as causes of the pain (Waddell 1998). Plain films should be obtained and evaluated for the presence of pars defects and spondylolisthesis. If no radicular pain is present, conservative therapy is usually instituted based on the plain films findings. If alternate diagnoses need to be excluded, MRI is probably the best single test. Although a bone scan is usually positive in cases of spondylolysis, it may miss some instances (particularly without SPECT) and does not discriminate between the various causes of pain possible in these patients. We have yet to encounter a case wherein a high-quality MRI was negative and the patient was later shown to have spondylolysis, either by nuclear medicine, CT, or clinical follow-up studies.

The findings of spondylolysis may be quite subtle on MRI, and the interpreting physician must keep in mind that ancillary findings (including pedicle marrow signal intensity changes, a subtle bulbous appearance of the pars on axial images, and a slightly widened spinal canal) may be the only clue that spondylolysis is present (Figs. 8–3 to 8–5). If these findings are present in an adolescent with the appropriate pain diagram, the diagnosis of spondylolysis

*This may be unlikely nowadays: acetaminophen has replaced salicylates for treatment of pain in adolescents because of Reye's syndrome, and apparently acetaminophen does not have the same palliative effect in the treatment of osteoid osteoma.

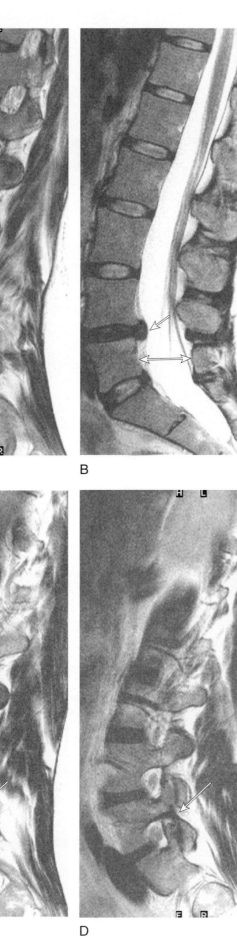

A

B

C

D

FIGURE 8–12

Increased central canal ratio in spondylolysis. A 27-year-old woman with central low back pain. *A,* Right parasagittal T2WI at the level of the pedicles demonstrates discontinuity of the pars *(arrow). B,* Sagittal T2WI shows moderate L4–5 disc dehydration as well as a 6.6-mm disc extrusion *(arrow).* Note anteroposterior (AP) widening of the central canal at L5 without spondylolisthesis *(double-headed arrow)* (L5:L1 ratio is 1.76 with a cutoff value of 1.25). *C* and *D,* Sequential left parasagittal T2WIs through the left pedicle demonstrates an intact left pars *(arrows).*

(continued)

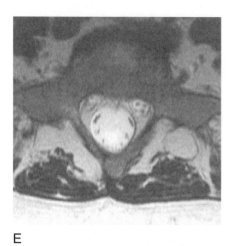

E

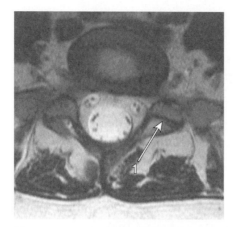

F

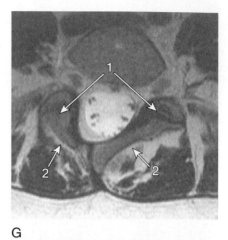

G

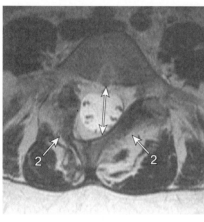

H

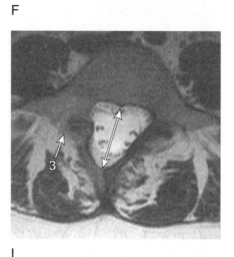

I

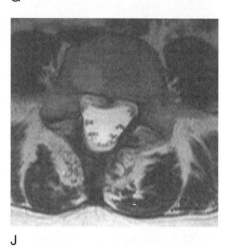

J

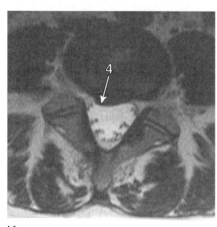

K

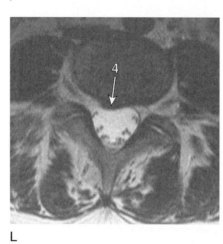

L

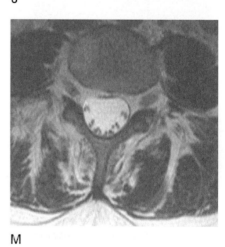

M

FIGURE 8–12 *(continued)*

E–M, Axial T2WIs from the L5–S1 facet joints *(arrow 1)* to the L4–5 disc demonstrate dysplasia of the posterior elements *(arrow 2),* AP widening of the central canal *(double-headed arrow),* right spondylolysis *(arrow 3),* and a right central disc extrusion *(arrow 4).* The disc extrusion produces no neural compression.

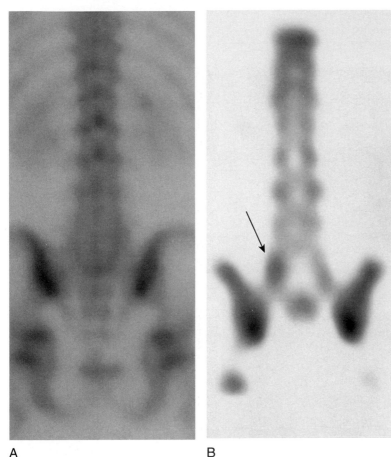

A

B

FIGURE 8–13

Pars defect with normal planar bone scan but positive SPECT study. A 13-year-old child with central low back pain. *A,* Planar bone scan that fails to reveal any focal abnormality of the lumbar spine. *B,* Coronal SPECT image demonstrates increased radiotracer activity within the right pars *(arrow).* SPECT studies are more sensitive in the detection of pars defects than are planar studies.

should be made, even in the absence of a definite gap within the pars or spondylolisthesis. In cases of radiculopathy, MR has the ability to diagnose the cause of neural impingement, including spinal canal, subarticular, and foraminal stenosis and disc herniation (Grenier 1989) and also fibroproliferative changes along the pars margins (Major 1999). MR is also able to evaluate not only the disc margin but also disc height and hydration, thus allowing the diagnosis of disc degeneration.

CT evaluation of pars abnormalities, particularly with 1-mm cuts through the level of the suspected pars and sagittal reconstructions, is much more easily interpreted than is MRI (Figs. 8–3 and 8–4). In addition, the degree of bony proliferation and healing may be directly assessed (Figs. 8–1 to 8–4). For many of the studies published in the literature, CT forms the reference standard. Note that prior to actual lysis of the pars, however, CT findings may be subtle or absent and consist only of equivocal "cystic lucencies" within the pedicle and pars. These cases are the equivalent of the stress reaction seen elsewhere in the skeleton and may be the most important not to miss, because treatment at this time may prevent progression to full-fledged spondylolysis (Harvey 1998).

Both CT and MR, as cross-sectional imaging studies, allow the differentiation of the much more frequently encountered open-arch lytic/dysplastic spondylolisthesis (Wiltse Type II) from the uncommon closed-arch dysplastic

spondylolisthesis (Wiltse Type I). As noted earlier, imaging findings in these two types overlap (Grobler 1993), but when dysplastic changes are *not* accompanied by AP elongation of the central canal, considerable neural compression may result, and this may alter the management strategy.

CLINICAL SCENARIO 2: THE PATIENT IS MIDDLE-AGED OR OLDER, PRESENTS WITH LOW BACK PAIN, AND HAS SPONDYLOLYSIS ON IMAGING

Because spondylolysis nearly always has its onset during adolescence, it has been stated to rarely, if ever, be the sole cause of back pain in patients older than 40 years of age (MacNab 1990). However, although spondylolysis is rarely the sole cause of back pain in patients older than 40, collateral pain-producing pathology may accompany spondylolysis. This collateral pathology may become symptomatic in middle age and beyond. As noted earlier, such collateral pathology includes the following:

1. Increased spondylolisthesis secondary to degenerative narrowing of the disc below the pars defect (Floman 2000). This may result in exacerbation of foraminal stenosis, not only because of further slippage of the upper on the lower level but also because of decreased disc height (furthering up-down stenosis) (Figs. 8–18 and 8–23).

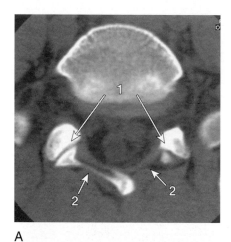
A

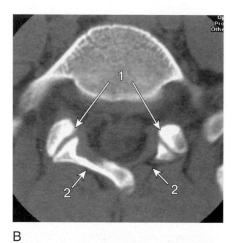
B

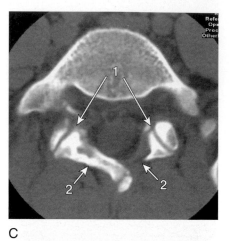
C

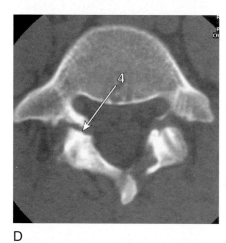
D

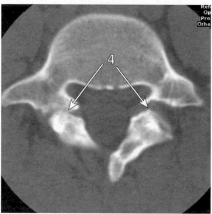
E

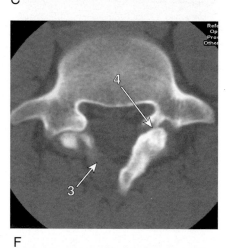
F

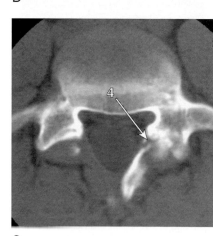
G

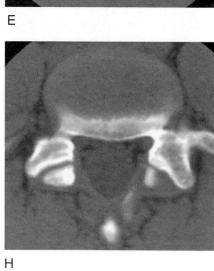
H

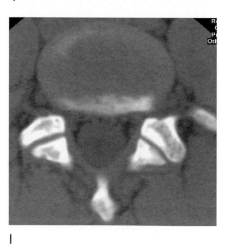
I

FIGURE 8–14

Pars defects with accompanying posterior element anomalies. A 24-year-old man with central low back pain. *A–I,* Sequential 3-mm axial CT images from the S1 through the L4–5 disc demonstrates hypoplasia of the facets *(arrow 1),* asymmetry of the laminae *(arrow 2),* and an osseous posterior cleft *(arrow 3)* below the level of the bilateral pars defects *(arrow 4).*

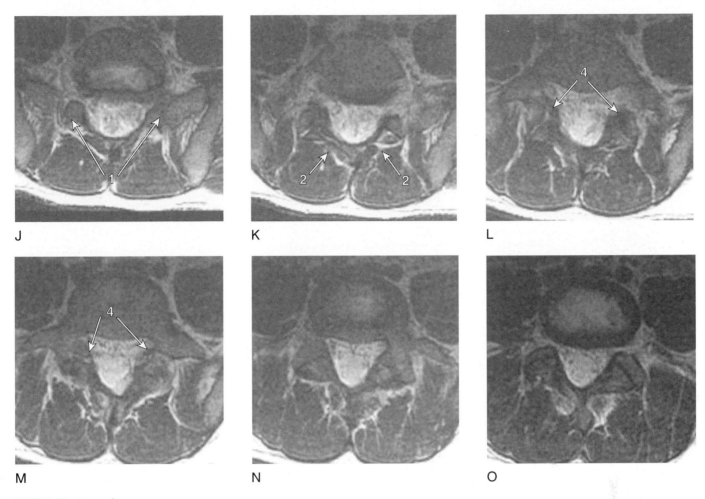

FIGURE 8–14 *(continued)*

J–O, Sequential T2WI (5-mm slices) demonstrate the same abnormalities, but it is much harder to appreciate them on this somewhat older scan with 256 × 256-image matrix size and 5-mm thick slices.

2. Disc herniation. This is more frequently seen above the level of the pars defect (Fig. 8–12) but may also occur below the level of the defect (Figs. 8–10, 8–19, and 8–24), or at both levels. As noted earlier, the increased AP canal diameter may protect the patient from neural compression from central disc herniations at the level of spondylolisthesis. Unfortunately, foraminal disc herniations are usually superimposed on foraminal stenosis and cause more impingement than would otherwise be the case (Fig. 8–20).

3. Internal disc disruption. Full-thickness annular fissures and accompanying disc dehydration and loss of height frequently coexist with spondylolysis, both below and above the level of the lysis (Figs. 8–6, 8–10, and 8–21). Grobler and Wiltse (1997) advocate evaluation of the level above the lysis with discography as part of surgical planning for possible inclusion in the fusion.

4. Proliferative changes associated with the pars defects.
   a. Fibroproliferative changes may cause radicular symptoms because of lateral recess or foraminal stenosis (Major 1999) (Fig. 8–25).
   b. Retrodural cysts may cause spinal canal stenosis. A posterior channel may connect the left and right pars

defects, and this channel may expand with fluid, resulting in spinal canal stenosis (Duprez 1999) (Fig. 8–15).

Of course, patients with spondylolysis may have unrelated pathology as well, with disc degeneration remote from the spondylolysis defects (Fig. 8–26), degenerative spondylolisthesis, spinal stenosis (Fig. 8–15), synovial cysts (Fig. 8–16), compression fracture (Fig. 8–27), or some other process causing low back pain with or without radiculopathy. For both the collateral pathology and for unrelated but still causative pathology resulting in low back pain with or without radiculopathy, MRI is the study of choice. It is the best single test to evaluate the many abnormalities that may cause such symptoms and may often supplant multiple other studies, particularly in difficult cases (Duprez 1999).

Reporting

MAGNETIC RESONANCE IMAGING

The MRI report in spondylolysis, as in reports on other processes, should contain a body and a conclusion. The

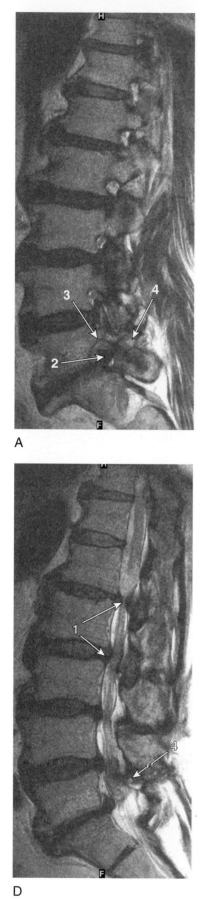

A

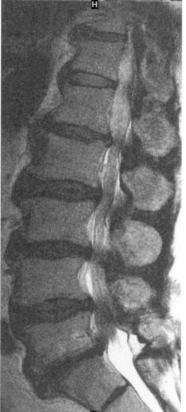

B

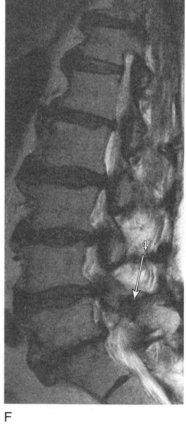

C

D

E

F

FIGURE 8–15   *See legend on opposite page*

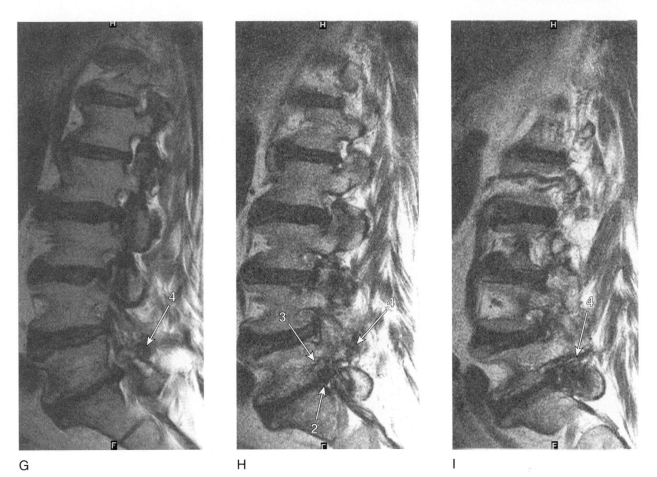

G   H   I

FIGURE 8–15

Pars defects with accompanying retrodural cysts. A 70-year-old woman with low back and left buttock pain. *A–I,* Sagittal T2WIs (right to left) demon-strate multiple degenerative findings with a similar appearance from L1–2 through L4–5, with disc dehydration and extensive degenerative disc bulging at all these levels that combine with facet arthropathy to cause severe spinal canal stenosis (worst at L1–2 and L2–3) (*arrow 1*). At the L5–S1 level, there is severe loss of disc height and hydration as well as a disc contour abnormality (best termed an *extrusion* given the appearance within the foramina) (*arrow 2*), associated with severe foraminal stenosis and compression of the exiting L5 ganglia (*arrow 3*). In addition to these extensive degenerative changes, there are bilateral L5 pars defects with fibroproliferative changes along the margins (*arrow 4*).   (*continued*)

body should contain a description of the examination results, whereas the conclusion should offer one or more diagnoses that may produce the described findings. When spondylolysis is obvious and no other diagnosis is consid-ered, however, the body of the report should simply state that the spondylolysis is present. There is a widely used grading system developed by Meyerding (1932). In this sys-tem, the superior margin of the sacrum is divided into four equal segments in the AP direction. The position of the pos-teroinferior corner of the upper vertebral body at the level of the slip is noted, and if in the posteriormost of the four quarters, a Grade I slip is present; if in the second quarters, a Grade II slip is noted, and so forth. If the upper vertebral body is completely dislocated over the lower, this is called *spondyloptosis.* As an alternative or addition to Meyerding's grading system, one may simply provide an explicit per-centage of slip (Wiltse 1983).

When spondylolysis is less obvious, the body should contain descriptive terminology. The report should note whether the pars cortical margin appears continuous or

not, the presence of changes of marrow signal intensity in the pars and adjacent pedicle, the presence of a thickened or otherwise abnormal appearance of the pars on axial views, and whether there is central canal widening. If the canal ratio described by Ulmer and colleagues (Ulmer 1994) is used, the cutoff for the diagnosis of spondylolysis is 1.25, but this value is not widely known and needs to be incorporated (along with the reference) in the report. Ancillary studies including CT scan (see later), nuclear medicine (see later), and diagnostic/therapeutic injection may be suggested.

Infiltration of the pars defect with anesthetic and steroid may not only provide pain relief but may also predict surgi-cal results: Suh and associates (1991) found that patients who responded to preoperative lidocaine injections had better pain relief, level of function, and likelihood of return to work than those who did not.

The report needs to explicitly mention the presence or absence of ancillary pathology. This includes mention of the disc status (height, hydration, and disc contour) and foram-

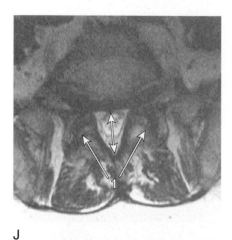

J

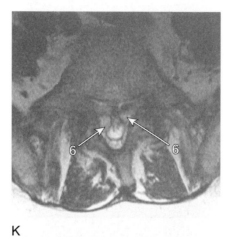

K

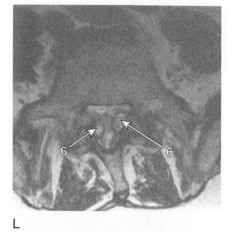

L

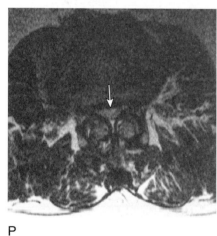

M

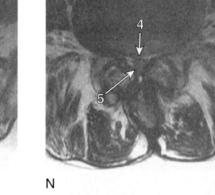

N

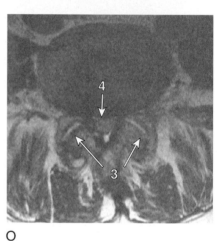

O

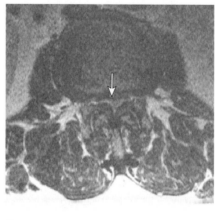

P

Q

FIGURE 8–15 (*continued*)

J–O, Sequential axial T2WI from the L5–S1 facets through the L4–5 disc show degenerative changes of the L5–S1 facet joints (*arrow 1*), anteroposterior elongation of the central canal (*double-headed arrow*), bilateral pars defects with fibroproliferative changes along the margins (*arrow 2*), and L4–5 severe facet arthropathy (*arrow 3*), disc bulging (*arrow 4*), and spinal canal stenosis (*arrow 5*). In addition, there are bilateral cysts projecting off the medial aspects of the pars defects narrowing the spinal canal (*arrow 6*). These lesions resemble synovial cysts but arise from the pars defects rather than the facet joints. *P* and *Q*, Axial T2WIs at L2–3 and L1–2 show severe spinal canal stenosis (*arrows*) at these levels from a combination of degenerative disc bulging and facet arthropathy.

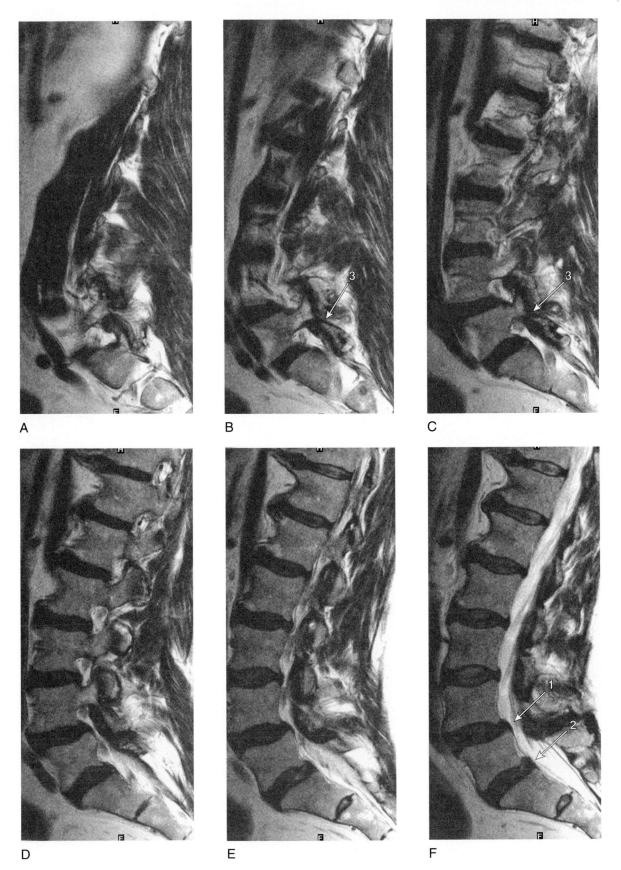

FIGURE 8–16

Combined lytic and degenerative spondylolisthesis. A 65-year-old woman with low back and left leg pain. *A–L*, Sequential sagittal T2WIs demonstrate multilevel degenerative changes, including T12–L1 through L3–4 mild disc dehydration and anterior osteophytic spurring and L4–5 and L5–S1 moderate disc dehydration. At L4–5, there is 20% degenerative spondylolisthesis (*arrow 1*) and at L5–S1 there is 15% lytic spondylolisthesis (*arrow 2*). There is

(continued)

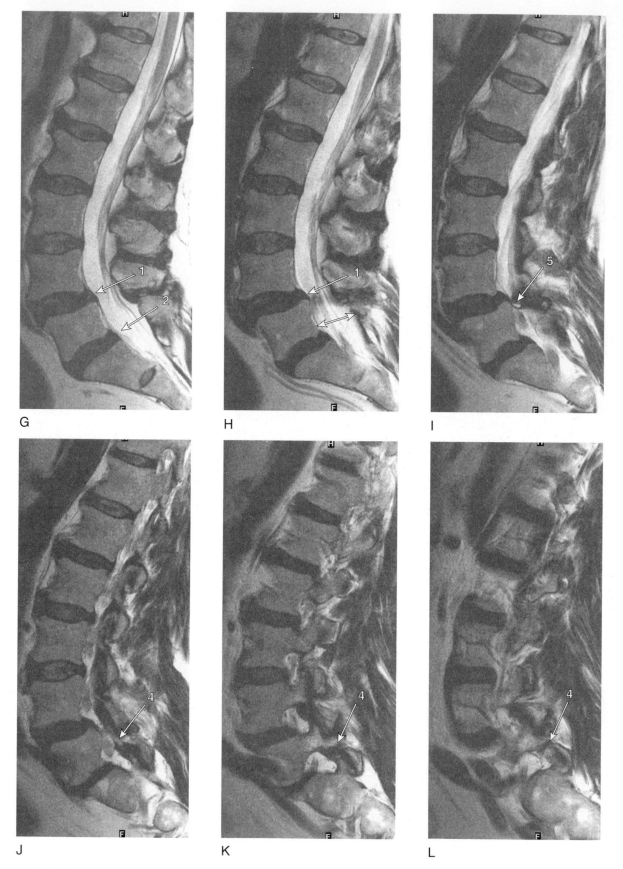

FIGURE 8–16 *(continued)*

anteroposterior (AP) elongation of the central spinal canal at the L5–S1 level *(double-headed arrow)*. The right pars demonstrates continuous marrow *(arrow 3)*. On the left side, there is discontinuity signal intensity within the marrow *(arrow 4)*. At the L4–5 level, a synovial cyst projects off the anterior aspect of the left facet joint *(arrow 5)*.

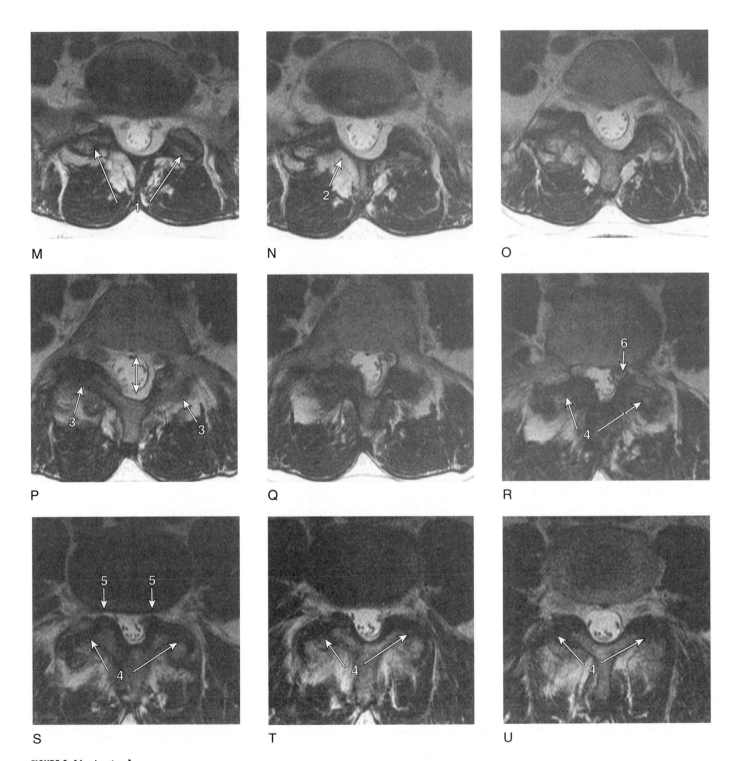

FIGURE 8–16 (*continued*)

M–U, Sequential axial T2WIs from the L5–S1 facet joints (*arrow 1*) to the L4–5 disc demonstrate dysplastic changes of the posterior elements below the level of the pars defects (*arrow 2*), with an abnormal appearance of the right L5–S1 facet joint and asymmetry of the laminae. There are fibroproliferative changes along the pars defects at the level of the transverse processes (*arrow 3*), along with AP elongation of the central canal (*double-headed arrow*). The L4–5 facet joints demonstrate severe facet arthropathy (*arrow 4*) with severe bilateral subarticular recess stenosis (*arrow 5*). In addition, there is a synovial cyst (*arrow 6*) projecting off the anterior aspect of the left L4–5 facet joint, further narrowing the left subarticular recess and compressing the traversing left L5 nerve root.

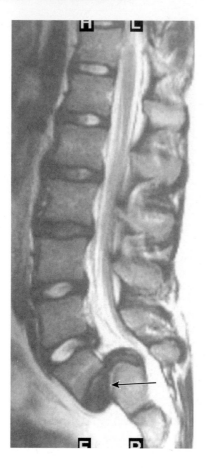

FIGURE 8–17

Spondyloptosis. A 14-year-old boy with known spondyloptosis. Sagittal T2WI shows at least 80% spondylolisthesis of L5 on S1 with rounding of the superior margin of the S1 vertebral body (*arrow*).

COMPUTED TOMOGRAPHY

Reporting of CT is generally more straightforward than reporting of MR, since CT is, in most cases, the reference standard for whether spondylolysis is "really there" or not. As in MRI reporting, the percentage of associated spondylolisthesis should be reported (this requires sagittal reconstruction of the axial images or a high-quality digital scout film). The report should include an assessment of the degree of healing and whether there is any bony bridging across the spondylolysis, as well as measurement of the size of the gap. Ancillary pathology (such as disc herniations and foraminal stenosis) should be reported as discussed in the recommendations of Chapter 2. CT may demonstrate few findings in those rare cases in which the process is quite early and has not yet resulted in any bony discontinuity.

NUCLEAR MEDICINE

Bone scan images are generally relatively easy to describe, having only a few possibilities: normal radiotracer uptake, increased radiotracer uptake, and decreased radiotracer uptake. Areas of abnormal uptake should be localized to the extent possible given the anatomic resolution of the technique: planar images do not allow nearly as exact localization as do SPECT images. Any focus of increased radiotracer localization carries a differential diagnosis, and the other possible disease processes (generally, osteoid osteoma and facet fracture in the young; metastatic disease, facet arthropathy and facet fracture in the middle-aged and elderly) should be mentioned. Note that if other imaging modalities have already been obtained allowing certain diagnosis, and the nuclear medicine study is done merely to assess "disease activity," then a statement such as "increased radiotracer localization in the left L5 pars consistent with the diagnosis of spondylolysis as seen on the patient's recent MR study and corresponding to active disease" may be made. Nuclear medicine has the advantage of being predictive of surgical outcome (Raby 1993).

Conclusion

Spondylolysis has many features that may be detected with modern, high-resolution MRI. If plain films do not allow complete disease characterization, MR is probably the method of choice for evaluation, since it allows the most complete characterization of the ancillary pathology seen in spondylolysis, particularly in the middle-aged or elderly. CT is also frequently performed in spondylolysis, either to confirm the sometimes subtle findings encountered at MRI, or to better assess the bony anatomy, including healing of the pars defects. Nuclear medicine offers the ability to characterize disease activity and has been shown to correlate to surgical outcome (Raby 1993). Although to our knowledge no study has yet been published to establish the fact, we believe that the presence of T1 and T2 prolongation (Ulmer Type I) (Ulmer 1995a) offers the same information. In summary, we believe that MR is the one imaging study that best answer the clinician's two main questions regarding spondylolysis (Harvey 1998): Is spondylolysis present? If so, is it the cause of the patient's symptoms?

inal size (degree of stenosis and any associated neural impingement). We describe our recommendations for reporting degenerative abnormalities in Chapter 2. If it seems likely that the ancillary pathology is the cause of the patient's pain (rather than the spondylolysis per se), note should be made of this fact in the report.

With respect to types of spondylolysis, Wiltse's classification system is widely but not universally known. We do not generally incorporate the Wiltse type in our reports but rather use the explicit descriptors, for example, *lytic,* (or *isthmic*), *dysplastic,* and *degenerative.* As noted earlier, there is overlap of the imaging characteristics of lytic and dysplastic spondylolisthesis, occasionally warranting the term *lytic/dysplastic.* There are two other classifications of types with respect to spondylolysis/spondylolisthesis in the literature. Ulmer and colleagues (1995a) classify marrow signal intensity changes as Modic's subchondral marrow changes (Modic 1988) (see earlier), and Udeshi and Reeves (1999) classify the appearance of the marrow in the pars into four types. Neither of these systems is widely enough known at present to merit use without explicit reference within the report, and the clinical usefulness of using these typing systems (rather than just reporting the changes) is probably limited.

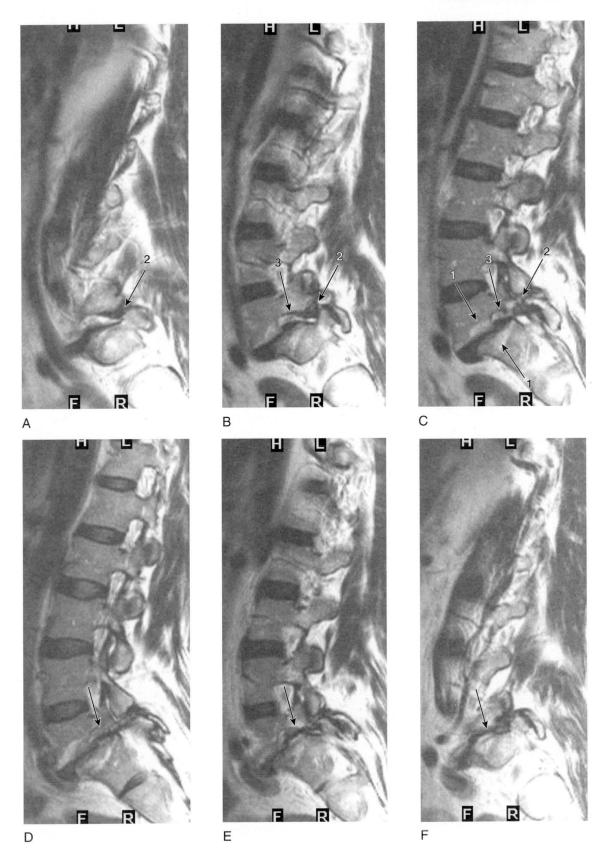

FIGURE 8–18

Lytic spondylolisthesis with associated foraminal stenosis. A 52-year-old woman with severe left leg pain after walking for 15 minutes. *A–C,* Sequential right parasagittal T2WIs through the level of the right foramen demonstrate severe loss of disc height and hydration, subchondral T2 prolongation *(arrow 1),* and 40% spondylolisthesis. There is a pars defect *(arrow 2)* with fibroproliferative changes. Forward descent of L5 on S1 has led to severe up-down foraminal stenosis and L5 ganglionic compression *(arrow 3),* exacerbated by loss of height of the L5–S1 disc. *D–F,* Sequential left parasagittal T2WIs show similar changes on the left side, with even more severe up-down foraminal stenosis and left ganglionic compression *(arrow).*   *(continued)*

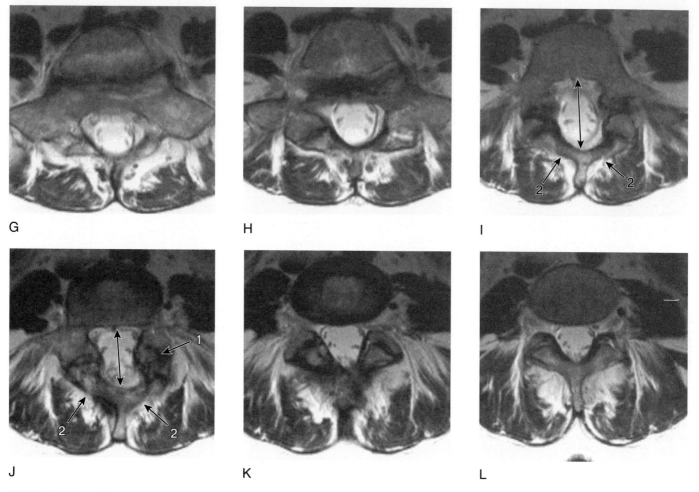

G

H

I

J

K

L

FIGURE 8–18   *(continued)*

G–L, Sequential axial T2WIs from the L5–S1 facets to the L4–5 disc level show bilateral spondylolysis defects with fibroproliferative changes along the pars margins *(arrow 1)* and posterior element dysplasia with asymmetry of the laminae *(arrow 2)* and an off-center location of the spinous process. Note the anteroposterior elongation of the central canal at the level of the slip *(double-headed arrow)*.

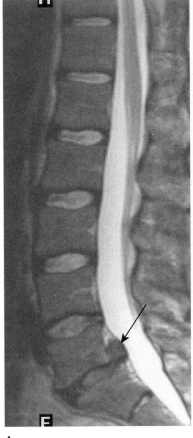

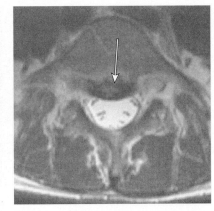

B

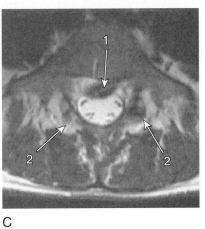

A

C

FIGURE 8–19

Spondylolysis with accompanying disc herniation. A 39-year-old man with central low back pain. *A,* Sagittal T2WI shows L4–5 mild disc dehydration and L5–S1 moderate loss of disc height and moderate disc dehydration. The L5:L1 ratio measure 1.3, and there is 15% spondylolisthesis of L5 on S1, although this is easy to overlook because of the 9-mm cranially dissecting disc extrusion at this level (*arrow*). *B,* Axial T2WI at the L5–S1 level demonstrates the central disc extrusion (*arrow*) that causes no neural compression, at least partially because of the anteroposterior widening of the spinal canal (the patient has an inherently large spinal canal, as well). *C,* Axial T2WI just above *B* demonstrates the cranially extruded disc herniation (*arrow 1*) as well as bilateral pars defects (*arrow 2*).

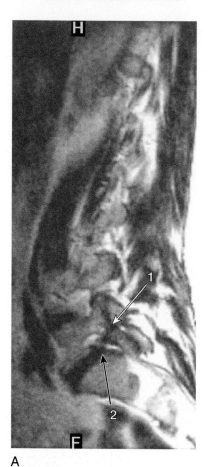

A

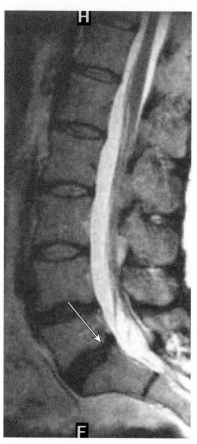

B

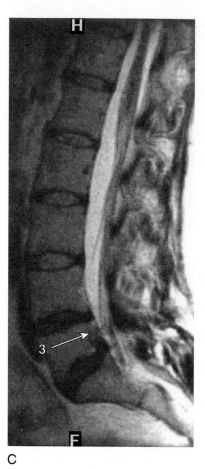

C

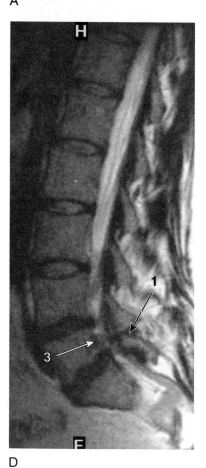

D

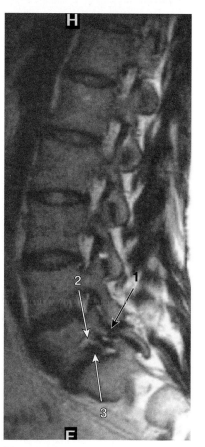

E

FIGURE 8–20

Spondylolysis with accompanying disc herniation. A 38-year-old man with chronic low back pain and new left hip and lateral thigh pain. *A,* Right parasagittal T2WI through the neural foramen demonstrates spondylolysis *(arrow 1)* and severe up-down foraminal stenosis with mild flattening of the exiting right L5 ganglion *(arrow 2).* *B,* Sagittal T2WI demonstrates moderate disc dehydration at L4–5 and L5–S1, along with 5% lytic spondylolisthesis of L5 on S1 *(arrow).* *C–E,* Sequential left parasagittal T2WIs through the left neural foramen demonstrate a left pars defect *(arrow 1)* and severe up-down foraminal stenosis *(arrow 2).* In addition, there is abnormal soft tissue dissecting along the dorsal margin of the L5 vertebral body and extending into the foramen *(arrow 3)* from a disc extrusion, exacerbating L5 ganglionic compression.

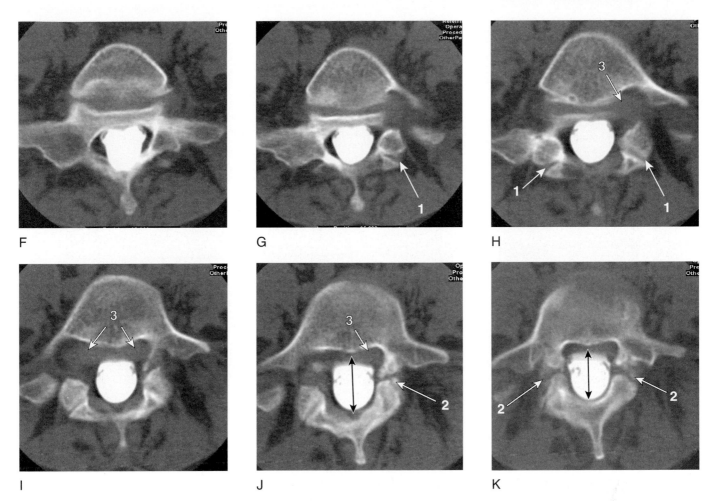

FIGURE 8–20 *(continued)*

F–K, Sequential 3-mm CT-myelogram slices from the L5–S1 facet joints through the L4–5 disc demonstrate hypoplastic L5–S1 facet joints *(arrow 1),* bilateral pars defects *(arrow 2),* and anteroposterior elongation of the central canal *(double-headed arrow).* Asymmetric soft tissue fills the anterior epidural fat, particularly at the level of the transverse processes *(arrow 3),* and the left neural foramen is completely filled with soft tissue representing herniated disc material *(arrow 3).*

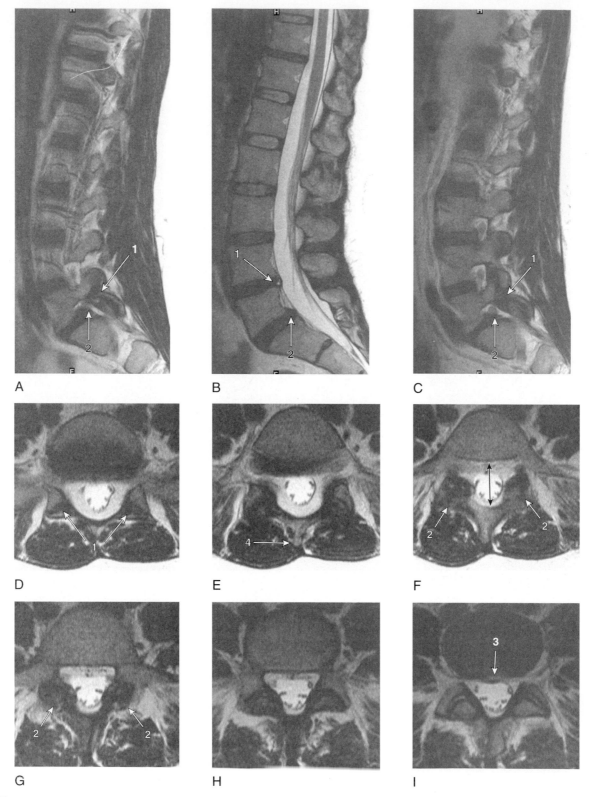

FIGURE 8–21

Disc degeneration above the level of pars defects. A 42-year-old woman with lower right leg and ankle tingling and burning. *A,* Right parasagittal T2WIs through the neural foramen demonstrate a right pars defect (*arrow 1*) along with severe up-down foraminal stenosis and moderate compression of the exiting L5 ganglion (*arrow 2*). *B,* Sagittal T2WI demonstrates L2–3 and L3–4 mild disc dehydration, L4–5 moderate disc dehydration with a focus of T2 prolongation in the posterior disc (*arrow 1*), and L5–S1 moderate disc dehydration with 10% lytic spondylolisthesis (*arrow 2*). *C,* Left parasagittal T2WIs through the foramen demonstrate a left pars defect (*arrow 1*) along with severe up-down foraminal stenosis but only mild flattening of the exiting L5 ganglion (*arrow 2*). *D–I,* Sequential axial T2WIs from the L5–S1 facet joints through the L4–5 disc demonstrate an atrophic appearance of the L5–S1 facet joints (*arrow 1*), extensive fibroproliferative changes along bilateral pars defects (*arrow 2*), anteroposterior elongation of the central canal (*double-headed arrow*), and a central focus of T2 prolongation, with a minimal (2- to 3-mm) associated midline disc protrusion (*arrow 3*). The laminae are minimally asymmetric, and there is an off-center position of the spinous process (*arrow 4*).

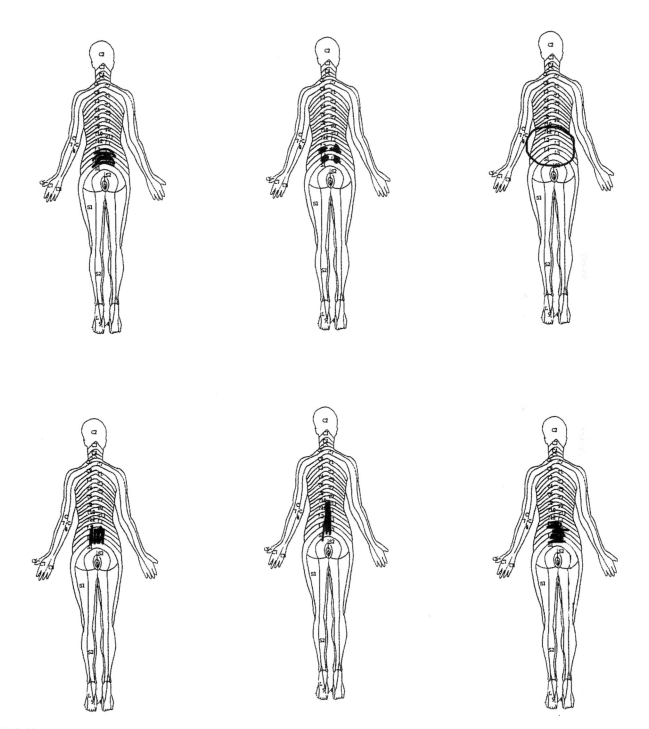

FIGURE 8–22

Clinical Scenario 1. **These pain diagrams are typical of symptomatic spondylolysis.** The six pain diagrams were created by young patients with symptomatic spondylolysis.

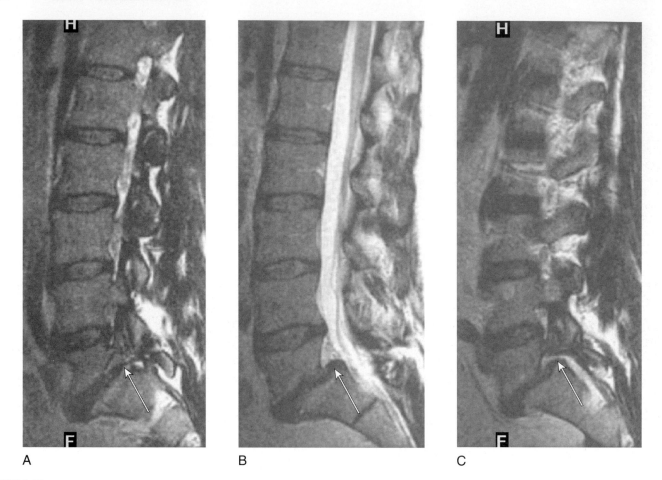

A   B   C

FIGURE 8–23

Disc degeneration exacerbating foraminal stenosis in spondylolysis with spondylolisthesis. A 51-year-old man with a 9-year history of intermittent bilateral leg burning and tingling. *A,* Right parasagittal T2WI at the level of the foramen demonstrates severe up-down foraminal stenosis with compression of the exiting right L5 ganglion *(arrow).* The up-down stenosis from the patient's spondylolisthesis is exacerbated secondary to loss of disc height and degenerative disc bulging. *B,* Sagittal T2WI demonstrates L5–S1 severe loss of disc height and disc dehydration, with 25% lytic spondylolisthesis *(arrow).* *C,* Left parasagittal T2WI shows similar findings to the right side, with severe up-down foraminal stenosis exacerbated from loss of disc height and degenerative disc bulging *(arrow).*

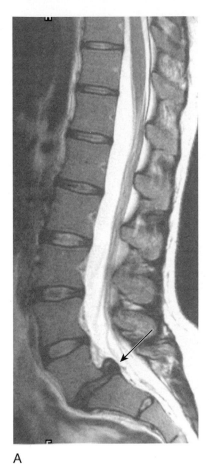

A

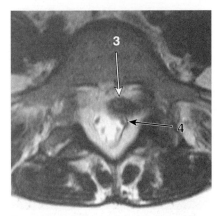

B

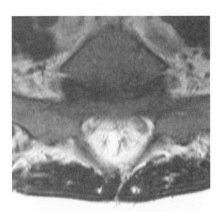

D

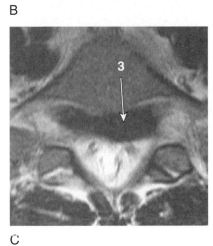

C

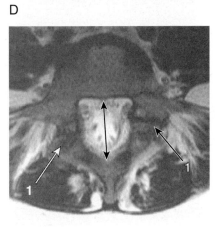

E

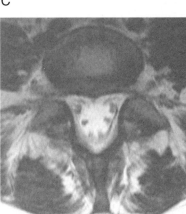

F

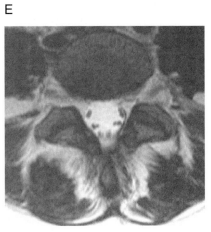

G

FIGURE 8–24

Spondylolysis with disc herniation. A 29-year-old woman with central low back pain. *A,* Sagittal T2WI shows 25% lytic spondylolisthesis with moderate loss of disc height and dehydration as well as a cranially dissecting 9-mm disc extrusion *(arrow)*. *B–G,* Sequential axial T2WIs from the S1 pedicles through the L4–5 disc show bilateral pars defects *(arrow 1)* as well as anteroposterior elongation of the central canal *(double-headed arrow)*. The disc extrusion *(arrow 3)* lies along the anterior aspect of the right S1 nerve root *(arrow 4)*, with minimal neural compression because of the capacious central canal.

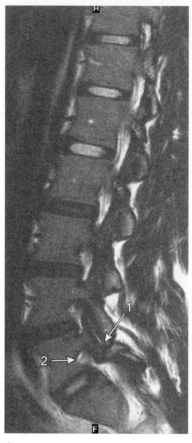

A

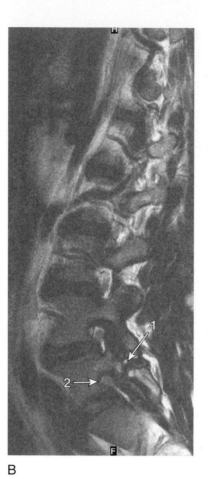

B

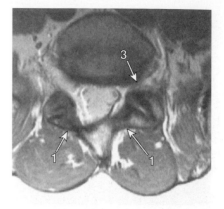

C

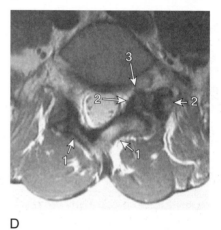

D

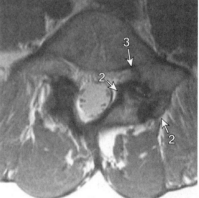

E

FIGURE 8–25

Spondylolysis with fibroproliferative changes contributing to radicular symptoms. A 32-year-old man with low back and left leg pain. *A*, Sagittal T2WI at the level of the right neural foramen demonstrates mild fibroproliferative changes along the right L5 pars defect (*arrow 1*) with moderate front-back foraminal stenosis and mild right L5 flattening (*arrow 2*). *B*, Sagittal T2WI at the level of the left neural foramen demonstrates a left pars defect (*arrow 1*) somewhat more pronounced anteroposterior narrowing of the neural foramen and compression of the left L5 ganglion (*arrow 2*). *C–E*, Sequential axial MRI examinations through the L5–S1 foraminal level shows marked asymmetry of the laminae (*arrow 1*). There are marked left fibroproliferative changes along the pars margins (*arrow 2*), with associated narrowing of the left neural foramen (*arrow 3*).

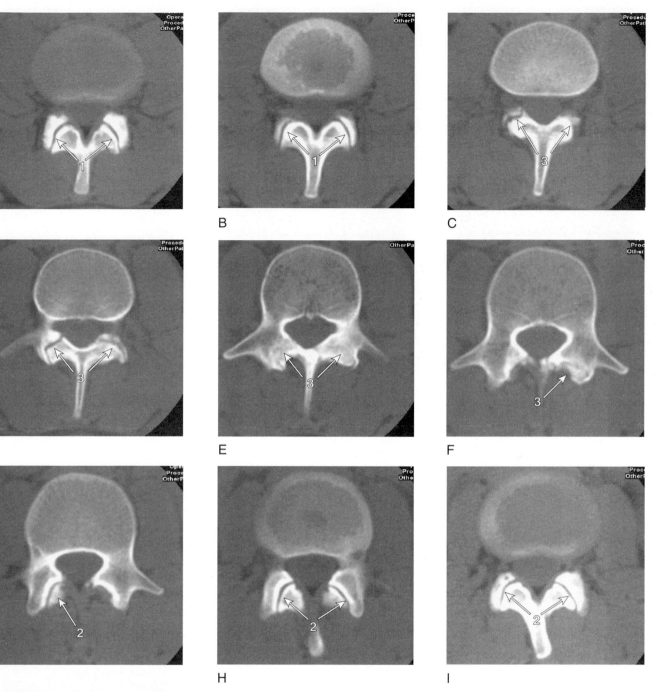

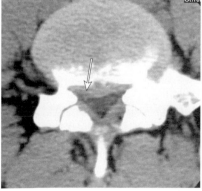

FIGURE 8–26

Spondylolysis with another (physically remote) cause of pain. A 22-year-old man with right leg pain. *A–I,* Sequential 3-mm CT slices from the L2–3 facet joints *(arrow 1)* through the L1–2 facet joints *(arrow 2)* with partially healed bilateral L2 pars defects *(arrow 3). J,* CT at L4–5 shows a right central disc protrusion *(arrow)* superimposed on an inherently small spinal canal with severe subarticular recess narrowing and compression of the traversing right L5 nerve root, most likely representing the symptom producing lesion in this man with healed higher-level pars defects and left lower extremity symptoms.

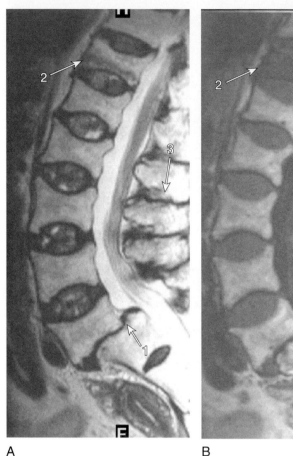

A
B

FIGURE 8–27

Spondylolysis with another (physically remote) cause of pain. A 79-year-old woman with central low back pain. *A,* Sagittal T2WI demonstrates severe loss of disc height and hydration at L5–S1, along with 30% lytic spondylolisthesis (*arrow 1*). Note the band of T2 inhomogeneity along the inferior margin of the T12 vertebrae (*arrow 2*). The vertebral bodies are bowed, and there is apposition of spinous processes posteriorly (Baastrup's disease) (*arrow 3*). *B,* Sagittal T1WI shows T1 prolongation corresponding to inhomogeneity of signal intensity seen on *A* and indicating an acute or subacute vertebral body fracture.

References

Akari T, Harata S, Nakano K, Satoh T. Reactive sclerosis of the pedicle associated with contralateral spondylolysis. Spine 1992; 17:1424–1425.

Campbell RSD, Grainger AJ. Optimization of MRI pulse sequences to visualize the normal pars interarticularis. Clin Radiol 1999; 54:63–68.

Dai LY. Disc degeneration in patients with lumbar spondylolysis. J Spinal Disord 2000; 13:478–486.

Duprez T, Mailleaux P, Bodart A, Coulier B, Malghem J, Maldague B. Retrodural cysts bridging a bilateral lumbar spondylolysis: a report of two symptomatic cases. J Comput Assist Tomogr 1999; 23:534–537.

Elliott S, Hutson MA, Wastie ML. Bone scintigraphy in the assessment of spondylolysis in patients attending a sports injury clinic. Clin Radiol 1988; 39:269–272.

Floman Y. Progression of lumbosacral isthmic spondylolisthesis in adults. Spine 2000; 25:342–347.

Garber JE, Wright AM. Unilateral spondylolysis and contralateral pedicle fracture. Spine 1986; 11:63–66.

Ghelman B, Doherty JH. Demonstration of spondylolysis by arthrography of the apophyseal joint. AJR Am J Roentgenol 1978; 130:986–987.

Grenier N, Kressel HY, Schiebler ML, Grossman RI. Isthmic spondylolysis of the lumbar spine: MR imaging at 1.5 T. Radiology 1989; 170:489–493.

Grobler LJ, Robertson PA, Novotny JE, Pope MH. Etiology of spondylolisthesis: assessment of the role played by lumbar facet joint morphology. Spine 1993; 18:80–91.

Grobler LJ, Wiltse LL. Classification, and nonoperative and operative treatment of spondylolisthesis. In Frymoyer JW (ed). The Adult Spine: Principles and Practice, 2nd ed. Philadelphia, Lippincott-Raven, 1997.

Grogan JP, Hemminghytt S, Williams AL, Carrera GF, Haughton VM. Spondylolysis studied with computed tomography. Radiology 1982; 145:737–742.

Guillodo Y, Botton E, Saraux A, Le Goff P. Contralateral spondylolysis and fracture of the lumbar pedicle in an elite female gymnast. Spine 2000; 25:2541–2543.

Harvey CJ, Richenberg JL, Saifuddin A, Wolman RL. Pictorial review: the radiological investigation of lumbar spondylolysis. Clin Radiol 1998; 53:723–728.

Ikata T, Miyake R, Katoh S, Morita T, Murase M. Pathogenesis of sports-related spondylolisthesis in adolescents: radiographic and magnetic resonance imaging study. Am J Sports Med 1996; 24:94–98.

Jinkins JR, Matthes JC, Sener RN, Venkatappan S, Rauch R. Spondylolysis, spondylolisthesis, and associated nerve root entrapment in the lumbosacral spine: MR evaluation. AJR Am J Roentgenol 1992; 159:799–803.

Jinkins JR, Rauch A. Magnetic resonance imaging of entrapment of lumbar nerve roots in spondylotic spondylolisthesis. J Bone Joint Surg Am 1994; 76:1643–1648.

Johnson DW, Farnum GW, Latchaw RE, Erba SM. MR imaging of the pars interarticularis. AJR Am J Roentgenol 1989; 152:327–332.

Lowe J, Schachner E, Hirschberg E, Shapiro Y, Libson E. Significance of bone scintigraphy in symptomatic spondylolysis. Spine 1984; 9:653–655.

MacNab I, McCullouch J. Backache, 2nd ed. Baltimore, Williams & Wilkins, 1990.

Major NM, Helms CA, Richardson WJ. MR imaging of fibrocartilaginous masses arising along the margins of spondylolysis defects. AJR Am J Roentgenol 1999; 173:673–676.

Maldague B, Mathurin P, Malghem J. Facet joint arthrography in lumbar spondylolysis. Radiology 1981; 140:29–36.

McAfee PC, Yuan HA. Computed tomography in spondylolisthesis. Clin Orthop 1982; 166:62–71.

Meyerding HW. Spondylolisthesis. Surg Gynecol Obstet 1932; 54:371–377.

Modic MT, Steinberg PM, Ross JS, Masaryk TJ, Carter JR. Degenerative disk disease: assessment of changes in vertebral body marrow with MR imaging. Radiology 1988; 166:193–199.

Raby N, Mathews S. Symptomatic spondylolysis: correlation of CT and SPECT with clinical outcome. Clin Radiol 1993; 48:97–99.

Redla S, Kisdar T, Saifuddin A, Taylor BA. Imaging features of cervical spondylolysis with emphasis on MR appearances. Clin Radiol 1999; 54:815–820.

Rossi F. Spondylolysis, spondylolisthesis, and sports. J Sports Med Phys Fitness 1978; 18:317–340.

Rothman SLG, Glenn WV. CT multiplanar reconstruction in 253 cases of lumbar spondylolysis. AJNR Am J Neuroradiol 1984; 5:81–90.

Sagi HC, Jarvis JG, Uhthoff HK. Histomorphic analysis of the development of the pars interarticularis and its association with isthmic spondylolysis. Spine 1998; 23:1635–1640.

Sener RN, Matthes JC, Venkatappan S, Jinkins JR. Posterior dislocation of the neural arch of L5 due to spondylolysis. Neuroradiology 1991; 33:463.

St. Amour TE, Hodges SC, Laakman RW, Tarnas DE. Spondylolysis with spondylolisthesis. In St. Amour TE, Hodges SC, Laakman RW, Tarnas DE (eds). MRI of the Spine. New York, Raven Press, 1994.

Suh PB, Esses SI, Kostuik JP. Repair of pars interarticularis defect: the prognostic value of pars infiltration. Spine 1991; 16:S445–S448.

Szypryt EP, Twining P, Mullholland RC, Worthington BS. The prevalence of disc degeneration associated with neural arch defects of the lumbar spine assessed by magnetic resonance imaging. Spine 1989; 14:977–981.

Teplick JG, Laffey PA, Berman A, Haskin ME. Diagnosis and evaluation of spondylolisthesis and/or spondylolysis on axial CT. AJNR Am J Neuroradiol 1986; 7:479–491.

Udeshi UL, Reeves D. Routine thin slice MRI effectively demonstrates the lumbar pars interarticularis. Clin Radiol 1999; 54:615–619.

Ulmer JL, Elster AD, Mathews VP, King JC. Distinction between degenerative and isthmic spondylolisthesis on sagittal images: importance of increased anteroposterior diameter of the spinal canal ("wide canal sign"). AJR Am J Roentgenol 1994; 163:411–416.

Ulmer JL, Elster AD, Mathews VP, Allen AM. Lumbar spondylolysis: reactive marrow changes seen in adjacent pedicles on MR images. AJR Am J Roentgenol 1995a; 164:429–433.

Ulmer JL, Mathews VP, Elster AD, King JC. Lumbar spondylolysis without spondylolisthesis: recognition of isolated posterior element subluxation on sagittal MR. AJNR Am J Neuroradiol 1995b; 16:1393–1398.

Ulmer JL, Mathers VP, Elster AD, Mark LP, Daniels DL, Mueller W. MR imaging of lumbar spondylolysis: the importance of ancillary observations. AJR Am J Roentgenol 1997; 169:233–239.

Waddell G. The Back Pain Revolution. New York, Churchill Livingstone, 1998.

Wiltse LL, Fonseca AS, Amster J, Dimartino P, Ravessoud FA. Relationship of the dura, Hofmann's ligaments, Batson's plexus, and a fibrovascular membrane lying on the posterior surface of the vertebral bodies and attaching to the deep layer of the posterior longitudinal ligament: an anatomical, radiologic, and clinical study. Spine 1993; 18:1030–1043.

Wiltse LL, Newman PH, Macnab I: Classification of spondylolysis and spondylolisthesis. Clin Orthop 1976; 117:23–29.

Wiltse LL, Widell EH, Jackson DW. Fatigue fracture: the basic lesion in isthmic spondylolisthesis. J Bone Joint Surg Am 1975; 57:17–22.

Wiltse LL, Winter RB. Terminology and measurement of spondylolisthesis. J Bone Joint Surg Am 1983; 65:768–772.

Yamane T, Yoshida T, Mimatsu K. Early diagnosis of lumbar spondylolysis by MRI. J Bone Joint Surg Br 1993; 75:764–768.

Miscellaneous Diseases of the Spine

DONALD L. RENFREW • PETER BOVE • MICHAEL W. HAYT

Arthropathies Affecting the Spine

RHEUMATOID ARTHRITIS OF THE SPINE

Definition. Rheumatoid arthritis is an inflammatory arthropathy characterized by synovial overgrowth, erosions, and occasionally fusion.

Imaging Findings. At the craniocervical junction, rheumatoid arthritis may result in a pannus (inflammatory thickening of the synovium) with associated erosion of the dens (Fig. 9–1) (Bundschuh 1988, St. Amour 1994, Wolfe 1987). When erosive change has weakened or destroyed the

transverse ligament, there is associated atlantoaxial subluxation, although subluxation may be reduced and less well seen in the supine position (which is generally how the patients are examined in magnetic resonance imaging [MRI]) (Oostveen 1998). Erosion of the transverse ligament, along with erosion of the occiput–C1 and C1–2 joints, also results in cranial settling, wherein the dens ascends relative to the skull base (Bundschuh 1987, Oostveen 1998) (Fig. 9–2). Pannus, atlantoaxial subluxation, and cranial settling all may be associated with neural compression (Bundschuh 1988, Aisen 1987, Larsson 1989). In the subaxial spine, rheumatoid arthritis may result in

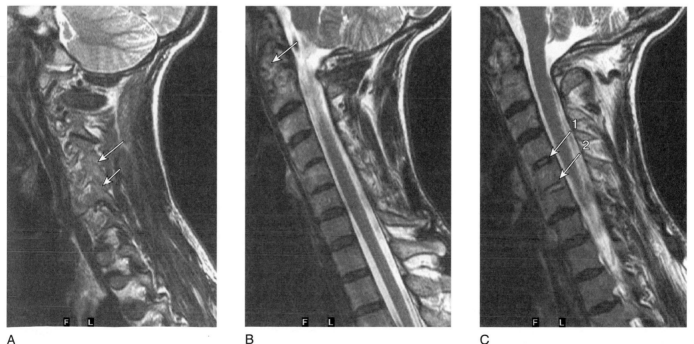

A   B   C

FIGURE 9–1

Rheumatoid arthritis of the cervical spine with erosion of the dens and subaxial disease. A 43-year-old patient with neck and back pain and a history of rheumatoid arthritis. *A,* Right parasagittal T2WI demonstrates multilevel facet joint abnormality with fusion across the C4–5 and C5–6 facet joints (*arrows*). The patient's contralateral facets (not shown) were also fused. *B,* Sagittal T2WI demonstrates erosion of the dens (*arrow*). *C,* Left parasagittal T2WI demonstrates T2 prolongation along the C4–5 (*arrow 1*) and C5–6 (*arrow 2*) discs, consistent with rheumatoid discitis.

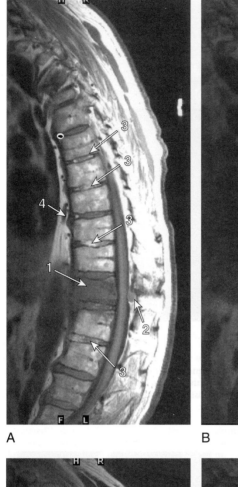

A

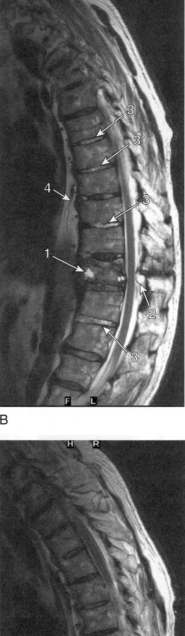

B

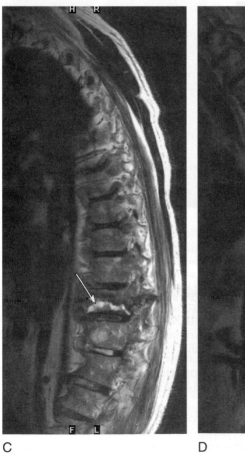

C

D

FIGURE 9–5

Ankylosing spondylitis with fracture of the thoracic spine. A 67-year-old patient with known ankylosing spondylitis and trauma 1 month previously. *A,* Sagittal T1WI demonstrates extensive T1 prolongation of the T11 vertebral body (*arrow 1*), along with an abnormal focus of T1 prolongation posteriorly at the same level (*arrow 2*). There is abnormal, fatty degeneration of multiple intervertebral discs (*arrows 3*) consistent with long-standing fusion. There are flowing syndesmophytes anteriorly (*arrow 4*). *B,* Sagittal T2WI demonstrates foci of T2 prolongation within the T11 vertebral body (*arrows 1*), the rounded focus posteriorly which also demonstrates T2 prolongation (*arrow 2*), fatty degeneration of the intervertebral discs (*arrows 3*), and flowing anterior syndesmophytes (*arrows 4*). *C,* Right parasagittal T2WI demonstrates a horizontal band of T2 prolongation (*arrow*) consistent with either fluid or granulation tissue along a plane of motion. *D,* Left parasagittal T2WI demonstrates a plane of T2 prolongation (*arrow*) within the left pars interarticularis, consistent with a fracture plane through the posterior elements.

9 Miscellaneous Diseases of the Spine

DONALD L. RENFREW • PETER BOVE • MICHAEL W. HAYT

Arthropathies Affecting the Spine

RHEUMATOID ARTHRITIS OF THE SPINE

Definition. Rheumatoid arthritis is an inflammatory arthropathy characterized by synovial overgrowth, erosions, and occasionally fusion.

Imaging Findings. At the craniocervical junction, rheumatoid arthritis may result in a pannus (inflammatory thickening of the synovium) with associated erosion of the dens (Fig. 9–1) (Bundschuh 1988, St. Amour 1994, Wolfe 1987). When erosive change has weakened or destroyed the transverse ligament, there is associated atlantoaxial subluxation, although subluxation may be reduced and less well seen in the supine position (which is generally how the patients are examined in magnetic resonance imaging [MRI]) (Oostveen 1998). Erosion of the transverse ligament, along with erosion of the occiput–C1 and C1–2 joints, also results in cranial settling, wherein the dens ascends relative to the skull base (Bundschuh 1987, Oostveen 1998) (Fig. 9–2). Pannus, atlantoaxial subluxation, and cranial settling all may be associated with neural compression (Bundschuh 1988, Aisen 1987, Larsson 1989). In the subaxial spine, rheumatoid arthritis may result in

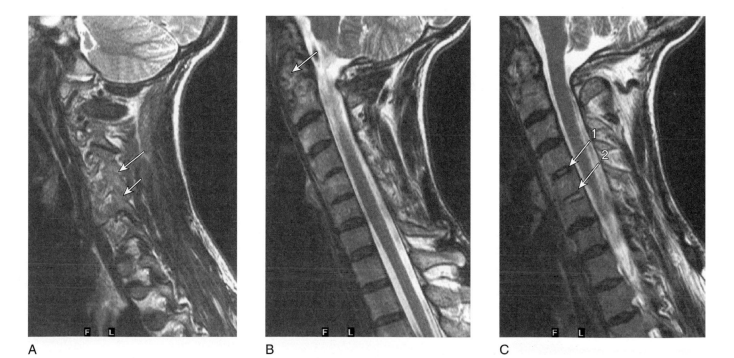

A B C

FIGURE 9–1

Rheumatoid arthritis of the cervical spine with erosion of the dens and subaxial disease. A 43-year-old patient with neck and back pain and a history of rheumatoid arthritis. *A,* Right parasagittal T2WI demonstrates multilevel facet joint abnormality with fusion across the C4–5 and C5–6 facet joints (*arrows*). The patient's contralateral facets (not shown) were also fused. *B,* Sagittal T2WI demonstrates erosion of the dens (*arrow*). *C,* Left parasagittal T2WI demonstrates T2 prolongation along the C4–5 (*arrow 1*) and C5–6 (*arrow 2*) discs, consistent with rheumatoid discitis.

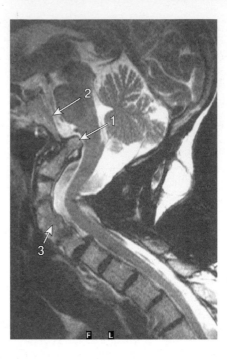

FIGURE 9–2

Rheumatoid arthritis of the cervical spine with cranial settling and subaxial disease. A 56-year-old patient with long-standing rheumatoid arthritis after multiple surgical procedures, including posterior decompression through the upper cervical spine. Sagittal T2WI demonstrates cranial settling with superior migration of the dens (*arrow 1*) relative to the clivus (*arrow 2*). There is "stair-step" deformity of C4–5, C5–6, and C6–7, with associated fusion of C4–5 (*arrow 3*). There is accentuation of cervical lordosis and pronounced angulation of the mid-cervical cord, but no T2 prolongation within the brain stem or cord is present.

erosion or fusion of the facet joints (Wolfe 1988) (Fig. 9–1). It may also result in inflammatory discitis, with findings of T1 and T2 prolongation, usually in multiple discs (St. Amour 1994) (Figs. 9–1 and 9–2). The spine may assume a "stair-step" appearance, with multilevel subluxations.

Differential Diagnosis. Atlantoaxial subluxation may also be seen in ankylosing spondylitis, Down syndrome, retropharyngeal abscess, and ossification of the posterior longitudinal ligament (Takasita 2000). Fusion of the facet joints may occur with other inflammatory arthropathies, on a congenital/developmental basis, or as a result of fusion surgery.

Clinical Significance. There is often striking discordance between imaging findings and clinical manifestations in rheumatoid arthritis (Bundschuh 1988, Oostveen 1998). Rheumatoid arthritis of the spine is generally treated conservatively (St. Amour 1994). When neurologic compromise is evident on MRI examination (either at the skull base from panus formation, atlantoaxial subluxation, or cranial settling, or in the subaxial spine from stair-step deformity with multilevel subluxations), decompression may be undertaken.

Reporting. The report of cervical spine imaging in any patient with known rheumatoid arthritis should include mention of the craniocervical relationships and any neural compression or areas of T2 prolongation within the spinal cord or medulla. Supine extension MRI may underestimate the degree of neural compression because of worsening atlantoaxial subluxation in flexion (Oostveen 1998). Similarly, in the subaxial spine, the degree of cord compression may be underestimated because of increased subluxation along abnormal facet joints in flexion. In addition to the usual grading of spinal canal and neural foraminal stenosis (see Chapter 2), the report should specific mention of disc abnormalities related to rheumatoid arthritis (rheumatoid discitis) and facets (synovial overgrowth or fusion).

ANKYLOSING SPONDYLITIS

Definition. Ankylosing spondylitis is a seronegative[*] spondyloarthropathy that preferentially involves the sacroiliac joints and spine, usually beginning at the thoracolumbar junction and sometimes progressing to involve the entire spine.

Imaging Findings. Sacroiliitis progressing to fusion, "squaring" of the vertebral bodies with resorption along the vertebral body margins, ossification of the anterior annular fibers and anterior longitudinal ligament, atlantoaxial subluxation, and dural ectasia (Bilgen 1999, St. Cloud 1994) (Figs. 9–3 and 9–4) all are findings of ankylosing spondylitis. Some patients with ankylosing spondylitis undergo multilevel autofusion and, with or without trauma, undergo fracture of the fused segments. These fractures are usually quite unstable and may proceed to a pseudarthrosis (St. Amour 1994, Bilgen 1999) (Figs. 9–4 and 9–5).

Differential Diagnosis. The combination of resorption of the margins of the vertebral bodies and calcification/ossificiation of the anterior longitudinal ligament and peripheral annular fibers results in a characteristic plain film appearance called the "bamboo spine." Similar multilevel fusion may accompany juvenile rheumatoid arthritis. Fractures through a multilevel fusion may follow ankylosing spondylitis but may also be seen following degenerative stiffening or fusion of the spine, as well as postoperative fusion of the spine. Lesions similar to the arachnoid diverticula seen in ankylosing spondylitis may be seen on an idiopathic basis (see section, "Spinal Meningeal Cysts") or accompany Marfan's syndrome (Ahn 2000).

Clinical Significance. Ankylosing spondylitis may be associated with significant disability. Back pain may be the primary disabling condition, but patients may also develop myelopathy from atlantoaxial instability, neural compression from complicating fractures, and cauda equina syndrome from adhesive arachnoiditis (Bilgen 1999).

Reporting. Imaging (computed tomography [CT] and MRI) of the spine in cases of ankylosing spondylitis generally is directed at evaluation of possible complications such as atlantoaxial subluxation, stenosis, and fracture. Dural diverticula may be associated with arachnoiditis in some cases. Correlation with whether the patient presents with acute local pain following trauma or whether the patient has radicular symptoms helps in directing attention to the imaging findings of these complications.

---

[*]That is, the patient is serum rheumatoid factor negative.

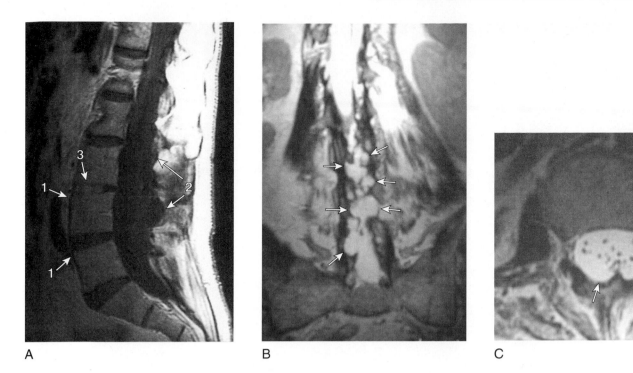

FIGURE 9–3

Ankylosing spondylitis with dural ectasia. *A,* Sagittal T1WI demonstrates squaring of the vertebral bodies anteriorly *(arrows 1)* and expansion of the spinal canal with posterior diverticula *(arrows 2).* There is autofusion along the L3–4 level with fatty degeneration of the disc *(arrow 3).* *B,* Coronal T2WI demonstrates the multiple posterior arachnoid diverticula *(arrows).* *C,* Axial T2WI demonstrates erosion of laminae posteriorly by the expanded spinal canal.

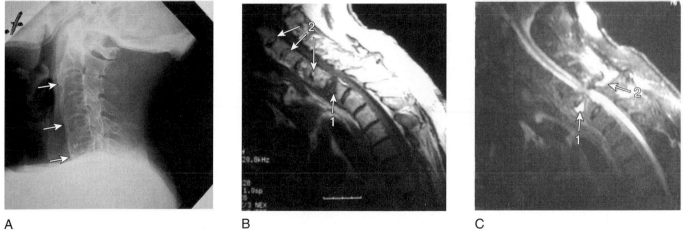

FIGURE 9–4

Ankylosing spondylitis with fracture of the cervical spine. *A,* Lateral plain film examination demonstrates ossification of the anterior longitudinal ligament and anterior annular fibers along with squaring of the vertebral body margins *(arrows).* *B,* Sagittal T1WI of the cervical spine shows T1 prolongation along the superior C7 vertebral body and deformity of C7 consistent with acute fracture *(arrow 1).* There is also fatty replacement of multiple cervical intervertebral discs *(arrows 2)* secondary to autofusion across these levels. *C,* Sagittal T2WI demonstrates T2 prolongation along the C7 vertebral body consistent with acute fracture *(arrow 1).* There is also T2 prolongation posteriorly at the C7 level *(arrow 2),* consistent with acute injury posteriorly as well.

DIALYSIS SPONDYLOARTHROPATHY

Definition. Dialysis spondylitis that develops in patients with chronic renal failure. This spondylitis may be relatively rapid and destructive.

Imaging Findings. Many patients undergoing dialysis develop superficial corner erosions of the vertebral bodies (Sundaram 1987) that are generally asymptomatic; some

patients develop a much more aggressive and rapidly developing form of erosive spondyloarthropathy that may resemble infectious spondylitis (Sundaram 1987, Kaplan 1987; Rafto 1988) (Fig. 9–6).

Differential Diagnosis. The erosive changes across the level of the disc, along with disc narrowing, may closely resemble infectious spondylitis (Kaplan 1987) and in many

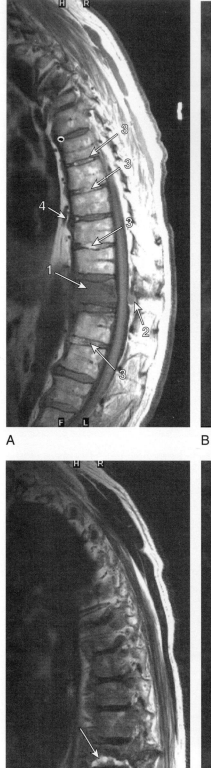

A

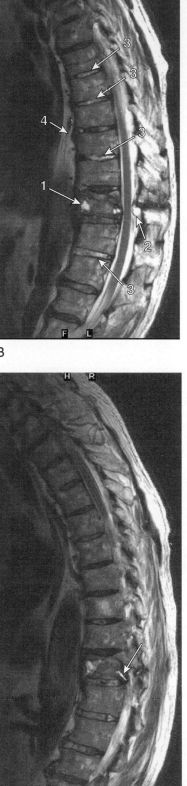

B

C

D

FIGURE 9–5

Ankylosing spondylitis with fracture of the thoracic spine. A 67-year-old patient with known ankylosing spondylitis and trauma 1 month previously. *A*, Sagittal T1WI demonstrates extensive T1 prolongation of the T11 vertebral body (*arrow 1*), along with an abnormal focus of T1 prolongation posteriorly at the same level (*arrow 2*). There is abnormal, fatty degeneration of multiple intervertebral discs (*arrows 3*) consistent with long-standing fusion. There are flowing syndesmophytes anteriorly (*arrow 4*). *B*, Sagittal T2WI demonstrates foci of T2 prolongation within the T11 vertebral body (*arrows 1*), the rounded focus posteriorly which also demonstrates T2 prolongation (*arrow 2*), fatty degeneration of the intervertebral discs (*arrows 3*), and flowing anterior syndesmophytes (*arrows 4*). *C*, Right parasagittal T2WI demonstrates a horizontal band of T2 prolongation (*arrow*) consistent with either fluid or granulation tissue along a plane of motion. *D*, Left parasagittal T2WI demonstrates a plane of T2 prolongation (*arrow*) within the left pars interarticularis, consistent with a fracture plane through the posterior elements.

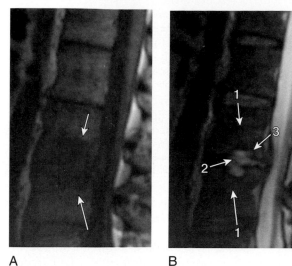
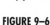

FIGURE 9–6

Dialysis spondyloarthropathy. *A,* Sagittal T1WI demonstrates T1 prolongation in the subchondral marrow adjacent to a thoracic disc (*arrows*). *B,* Sagittal T2WI demonstrates T2 prolongation along the subchondral marrow as well (*arrows 1*), and also T2 prolongation within the disc, particularly along its posterior margin (*arrow 2*). There is erosive change of the end plates (*arrow 3*). Biopsy demonstrated evidence of dialysis spondyloarthropathy, with no infectious organisms cultured and no histologic evidence of acute infection.

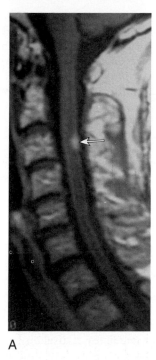
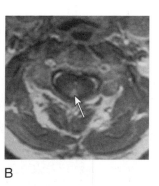

FIGURE 9–8

Multiple sclerosis with enhancing cord lesions. *A,* Sagittal T1WI following contrast enhancement demonstrates a focus of intense contrast enhancement in the dorsal spinal cord at the C3 level (*arrow*). *B,* Axial T1WI following contrast enhancement also demonstrates the contrast-enhancing plaque within the posterior spinal cord (*arrow*).

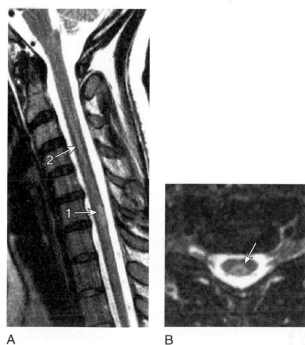

FIGURE 9–7

Multiple sclerosis of the cervical spinal cord. A 30-year-old patient with known multiple sclerosis and paresthesias sent for evaluation of cord lesions. *A,* Sagittal gradient-recalled echo T2WI demonstrates somewhat well-defined foci of T2 prolongation measuring 15 to 20 mm in length and 5 to 6 mm in diameter in the lower cervical spine (*arrow 1*). Additional, ill-defined T2 prolongation is seen in the more superior cervical spinal cord (*arrow 2*), although this finding is difficult to differentiate from artifact . *B,* Axial fast spin-echo T2WI demonstrates a large, confluent focus of T2 prolongation in the posterior spinal cord (*arrow*).

cases require biopsy, since hemodialysis patients are immunocompromised and infection needs to be excluded as the cause of the abnormality.

Clinical Significance. Infectious spondylitis is treated with antibiotics (with surgery as necessary), whereas dialysis spondyloarthropathy generally has no specific treatment.

Reporting. The findings of subchondral marrow changes, erosion of the end plates, and T2 prolongation within the intervertebral disc are nonspecific, and both infection and dialysis spondyloarthropathy need to be mentioned in the report.

Multiple Sclerosis

Definition. Multiple sclerosis is a demyelinating disease of the brain and spinal cord.

Imaging Findings. Multiple sclerosis of the spinal cord may demonstrate one or several of multiple imaging findings (Glasier 1995, Tartaglino 1995, Trop 1998). Often, multiple sclerosis presents with one or more foci of T2 prolongation (possibly with accompanying T1 prolongation) within the spinal cord (Fig. 9–7). Early in the course of the disease, images may demonstrate cord edema and swelling, whereas later in the course of the disease there may be cord atrophy. Active lesions demonstrate contrast enhancement (Fig. 9–8). Multiple sclerosis may present with a single large lesion mimicking neoplasm (Glasier 1995).

Differential Diagnosis. Multiple small, variably sized foci of T2 prolongation may represent multiple sclerosis plaques, vasculitis, Lyme disease, metastatic deposit, or granulomatous disease. Metastatic deposit and granulomatous disease usually demonstrate additional lesions in the intramedullary-intradural or extramedullary compartments. When multiple sclerosis presents with a single, large plaque with associated cord edema, the differential diagnosis includes acute disseminating encephalomyelitis (ADEM) and neoplasm. ADEM and multiple sclerosis may have identical imaging findings; in ADEM, there may be a history of viral illness or inoculation, and the disease usually remits after a single instance. Neoplasms tend to be less fusiform and more globular than multiple sclerosis plaques. Atrophy of the cord without focal lesions is a nonspecific finding that may be seen late in multiple sclerosis but also following trauma, cord ischemia, or compression (St. Amour 1994).

Clinical Significance. Approximately 10% of patients with multiple sclerosis will present with symptoms related to cord abnormality. Multiple sclerosis has protean manifestations including numbness, dysesthesias, burning sensations, hemiparesis, constipation, and urinary retention or incontinence. The amount of disease indicated on T2-weighted image (T2WI) is a poor predictor of disability, and MRI frequently shows lesions that are not evident clinically (Trop 1998). Approximately 90% to 95% of patients have an initially relapsing-remitting course of disease, with about two thirds of these patients later developing progression of the disease (Miller 1991). Other patients are more fortunate, with little disability from the disease even after several years of remissions and exacerbations.

Reporting. Patients undergoing imaging for multiple sclerosis fall into one of two categories: those being evaluated for known multiple sclerosis, and those in whom the diagnosis may not be suspected. If a patient with suspected multiple sclerosis but no prior spine studies is undergoing evaluation, the report should describe all cord lesions with the level, size, and contrast enhancement pattern. The entire cord needs to be evaluated from the cervicomedullary junction through the conus, although most lesions occur in the cervical spine. For follow-up of known lesions (done for either treatment evaluation or for evaluation of new symptoms), the report should include a direct comparison with the prior study or studies and include a description of whether the plaques are stable, increasing, or decreasing in size as well as any change in contrast enhancement pattern. If the diagnosis was not suspected prior to imaging, then the report should describe the level, size, and imaging characteristics of the lesions; in almost all cases, such patients should undergo simultaneous or prompt MRI of the brain to evaluate for characteristic intracranial lesions. Although imaging findings are highly characteristic, correlation with the clinical history (of multiple lesions in time and space), cerebrospinal fluid (CSF) analysis, and evoked potentials is a necessary part of the complete evaluation of these patients.

Vascular Malformations

Definition. Vascular malformations of the cord are most often the result of anomalous arteriovenous shunting. Spinal arteriovenous malformations (AVMs) are a heterogeneous group of lesions generally divided into (1) arteriovenous fistulas, (2) intramedullary AVMs, and (3) intradural perimedullary fistulae. Advances in neuroimaging, interventional neuroradiology, and neurosurgical technique have better delineated the underlying pathophysiology of these lesions with ongoing refinement and revision of classification schemes. One of the more commonly used classification schemes is that proposed by Anson and Spetzler (1992), who type spinal AVMs as in the following discussion.

Type I AVMs are synonymous with dural arteriovenous fistulae (DAVFs), the most frequently encountered AVM of the cord (Wong 1999). The lesions arise outside the cord as high pressure, slow-flow shunts typically fed by a transdural vessel emptying directly into a spinal medullary vein. Venous hypertension transmitted back to the cord, rather that vascular steal, is considered to be the primary cause of symptoms in DAVFs.

Types II and III AVMs represent intramedullary high-pressure, high-flow vascular malformations. Type II, or glomus, AVMs are characterized as compact vascular masses that can occur throughout the cord. The lesions are fed by vessels from the anterior or posterior spinal arteries, demonstrate a nidus, and, internally, have no intervening cord parenchyma (Wong 1999). Type III, or juvenile, AVMs are similar to Type II but are larger, sprawling malformations. They may span several segments, internally entrap portions of the cord, and show large extramedullary components (Wong 1999). They are also supplied by branches of the anterior or posterior spinal arteries. Both Types II and III AVMs may have multiple feeders and tend to develop varicosities and feeding pedicle aneurysms. Vascular steal, venous hypertension, and mass effects lead to myelopathic changes and progressive neurologic deterioration.

Type IV AVMs are intradural perimedullary AVMs that lack a nidus (as seen in Types II and III) and result from a direct fistula connecting the spinal arteries to a draining vein (Wong 1999). They arise from feeders of the spinal arteries, occur typically on the ventral cord surface and often near the conus. These lesions are further subdivided by flow rate and vascular engorgement. Because of their superficial location, smaller, slower-flowing lesions may be obscured by CSF flow pulsation.

Spinal cavernous malformations are a less common type of vascular malformation distinct from spinal AVMs. These lesions lack an arteriovenous shunt. They are slow-flow lesions, most often intramedullary, with no feeding vessels or large draining veins. Pathologically spinal cavernous malformations have a "mulberry-like" appearance formed by focally enlarged capillary and sinusoidal spaces. They are indistinguishable from similar lesions more commonly found in the brain.

Imaging Findings. Plain films of the spine are rarely helpful in the evaluation of spinal AVMs. Myelography, although sensitive in the detection of extramedullary AVMs, is much more limited in detecting intramedullary lesions and myelopathic changes. Although CT, with or without myelography, can show focal cord widening, atrophy, and ectatic vessels, it is time intensive and exposes patients to high radiation doses. MR is the modality of choice when screening for spinal vascular malformations.

In cases of Type I AVMs findings may be subtle and the radiologist must carefully examine the cord for both direct and indirect changes. Typical MR findings with Type I AVMs include spinal cord enlargement, central cord T2 prolongation, cord T1 prolongation, scalloping of the cord surface, serpentine perimedullary flow voids, and dilated perimedullary veins on administration of contrast agent (Gilbertson 1995, Jones 1997, Larsson 1991, Terwey 19989). The most sensitive sign of a DAVF is intramedullary T2 hyperintensity; however, this finding is nonspecific (Gilbertson 1995) and can be seen in a variety of cord processes. Dilated branches of the spinal arteries and coronal venous plexus create the more specific finding of serpentine flow voids about the cord on T2 images, and a "sawtooth" or scalloped appearance on T1 images (Fig. 9–9). Note should be made that pulsating CSF and flow artifact is an important mimicker of this characteristic finding. Use of cardiac gated imaging and follow-up with conventional myelography in cases of equivocal MRI results has been advocated (Halbach 1993, Rosenblum 1987).

In cases of Types II, III, and IV AVMs the malformation is often more clearly seen as an intramedullary or extramedullary collection of ectatic, entangled vessels on multiple sequences. MR is quite sensitive in delineating areas of vascular ectasia, cord expansion, edema, hemorrhage, and extramedullary extension (Hurst 1996) (Fig. 9–10). In all cases of AVMs intravascular gadolinium often improves conspicuity of abnormal vessels, particularly in smaller,

more subtle lesions. Because CSF pulsation may also obscure Type VI AVMs, cardiac gating and myelography should be considered in cases of high clinical suspicion but uncertain MR results (Halbach 1993, Rosenblum 1987). Although MR is quite sensitive in identifying AVMs and myelopathic sequelae, locating of the exact level of the nidus, the number and size of feeding vessels, aneurysms, varices, routes of drainage and paths of collateral supply are necessary in therapeutic considerations. Ultimately, this information is only clearly provided by arteriography, which has the added advantage of possible concomitant embolotherapy.

Cavernous malformations are best evaluated with MRI because they are considered to be arteriographically occult. Imaging characteristics are similar to those of cerebral cavernous malformations and typically demonstrate a well-circumscribed intramedullary lesion with different stages of blood breakdown products (Fig. 9–11). Often a dark hemosiderin ring with "blooming" on gradient-echo images is present. Gradient-recalled sequences can be particularly sensitive in detecting spinal cavernous malformations (Labauge 1998). Prominent surrounding vessels and flow voids are not seen. Multiple lesions may occur throughout the neuraxis, thus imaging of the entire cord and brain should be considered (Bourgouin 1992).

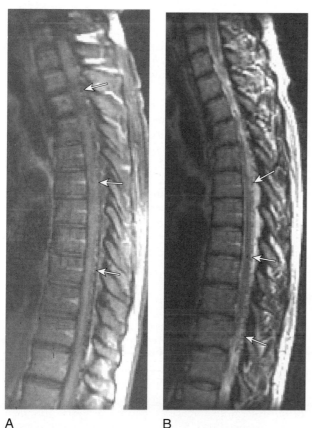

A   B

FIGURE 9–9

Dural arteriovenous malformation. *A,* Sagittal T1WI demonstrates multiple superficial flow voids created by dilated spinal veins and coronal venous plexus, with a "sawtooth" appearance. *B,* Sagittal T2WI again demonstrates dilated spinal veins *(arrows).*

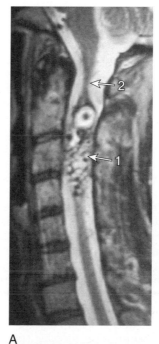
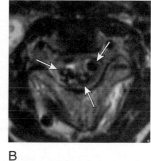

A   B

FIGURE 9–10

Intramedullary arteriovenous malformation (AVM). *A,* Sagittal T1WI demonstrates a typical intramedullary AVM, with the characteristic tangle of flow voids from prominent vessels *(arrow).* There is atrophy at the cervicomedullary junction *(arrow 2),* likely due to chronic ischemia from vascular steal or previous infarct. *B,* Axial T2WI demonstrates multiple flow voids *(arrows)* within the spinal canal.

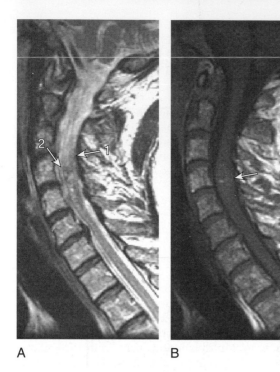
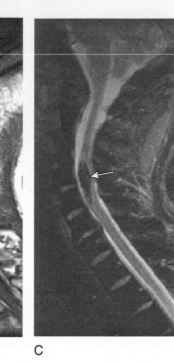

A   B   C

FIGURE 9–11

Cavernous malformation of the cervical cord with recent hemorrhage. *A,* Sagittal T2WI shows cord expansion and heterogeneous signal changes (*arrow 1*). There is a subtle intramedullary hemosiderin ring (*arrow 2*), indicative of past bleeding. *B,* Sagittal T1WI reveal vague high signal within the cord (*arrow*). *C,* Sagittal gradient-echo images illustrate focal hematomyelia (*arrow*).

Differential Diagnosis. Separation of highly vascular tumors with prominent feeding vessels from vascular malformations may be difficult or impossible. Other disease processes can lead to similar changes of cord ischemia, edema, expansion, or hemorrhage. Typically, most other spinal tumors lack the high flow rates and degree of entangled, serpiginous flow voids characteristic of AVMs. Impedance of normal cord drainage from masses, traumatic, degenerative, or congenital spinal changes can produce prominent collateral drainage routes and degrees of venous engorgement similar to that of AVMs. In cases of intracranial subarachnoid hemorrhage without known source, examination for spinal AVMs should be considered.

Although characteristic, the appearance of spinal cavernous malformations is not considered pathognomonic. Particularly with acute hematomyelia more indicative imaging findings can be obscured. Hemorrhagic neoplasms and AVMs should be considered in the differential of spinal cavernous malformations.

Clinical Significance. Presentation with acute hemorrhage can occur in all spinal vascular malformations, although it is more typical in high-flow Types II, III, and IV AVMs. Subarachnoid hemorrhage is the most frequent of Type II AVMs, whereas chronic pain and neurologic deterioration from vascular compromise and mass effects is more common in Types III and IV AVMs. Hemorrhage is less common in Type I AVMs and has been seen with cervical cord–based lesions. In cases of unexplained intracranial subarachnoid hemorrhage, evaluation form possible spinal AVM should be considered. Usually, once a vascular malformation is identified on MRI, it will undergo further evaluation with arteriography and possible endovascular therapy. In all cases the early identification of suspect lesions and diagnosis of AVM are key to effective intervention. Long-standing effects of cord ischemia, edema, and chronic hemorrhage are often fixed or poorly reversible.

Presentations of spinal cavernous malformations range from asymptomatic to fulminant. Chronic hemorrhage leads to slowly progressive sensorimotor symptoms, whereas acute hematomyelia is the chief cause of sudden neurologic decline. Small, asymptomatic lesions may be found incidentally and are typically not treated. Whole neuraxis imaging in such cases to uncover additional lesions may be beneficial.

Reporting. Although MRI is relatively sensitive to the discovery of vascular malformations, it has a limited ability to categorize the malformations by type (St. Amour 1994). The report should describe the location of all portions, intraspinal and extraspinal, of the lesion, the extent of cord changes, and evidence of hemorrhage. Arteriography generally is necessary to identify the dominant feeding vessels, aneurysms, draining veins, and exact location of fistula or nidus. Conversely, other than excluding the possibility of an underlying AVM, arteriography plays little role in the characterization of cavernous malformations.

Spinal Meningeal Cysts

Definition. Spinal meningeal cysts are Arachnoid-lined fluid collections either herniated through the dura as diverticula (extradural arachnoid cysts) or within the dura (intradural arachnoid cysts). Nomenclature is confusing, because these lesions have been termed *meningeal cysts*, *meningeal diverticula*, *meningoceles*, *leptomeningeal cysts*, *occult intrasacral meningoceles*, *perineural cysts*, and *Tarlov cysts* (St. Amour 1994). Furthermore, most of these lesions are diverticula with communication to the subarachnoid space rather than true cysts (a noncommunicating fluid collection). The term *cyst* is embedded in the literature, however. Nabors and associates (1988) proposed a classification system based on radiographic, surgical, and histologic

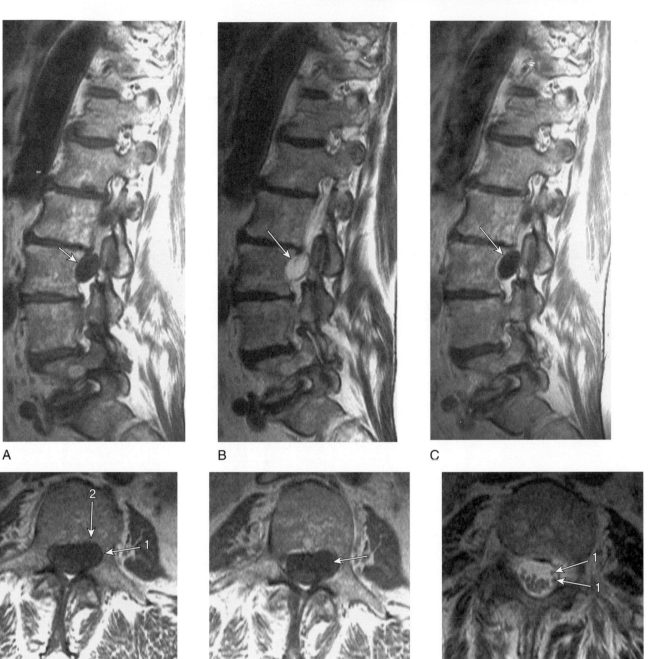

A

B

C

D

E

F

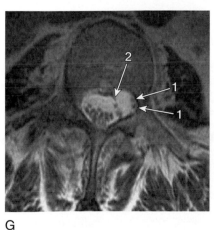

G

FIGURE 9–12

Nabors Type II meningeal cysts, also known as *nerve root diverticula.* A 71-year-old woman with right lateral thigh and right L5–S1 foraminal stenosis (not shown). *A,* Left parasagittal T1WI demonstrates multilevel degenerative changes (incompletely demonstrated on the limited images presented here); the patient had scoliosis apex to the left at the L3 level, so the scan includes the left side of the spinal canal at L3 but is at the level of the pedicles above (at L1) and below (at L5). An 18 × 10-mm smoothly marginated oval focus of T1 prolongation lies along the posterior, upper margin of the L3 vertebral body *(arrow),* where there is associated minimal bony remodeling. *B,* Left parasagittal T2WI demonstrates the lesion to have signal intensity isointense to cerebrospinal fluid *(arrow). C,* Left parasagittal T1WI following contrast administration demonstrates no contrast enhancement of the lesion *(arrow). D,* Axial T1WI prior to administration of contrast material at the level of the L3 pedicle shows thinning of the medial aspect of the L3 pedicle *(arrow 1)* and slight scalloping of the dorsal margin of the L3 vertebral body *(arrow 2). E,* Axial T1WI following contrast administration shows no contrast enhancement of the cyst *(arrow). F* and *G,* Adjacent axial T2WIs through the lower and mid-L3 pedicle demonstrate the body remodeling and also nerve roots *(arrow 1)* within the lesion. Note the dura separating the diverticulum from the thecal sac *(arrow 2).*

results in 22 cases; imaging alone may not allow specific typing (St. Amour 1994) but should allow confident diagnosis of a meningeal cyst. Meningeal cysts may form secondary to congenital holes in the dura with herniation of arachnoid through the defect and subsequent expansion. Nabors and associates (1994) classify such cysts, which do not contain nerve fibers, as Type I. Type II cysts contain nerve fibers and are either meningeal diverticula that arise proximal to the posterior root ganglion (Fig. 9–12) or perineural or Tarlov dorsal cysts, which are expansions of the perineural space beyond where the dura joins the nerve sleeve (Fig. 9–13). Type III cysts are intradural arachnoid cysts.

Imaging Findings. MRI demonstrates characteristics of a cyst, with signal intensity largely following that of CSF and lack of contrast enhancement. The lesions may demonstrate hyperintensity on T2WI relative to CSF secondary to lack of pulsation artifacts with the cyst. Type II perineural or Tarlov cysts frequently involve the sacral nerve roots and may cause extensive bony remodeling (Fig. 9–13). Type II meningeal diverticula may also expand bone (Figs. 9–12 and 9–13). Type I cysts of the thoracic spine are associated with expansion of the spinal canal, flattening of the spinal cord, and myelopathic symptoms (Fig. 9–14).

Differential Diagnosis. Cysts may superficially resemble solid masses such as meningiomas, schwannomas, or

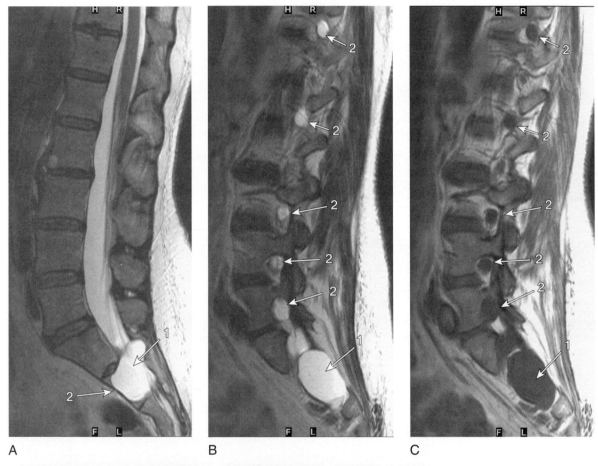

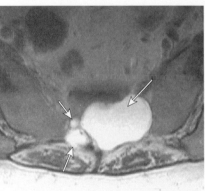
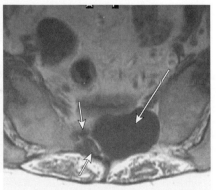

FIGURE 9–13

Multiple perineural cysts (Nabors Type II). A 68-year-old woman with low back pain, difficulty walking, and bowel incontinence. *A,* Sagittal T2WI demonstrates a large perineural cyst (*arrow 1*) with extensive bony remodeling of the S1 vertebra (*arrow 2*). *B,* Right parasagittal T2WI through the level of the pedicles demonstrates not only the sacral perineural cysts (*arrow 1*) but also multiple additional either perineural cysts or nerve root diverticula through the lumbar spine (*arrows 2*). *C,* Right parasagittal T1WI (matching *B*) demonstrates T1 prolongation through the S1 perineural cysts (*arrow 1*) as well as the lumbar lesions (*arrows 2*). *D,* Axial T2WI through the sacrum demonstrates perineural cysts with extensive sacral bony remodeling. Note T2 prolongation with the cysts (*arrows*). *E,* Axial T1WI (matching *D*) demonstrates T1 prolongation with the cysts (*arrows*).

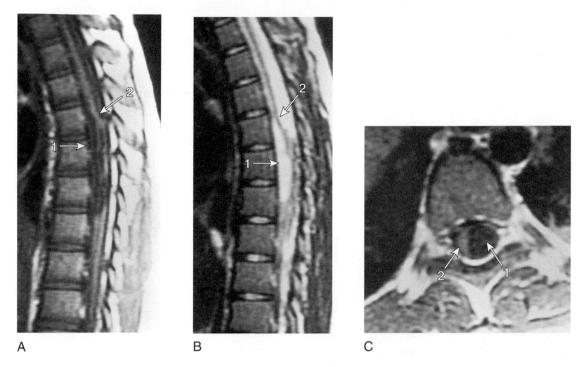

FIGURE 9–14

Thoracic arachnoid cyst. *A,* Sagittal T1WI demonstrates a large focus of T1 prolongation *(arrow 1)* anterior to the spinal cord *(arrow 2)* displacing it posteriorly. *B,* Sagittal T2WI demonstrates the same lesion shows T2 prolongation *(arrow 1)* and posterior deviation and distortion of the spinal cord *(arrow 2).* *C,* Axial T1WI demonstrates the large cyst to occupy most of the left side of the spinal canal *(arrow 1),* flattening the cord along the right side of the spinal canal *(arrow 2).*

neurofibromas. However, the T1 prolongation is greater with cysts, and there is a lack of contrast enhancement that usually allows confident diagnosis.

Clinical Significance. Type II cysts are usually asymptomatic, although, if large, they may be associated with symptoms ranging from low back pain to lower extremity dysesthesias or even bowel and bladder complaints (Fig. 9–13). Such cysts may be treated with percutaneous injection (Patel 1997). Type I cysts are more frequently symptomatic (at least when diagnosed), particularly in the thoracic spine. These usually require surgical treatment.

Reporting. Description of these lesions is generally straightforward, and the report may note that although the imaging characteristics may be impressive, the lesions are generally asymptomatic.

Epidural Lipomatosis

Definition. Excessive deposition of lipid within the epidural space of the thoracic or lumbar spine.

Imaging Findings. In the lumbar canal, fat surrounds and compresses the central thecal sac (Fig. 9–15). In the thoracic spine, excessive (>6 mm) fat is seen posterior to the spinal cord (Quint 1988) (Fig. 9–16).

Differential Diagnosis. Lipomas of the epidural space demonstrate fat signal and are focal rather than diffuse (St. Amour 1994). In the thoracic spine, epidural *lipomatosis* usually occurs *posteriorly,* whereas epidural *lipomas* usually occur *anteriorly* (St. Amour 1994). Other tissues (e.g., epidural tumor, abscess) that may diffusely involve the

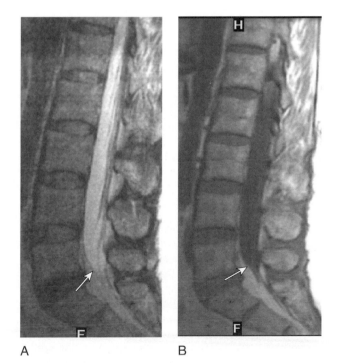

FIGURE 9–15

Lumbar epidural lipomatosis. A 60-year-old patient with low back and bilateral leg pain. *A,* Sagittal T2WI demonstrates tapering of the distal thecal sac, which is surrounded by fat *(arrow).* Because of the similar signal intensity of fat and cerebrospinal fluid on T2WI, this finding is subtle. *B,* Sagittal T1WI also demonstrates a tapered distal thecal sac *(arrow)* that is quite narrowed at the L5–S1 disc level secondary to surrounding fat. This finding is much more conspicuous on T1WI than on T2WI.

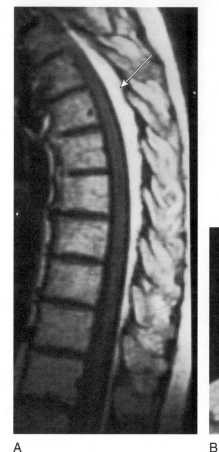

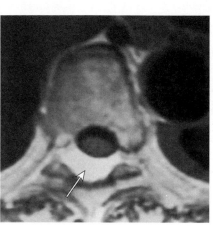

A   B

FIGURE 9-16

Thoracic epidural lipomatosis. *A,* Sagittal T1WI demonstrates extensive epidural fat *(arrow)* posterior to the spinal thoracic cord. *B,* Axial T1WI also demonstrates extensive epidural fat *(arrow)* posterior to the spinal cord.

epidural space demonstrate different imaging characteristics. In particular, these tissues generally display T1 prolongation rather than the T1 shortening seen with fat.

Clinical Significance. Epidural lipomatosis is usually secondary to exogenous steroid administration (Gero 1989, Quint 1988, Roy-Camille 1991, St. Amour 1994). Patients develop nonspecific symptoms including back pain, radiculopathy, or myelopathic symptoms (Fessler 1992, Randall 1986). In patients with rapidly developing or severe neurologic symptoms (foot drop, paresthesias, cauda equina syndrome) surgery probably will be considered and may be undertaken early. Patients with a more gradual onset of symptoms are generally treated conservatively with, if possible, tapering of the steroids: several reports have indicated improvement of symptoms and decreased epidural fat on imaging in patients following reduction of steroid dosage (St. Amour 1994, Quint 1988).

Reporting. The report should state the level and severity of the spinal canal narrowing associated with the epidural lipomatosis. It may be difficult to definitely ascribe symptoms to what appears to be overabundant fat within the epidural space, and a given patient's symptoms may be secondary to concurrent degenerative changes rather than the epidural lipomatosis itself. In addition, correlation with any history of steroid use is necessary: the diagnosis of epidural lipomatosis is unlikely (although possible) in the absence exogenous steroids (Gero 1989).

Paget's Disease

Definition. Paget's disease is a disease of unknown etiology (possibly a viral infection of osteoblasts) resulting in bone resorption followed by bone repair (Resnick 1988). The repair is imperfect, however, resulting in a number of characteristic abnormalities including bony enlargement, sclerosis, and trabecular and cortical thickening.

Imaging Findings. There are multiple imaging findings within the spine, including bony enlargement with or without resultant stenosis, abnormal signal intensity within the marrow (Fig. 9–17), basilar invagination, and thickening of the bony cortex or trabeculae (Hayes 1989, Roberts 1989, St. Amour 1994). Bone marrow signal intensity within areas of Paget's disease varies greatly, demonstrating T1 prolongation/T2 prolongation in areas of fibrovascular tissue (and thus mimicking tumor, fracture, and other causes of increased free water in the marrow), T1 prolongation/T1 shortening in areas of sclerotic bone (and mimicking blastic metastatic deposits, Modic Type III changes, and other causes of decreased free water in the marrow), and T1 shortening/T2 prolongation in areas of fat deposition. If cortical and trabecular thickening and bony enlargement are not present or prominent, these marrow patterns may be quite confusing. Two descriptive terms used in describing the plain film appearance of Paget's disease in the spine are a *picture frame* vertebral body, referring to the thickened

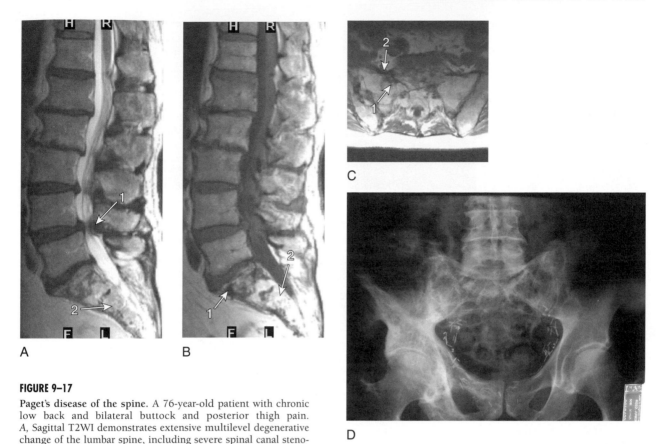

FIGURE 9–17

Paget's disease of the spine. A 76-year-old patient with chronic low back and bilateral buttock and posterior thigh pain. *A,* Sagittal T2WI demonstrates extensive multilevel degenerative change of the lumbar spine, including severe spinal canal stenosis at L4–5 secondary to degenerative disc bulging and facet arthropathy *(arrow 1).* There is extensive abnormal signal intensity with the sacrum, with an inhomogeneous appearance of mixed T2 shortening and prolongation *(arrow 2). B,* Sagittal T1WI demonstrates inhomogeneity as well, with foci of T1 prolongation *(arrow 1)* in the more superior sacrum and T1 shortening *(arrow 2)* in the inferior sacrum. *C,* Axial T1WI through the upper sacrum demonstrates diffuse textural abnormality. There is thickening of trabeculae *(arrow 1)* and the anterior cortex of the sacrum *(arrow 2). D,* Anteroposterior plain film of the pelvis demonstrates typical cortical and trabecular thickening of Paget's disease.

cortex around the margins of the vertebral body, and the *ivory* vertebral body, referring to relatively uniform sclerosis of the vertebral body.

Differential Diagnosis. Abnormal marrow signal intensity (usually T1 and T2 prolongation) may be seen in any of several marrow replacement processes (see Chapter 4); the differentiation of these processes from Paget's disease rests on recognition of the thickened cortex and trabeculae as well as correlation with clinical history and correlation with classic findings on plain films (Fig. 9–17). Few processes may result in enlargement of bone. Occasionally, slow-growing primary tumors expand rather than destroy bone, and these lesions are not associated with trabecular or cortical thickening; AVMs resulting in increased blood flow to a vertebra may also result in increased size of a vertebral body, but, again, usually no trabecular or cortical thickening is present.

Clinical Significance. Paget's disease is often asymptomatic in the pelvis or skull, but Paget's disease of the spine may be associated with symptomatic spinal stenosis. The reformed bone in Paget's disease is weaker than normal bone and thus more prone to fracture. Rarely, Paget's disease may undergo malignant degeneration, and in these cases there may be an associated soft tissue mass.

Reporting. Making the diagnosis of Paget's disease on the basis of the MRI alone may be difficult because the

imaging findings may be far less characteristic than those seen on plain films. In those cases where the disease is suspected, correlation with the clinical history and plain films is essential. If the patient is known to have Paget's disease, an assessment of whether this represents the symptom producing lesion or not is important: the Paget's disease may be an incidental finding, or it may be the cause of the patient's pain from stenosis, fracture through weakened bone, or malignant degeneration (Boutin 1998).

Idiopathic Spinal Cord Herniation

Definition. Anterior displacement of the thoracic spinal cord, apparently through a congenital defect of the dura (Miyaguchi 2001, Wada 2000).

Imaging Findings. MRI and CT-myelogram images demonstrate anterior displacement of the spinal cord, absence of ventral subarachnoid space, and an "empty canal" behind the cord (Miyaguchi 2001, Wada 2000) (Fig. 9–18).

Differential Diagnosis. Thoracic arachnoid cysts may demonstrate CSF signal intensity and displace and flatten the spinal cord but will usually not cause the drastic and abrupt curvature of the spinal cord seen in idiopathic spinal cord herniation. Although dorsally located tumors may cause anterior displacement of the spinal cord, tumors

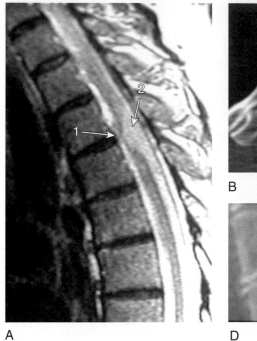

A

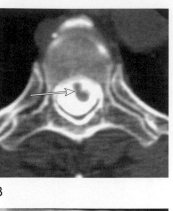

B

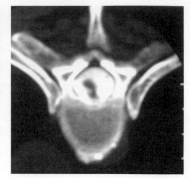

C

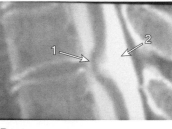

D

FIGURE 9–18

Idiopathic herniation of the spinal cord. *A,* Sagittal T2WI demonstrates abrupt anterior displacement and flattening of the spinal cord *(arrow 1)* along with expansion of the subarachnoid space posteriorly *(arrow 2).* *B,* Axial CT-myelogram done in a supine position demonstrates an abnormal configuration of the spinal cord *(arrow 1),* with a portion of the cord herniated through an anterior dural defect. *C,* Axial CT-myelogram done in a prone position shows a fixed position of the spinal cord without change from study done in the supine position *(B). D,* Sagittal reconstruction from CT-myelogram shows abrupt anterior deviation of the spinal cord *(arrow 1)* and expansion of the posterior subarachnoid space *(arrow 2).*

demonstrate contrast enhancement and also do not follow CSF signal intensity exactly on all imaging sequences.

Clinical Significance. Idiopathic spinal cord herniation may cause muscle atrophy and weakness in the lower extremity, occasionally with contralateral sensory deficit (Brown-Sequard syndrome).

Reporting. Suspecting this rare diagnosis relies on knowledge of its specific and peculiar appearance (Fig. 9–18). The level of the lesion, degree of spinal cord flattening, and any associated disc abnormality should be reported (Miyaguchi 2001).

References

Arthropathies Affecting the Spine

Ahn NU, Sponseller PD, Ahn UM, Nallamshetty L, Kuszyk BS, Zinreich SJ. Dural ectasia is associated with back pain in Marfan syndrome. Spine 2000; 25:1562–1568.

Aisen AM, Martel W, Ellis JH, McCune WJ. Cervical spine involvement in rheumatoid arthritis: MR imaging. Radiology 1987; 165:159–163

Bilgen IG, Yunten N, Usten EE, Oksel F, Gumusdis G. Adhesive arachnoiditis causing cauda equina syndrome in ankylosing spondylitis: CT and MRI demonstration of dural calcification and a dorsal dural diverticulum. Neuroradiogy 1999; 41:508–511.

Bundschuh C, Modic MT, Kearney F, Morris R, Deal C. Rheumatoid arthritis of the cervical spine: surface-coil MR imaging. AJR Am J Roentgenol 1988; 151:181–187.

Kaplan P, Resnick D, Murphy M, Heck L, Phalen J, Egan D, Rutsky E. Destructive non-infectious spondyloarthropathy in hemodialysis patients: a report of four cases. Radiology 1987; 162: 241–244.

Larsson EM, Holtas S, Zygmunt S. Preoperative and postoperative MR imaging of the craniocervical junction in rheumatoid arthritis. AJR Am J Roentgenol 1989; 152:561–566.

Oostveen JCM, Roozeboom AR, van de Laar MAFJ, Heeres J, den Boer JA, Lindeboom SF. Functional turbo spin-echo magnetic resonance imaging versus tomography for evaluating cervical spine involvement in rheumatoid arthritis. Spine 1998; 23:1237–1244.

Rafto SE, Dalinka MK, Schiebler ML, Burk DL, Kricun ME. Spondyloarthropathy of the cervical spine in long-term hemodialysis. Radiology 1988, 166:201–204.

St. Amour TE, Hodges SC, Laakman RW, Tamas DE. Rheumatoid arthritis. In St. Amour TE, Hodges SC, Laakman RW, Tamas DE (eds). MRI of the Spine. New York, Raven Press, 1994.

Sundaram M, Seelig R, Pohl D. Vertebral erosions in patients undergoing maintenance hemodialysis for chronic renal failure. Am J Roentgenol 1987; 149: 323–327

Takasita M, Matsumoto H, Uchinou S, Tsumura H, Torisu T. Atlantoaxial subluxation associated with ossification of posterior longitudinal ligament of the cervical spine. Spine 2000; 25:2133–2136.

Wolfe BK, O'Keefe D, Mitchell DM, Tchang SPK. Rheumatoid arthritis of the cervical spine: early and progressive radiographic features. Radiology 1987; 165:145–148.

Demyelinating Disease

Glasier CM, Robbins MB, Davis PC, Ceballos E, Bates SR. Clinical, neurodiagnostic, and MR findings in children with spinal and brain stem multiple sclerosis. AJNR Am J Neuroradiol 1995; 16:87–95.

Miller DH, Barkhof F, Kappos L, Scotti G, Thompson AJ. Magnetic resonance imaging in monitoring the treatment of multiple sclerosis: concerted action guidelines. J Neurol 1991; 54:683–688.

St. Amour TE, Hodges SC, Laakman RW, Tamas DE. Multiple sclerosis. In St. Amour TE, Hodges SC, Laakman RW, Tamas DE (eds). MRI of the Spine. New York, Raven Press, 1994.

Tartaglino LM, Friedman DP, Flanders AE, Lubin FD, Knobler RL, Leim M. Multiple sclerosis in the spinal cord: MR appearance and correlation with clinical parameters. Radiology 1995; 195:725–732.

Trop I, Bourgouin PM, Lapierre Y, Duquette P, Wolfson CM, Duong HD, Trudel GC. Multiple sclerosis of the spinal cord: diagnosis and follow-up with contrast-enhanced MR and correlation with clinical activity. AJNR Am J Neuroradiol 1998; 19:1025–1033.

Vascular Malformations

Anson JA, Spetzler RF. Classification of spinal arteriovenous malformations and implications for treatment. Barrows Neurol Instit Q 1992; 8:2–8.

Bourgouin PM, Tampieri D, Johnston W, Steward J, Melancon D, Ethier R: Multiple occult vascular malformations of the brain and spinal cord: MRI diagnosis. Neuroradiology 1992; 34:110–111.

Gilbertson JR, Miller GM, Goldman MS, March WR: Spinal dural arteriovenous fistulas: MR and myelographic findings. AJNR Am J Neuroradiol 1995; 16:2049–2057.

Halbach VV, Higashida RT, Dowd CF: Treatment of giant intradural (perimedullary) arteriovenous fistulas: clinical study. Neurosurgery 1993; 33:972–980.

Hurst RW: Spinal vascular disorders. In Atlas SW (ed). Magnetic Resonance Imaging of the Brain and Spine, 2nd ed. Philadelphia, Lippincott-Raven, 1996, pp 1387–1412.

Jones BV, Ernst RJ, Tomsick TA, Tew J Jr: Spinal dural arteriovenous fistulas: recognizing the spectrum of magnetic resonance imaging findings. J Spinal Cord Med 1997; 20:42–48.

Larsson EM, Desai P, Hardin CW, Story J, Jinkins JR: Venous infarction of the spinal cord resulting from dural arteriovenous fistula: MR imaging findings. AJNR Am J Neuroradiol 1991; 12:739–743.

Labauge P, Laberge S, Brunereau L, Levy C, Tournier-Lasserve E. Hereditary cerebral cavernous angiomas: clinical and genetic features in 57 French families. Lancet 1998; 352:1892–1897.

Rosenblum B, Oldfield EH, Doppman JL, et al: Spinal arteriovenous malformations: a comparison of dural arteriovenous fistulas and intradural AVMs in 81 patients. J Neurosurg 1987; 67:795–802.

St. Amour TE, Hodges SC, Laakman RW, Tamas DE. Vascular malformations. In St. Amour TE, Hodges SC, Laakman RW, Tamas DE (eds). MRI of the Spine. New York, Raven Press, 1994.

Terwey B, Becker H, Thron AK, Vahldiek G: Gadolinium-DTPA–enhanced MR imaging of spinal dural arteriovenous fistulas. J Comput Assist Tomogr 1989; 13:30–37.

Wong JH, Kim JH, Awad IA: Pathological features of spinal vascular malformations. In Barrow DL, Awad IA (eds): Spinal Vascular Malformations. Park Ridge, IL, American Association of Neurological Surgeons, 1999, pp 9–21.

Spinal Meningeal Cysts

Nabors MW, Pait TG, Byrd EB, Karim NO, Davis DO, Kobrine AI, Rizzoli HV. Updated assessment and current classification of spinal meningeal cysts. J Neurosurg 1988; 68:366–377.

Patel MR, Louie W, Rachlin J. Percutaneous fibrin glue therapy of meningeal cysts of the sacral spine. AJR Am J Roentgenol 1997; 168:367–370.

St. Amour TE, Hodges SC, Laakman RW, Tamas DE. Arachnoid (meningeal) cysts. In St. Amour TE, Hodges SC, Laakman RW, Tamas DE (eds). MRI of the Spine. New York, Raven Press, 1994.

Epidural Lipomatosis

Fessler RG, Johnson DL, Brown FD, Erickson RK, Reid SA, Kranzler L. Epidural lipomatosis in steroid-treated patients. Spine 1992; 17:183–199.

Gero BT, Chynn KY. Symptomatic spinal epidural lipomatosis without exogenous steroid intake. Neuroradiology 1989; 31:190–192.

Quint DJ, Boulos RS, Sanders WP, Mehta BA, Patel SC, Tiel RL. Epidural Lipomatosis. Radiology 1988; 169:485–490.

Randall BC, Muraki AS, Osborn RE, Brown F. Epidural lipomatosis with lumbar radiculopathy: CT appearance. J Comput Assist Tomogr 1986; 10:1039–1041.

Roy-Camille R, Mazel CH, Husson JL, Saillant G. Symptomatic spinal epidural lipomatosis induced by a long-term steroid treatment: review of the literature and report of two additional cases. Spine 1991; 16:1365–1371.

St. Amour TE, Hodges SC, Laakman RW, Tamas DE. Epidural lipomas, angiolipomas, and epidural lipomatosis. In St. Amour TE, Hodges SC, Laakman RW, Tamas DE (eds). MRI of the Spine. New York, Raven Press, 1994.

Paget's Disease

Boutin RD, Spitz DJ, Newman JS, Lenchik L, Steinbach LS. Complications in Paget disease at MR imaging. Radiology 1998; 209:641–651.

Hayes CW, Jensen ME, Conway WF. Non-neoplastic lesions of vertebral bodies: findings in magnetic resonance imaging. Radiographics 1989; 9:883–903.

Resnick D. Paget disease of bone: current status and a look back to 1943 and earlier. AJR Am J Roentgenol 1988; 150:249–256.

Roberts MC, Kressel HY, Fallon MD, Zlatkin MB, Dalinka MK. Paget disease: MR imaging findings. Radiology 1989; 173:341–345.

St. Amour TE, Hodges SC, Laakman RW, Tamas DE. Differential diagnosis of extradural tumors. In St. Amour TE, Hodges SC, Laakman RW, Tamas DE (eds). MRI of the Spine. New York, Raven Press, 1994.

Idiopathic Spinal Cord Herniation

Miyaguchi M, Nakamura H, Shakudo M, Inoue Y, Yamano Y. Idiopathic spinal cord herniation associated with intervertebral disc extrusion: a case report and review of the literature. Spine 2001; 26:1090–1094.

Wada E, Yonenobu K, Kang J. Idiopathic spinal cord herniation: report of three cases and review of the literature. Spine 2000; 25:1984–1988.

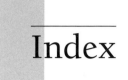

Index

Note: Page numbers followed by f and t indicate figures and tables, respectively. Page numbers followed by n indicate footnotes.

A

Abscess
  epidural, 266, 268, 273f, 277
  paraspinal, 266, 275, 277
  retropharyngeal, 354
  with infectious spondylitis, 268, 271, 273f
Acute disseminating encephalomyelitis (ADEM), 358
Age, and tumor characteristics, 211
Aging
  bone marrow changes with, 208, 221f
  vertebral body wedge deformity with, 237
Allograft, bone, 132
Anatomy
  of cervical spine, 7–9, 7f–9f
  of lumbar spine, 1–6, 1f–6f
  of thoracic spine, 6–7, 6f–7f
Aneurysmal bone cysts, imaging characteristics of, 211
Angiolipoma, 204f
  epidural lesion caused by, 204, 209f–210f
Ankylosing spondylitis, 354, 355f, 356f
Annular fissure, 19–22, 27f, 28f
  in disc bulges, 29
Anterior longitudinal ligament, ossification of, 354
Arachnoid cyst(s)
  differential diagnosis of, 296, 300–301
  extradural, 360
  intradural, 360
  thoracic, 362, 363f
Arachnoiditis, postoperative, 162, 184f–187f
Arteriovenous fistulas, 358–360
Arteriovenous malformations
  dural, 359, 359f
  intramedullary, 358–360, 359, 359f
  spinal, 358–360
    classification of, 358
Arthritis, rheumatoid. See Rheumatoid arthritis.
Arthropathy
  facet. See Facet joint(s), disease of.
  spinal involvement in, 353–357
Astrocytoma, 192, 193f, 197
Athletes, spondylolysis in, 305
Atlantoaxial subluxation, 353, 354
Autograft, bone, 132

B

Baastrup's disease, 66, 67f
Back pain. See also Degenerative disease; Pain.
  in degenerative disease, 22–25
  in infectious spondylitis, 259
  prevalence of, 11
  treatment of, success of, factors affecting, 15
Bamboo spine, 354
Block vertebrae, 283t

C

Bone
  cortex of, post-traumatic interruption of, 234f, 235–236, 236t, 237f–239f
  malalignment of, after fracture, 242–245, 245f
Bone fragments
  abnormal, 236, 236t, 237–242
    with fractures, 237
    with osteophytic spurring, 237
    with un-united ossification center, 237
  in spondylolysis, 314–317
Bone graft(s), 132, 136f, 137f
  pseudarthrosis through, 157, 164f–168f
  resorption of, 157, 169f–170f
Bone island. See Enostosis.
Bone marrow
  abnormalities of, in spondylolysis, 308, 323f
  fatty, 208, 221f, 222f
    adjacent to pars defect, 308, 323f
  myeloid depletion pattern in
    after radiation therapy, 208, 215f, 220f
    in myelofibrosis, 208, 221f
  signal intensity of
    abnormal, with reconversion pattern, 211, 222f–223f
    in infectious discitis, 259f–262f, 261–264
    with wedge fractures of vertebral bodies, 237, 242f, 243f
  subchondral. See Subchondral bone marrow.
  yellow, conversion of, to red marrow, 211, 222f–223f
Bone scan(s)
  in degenerative disease, 16
  in postoperative patient, 137
  in spondylolysis, 305–306, 306t, 306f–307f, 315f, 327f–329f
    reporting of, 338
  in trauma patient, 233, 237, 241f, 242, 251f, 252
  of tumors, 192, 217
  of wedge fractures of vertebral bodies, 236–237, 241f
Bony spurs, in spondylolysis, 314–317
Brain tumor, drop metastases from, 197, 200, 200f
Bright disc sign, 211, 219f, 223f
Butterfly vertebrae, 283t, 300, 302f

C

Calcification. See also Ossification.
  of intervertebral disc, 19, 20f
  of ligamentum flavum, 66–68, 68f
  of posterior longitudinal ligament, 66–68, 68f
Cauda equina syndrome, 37–38, 46
  in ankylosing spondylitis, 354
Caudal regression syndrome, 282t, 283t, 284
  blunted conus in, 284, 290f
  occult, 283t, 296–298

Caudal regression syndrome (*Continued*)
  with tethered cord and lipomyelomeningocele, 295f, 296
Cavernous angioma, 197
Cavernous malformations, spinal, 358, 359, 360f
Cerebellar tonsils, abnormally low position of, 283t
Cerebrospinal fluid (CSF)
  and neural elements, outside normal spinal canal, 282t
  in herniated meninges, outside normal spinal canal, 282t
  in spinal cord and paralleling long axis of cord, 282t
Cervical spine
  anatomy of
    on axial gradient-echo image, 8–9, 9f
    on axial images, 8–9, 9f
    on sagittal images, 7–8, 7f–8f
  degenerative disease in, 74, 77f
  disc contour abnormalities in, 48f
  disc degeneration in, 15f
  disc extrusion in, 18f
  disc herniation in, 18f, 39–42, 45f, 47f, 48f
    size of, 30, 30t
    unusual findings with, 37
  facet arthropathy of, asymmetric, 64, 64f
  fractures of
    imaging of, 233, 234f, 235f
    in ankylosing spondylitis, 354, 355f
  lumbar spine and, differences between, 39–40
  magnetic resonance imaging of, 16–18, 18f
    fast spin-echo image in, 18, 18f
    gradient-echo image in, 8–9, 9f, 18, 18f
  nerves of, numbering of, 42
  paracentral disc extrusion in, 45f
  rheumatoid arthritis of, 353f, 353–354, 354f
  segmentation anomalies of, 297f
    complex, with scoliosis, 299f
  spondylolysis in, 305
  spondylotic myelopathy and, 54–56, 60f
Chemotherapy, diffuse abnormal marrow after, 208, 215f
Chiari malformation, 197
  type I, 283t
  type II, 283t, 284
Claustrophobia, sedation for, 98
Computed tomography (CT)
  discontinuity of bony cortex on, 236, 239f
  facet joint grading scheme with, 63f
  of congenital and developmental anomalies, 281
  of degenerative disease, 16, 17f
  of gas collections, 143, 147f
  of postoperative patient, 132–137
  of sacral insufficiency fractures, 252–253, 254f, 255f
  of spinal metastases, 214
  of spondylolysis, 306, 306t, 306f–307f, 308, 309f–321f, 329
    reporting of, 338

To My Sweet Sweet Cui
for this 7th birthday!
Because she loves to read
here is another book to
keep her interested and
expand her imagination.
I hope you enjoy this book.
Love, Auntie Jessica (F)
2/15/2002

101
BEDTIME
STORIES

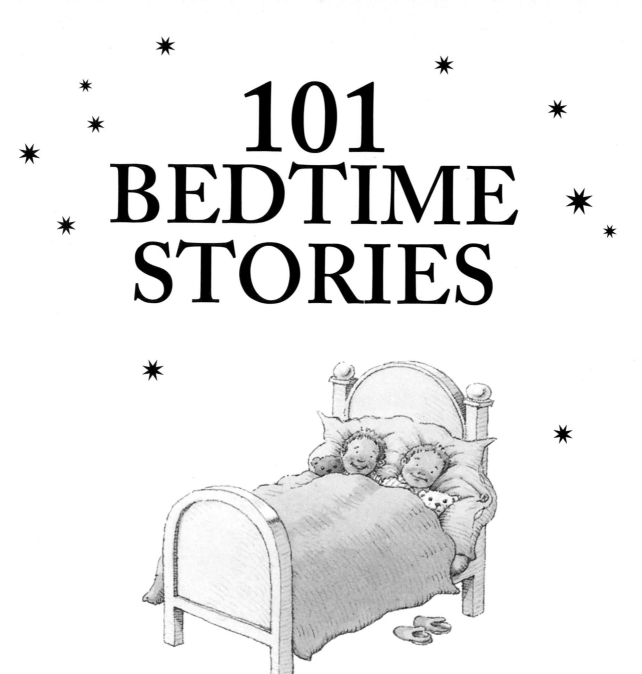

OVER 100 FAVORITE
STORIES & RHYMES

BORDERS

Contents

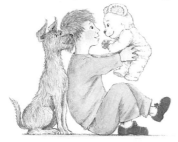
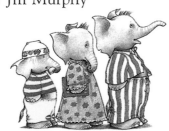

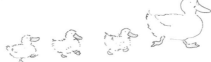
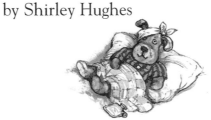
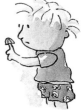
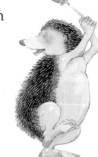

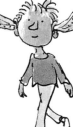
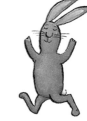
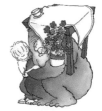
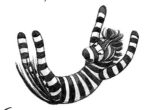
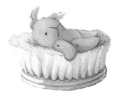
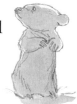
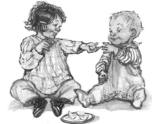

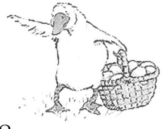
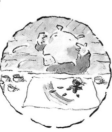

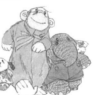
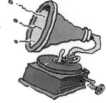
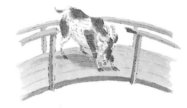
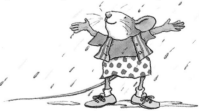

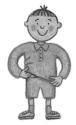
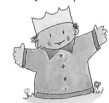
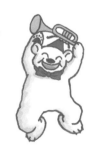
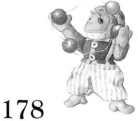
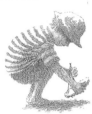
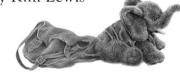

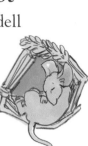
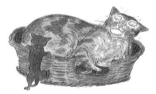
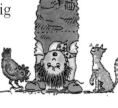
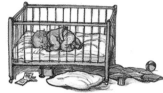
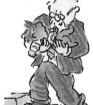
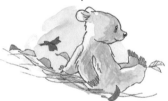
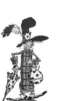
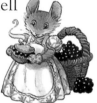
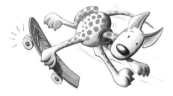

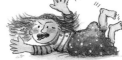
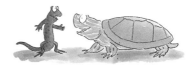
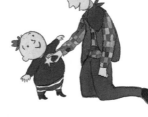
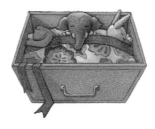
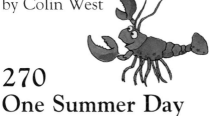
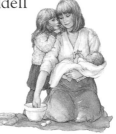

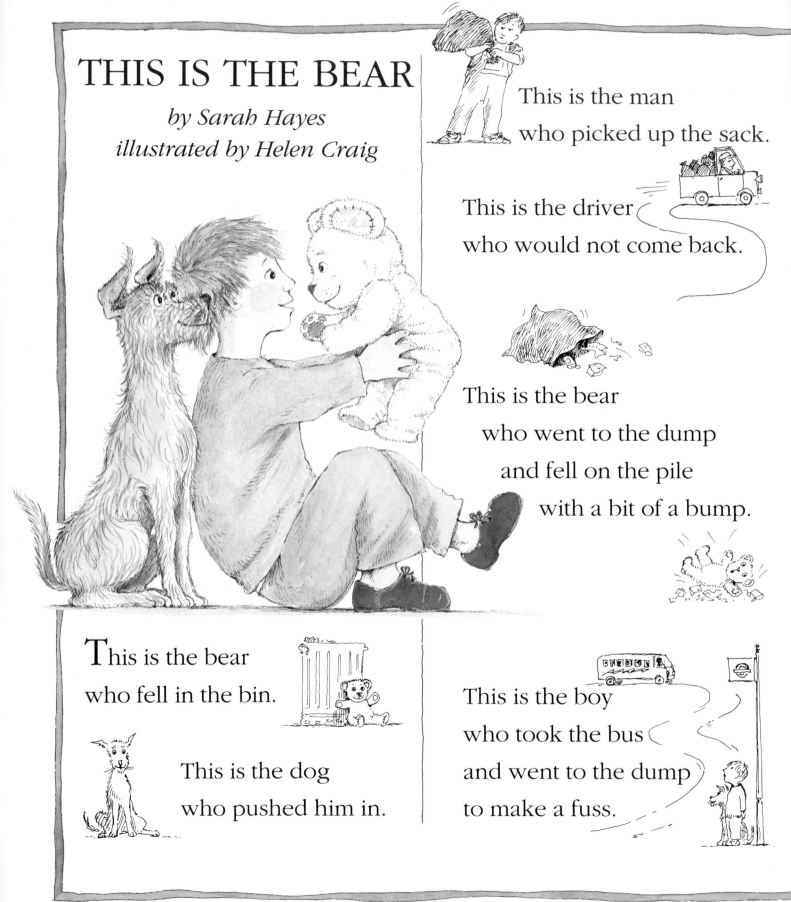

THIS IS THE BEAR

by Sarah Hayes
illustrated by Helen Craig

This is the man
who picked up the sack.

This is the driver
who would not come back.

This is the bear
who went to the dump
and fell on the pile
with a bit of a bump.

This is the bear
who fell in the bin.

This is the dog
who pushed him in.

This is the boy
who took the bus
and went to the dump
to make a fuss.

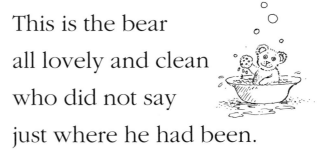

This is the man
in an awful grump
who searched and searched
and searched the dump.

This is the bear
all lovely and clean
who did not say
just where he had been.

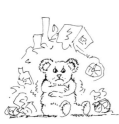

This is the bear
all cold and cross
who did not think
he was really lost.

This is the boy
who knew quite well,
but promised his friend
he would not tell.

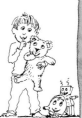

This is the dog
who smelled the smell
of a bone and a tin
and a bear as well.

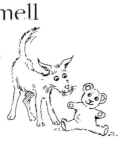

And this is the boy
who woke up in the night
and asked the bear
if he felt all right –
and was very surprised
when the bear shouted out,
"How soon can we have
another day out?"

This is the man
who drove them home –
the boy, the bear
and the dog with a bone.

Daisy Dare

by Anita Jeram

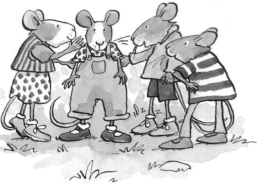

Daisy Dare did things her friends were far too scared to do.

"Just dare me," she said. "Anything you like. I'm never, *ever* scared!"

So they dared her to walk the garden wall.

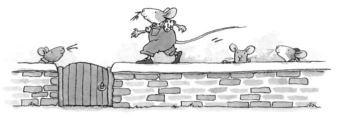

They dared her to eat a worm.

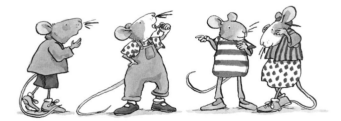

They dared her to stick out her tongue at Miss Crumb.
And she did!

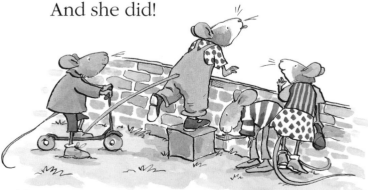

One day, Daisy's friends thought of a really scary dare to do. They whispered it to Daisy.

"I'm not doing that!" she said.

"Daisy Dare-not!" they laughed.

Daisy took a deep breath. "All right," she said. "I'll do it."

This was the dare: to take the bell off the cat's collar.

The cat was asleep. That was good. The bell slipped off easily. That was good too. But Daisy's hands trembled so much that the bell tinkled, the cat woke up and that was very, very bad!

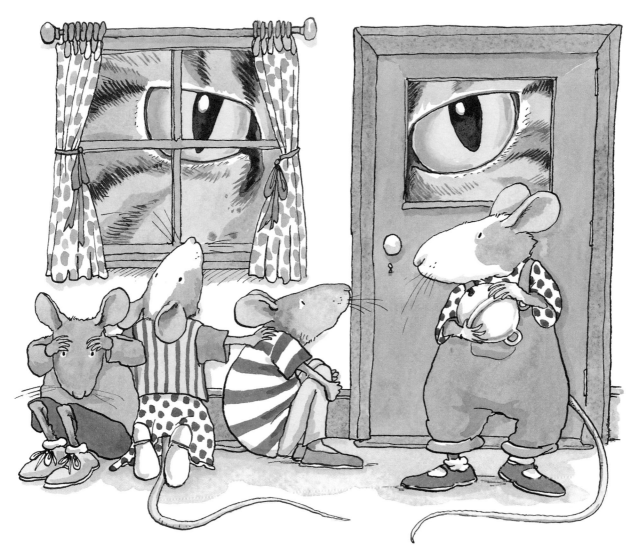

Daisy ran and ran as fast as she could, back to her friends, through the garden gate, and into the house where the cat couldn't follow.

"Phew!" said Billy.

"Wow!" gasped Joe.

"You're the bravest, most daring mouse in the whole world!" shouted Contrary Mary.

Daisy Dare grinned with pride.

"Just dare me," she said. "Anything you like… I'm only *sometimes* scared!"

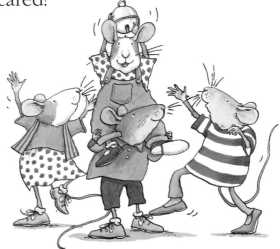

11

Chi-li the Panda

by Derek Hall • illustrated by John Butler

Chi-li loves to play with his mother. Sometimes she gives him a piggy-back and then he feels as tall as a grown-up panda.

Soon, it is dinner time. The grown-ups eat lots of bamboo shoots, crunching the juicy stems. Chi-li likes to chew the soft leaves.

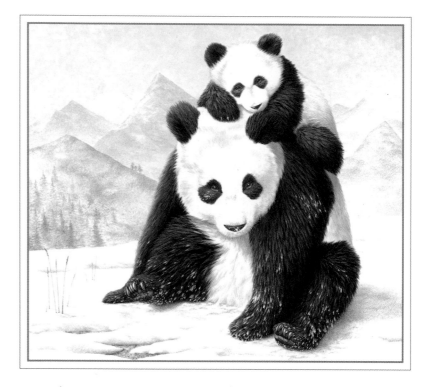

The grown-ups eat for such a long time, they always fall asleep afterwards. Chi-li scampers off to play. He rolls over and over in the snow and tumbles down a hill.

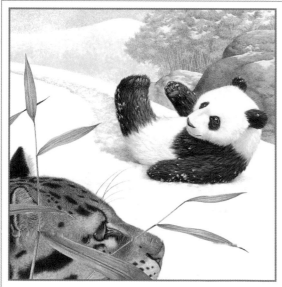

When Chi-li stops at the bottom he cannot see his mother any more. But he sees a leopard! Chi-li is very frightened.

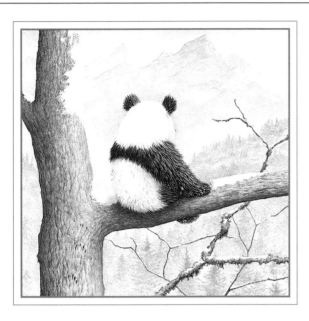

He scrambles over to the nearest tree and climbs up. Chi-li has never climbed before, and it is so easy! He digs his claws into the bark and goes up and up.

Soon, he is near the top. Chi-li feels so good up here. And he can see such a long way over the mountains and trees and snow of China.

Chi-li hears his mother crying. She is looking for him. He starts to climb down. But going down is harder than climbing up, and he slips. Plop! He lands in the snow.

Chi-li's mother is so happy. She gathers him up in her big furry arms and cuddles him. It is lovely to be warm and safe with her again.

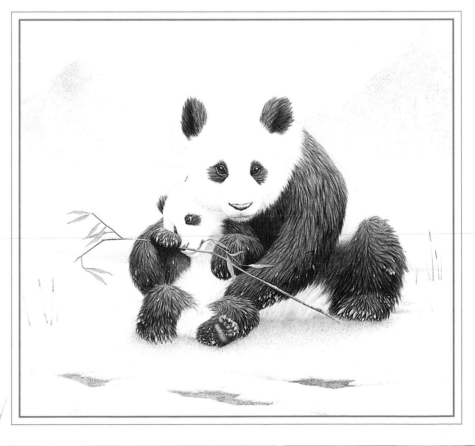

FIVE MINUTES' PEACE

by Jill Murphy

The children were having breakfast. This was not a pleasant sight.
Mrs Large took a tray from the cupboard.
She set it with a teapot, a milk jug, her favourite cup and saucer, a plate of marmalade toast and a leftover cake from yesterday. She stuffed the morning paper into her pocket and sneaked off towards the door.
"Where are you going with that tray, Mom?" asked Laura.
"To the bathroom," said Mrs Large.

"Why?" asked the other two children.
"Because I want five minutes' peace from you lot," said Mrs Large. "That's why."

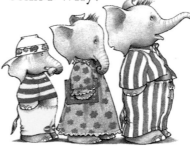

"Can we come?" asked Lester as they trailed up the stairs behind her.
"No," said Mrs Large, "you can't."
"What shall we do then?" asked Laura.
"You can play," said Mrs Large. "Downstairs. By yourselves. And keep an eye on the baby."
"I'm not a baby," muttered the little one.

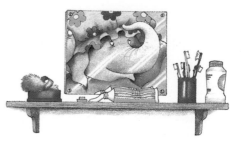

Mrs Large ran a deep, hot bath. She emptied half a bottle of bath foam into the water, plonked on her bath-hat and got in.
She poured herself a cup of tea and lay back with her eyes closed.
It was heaven.

"Can I play you my tune?" asked Lester.

Mrs Large opened one eye.

"Must you?" she asked.

"I've been practising," said Lester. "You told me to. Can I? Please, just for one minute."

"Go on then," sighed Mrs Large.

So Lester played. He played "Twinkle, Twinkle, Little Star" three and a half times. In came Laura. "Can I read you a page from my reading book?" she asked.

"No, Laura," said Mrs Large. "Go on, all of you, off downstairs."

"You let Lester play his tune," said Laura. "I heard. You like him better than me. It's not fair."

"Go on then. Just one page."

So Laura read. She read four and a half pages of "Little Red Riding Hood".

In came the little one with a trunkful of toys. "For you!" he beamed, flinging them all into the bath water.

"Thank you, dear," said Mrs Large weakly.

"Can I see the cartoons in the paper?" asked Laura.

"Can I have the cake?" asked Lester.

"Can I get in with you?" asked the little one.

Mrs Large groaned.

In the end they all got in. The little one was in such a hurry that he forgot to take off his pyjamas.

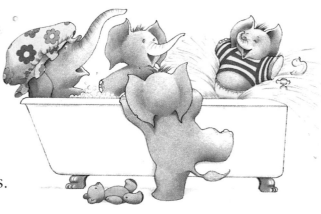

Mrs Large got out. She dried herself, put on her dressing-gown and headed for the door.

"Where are you going now, Mom?" asked Laura.

"To the kitchen," said Mrs Large.

"Why?" asked Lester.

"Because I want five minutes' peace from you lot," said Mrs Large. "That's why." And off she went downstairs, where she had three minutes and forty-five seconds of peace before they all came to join her.

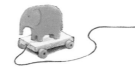

15

Tell Us a Story

by Allan Ahlberg
illustrated by
Colin McNaughton

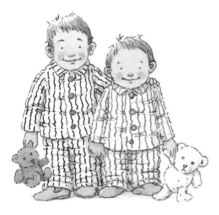

Two little boys
climbed up
to bed.

"Tell us a story, Dad,"
they said.
"Right!" said Dad.

The Pig

"There was once a pig
who ate too much
and got so big
he couldn't sit down,
he couldn't bend.

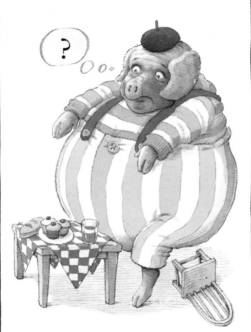

So he ate standing up
and got bigger –
The End!"

'That story's no good,
Dad," the little boys said.
"Tell us a better one
instead."
"Right!" said Dad.

The Cat

"There was once a cat
who ate so much
and got so fat

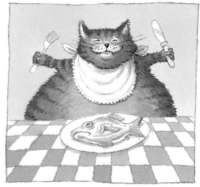

he split his fur
which he had to mend
with a sewing machine
and a zip – The End!"

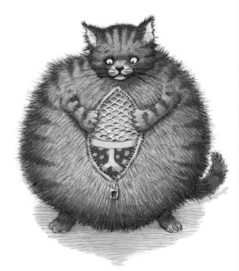

"That story's too mad,
Dad," the little boys said.
"Tell us another one
instead."
"Right!" said Dad.

The Horse

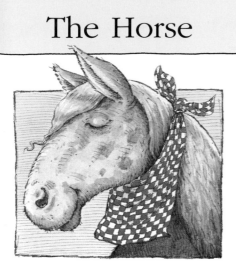

"There once was a horse who ate too much and died, of course – The End!"

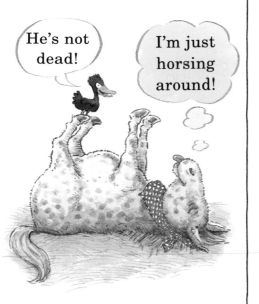

He's not dead!

I'm just horsing around!

"That story's too sad, Dad," the little boys said. "Tell us a nicer one instead." "Right!" said Dad.

The Cow

"There once was a cow who ate so much that even now she fills two fields

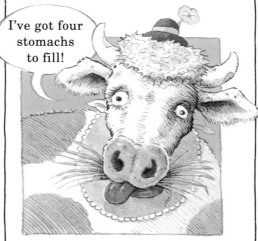

I've got four stomachs to fill!

and blocks a road, and when they milk her she has to be towed! She wins gold cups and medals too, for the creamiest milk and the *loudest* moo!"

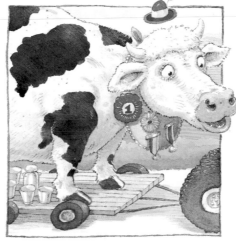

"Now that's the end," said Dad. "No more." And he shut his eyes and began to snore.

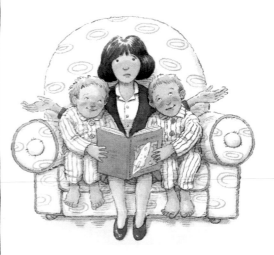

Then the two little boys climbed out of bed and crept downstairs

to their Mom instead.

The End

17

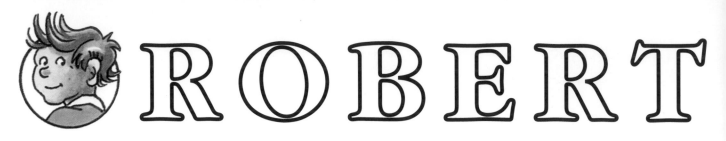

ROBERT

by Philippe

Robert lived with his mother and father in a big house. He had no brothers or sisters but he had lots of toys to play with. One day his mother came into his room. "Robert," she said, "be a little angel and run down to the shops for some biscuits. Aunt Susie is coming to tea."

On the way Robert met Mrs French. "Going shopping for your mummy?" she said. "What a good little boy you are."

At the flower stall the lady said, "That's Mrs Waters' little Robert. Isn't he a little darling?"

Mr Brown in the shop said, "Hello, little man. What can I do for you?"

"Little again!" Robert thought crossly. "Why do they all say I'm little?"

When Robert got home Aunt Susie was there.

"You little sweetie, my favourite biscuits!" she cooed. "Here, help yourself, my pet. I know what hungry tummies little boys like you always have."

"I am *not* little!" Robert screamed

I AM NOT LITTLE!!

THE GREAT

Dupasquier

furiously and he marched up to his room and slammed the door. From that moment on, Robert was a different boy. He was always staring into the mirror. "What rubbish," he'd say, "I'm not little. I'm *not*." He sulked. He did all kinds of silly things, trying to make himself look bigger.

Robert's behaviour got worse and worse. His parents were at their wits' end.

They tried everything. In the end they sent for the doctor. But that was no good. Robert bit him.

That night he dressed up as a horrible monster. "I'm a giant. I'm going to gobble you all up!" he shouted.

"This can't go on," said Mr Waters. "What the boy needs is a change."

So the next day they went on a trip to the zoo.

Robert was as horrid as ever. "I hate zoos," he said.

19

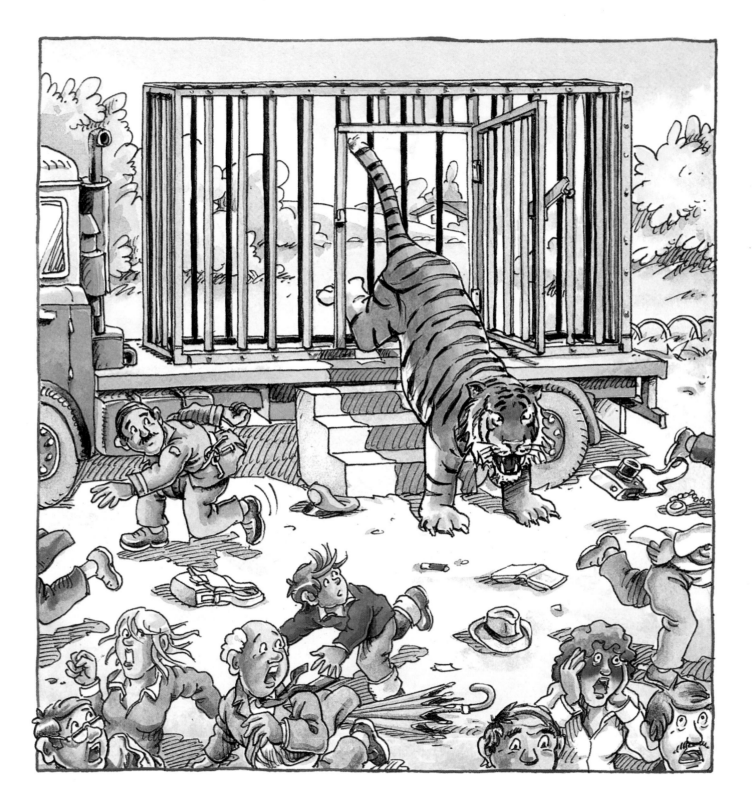

He hated the parrots; he hated the giraffes; he didn't even like the monkeys. Then a great big truck came into the zoo. On the truck was a cage and in the cage was an enormous tiger.

The keeper got up to check the bolts. "Keep back," he warned. "This fellow eats people for breakfast."

Just then a terrible thing happened. The tiger jumped at the cage door. The keeper fell over backwards. The door flew open.

The tiger leapt out. People were screaming and running everywhere. But Robert was left behind. He was standing in front of the cage. All by himself. Except for the tiger.

The tiger crouched, ready to spring. Someone screamed, "It's going to eat the little boy!"

But Robert had seen the open cage. The tiger pounced; Robert dashed inside. The tiger was right behind him. But before the tiger could reach him Robert squeezed out through the bars on the other side. No sooner had his feet touched the ground than he quickly ran round the truck. SLAM!

He had the cage door shut and bolted. The tiger was trapped.

The crowd couldn't believe it. Everyone cheered. Robert was a hero! They carried him round the zoo in triumph.

Next time he went shopping nobody called Robert little.

"My, what a big boy you are," Mrs French called as he passed.

"Stronger than a tiger," said the lady at the flower stall.

Everyone he met seemed to know about his great adventure.

"Here comes Robert the Great. Aren't we all proud of our big boy then?" said Aunt Susie the next time she came to tea.

"I'm not really big," Robert said, "or I couldn't have got through the bars of the cage, could I, Aunt Susie?"

TERRIBLE, TERRIBLE

There once was a terrible tiger, so terrible to see.
There once was a terrible tiger, as fierce as fierce can be.
There once was a terrible tiger that looked down from a tree.
There once was a terrible tiger that came creeping after me.
There once was a terrible tiger with teeth as sharp as sharp could be.
That terrible, terrible tiger – will he eat ME?
That terrible, terrible tiger, he roared … and leapt at me.

TIGER
by Colin and Jacqui Hawkins

I cuddled that terrible tiger.
He's really my kitten, you see.

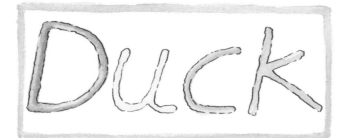

DUCK

by David Lloyd

illustrations by Charlotte Voake

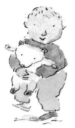

There was a time, long ago, when Tim called all animals duck.
"Duck," Tim said.
"Horse," said Granny.
"Duck," Tim said.
"Sheep," said Granny.
"Duck," Tim said.
"Speckled hen," said Granny.
So Granny took Tim to the pond.
"Duck," she said.
Tim looked and looked.
"Duck," he said.
Granny kissed him.

A little later
Tim saw a tractor.
"Truck," he said.
A little later
Tim saw a bus.
"Truck," he said.
A little later
Tim saw an old car.
"Truck," he said.
So Granny showed Tim a truck.
"Truck," she said.
Tim looked and looked.
"Truck," he said.
Granny kissed him.

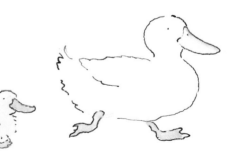

24

For some time 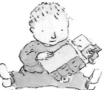 after this Tim never said a single word. He just looked and looked. He looked at his train. He looked at his truck. But he never said a single word. Then Granny took Tim to the pond again. Tim saw the duck.

He looked and looked. The duck said, "Quack!" "Duck," Tim said. "Duck," Granny said. Granny kissed Tim. Tim kissed Granny.

25

We Love Them

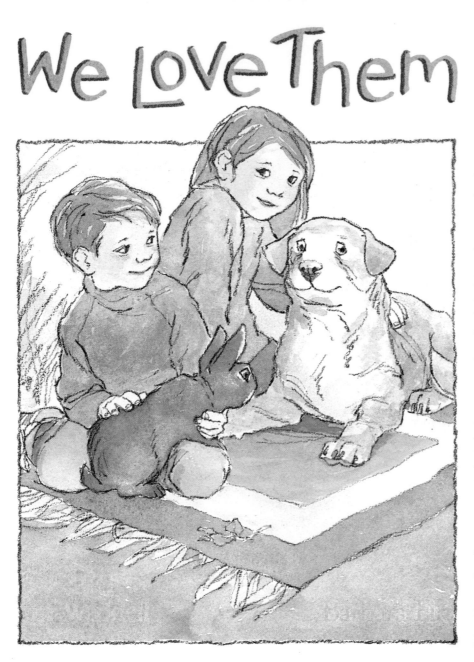

by Martin Waddell
illustrated by Barbara Firth

It lay with Ben. Ben licked it. Becky said that Ben thought it was a little dog, and it thought Ben was a big rabbit. They didn't know they'd got it wrong. Becky said we wouldn't tell them.

We called our rabbit Zoe. She stayed with Ben. She played with Ben.

We loved them.

Zoe wasn't little for very long. She got big…and bigger… and bigger still, but not as big as Ben.

But Ben was old…and one day Ben died. We were sad and Zoe was sad. She wouldn't eat her green stuff. She sat and sat.

I n all the white fields there was one rabbit. It was lost. It was small. It lay in the snow.

Ben found it. Ben barked. We picked it up and took it home. Becky thought it would die, but it didn't.

26

There was no Ben for our rabbit, until one day… in the pale hay …there was a puppy.

We took it home. It lay down with Zoe. Becky said our puppy thought Zoe was a dog. And Zoe thought our puppy

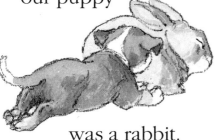

was a rabbit. They didn't know they'd got it wrong. Becky said we wouldn't tell them.

The puppy stayed. The puppy played. We loved him, just like we loved Ben.

We called our puppy Little Ben. But Little Ben got big… and bigger… and bigger

still. He got bigger than our rabbit but not as big as old Ben.

Zoe still thinks Little Ben is a rabbit, and Becky says that Zoe doesn't mind.

Becky says that Zoe likes big rabbits.

Zoe and little Ben play with us in the green fields. They are our dog and our rabbit.

We love them.

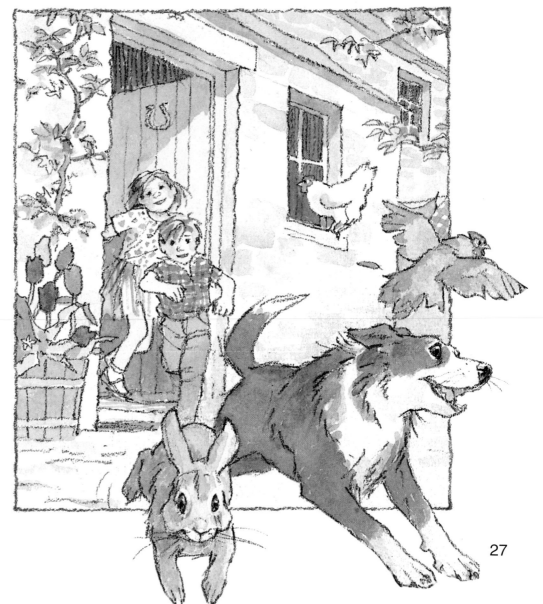

27

Out and About

by Shirley Hughes

The Grass House

The grass house
Is my private place.
Nobody can see me
In the grass house.
Feathery plumes
Meet over my head.
Down here,
In the green, there are:
Seeds
Weeds
Stalks
Pods
And tiny little flowers.

Only the cat
And some busy, hurrying ants
Know where my grass house is.

Mudlarks

I like mud.
The slippy, sloppy, squelchy kind,
The slap-it-into-pies kind.
Stir it up in puddles,
Slither and slide.
I *do* like mud.

Wind

I like the wind.
The soft, summery, gentle kind,
The gusty, blustery, fierce kind.
Ballooning out the curtains,
Blowing things about,
Wild and wilful everywhere.
I *do* like the wind.

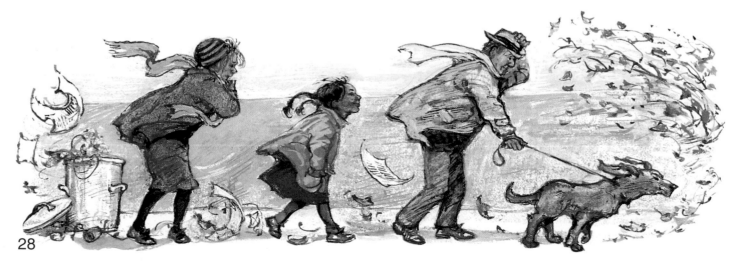

Seaside

Sand in the sandwiches,
Sand in the tea,
Flat, wet sand running
Down to the sea.
Pools full of seaweed,
Shells and stones,
Damp bathing suits
And ice-cream cones.
Waves pouring in
To a sand-castle moat.
Mend the defences!
Now we're afloat!
Water's for splashing,
Sand is for play,
A day by the sea
Is the best kind of day.

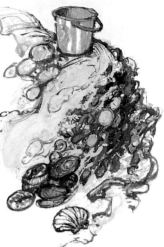

Sand

I like sand.
The run-between-your-fingers kind,
The build-it-into-castles kind.
Mountains of sand meeting the sky,
Flat sand, going on for ever.
I *do* like sand.

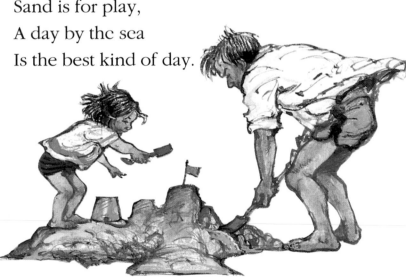

Water

I like water.
The shallow, splashy, paddly kind,
The hold-on-tight-it's-deep kind.
Slosh it out of buckets,
Spray it all around.
I *do* like water.

Sick

Hot, cross, aching head,
Prickly, tickly, itchy bed.
Piles of books and toys and puzzles
Heavy on my feet,
Pillows thrown all anyhow,
Wrinkles in the sheet.
Sick of medicine, lemonade,
Soup spooned from a cup.
When will I be *better?*
When can I *get up?*

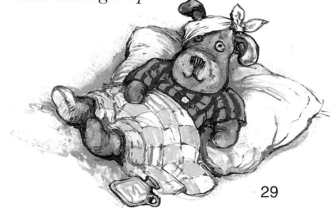

29

Beaky

by Jez Alborough

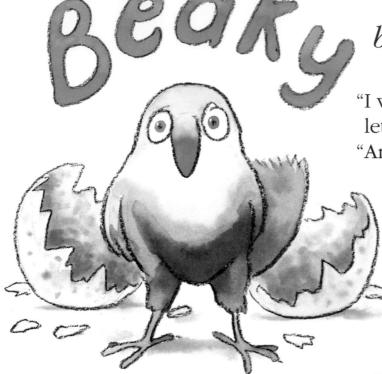

"I will call you Beaky. Come on, let's go for a walk."

"Am I a frog?" asked Beaky as they hopped along. Frog laughed.

"If you were a frog," he said, "then you would be able to hop as high as me and you wouldn't have those funny fluffy flaps."

"If I'm not a frog," said Beaky, "then what am I?"

"I don't know," puzzled Frog, "I've never seen anything like you before; but you must be something…everything is something!"

Before long they found Snake.

"What's he doing?" asked Beaky.

"Slithering," said Frog. "Precisely," said Snake. "It's simply splendid to slither, you should try a slither yourself."

An egg tumbled down through the leaves and branches and shattered into pieces on the rain forest floor.

Out popped a fluffy creature with a bright blue beak and a curly orange tail.

"Hello," croaked Frog, jumping out from behind a bush.

"I'm a frog, what are you?" The creature looked confused.

"Don't you know what you are?" asked Frog. The creature shook its head.

"Then you can be my friend," said Frog.

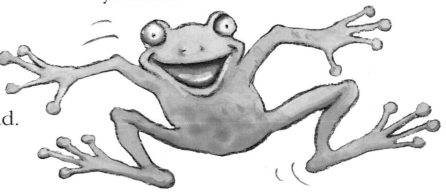

"Yes, have a try," said Frog, for he wondered whether Beaky might be some sort of snake. So Beaky lay on the earth and tried to slither. Nothing happened.

"Oh dear," said Frog. Snake laughed. "Too short," he said, and slithered off into the trees. Beaky and Frog hopped to the river where they found Fish gliding about in the water.

"What's he doing?" asked Beaky.

"I'm swimming," said Fish. "Come and join me, the water's lovely."

"Good idea," said Frog, thinking that Beaky might be some sort of fish. "Try a swim."

Beaky splished and splashed and flipped and flapped, but couldn't swim a stroke. "Oh dear," said Frog. Fish giggled. "Too fluffy," he said, and swam away.

"Everyone knows what they are except me," sighed Beaky. Just then he heard something singing softly, far away.

"Did you hear that?" he said excitedly. "Hear what?" said Frog.

"Listen!" said Beaky. "It came from up there." Frog looked up to the top of the trees, then he heard it too.

"Someone up there must be really happy," said Beaky, "to sing such a joyful song. Do you think I could ever be that happy?"

"Maybe," said Frog, "but not until we discover what you are." Then he had an idea.

"Let's climb up there," he said, "and see if we can find out." So up they went, but the higher they climbed the more frightened Frog became. So Beaky had to go on alone. On and on he struggled, all through the day and into the night until he could go no further.

"Now I'm lost," cried Beaky, "and I still haven't found out what I am. Maybe I should never have left the forest floor. Perhaps the song was just a dream." And with this thought, he slept. Beaky awoke the next morning to the sound of a familiar song. Looking round, he saw circling in the air a beautiful fluffy creature with a bright blue beak and a curly orange tail.

"What are you?" called Beaky.

"I'm a bird," sang the creature, "a bird of Paradise."

"A bird," said Beaky, "that's what I am."

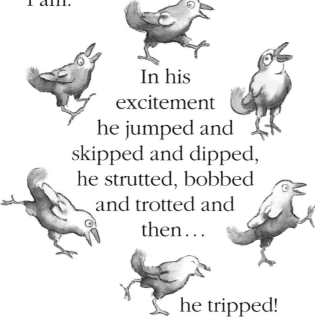

In his excitement he jumped and skipped and dipped, he strutted, bobbed and trotted and then...

he tripped!

Down and down he fell, crashing through leaves and branches, down towards the earth below.

"Flap your wings!" called the bird. "Flap your wings!"

Beaky opened wide his fluffy flaps. "My wings," he cried, "these are my *wings*." And with a *whoosh* he began to fly... up past a tree where Snake was slithering... down to the river where Fish was swimming... and back to the vine where Frog was still waiting.

"Frog," said Beaky, "look at me. I can't slither, or swim, or hop like you, but I can *fly!* "

At that moment Beaky heard the singing once more and it seemed to be calling him.

"I must go," he said, "but I'll come back and visit."

Then he flew up towards the treetops.

"Beaky," called Frog, "you haven't told me what you are."

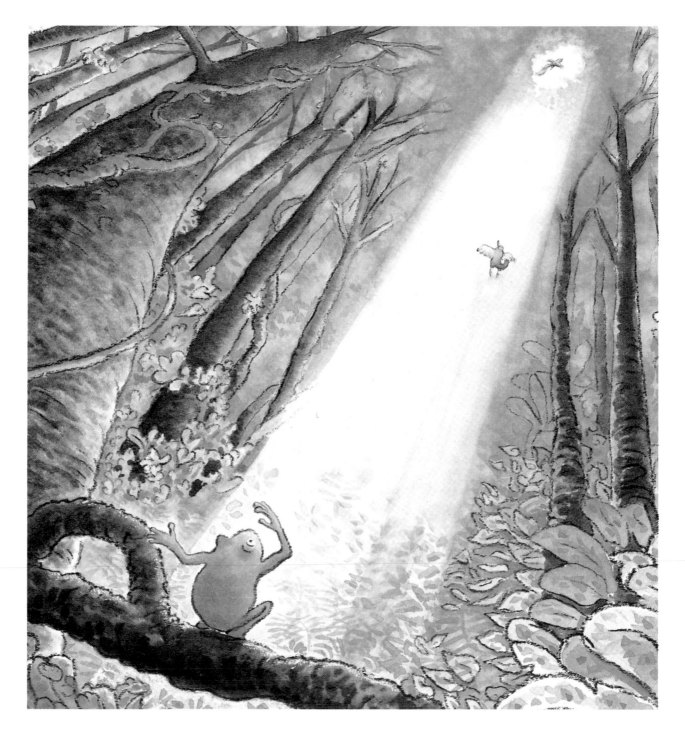

"I'm a bird," cried Beaky. "I'm a bird...a bird of Paradise!"

NONSENSE RHYMES

Gregory Griggs,
Gregory Griggs,
Had twenty-seven different wigs.
He wore them up,
He wore them down,
To please the people of the town;
He wore them east,
He wore them west;
But he never could tell
Which he liked best.

Old Mother Shuttle
Lived in a coal-scuttle,
Along with her dog and her cat;
What they ate I can't tell,
But 'tis known very well,
That not one of the party was fat.

Old Mother Shuttle
Scoured out her coal-scuttle,
And washed both her dog and her cat;
The cat scratched her nose,
So they came to hard blows
And who was the gainer by that?

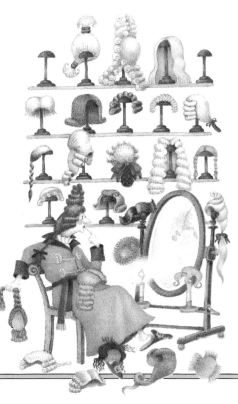

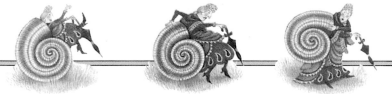

illustrated by Nicola Bayley

I dreamed a dream next Tuesday week,
Beneath the apple trees;
I thought my eyes were big pork pies,
    And my nose was Stilton cheese.
      The clock struck twenty minutes to six,
     When a frog sat on my knee;
   I asked him to lend me eighteen pence,
But he borrowed a shilling of me.

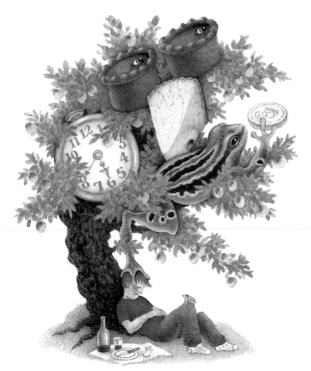

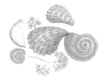

There was an old lady of Wales,
Who lived upon oysters and snails.
Upon growing a shell,
She exclaimed, "It is well,
I won't have to wear bonnets or veils."

35

MRS GOOSE'S

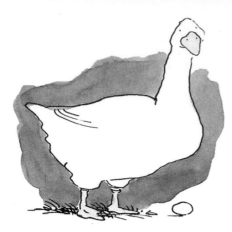

One day Mrs Goose found an egg and made a lovely nest to put it in. Mrs Goose sat on the egg to keep it safe and warm. Soon the egg started

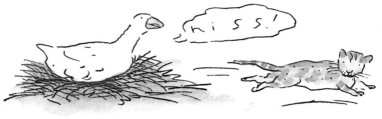

to crack open. The little bird inside was pecking at the shell. Mrs Goose's baby was very very small and fluffy and yellow.

Mrs Goose took her baby out to eat some grass. But her baby didn't want to eat grass.

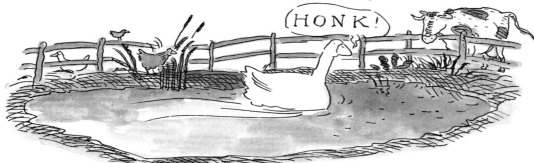

She ran off to look for something different.

Mrs Goose took her naughty baby to the pond.

The water looked cold and grey.

Poor Mrs Goose! Her baby would not swim!

BABY

by Charlotte Voake

The baby grew and grew and grew.

Mrs Goose's feathers were smooth and white.

Mrs Goose's baby had untidy brown feathers.

Mrs Goose had large webbed feet.

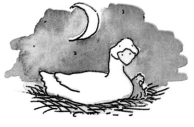

Her baby had little pointed toes.

The baby followed Mrs

Goose everywhere,

and cuddled up to her at night.

Mrs Goose guarded her

baby from strangers.

Mrs Goose's baby never did eat much grass.

The baby never did go swimming in the pond.

And everyone except Mrs Goose knew why.

Mrs Goose's baby was a

CHICKEN!

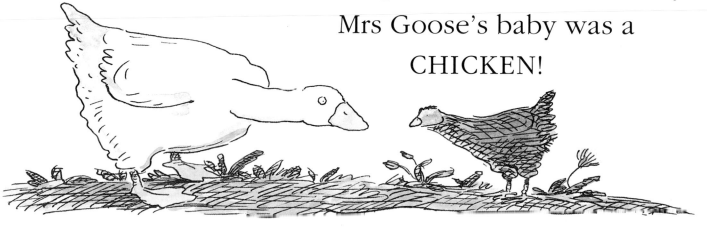

Sally and the Limpet

by Simon James

Not long ago, on a Sunday, Sally was down on the beach exploring, when she found a brightly coloured, bigger-than-usual limpet shell. She wanted to take it home but, as she pulled, the limpet made a little squelching noise and held on to the rock. The harder Sally tugged, the more tightly the limpet held on, until, suddenly, Sally slipped and fell – with the limpet stuck to her finger.

Though she pulled with all her might, it just wouldn't come off. So she ran over to her dad. He heaved and groaned, but the limpet made a little squelching noise and held on even tighter.

So, that afternoon, Sally went home in the car with a limpet stuck to her finger. When they got home, her dad tried using his tools.

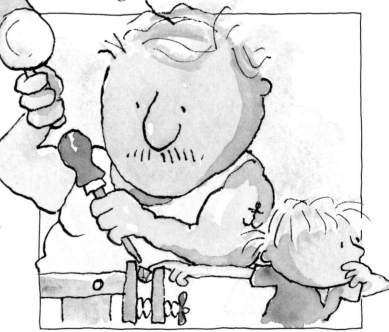

Her brother tried offering it lettuce and cucumber.

But, that night, Sally went to bed with a limpet stuck to her finger.

Next day it was school. All her friends tried to pull the limpet off her finger.

Mr Wobblyman, the nature teacher, said that limpets live for twenty years, and stay all their lives on the same rock.

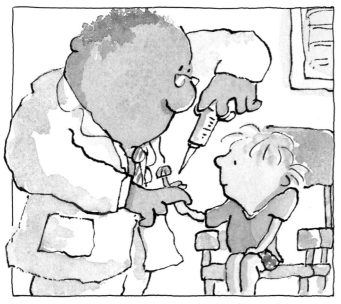

In the afternoon, Sally's mother took her to the hospital, to see the doctor. He tried chemicals, injections, potions and pinchers.

Sally was beginning to feel upset. Everyone was making too much fuss all around her. She kicked over the doctor's chair and ran. She ran through the endless corridors. She just wanted to be on her own. She ran out of the hospital and through the town. She didn't stop when she got to the beach. She ran through people's sandcastles. She even ran over a fat man.

When she reached the water, she jumped in with all her clothes on. Sally landed with a big splash and then just sat in the water.

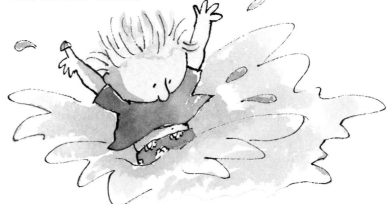

The limpet, feeling at home once more, made a little squelching noise and wiggled off her finger.

But Sally didn't forget what Mr Wobblyman, the nature teacher, had said. Very carefully, she lifted the limpet by the top of its shell. She carried it back across the beach, past the fat man she had walked on, and gently, so gently, she put the limpet back on the very same rock where she had found it the day before.

Then, humming to herself, she took the long way home across the beach.

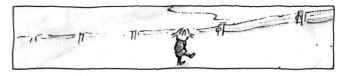

WHO'S 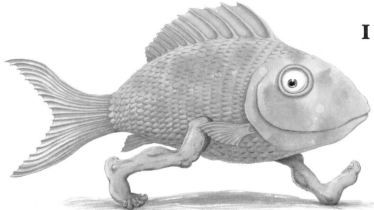 BEEN SLEEPING

I ONCE SAW A FISH UP A TREE

I once saw a fish up a tree,
  And this fish he had legs, believe me.
    Said the monster, "I'll swear,
    I'm just taking the air."
  Then he jumped down and ran off to sea.

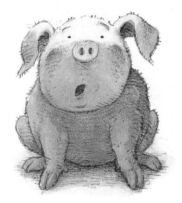

MOM IS HAVING A BABY!

Mom is having a baby!
I'm shocked! I'm all at sea!
What's she want another one for:
WHAT'S THE MATTER WITH ME!?

WHO'S BEEN SLEEPING IN MY PORRIDGE?

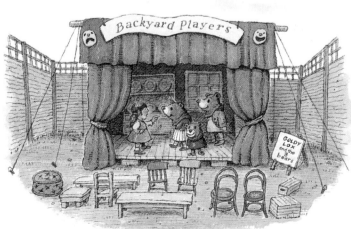

"Who's been sitting in my bed?"
  said the mommy bear crossly.
"Who's been eating my chair?"
  said the baby bear weepily.
"Who's been sleeping in my porridge?"
  said the papa bear angrily.
"Wait a minute," said Goldilocks.

"Why can't you guys just stick
  to the script? Now let's try
it again and this time no messing about."

IN 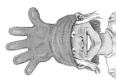 MY PORRIDGE?

by Colin McNaughton

ON YOUR HEAD BE IT!

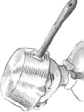

If you're poor and in distress,
Without a bean and penniless,
Your head is cold, your bonce is blue,
Then this is my headvice to you:
Wear a teapot, wear a shoe,
Lift it up, say "How de do!"
Wear a sock, wear a pan,
Wear a king-size baked-bean can.
Wear a saucer, wear a cup,
Wear a plantpot, downside up.
Wear a bucket, wear a bowl,
Wear the tube from a toilet roll.
Wear a lampshade, wear a vase,
Wear a fishbowl, man from Mars!

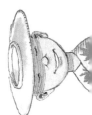

Wear a pie (not too hot!),
Wear a sooty chimneypot.
Wear a matchbox, wear a book,
For that literary look.
Wear an eggcup, plain or spotty,
Wear a washed-out baby's potty.
Wear a yellow traffic cone,
Wear a big brass bass trombone.
Wear an orange rubber glove,
Wear a housetrained turtle-dove.
Wear a ball, a loaf of bread,
A ripe banana – use your head!
Your head's in the sand if you can't see it.
If you catch cold, ON YOUR HEAD BE IT!

THE CROCODILE'S BRUSHING HIS TEETH

The crocodile's brushing his teeth, I'm afraid,
This certainly means we're too late.
The crocodile's brushing his teeth, I'm afraid,
He has definitely put on some weight.
The crocodile's brushing his teeth, I'm afraid,
It really is, oh, such a bore.
The crocodile's brushing his teeth, I'm afraid,
He appears to have eaten class four!

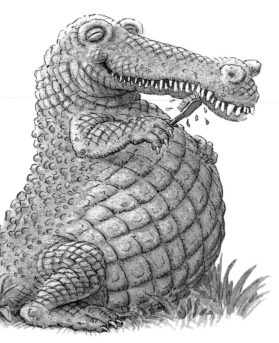

41

THE HAPPY HEDGEHOG

Deep in the heart of Dickon
Wood lived a happy hedgehog
named Harry.

Harry loved noise so he made
a big drum and he banged on
the drum tum-tum-te-tum.

A hedgehog called Helen
was out in the wood. She
heard tum-tum-te-tum
and she liked it. So she
made a drum and went
off to join in the drumming.
And so did a hedgehog
named Norbert and another
called Billy; they both made
drums and followed the tum-
tum-te-tums, until all of the
hedgehogs with drums were
gathered together at Harry's.
Tum-tum-te-tum went one
drum; that was Harry.
Diddle-diddle-dum went

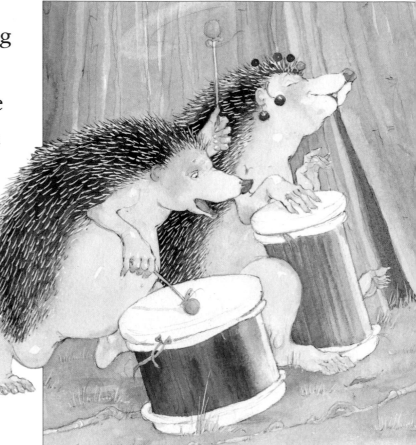

one drum; that was Helen.
Ratta-tat-tat went one drum;
that was Norbert.
And BOOM went one drum;
that was Billy.
Tum-tum-te-tum diddle-diddle-
dum ratta-tat-tat   BOOM
Tum-tum-te-tum diddle-diddle-

BAND

by **Martin Waddell**   *illustrated by* **Jill Barton**

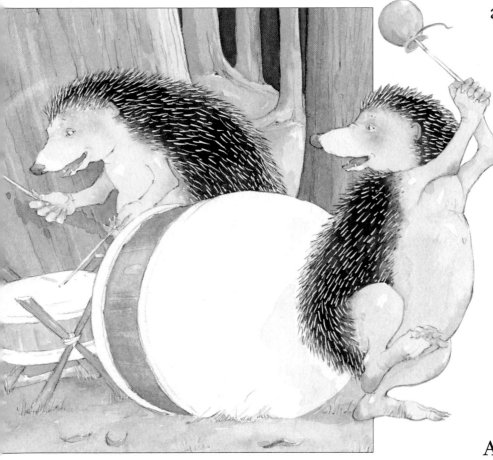

and the dove, the frog and the toad and the spider and the dog who was lost in the wood. Tum went the band and they STOPPED!

"We want to play too!" said the others. "But we haven't got drums. So what can we do?" And nobody knew except Harry.

Harry knew all about noise. So he said, "You can hum, you can hoot, you can buzz, you can whistle, you can clap, you can click, you can pop. We'll carry on with the drums."

And ...

dum ratta-tat-tat   BOOM
The whole wood was humming and tumming with drumming. **"STOP!"** cried the pheasant, the owl and the bee, the mole from his hole and a badger called Sam and his mother, and the fox and the crow, the deer

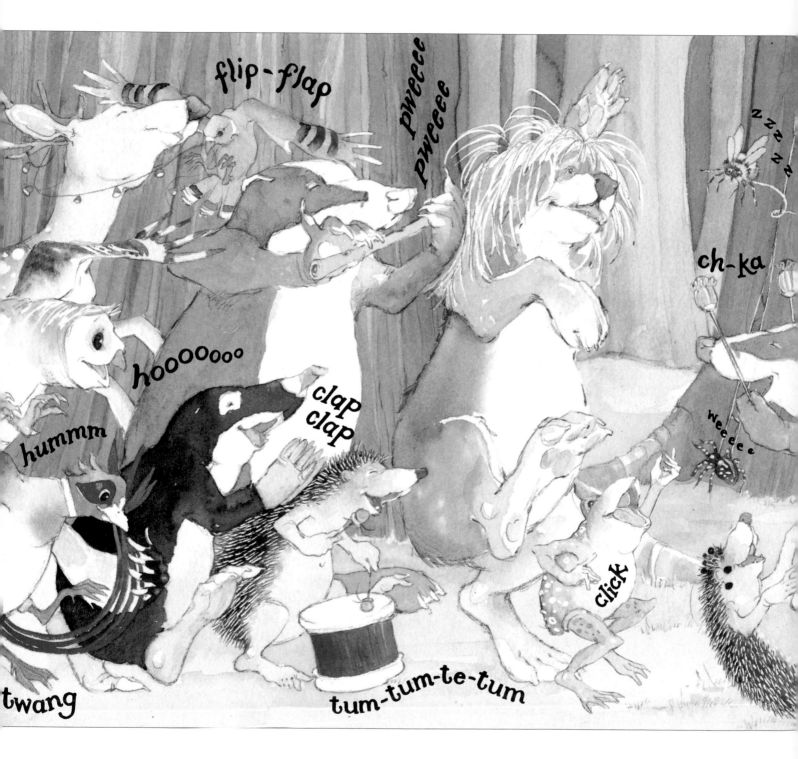

44

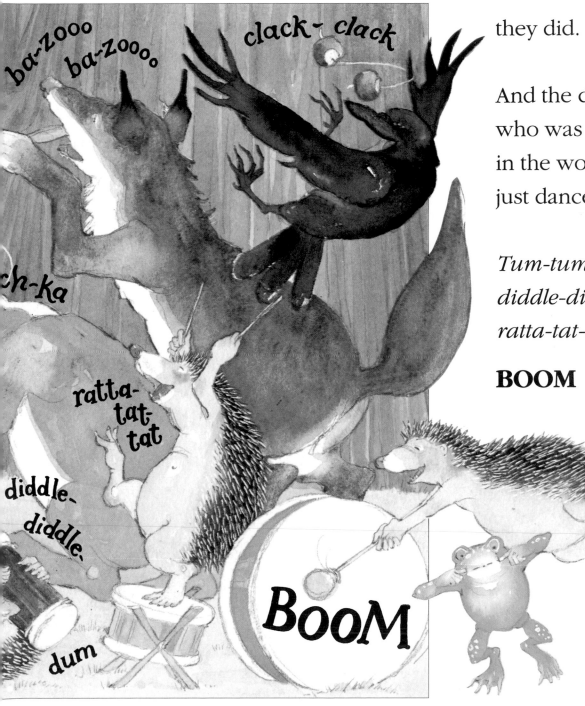

ba-zooo ba-zoooo

clack-clack

ch-ka

ratta-
tat-
tat

diddle-
diddle-
dum

BOOM

they did.

And the dog
who was lost
in the wood
just danced.

Tum-tum-te-tum
diddle-diddle-dum
ratta-tat-tat

BOOM

45

A Little Boy Came

from
HARD-BOILED LEGS

by **Michael Rosen**   illustrated by **Quentin Blake**

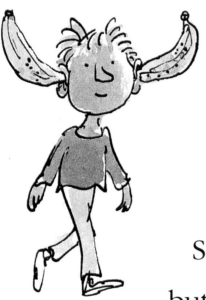

A little boy came down to breakfast

with bananas stuck in his ears.

Everyone said hello to him

but he didn't take any notice.

So his mom said, "Are you all right?"

but the little boy said nothing.

So his sister said,

"Are you all right?"

but the little boy

still said nothing.

Then his brother noticed that

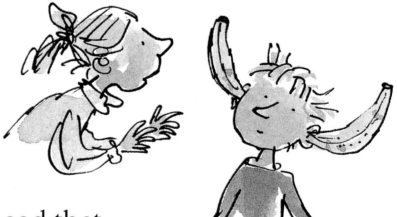

he had bananas stuck in his ears, so he said,

Down to Breakfast

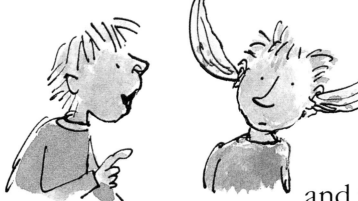

"Hey, you've
got bananas
stuck in your ears,"
and the little boy said, "What?"
So his brother said it again. "You've got bananas
stuck in your ears," and the little boy said, "What?"
So the brother shouted really loudly at him,
"YOU'VE GOT BANANAS STUCK IN YOUR EARS!"
And the little boy shouted back,
"I'M SORRY,
I CAN'T HEAR YOU.
I'VE GOT
BANANAS
IN MY EARS!"

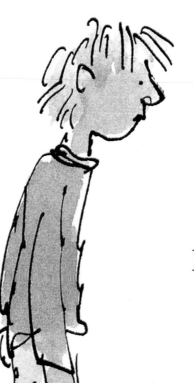

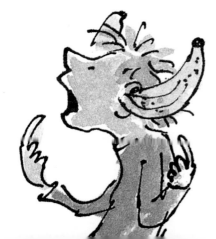

47

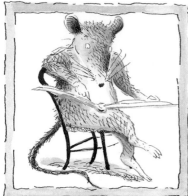

On Saturday night I lost my wife,
And where do you think I found her?
Up in the moon, singing a tune,
And all the stars around her.

Sally go round the sun,
Sally go round the moon,
Sally go round the chimney-pots
On a Saturday afternoon.

Moon

illustrated by Charlotte Voake

Hey diddle, diddle,
The cat and the fiddle,
    The cow jumped over the moon.
The little dog laughed
To see such sport,
    And the dish ran away with the spoon.

The man in the moon
Came tumbling down,
    And asked his way to Norwich.
He went by the south,
And burnt his mouth
    With supping cold pease-porridge.

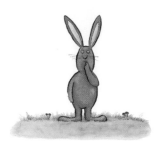

Daley B

Daley B didn't know
what he was.
"Am I a monkey?"
he said.
"Am I a koala?
Am I a porcupine?"

Daley B didn't know
where to live.
"Should I live in a cave?"
he said.
"Should I live in a nest?
Should I live in a web?"

Daley B didn't know
what to eat.
"Should I eat fish?"
he said.
"Should I eat potatoes?
Should I eat worms?"

Daley B didn't know
why his feet were so big.
"Are they for water
skiing?" he said.

"Are they for the mice
to sit on?
Are they to keep the
rain off?"

Daley B saw the birds
in the tree, and decided
he would live in a tree.
Daley B saw the
squirrels eating acorns,
and decided he would
eat acorns.
But he still didn't know
why his feet were so big.

One day, there was great
panic in the woodland.
All the rabbits gathered
beneath Daley B's tree.
"You must come down
at once, Daley B!"
they cried. "Jazzy D
is coming!"
"Who is Jazzy D?" asked
Daley B.

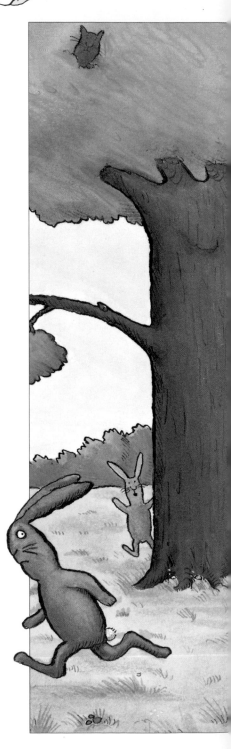

by Jon Blake *illustrated by* Axel Scheffler

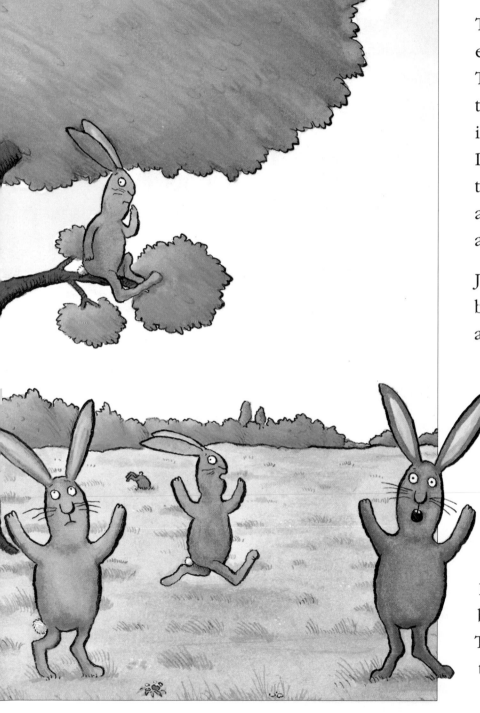

The rabbits were too excited to answer. They scattered across the grass and vanished into their burrows. Daley B stayed in his tree, and nibbled another acorn, and wondered about his big feet.

Jazzy D crept out of the bushes. Her teeth were as sharp as broken glass, and her eyes were as quick as fleas. Jazzy D sneaked around the burrows, but there was not a rabbit to be seen.

Jazzy D looked up. Daley B waved. Jazzy D began to climb the tree. The other rabbits poked out their noses, and trembled.

51

"Hello," said Daley B to Jazzy D. "Are you a badger? Are you an elephant? Are you a duck-billed platypus?"

Jazzy D crept closer.

"No, my friend," she whispered. "I am a weasel."

"Do you live in a pond?" asked Daley B.

"Do you live in a dam? Do you live in a kennel?"

Jazzy D crept closer still.

"No, my friend," she hissed, "I live in the darkest corner of the wood."

"Do you eat cabbages?" asked Daley B. "Do you eat insects? Do you eat fruit?"

Jazzy D crept right up to Daley B.

"No, my friend," she rasped, "I eat rabbits! Rabbits like you!"

Daley B's face fell. "Am I ... a rabbit?" he stammered.

Jazzy D nodded ... and licked her lips ...

and **leapt!**

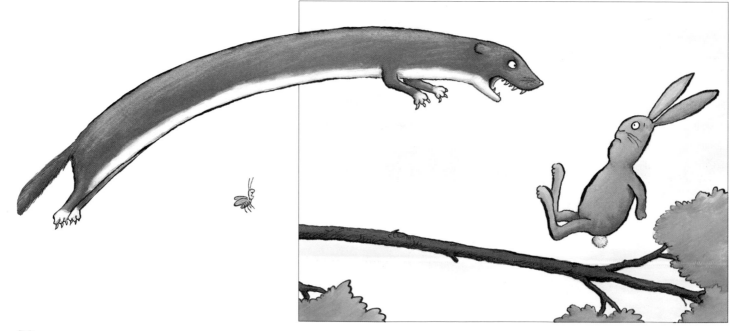

52

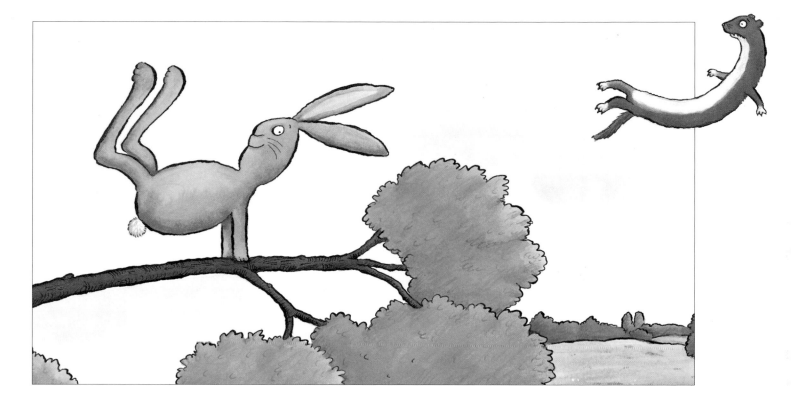

Daley B didn't have to think. Quick as a flash, he turned his back, and kicked out with his massive feet. Jazzy D sailed through the air, far far away, back where she came from.

The other rabbits jumped and cheered and hugged each other. "You're a hero, Daley B!" they cried.

"That's funny," said Daley B. "I thought I was a rabbit."

53

OWL BABIES

Once there were three baby owls:

Sarah... and Percy...

and Bill.

They lived in a hole
in the trunk of a tree
with their Owl Mother.

The hole had twigs and
leaves and owl feathers in it
It was their house.

BY MARTIN WADDELL   ILLUSTRATED BY PATRICK BENSON

One night they woke up and
their Owl Mother was GONE.
"Where's Mommy?" asked Sarah.
"Oh my goodness!" said Percy.
"I want my mommy!" said Bill.

The baby owls *thought*
(all owls think a lot) –
"I think she's gone hunting,"
said Sarah.
"To get us our food!" said Percy.
"I want my mommy!" said Bill.

But their Owl Mother didn't come.
The baby owls came out of their
house and they sat on the tree
and waited.

A big branch for Sarah,
a small branch for Percy,
and an old bit of ivy for Bill.
"She'll be back," said Sarah.
"Back *soon*!" said Percy.
"I want my mommy!" said Bill.

It was dark in the wood and
they had to be brave, for things
moved all around them.

"She'll bring us mice and things
that are nice," said Sarah.
"I suppose so!" said Percy.
"I want my mommy!" said Bill.

They sat and they thought
(all owls think a lot) –
"I think we should *all* sit on *my*
branch," said Sarah.
And they did, all three together.

"Suppose she got lost," said Sarah.
"Or a fox got her!" said Percy.
"I want my mommy!"
said Bill.
And the baby owls
closed their owl eyes
and wished their
Owl Mother
would come.

AND SHE CAME.
Soft and silent, she swooped
through the trees to Sarah and
Percy and Bill.
"Mommy!" they cried, and they
flapped and they danced, and they
bounced up and down on their
branch.
"WHAT'S ALL THE FUSS?"
their Owl Mother asked.
"You knew I'd come back."
The baby owls thought
(all owls think a lot) –
"I knew it," said Sarah.
"And I knew it!" said Percy.
"I love my mommy!"
    said Bill.

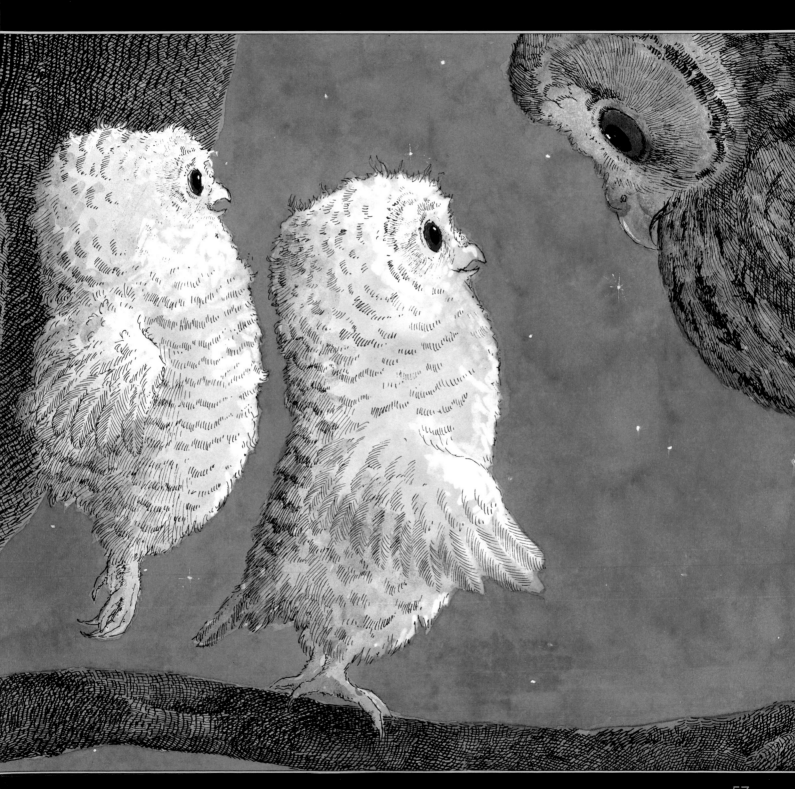

A Zoo in

Mom and I went to
the zoo.
I said, "Can I have a zoo
in our house?"
"Certainly not," said Mom.

But …

… on Monday a giraffe
was eating in
the kitchen.

On Tuesday
a hippopotamus was
splashing in the bath.

On Wednesday a monkey
was swinging in the hall.

On Thursday
a crocodile was washing
in the garden.

Our House

by Heather Eyles
illustrated by Andy Cooke

On Friday a lion was sleeping in the living room.

On Saturday all the animals came and we had a party.

On Sunday Mom sent them all back to the zoo.

"Phew," said Mom.

But …

… she forgot the gorilla.

Floss

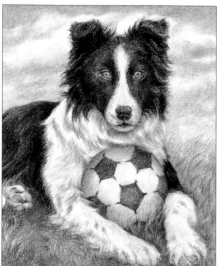

by *Kim Lewis*

Floss was a young border collie, who belonged to an old man in a town.

She walked with the old man in the streets, and loved playing ball with children in the park.

"My son is a farmer," the old man told Floss. "He has a sheepdog who is too old to work. He needs a young dog to herd sheep on his farm. He could train a Border collie like you."

So Floss and the old man travelled, away from the town with its streets and houses and children playing ball in the park. They came to the heather-covered hills of a valley, where nothing much grew except sheep. Somewhere in her memory, Floss knew about sheep. Old Nell soon showed her how to round them up. The farmer trained her to run wide and lie down, to walk on behind, to shed,

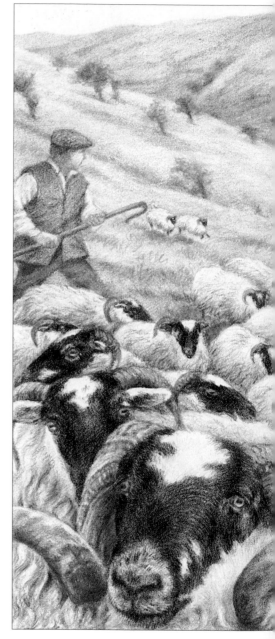

and to pen. She worked very hard to become a good sheepdog.

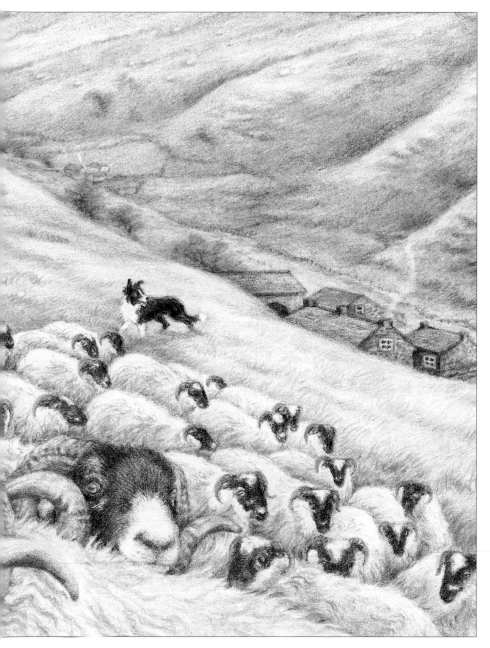

up balls in the park. The farmer took Floss on the hill one day, to see if she could gather the sheep on her own. She was rounding them up when she heard a sound. At the edge of the field the farmer's children were playing, with a brand new black and white ball.

Floss remembered all about children. She ran to play with their ball. She showed off her best nose kicks, her best passes. She did her best springs in the air.

"Hey, Dad, look at this!" yelled the children. "Look at Floss!"

But sometimes Floss woke up at night, while Nell lay sound asleep.

She remembered about playing with children and rounding

The sheep started drifting away. The sheep escaped through the gate and into the yard. There were sheep in the garden and sheep on the road.

"FLOSS! LIE DOWN!"

The farmer's voice was like thunder.

"You are meant for work on this farm, not play!" He took Floss back to the dog house. Floss lay and worried about balls and sheep. She dreamt about the streets of a town, the hills of a valley, children and farmers, all mixed together, while Nell had to round up the straying sheep. But Nell was too old to work every day, and Floss had to learn to take her place. She worked so hard to gather sheep well, she was much too tired to dream any more. The farmer was pleased and ran Floss in the dog trials.

"She's a good worker now," the old man said. The children still wanted

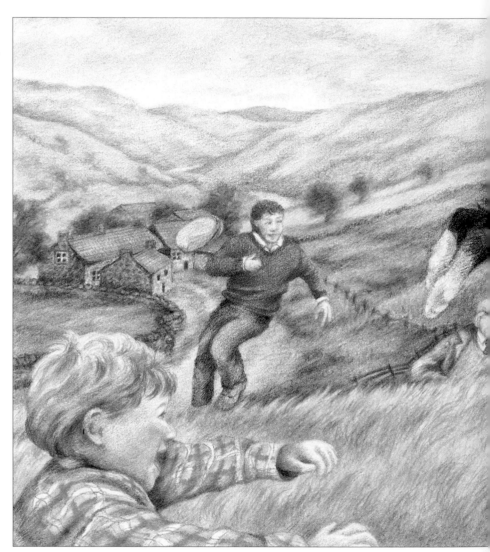

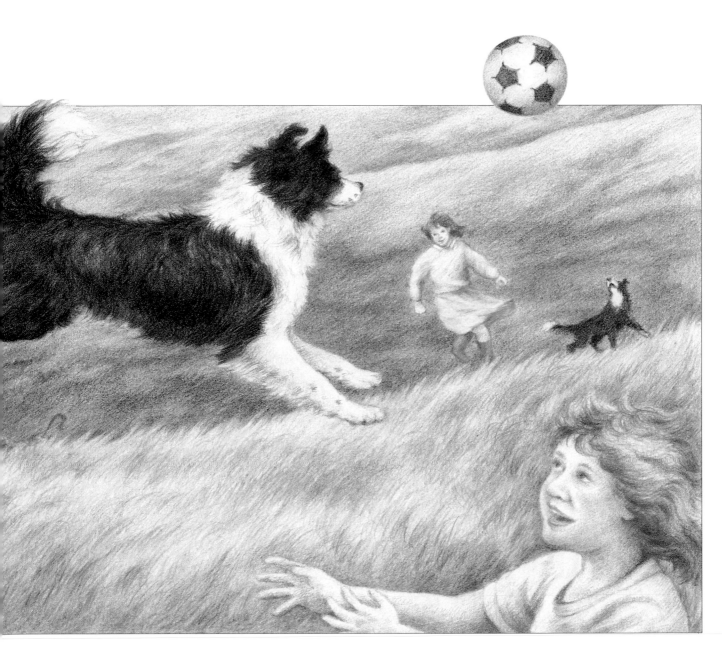

to play with their ball. "Hey, Dad," they asked, "can Old Nell play now?" But Nell didn't know about children and play. "No one can play ball like Floss," they said. "Go on, then," whispered the farmer to Floss. The children kicked the ball high in the air. Floss remembered all about children. She ran to play with their ball. She showed off her best nose kicks, her best passes. She did her best springs in the air.

TEN IN THE BED

There were **TEN** in the bed
and the little one said,
"Roll over, roll over!"
So they all rolled over
and Hedgehog fell out …

BUMP!

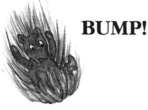

There were **NINE** in the bed
and the little one said,
"Roll over, roll over!"
So they all rolled over
and Zebra fell out …

OUCH!

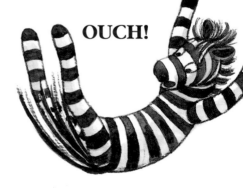

There were **EIGHT** in the bed
and the little one said,
"Roll over, roll over!"
So they all rolled over
and Ted fell out …

THUMP!

There were **SEVEN** in the bed
and the little one said,
"Roll over, roll over!"
So they all rolled over
and Croc fell out …

THUD !

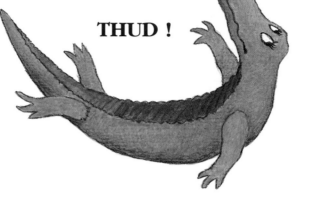

There were **SIX** in the bed
and the little one said,
"Roll over, roll over!"
So they all rolled over
and Rabbit fell out …

BONK!

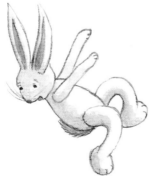

There were **FIVE** in the bed
and the little one said,
"Roll over, roll over!"
So they all rolled over
and Mouse fell out …

DINK!

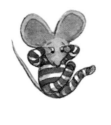

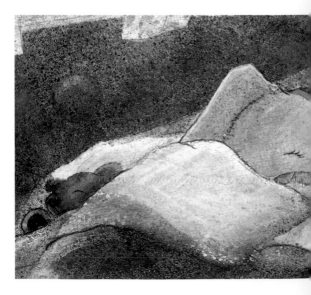

by Penny Dale

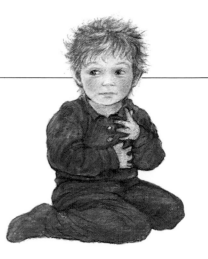

There were **FOUR** in the bed
  and the little one said,
    "Roll over, roll over!"
  So they all rolled over
  and Nelly fell out …

CRASH!

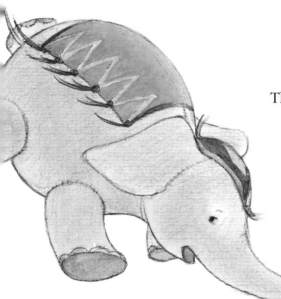

There were **THREE** in the bed
  and the little one said,
    "Roll over, roll over!"
  So they all rolled over
  and Bear fell out …

SLAM!

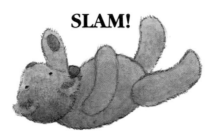

There were **TWO** in the bed
  and the little one said,
    "Roll over, roll over!"
  So they all rolled over
  and Sheep fell out …

DONK!

There was **ONE** in the bed
  and the little one said,
    "I'm cold! I miss you!"

So they all came back
  and jumped into bed –
  Hedgehog, Mouse, Nelly, Zebra,
  Ted, the little one, Rabbit, Croc,
    Bear and Sheep.

Ten in the bed,
  all fast asleep.

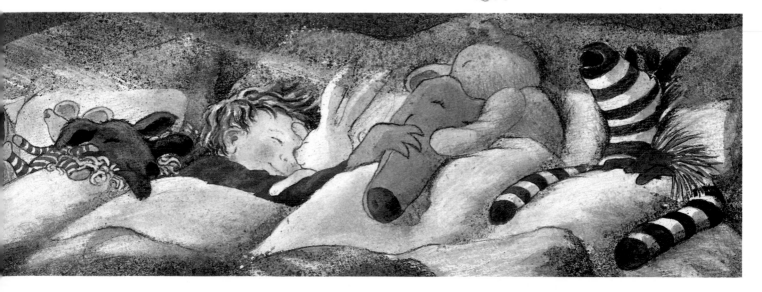

A Piece of Cake

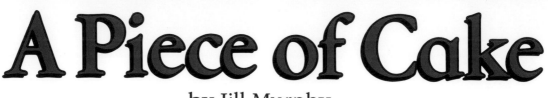

by Jill Murphy

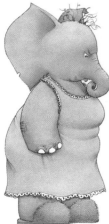

"I'm fat," said Mrs Large. "No you're not," said Lester. "You're our cuddly mommy," said Laura. "You're just right," said Luke. "Mommy's got wobbly bits," said the baby. "Exactly," said Mrs Large. "As I was saying – I'm fat."

"We must all go on a diet," said Mrs Large. "No more cakes. No more biscuits. No more crisps. No more sitting around all day. From now on, it's healthy living."

"Can we watch TV?" asked Lester, as they trooped in from school. "Certainly not!" said Mrs Large. "We're all off for a nice healthy jog round the park." And they were.

"What's for tea, Mom?" asked Laura when they arrived home.

"Some nice healthy watercress soup," said Mrs Large. "Followed by a nice healthy cup of water." "Oh!" said Laura. "That sounds ... nice."

"I'm just going to watch the news, dear," said Mr Large when he came home from work. "No you're not, dear," said Mrs Large. "You're off for a nice healthy jog round the park, followed by your tea – a delicious sardine with grated carrot." "I can't wait," said Mr Large.

It was awful. Every morning there was a healthy breakfast followed by exercises. Then there was a healthy tea followed by a healthy jog. By the time evening came everyone felt terrible. "We aren't getting any thinner, dear," said Mr Large.

"Perhaps elephants are meant to be fat," said Luke. "Nonsense!" said Mrs Large. "We mustn't give up now." "Wibbly-wobbly, wibbly-wobbly," went the baby.

One morning a parcel arrived. It was a cake from Granny. Everyone stared at it hopefully. Mrs Large put it into the cupboard on a high shelf. "Just in case we have visitors," she said sternly.

Everyone kept thinking about the cake. They thought about it during tea. They thought about it during the healthy jog. They thought about it in bed that night. Mrs Large sat up. "I can't stand it any more," she said to herself. "I must have a piece of that cake."

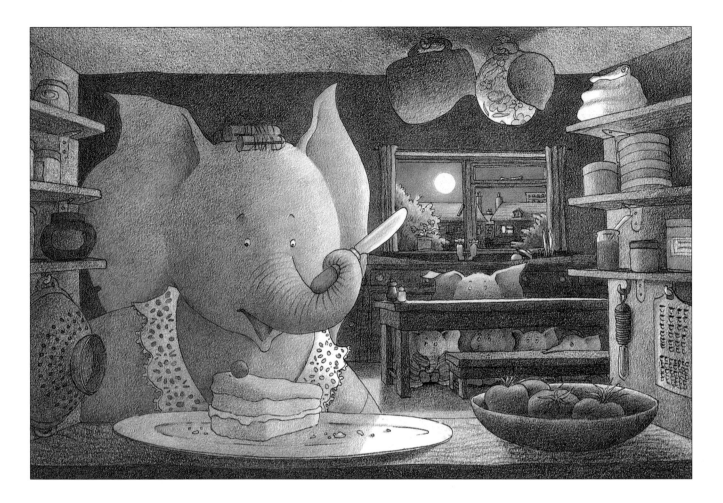

Mrs Large crept out of bed and went downstairs to the kitchen. She took a knife out of the drawer and opened the cupboard. There was only one piece of cake left!

"Ah ha!" said Mr Large, seeing the knife. "Caught in the act!"

Mrs Large switched on the light and saw Mr Large and all the children hiding under the table.

"There *is* one piece left," said Laura in a helpful way.

Mrs Large began to laugh. "We're all as bad as each other!" she said, eating the last piece of cake before anyone else did. "I do think elephants are meant to be fat," said Luke.

"I think you're probably right, dear," said Mrs Large. "Wibbly-wobbly, wibbly-wobbly!" went the baby.

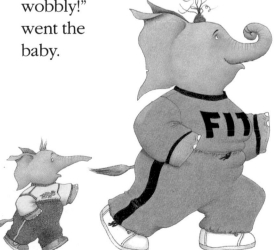

HORATIO'S BED

All night Horatio could not sleep.

He tossed and turned, 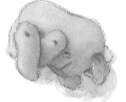 and wriggled, and rolled.

But he just could not
get comfortable.
I'll go and ask James
what's the matter,
he thought.
James was
busy drawing.
Horatio sat down.
"I couldn't sleep
all night," he said.
"Is it your bed?"
asked James.
"I haven't got
a bed," Horatio said.

"Then let's make you one,"
said James.
James took a clean sheet of paper
from his Useful Box and very
carefully drew a bed for Horatio.

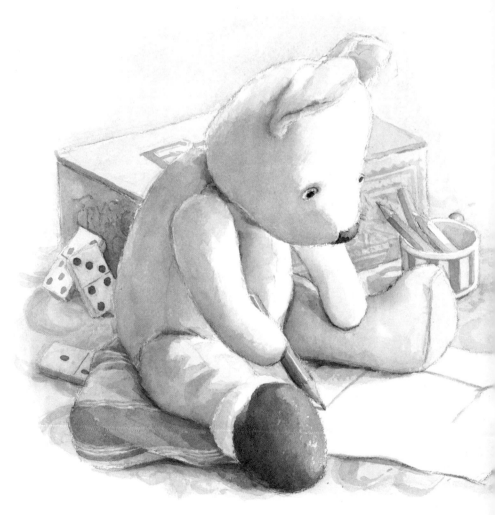

by Camilla Ashforth

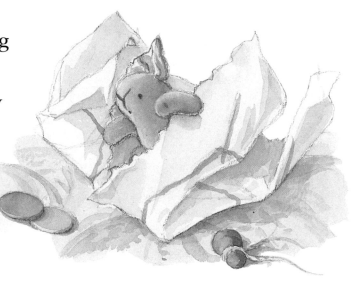

It was a big square bed with a leg at each corner. Then he took another sheet of paper and drew another bed for Horatio. This one was a big square bed with a leg at each corner too.

Horatio was very excited. He took one of James's drawings and tried to fold it into a bed. Then he climbed inside it and closed his eyes.

It wasn't very comfortable and when Horatio rolled over …

R R R I I I P P P !

James looked up. "That bed looks too hard to sleep on," he said and carried on with his drawing. Horatio thought for a moment. Then he pulled some feathers out of James's pillow and made a big square bed with them.

But when he lay on it the feathers tickled his nose. AAACHOO! AAACHOO! AAACHOO!

He sneezed and sneezed.

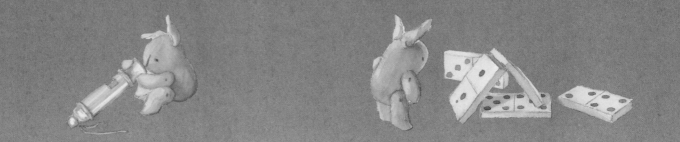

James put down his pencil and
blew away the feathers.
James sat Horatio down on
his Useful Box.
"You wait here a minute," he said,
"while I just finish drawing your
bed." He had already drawn five
square beds and was getting
rather good at them.
But when James turned away,
Horatio slipped down from the
Useful Box. He wanted to see
what James kept inside.
He made some steps up to the lid.
He pushed it open and leaned in.
There were all sorts of things –
buttons, brushes, keys and
clothes pegs, clock wheels,
clips and little bits of string.
Horatio looked for a bed.
He couldn't find anything that
looked like James's drawings.

But he did find a big red sock.
"Look, James!" he cried.
"I've found your other sock!"
James did not seem very pleased.
He didn't like anyone looking in
his Useful Box. Not even Horatio.
Very quietly and carefully he
started to put away his Useful Bits.
When he had finished, he closed
the lid and looked for Horatio.
"Now we can make you
a bed," he said.

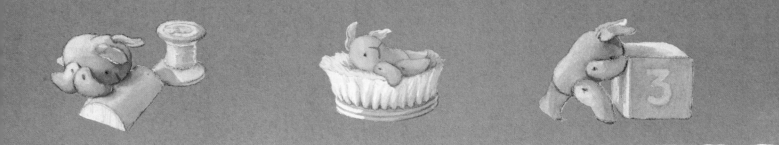

But there was no need, because
Horatio was fast asleep.
His bed was not
square and it did
not have a leg
at each corner.

But for little Horatio
it was just right.

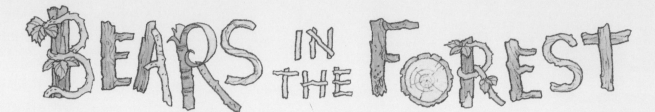

BEARS IN THE FOREST

by Karen Wallace illustrated by Barbara Firth

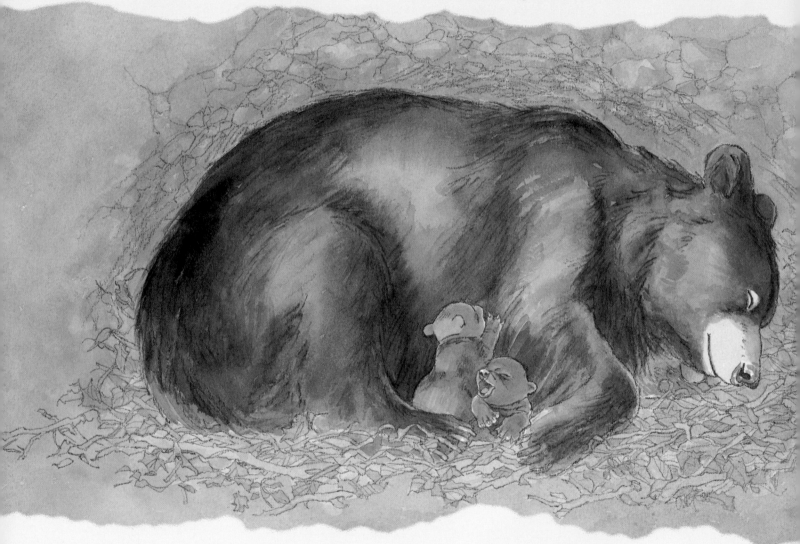

Deep in a cave, a mother bear sleeps. She is huge and warm. Her heart beats slowly. Outside it is cold and the trees are covered in snow. Her newborn cubs are blind and tiny. They find her milk and begin to grow.

Snow slips from the trees and melts on the ground. The ice has broken on the lake. Mother bear wakes. Her long sleep is over. She leads her cubs down to the lake shore. She slurps and slurps the freezing water.

Leaves burst from their buds. There are frogs' eggs in the lake. Mother bear snuffs the air for strange smells, listens for strange sounds. Her cubs know nothing of the forest. This is their first spring. Mother bear must take care.

The summer sun is hot. Mother bear sits in a tree stump. Angry bees buzz around her head, and stolen honey drops from her paws. Her two skinny bear cubs wrestle in the long grass. They squeal like little boys and roll over and over away from their mother. Mother bear growls.

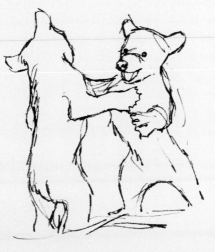

73

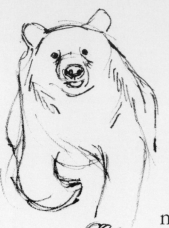

Come back! There are dangers in the forest! Her cubs do not hear her. Mother bear snorts. She is angry. She strides across the meadow and whacks them with a heavy paw.

Two frightened bear cubs scramble up the nearest tree. Mother bear waits below, still as a statue, listening to the forest. When she feels safe, she will call her cubs down. Mother bear must take care.

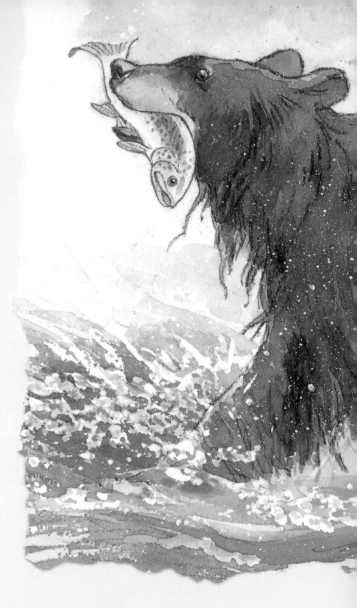

Soon the days grow shorter and squirrels start to hide acorns. Bushes are bright with berries. Seed pods flutter to the ground. Winter is coming. Mother bear and her cubs eat everything they can find.

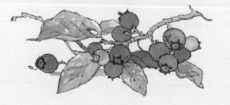

Icy winds blast the forest. Mother bear plods through the snow. Her cubs are fat. Their fur is thick. She chooses a shelter that is dark and dry, where they will sleep through the long winter months. When spring has woken the bears again, mother bear leads her cubs to

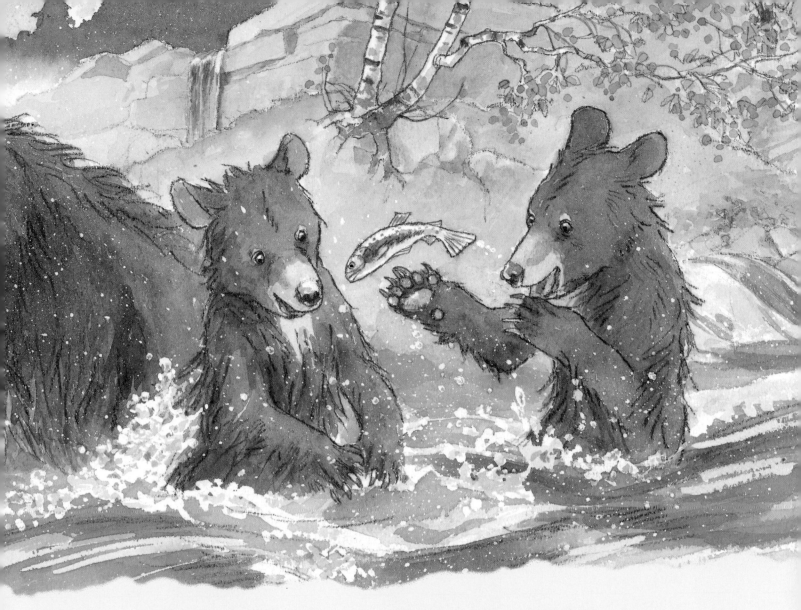

the river. She follows a trail worn deep in the ground. Hundreds of bears have walked this way before her. The river runs deep and fast. Mother bear wades in. Soon a silver trout flashes in her jaws. The cubs are hungry. They wade into the river and catch their own fish.

Mother bear gobbles berries. Her cubs are playing where she can't see them. They are almost grown. Soon they will leave her. Mother bear has taught them everything she knows.

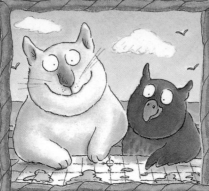

The Owl and the Pussy Cat

Illustrated by Louise Voce   Written by Edward Lear

The Owl and
   the Pussy Cat
      went to sea
In a beautiful
   pea-green boat,
They took some honey,
   and plenty of money,
Wrapped up in a
   five-pound note.
The Owl looked up
   to the stars above,
And sang
   to a small guitar,
"O lovely Pussy!
   O Pussy, my love,
What a beautiful
   Pussy you are,
You are, you are!
What a beautiful
   Pussy you are!"

Pussy said to the Owl,
   "You elegant fowl!
How charmingly
   sweet you sing!
O let us be married!
   too long we have
   tarried:
But what shall we
   do for a ring?"

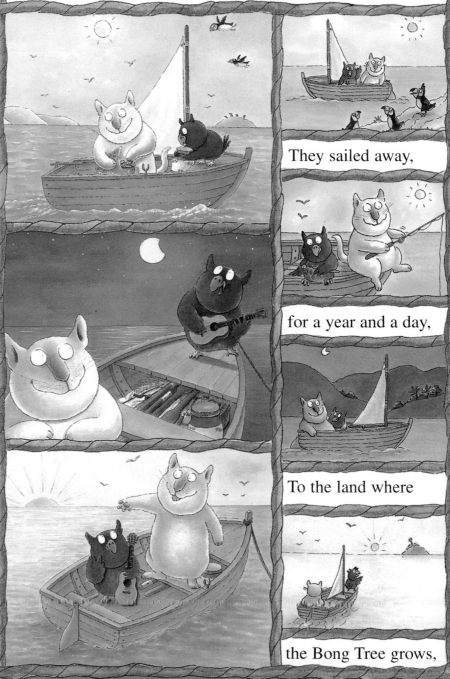

They sailed away,

for a year and a day,

To the land where

the Bong Tree grows,

76

And there in a wood
  a Piggy-wig stood
With a ring
  at the end of his nose,
His nose, his nose,
With a ring at the end
  of his nose.

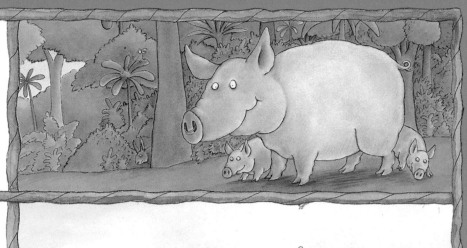

"Dear Pig,
  are you willing
  to sell for one shilling
Your ring?"
  Said the Piggy, "I will."
So they took it away,
  and were married
  next day
By the Turkey
  who lives on the hill.

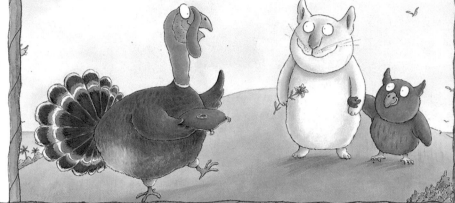

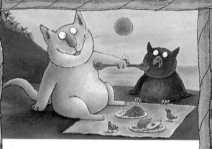

They dined on mince,
  and slices of quince,
Which they ate
  with a runcible spoon;
And hand in hand, on
  the edge of the sand,
They danced by the light
  of the moon,
The moon, the moon,
They danced by the light
  of the moon.

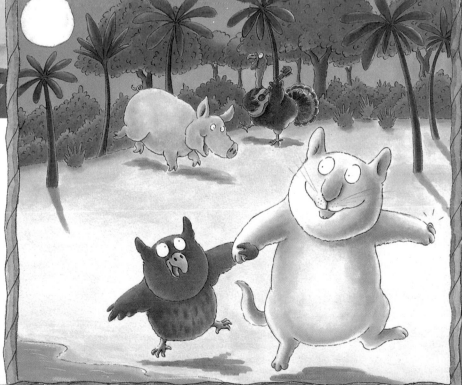

Let's Go Home, Little Bear

by Martin Waddell ✳ *illustrated by* Barbara Firth

Once there were two bears. Big Bear and Little Bear. Big Bear is the big bear and Little Bear is the little bear.

They went for a walk in the woods. They walked and they walked and they walked until Big Bear said, "Let's go home, Little Bear."

So they started back home on the path through the woods.

PLOD PLOD PLOD went Big Bear, plodding along.

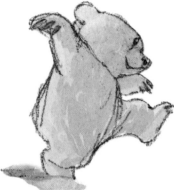

Little Bear ran on in front, jumping and sliding and having great fun.

And then … Little Bear stopped and he listened and then he turned round and he looked.

"Come on, Little Bear," said Big Bear, but Little Bear didn't stir.

"I thought I heard something!" Little Bear said.

"What did you hear?" said Big Bear.

"Plod, plod, plod," said Little Bear. "I think it's a Plodder!"

Big Bear turned round and he listened and looked.

No Plodder was there.

"Let's go home, Little Bear," said Big Bear. "The plod was my feet in the snow."

They set off again on the path through the woods.

PLOD PLOD PLOD went Big Bear with Little Bear walking beside him, just glancing a bit, now and again.

And then … Little Bear stopped and he listened and then he turned round and he looked.

"Come on, Little Bear," said Big Bear, but Little Bear didn't stir.

"I thought I heard something!" Little Bear said.

"What did you hear?" said Big Bear.

"Drip, drip, drip," said Little Bear. "I think it's a Dripper!"

Big Bear turned round, and he listened and looked.

No Dripper was there.

"Let's go home, Little Bear," said Big Bear.

"That was the ice as it dripped in the stream."

They set off again on the path through the woods.

PLOD PLOD PLOD went Big Bear with Little Bear closer beside him.

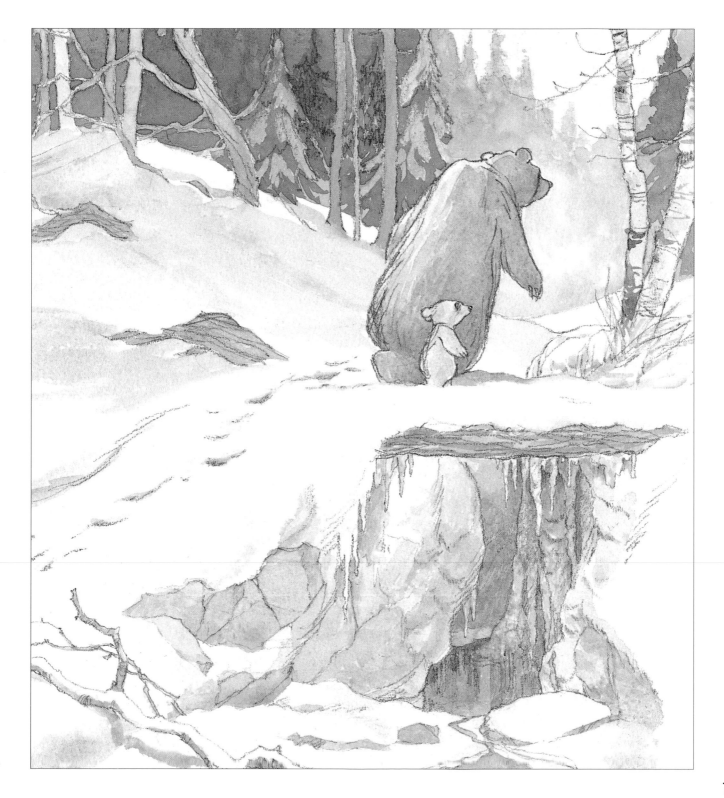

And then … Little Bear stopped and he listened and then he turned round and he looked.

"Come on, Little Bear," said Big Bear, but Little Bear didn't stir.

"I know I heard something this time!" Little Bear said.

"What did you hear?" said Big Bear.

"Plop, plop, plop," said Little Bear. "I think it's a Plopper."

Big Bear turned round, and he listened and looked.

No Plopper was there.

"Let's go home, Little Bear," said Big Bear.

"That was the snow plopping down from a branch."

PLOD PLOD PLOD went Big Bear along the path through the woods. But Little Bear walked slower and slower and at last he sat down in the snow.

"Come on, Little Bear," said Big Bear. "It is time we were both back home."

But Little Bear sat and said nothing.

"Come on and be carried," said Big Bear.

Big Bear put Little Bear high up on his back, and set off down the path through the woods.

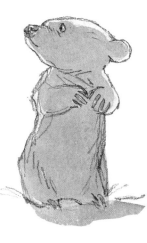

WOO WOO WOO "It's only the wind, Little Bear," said Big Bear and he walked on down the path.

CREAK CREAK CREAK "It's only the trees, Little Bear," said Big Bear and he walked on down the path.

PLOD PLOD PLOD "It is only the sound of my feet again," said Big Bear, and he plodded on and on and on until they came back home to their cave.

Big Bear and Little Bear went down into the dark, the dark of their own Bear Cave.

"Just stay there, Little Bear," said Big Bear, putting Little Bear in the Bear Chair with a blanket to keep him warm. Big Bear stirred up the fire from the embers and lighted the lamps and made the Bear Cave all cosy again.

"Now tell me a story," Little Bear said.

And Big Bear sat down in the Bear Chair with Little Bear curled on his lap. And he told a story of Plodders and Drippers and Ploppers and the sounds of the snow in the woods, and this Little Bear and this Big Bear plodding all the way...

HOME.

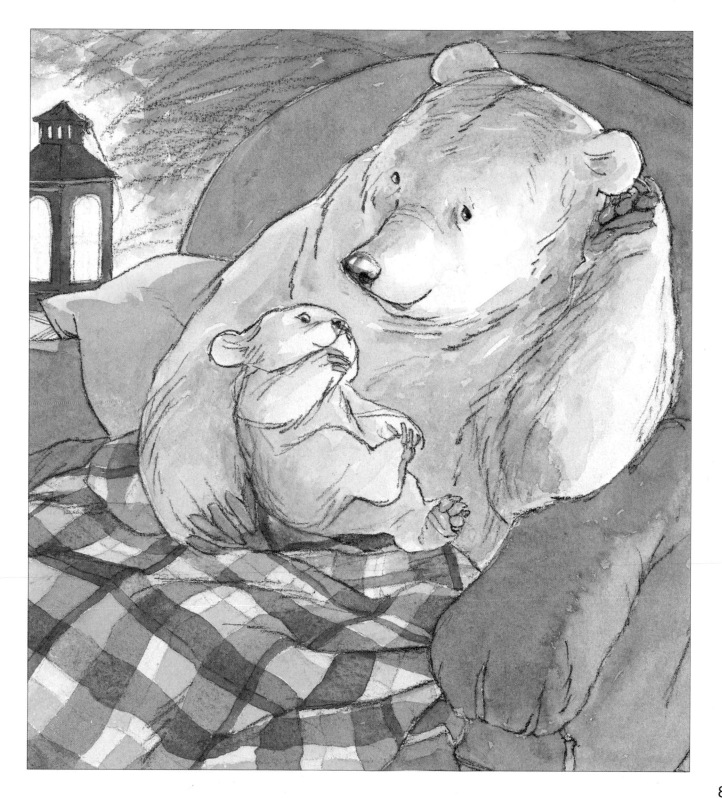

UNDER THE BED

by Michael Rosen   *illustrated by Quentin Blake*

Messing About

"Do you know what?"
said Jumping John.
"I had a bellyache
and now it's gone."

"Do you know what?"
said Kicking Kirsty.
"All this jumping
has made me thirsty."

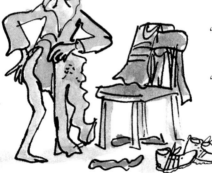

"Do you know what?"
said Mad Mickey.
"I sat in some glue
and I feel all sticky."

"Do you know what?"
said Fat Fred.
"You can't see me,
I'm under the bed."

After Dark

Outside after dark
trains hum and traffic lights wink
after dark, after dark.

In here after dark
curtains shake and cupboards creak
after dark, after dark.

Under the covers after dark
I twiddle my toes and hug my pillow
after dark, after dark.

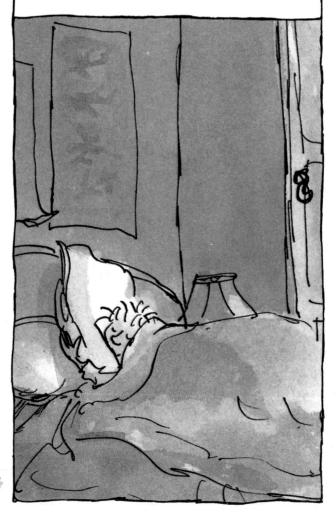

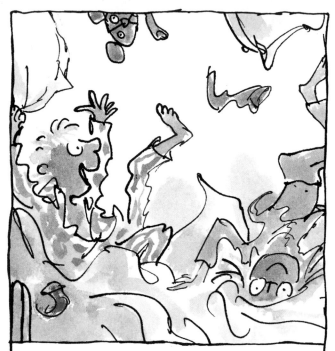

These Two Children

There were these two children
and they were in bed and it was
time they were asleep.

But they were making a huge noise,
shouting, yelling and screaming.
"Look at me!" "Look at you!"
"Let's go mad!" "Yes, let's go mad!"

Their dad heard them and
he shouted up to them,
"Stop the noise! Stop the noise!
If you don't stop the noise, I'm
coming upstairs and I'll give
you a bit of real trouble."

Everything went quiet.

A few minutes later one of the
children called out,
"Dad, Dad, when you come up to give
us a bit of real trouble, can you bring
us up a drink of water as well?"

Nat and Anna

Anna was in her room.
Nat was outside the door.
Anna didn't want Nat to come in.
Nat said, "Anna? Anna? Can I come in?"
Anna said, "I'm not in."

Nat went away.
Anna was still in her room.
Nat came back.
Nat said, "How did you say you're not in?
You must be in if you said you're not in."
Anna said, "I'm not in."
Nat said, "I'm coming in to see if you're in."
Anna said, "You won't find me because I'm not in."
Nat said, "I'm coming in."

Nat went in.
Nat said, "There you are. You are in."
Anna said, "Nat, where are you?
Where are you, Nat?"
Nat said, "I'm here."
Anna said, "I can't see you, Nat. Where are you?"
Nat said, "I'm here. Look."
Anna said, "Sorry, Nat. I can't see you."
Nat said, "Here I am. I'm going to scream, Anna.
Then you'll see me."
Anna said, "Where are you, Nat?"
Nat said, *"Yaaaaaaaaaaaaaaaaaaaa!"*
Anna said, "I can hear you, Nat. But I can't see you."
Nat said, "Right. I'm going out. Then you'll see me."

Nat went out.
Nat said, "Anna? Anna, can you see me now?"
Anna said, "No, of course I can't, you're outside."
Nat said, "Can I come in and see you then?"
Anna said, "But I'm not in."
Nat went away screaming.
He didn't come back.

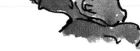

83

IN THE MIDDLE OF THE NIGHT

by Kathy Henderson
illustrated by Jennifer Eachus

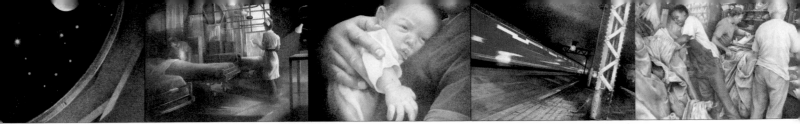

A long time after bedtime
when it's very very late
when even dogs dream
and there's deep sleep
breathing through the house

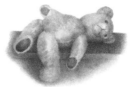

when the doors are locked
and the curtains drawn
and the shops are dark
and the last train's gone
and there's no more traffic
    in the street
because everyone's asleep

then

the window-cleaner comes
to the high-street shop fronts
and shines at the glass
in the street-lit dark

and a dust-cart rumbles past
on its way to the dump
loaded with the last
of the old day's rubbish.

On the twentieth floor
of the office-block
there's a lighted window
and high up there
another night cleaner's
vacuuming the floor
working nights on her own
while her children sleep at home.

And down in the dome
    of the observatory
the astronomer who's
    waited all day
    for the dark

is watching the good black sky
    at last
for stars and moons
and spikes of light
through her telescope
in the middle of the night
while everybody sleeps.

At the bakery
the bakers in their floury clothes
mix dough in machines
for tomorrow's loaves of bread

and out by the gate
rows of parked vans wait
for their drivers to come
and take the newly-baked
bread to the shops
for the time when the
bread-eaters wake.

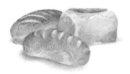

Across the town at the hospital
where the nurses watch in the
    dim-lit wards
someone very old shuts their eyes
and dies
breathes their very last breath
on their very last night.

Yet not far away on another floor
after months of waiting
a new baby's born
and the mother and the father
hold the baby and smile
and the baby looks up
and the world's just begun
but still everybody sleeps.

Now through the silent station
past the empty shops

and the office-blocks
past the sleeping streets
and the hospital
a train with no windows
goes rattling by

and inside the train the sorters sift
urgent letters and packets on the
    late night-shift
so tomorrow's post will arrive
    in time
at the towns and the villages
    down the line.

And the mother
with the wakeful child in her arms
walking up and down
and up and down
and up and down
the room
hears the train as it passes by
and the cats by the bins
and the night owl's flight
and hums hushabye and hushabye
we should be asleep now
you and I
it's late and time to close your eyes

it's the middle of the night.

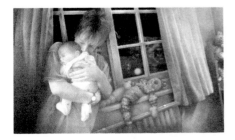

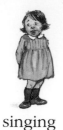
singing

Giving
by Shirley Hughes

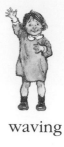
waving

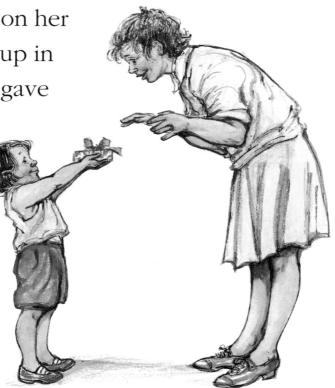

I gave Mom a present on her birthday, all wrapped up in pretty paper. And she gave me a big kiss.
I gave Dad a very special picture which I painted at playgroup. And he gave me a ride on his shoulders most of the way home.

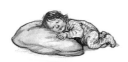
sleeping

telling

listening

thinking

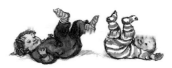
kicking

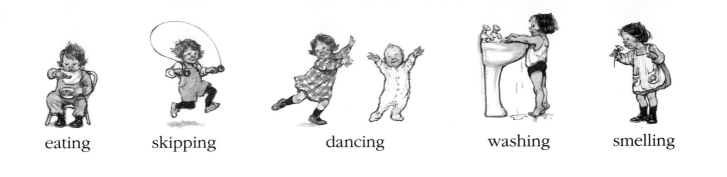

eating   skipping   dancing   washing   smelling

I gave the baby some
slices of my apple.
We ate them sitting
under the table.
At teatime the baby
gave me two of his
soggy crusts.

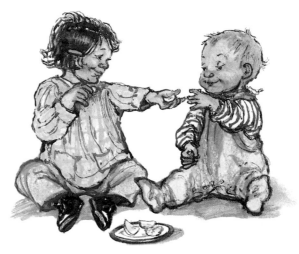

That wasn't much of a present!
You can give someone a cross look
or a big smile! You can give a tea party
or a seat on a crowded bus.

   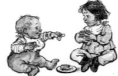 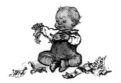

yawning   stroking   giving   writing   tearing

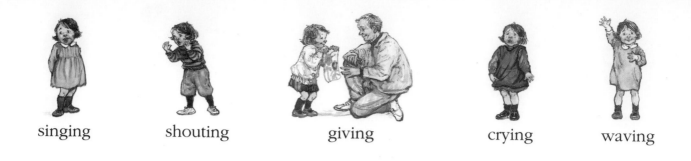

singing shouting giving crying waving

On my birthday Grandma and Grandpa gave me
a beautiful doll's pram. I said "Thank you"
and gave them each a big hug.
And I gave my dear Bemily a ride
in it, all the way down the garden
path and back again.
I tried to give
the cat a ride
too, but she
gave me a
nasty scratch!

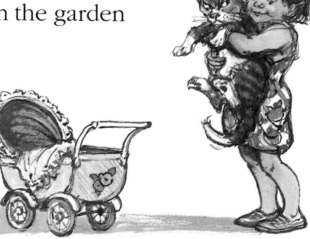

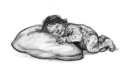 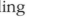 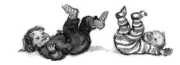

sleeping telling listening thinking kicking

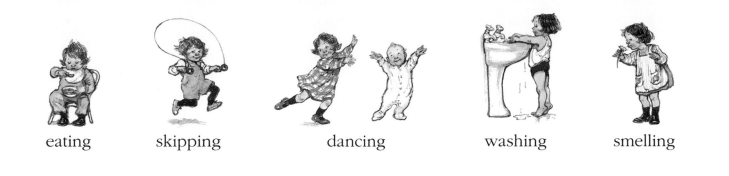

eating	skipping	dancing	washing	smelling

So Dad had to give my poor arm a kiss and a wash and a piece of sticking plaster. Sometimes, just when I've built a big castle out of bricks, the baby comes along and gives it a big swipe! And it all falls down. Then I feel like giving the baby a big swipe too. But I don't, because he is my baby brother, after all.

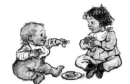

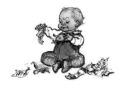

yawning	stroking	giving	writing	tearing

THE MOST OBEDIENT DOG

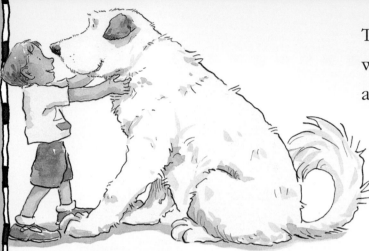

The most obedient dog in the world was waiting for something to happen, when Harry came up the path.

"Hello, boy," said Harry.

The most obedient dog in the world wagged his tail and started to follow.

"No … sit!" said Harry.

"I won't be long."

And then he was gone.

"Why are you sitting there?" asked a nosy bird. "Are you going to sit there all day?"

The most obedient dog in the world didn't answer. He just sat and waited for Harry.

Big, fat raindrops began to fall.

"I'm off," said the bird. And he flew away.

Everyone ran for cover, except the most obedient dog in the world. Thunder rumbled, lightning flashed and then the hailstones fell…

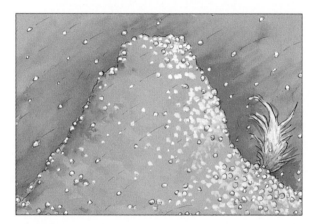

Quite a lot of hailstones! When the sun came out again the bird flew back. The most obedient dog in the world was still sitting there waiting for Harry.

IN THE WORLD by Anita Jeram

"What a strange dog," people said as they passed. Other dogs came to have a look. They sniffed and nuzzled and nudged and nipped, but they soon got bored and went away. The most obedient dog in the world sat … and sat … and sat … and sat. How long must he wait for Harry? Just then, a cat came by. "Quick!" said the bird, pulling his tail. "Why don't you chase it?" The dog's eyes followed the cat. His nose started to twitch, and his legs started to itch. He couldn't sit still any longer. He sprang to his feet …

and saw Harry! "Good boy!" said Harry. "You waited! Leave that cat. Let's go to the beach!" The dog looked at the cat, and he looked at Harry. Then he went to the beach with Harry. After all, he was …

the most obedient dog in the world!

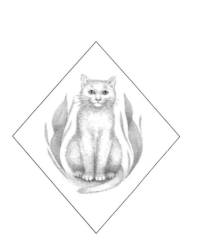

PARROT CAT

by Nicola Bayley

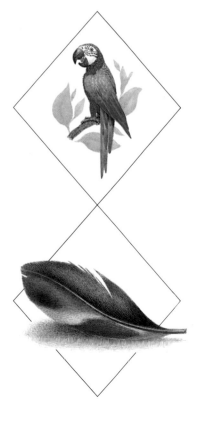

If I were a parrot
instead of a cat,

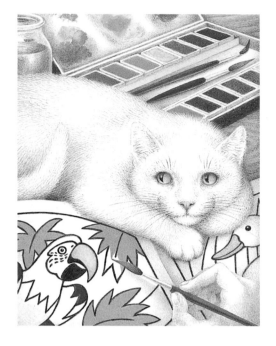

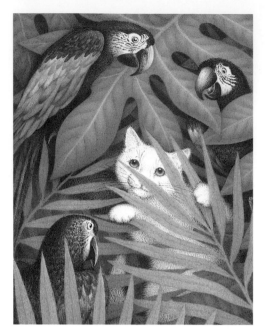

I would live
in the jungle,

I would fly
through the trees,

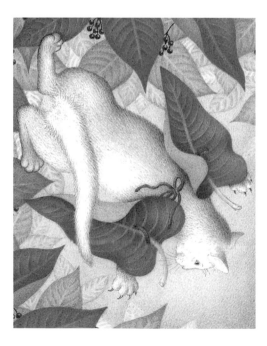

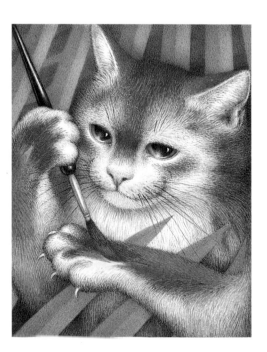

I would be coloured
so bright,

I would sit
on my nest,

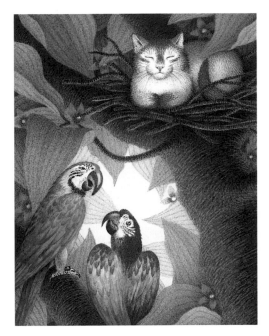

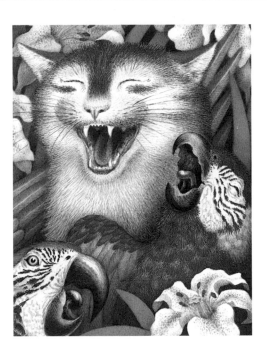

I would talk
and squawk,

and if a snake
ever came,

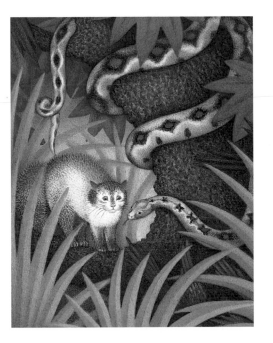

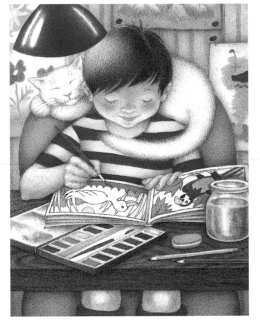

I would quickly turn
back into a cat again.

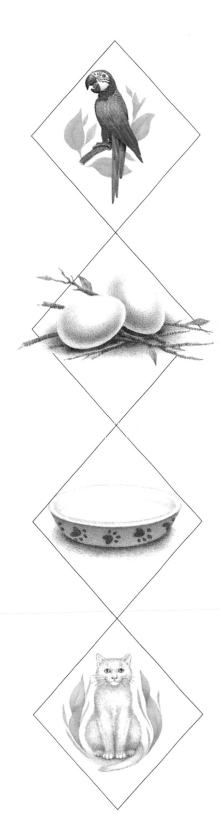

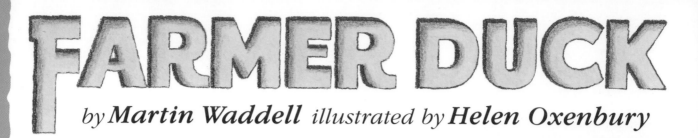

FARMER DUCK

by **Martin Waddell** illustrated by **Helen Oxenbury**

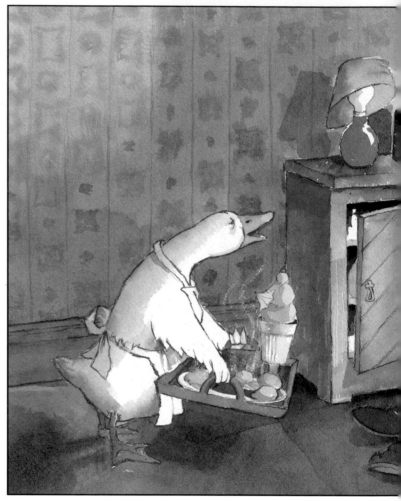

There once was a duck who had the bad luck to live with a lazy old farmer. The duck did the work. The farmer stayed all day in bed. The duck fetched the cow from the field.

"How goes the work?" called the farmer.

The duck answered,

"Quack!"

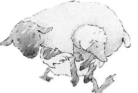

The duck brought the sheep from the hill.

"How goes the work?" called the farmer.

The duck answered,

"Quack!"

The duck put the hens in their house.

"How goes the work?" called the farmer.

The duck answered,

"Quack!"

The farmer got fat through staying in bed and the poor duck got fed up with working all day.

"How goes the work?"

"Quack!"

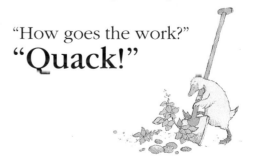

"How goes the work?"
"Quack!"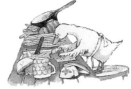

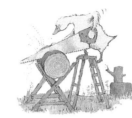 "How goes the work?"
"Quack!"

The poor duck was
sleepy and weepy
and tired.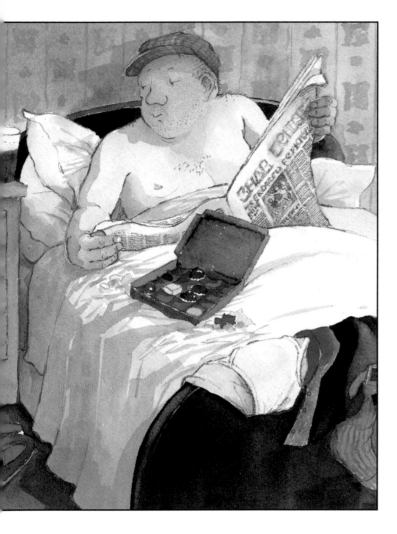
The hens and
the cow and the
sheep got very upset.
They loved the duck.
So they held a meeting under the
moon and they made a plan for the
morning.

"Moo!" said the cow.
"Baa!" said the sheep.
"Cluck!" said the hens.

And *that* was the plan!

"How goes the work?"
"Quack!"

"How goes the work?"
"Quack!"

"How goes the work?"
"Quack!"

It was just before dawn
and the farmyard was still. Through
the back door and into the house crept
the cow and the sheep and the hens.

They stole down the hall.
They creaked up the stairs.
They squeezed under
the bed of the farmer
and wriggled about.
The bed started to rock
and the farmer woke up,
and he called,
"How goes the work?" and…

"M o o!"
"B a a!"
"C l u c k!"

They lifted his bed
and he started to shout, and
they banged and they bounced
the old farmer about and about and
about, right out of the bed …
and he fled with the cow and the
sheep and the hens mooing and
baaing and clucking around him.

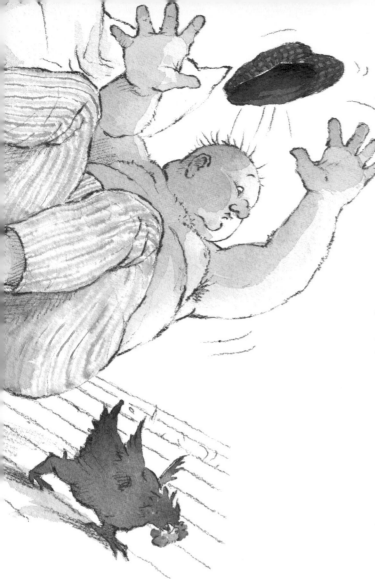

The duck awoke and waddled wearily into the yard expecting to hear, "How goes the work?" But nobody spoke!

Then the cow and the sheep and the hens came back.

"Quack?" asked the duck.

"Moo!" said the cow.

"Baa!" said the sheep.

"Cluck!" said the hens.

Down the lane... **"Moo!"**

through the fields... **"Baa!"**

over the hill... **"Cluck!"**

and he never came back.

Which told the duck the whole story.

Then mooing and baaing and clucking and quacking they all set to work on their farm.

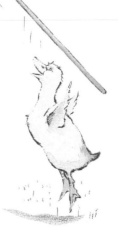

The FIBBS
by Chris Riddell

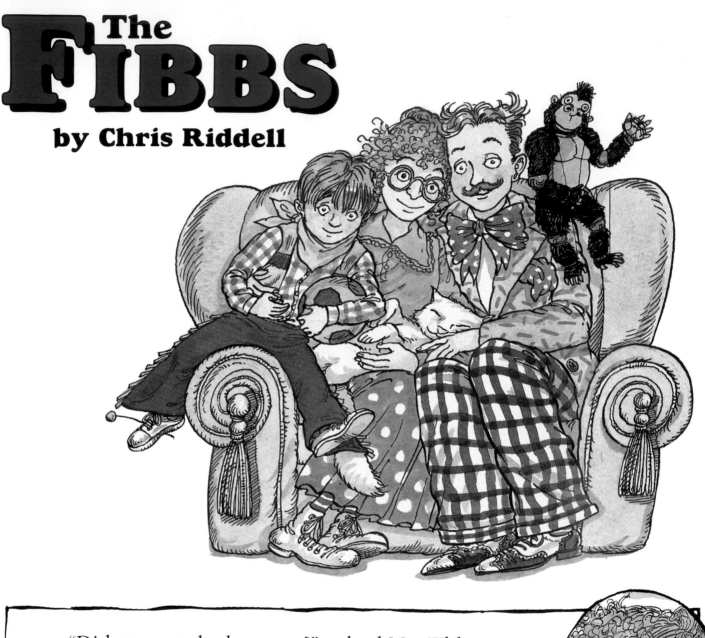

"Did you get the bananas?" asked Mrs Fibb
when Mr Fibb got back from the shops.

"Well, no," said Mr Fibb. "I meant to, but…"

"But what?" said Mrs Fibb.

"*You're never going to believe this,*" said Mr Fibb,
"but I had just come out of the greengrocer's …

when a giant hairy hand came down from the sky and grabbed me! There I was on top of an office block in the clutches of a giant gorilla. I could see police cars and fire engines down below, and a huge crowd gathered. Then from out of the clouds came fighter planes with their guns blazing and the gorilla got very angry. So before there was a nasty accident I decided to sort things out myself. 'Excuse me,' I said to the gorilla, 'would you care for a banana?' 'How kind,' said the gorilla and ate all the bananas in one mouthful. Then he gave me a lift home on his back. Still, never mind, we can have some of your chocolate cake instead."

"Well, no," said Mrs Fibb. "I was baking today, but..."

"But what?" said Mr Fibb.

"*You're never going to believe this,*" said Mrs Fibb, "but just after you left, something that looked like a giant tea saucer landed in the back garden.

And three little green people climbed
out of it and came into the kitchen.
'We come in peace, earth woman,' they said.
'What's cooking?'
'Nothing yet,' I said, 'but I'm
about to bake a chocolate cake.'

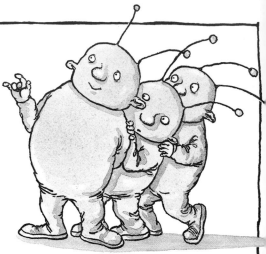

'Then we shall help you,' they said and straight away they began.
They mixed up flour and baked beans and washing-up liquid and
pepper and put it in the oven. Before you could say 'little green
Martians' the oven door opened
and a big spongy blob
jumped out and started
chasing the cat.
'That's the best cake
we've ever baked,' said
the little green people.
'You can keep it if you like.'
'No, thank you,' I said.
'I like earth cooking much
better.' So then I baked them
a big chocolate cake.

When they had all tasted a piece, they said,
'You must give us the recipe, earth woman.'
'Only if you take that nasty blob with you
when you go,' I replied. So they did. And they
took the rest of the chocolate cake, I'm afraid.
Still, never mind, at least we can have a cup of tea.
Now where's the teapot?"

"You're never going to believe this,"

said Tommy Fibb, running into the room, "but…"

"But what?" said Mr and Mrs Fibb.

"Well," said Tommy Fibb, "Mrs McBean

from next door accidentally kicked her football

through the window this morning … and it landed on the

table and smashed the teapot. I meant to tell you earlier, but…"

"You can't believe a word that child says," said Mrs Fibb.

"I don't know where he gets it from,"
said Mr Fibb.

My Old Teddy

by
DOM MANSELL

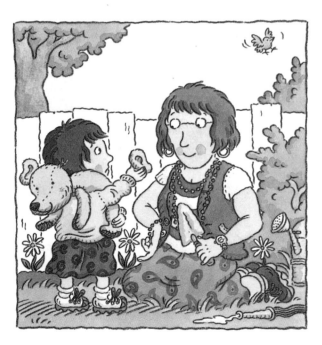

My old Teddy's leg came off.
Poor old Teddy!
I took him to the Teddy doctor.
She made Teddy better.

My old Teddy's ear came off.
Poor old Teddy!
I took him to the Teddy doctor.
She made Teddy better.

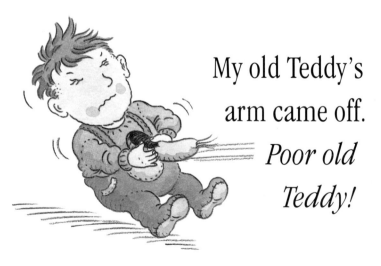

My old Teddy's
arm came off.
*Poor old
Teddy!*

I took him to the Teddy doctor.
She made Teddy better.

Then poor old Teddy's head
came off.

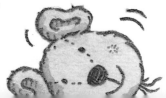

The Teddy doctor said,
"Teddy's had enough now.
Teddy has to rest."

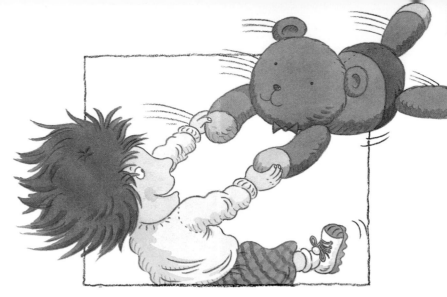

The Teddy doctor gave me … my new Teddy. I love new Teddy
very much, but I love poor
old Teddy best.

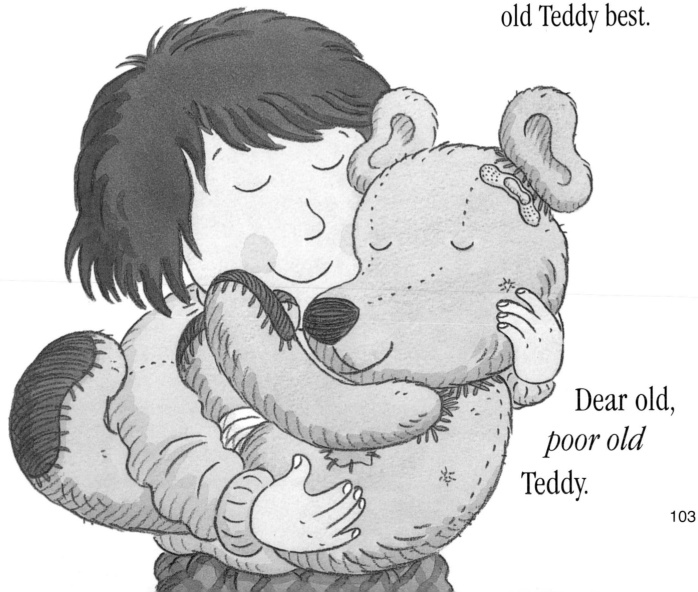

Dear old,
poor old
Teddy.

Little Pig's Tale

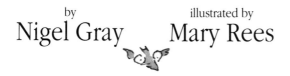

by
Nigel Gray

illustrated by
Mary Rees

On Monday, Little Pig's dad told him, "Next Sunday, it's your mom's birthday."

"Will she have a party?" asked Little Pig.

"No. I don't think she'll have a party," said Dad. "Will she have a birthday cake with lots of candles?"

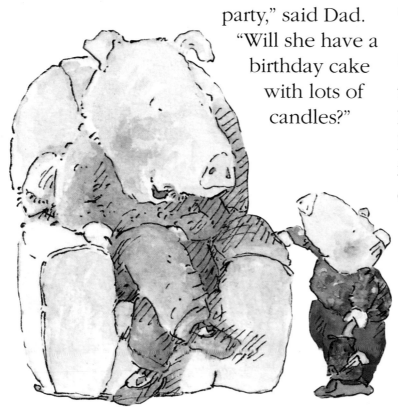

"No. I don't think she'll want a cake with lots of candles."

"Will we sing *Happy Birthday to You?*"

"Yes. We must sing *Happy Birthday to You.*"

"And will we give her presents?"

"Of course," said Dad. "I'll give her a present. And you should give her a present too."

"What will I give her?" asked Little Pig.

"I don't know," said Dad. "You'll have to think of something."

On Tuesday, Little Pig tried to think of something exciting. Perhaps his mom would like an aeroplane so she could fly high, high above the town … or a rocket so she could explore the moon … or a spaceship so she could venture into outer space… But Little Pig knew he couldn't really give her a spaceship, or a rocket, or even an aeroplane. For one thing, their garage was too small. He'd have to think of something else.

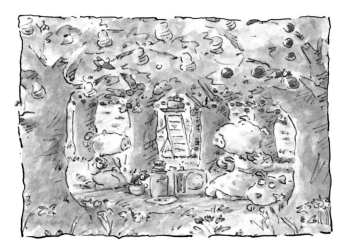

On Wednesday, Little Pig thought of flowers and fruit. He'd give his mom an orchard – an orchard with pears and plums, apples and apricots, with daffodils and crocuses growing in the lush grass under the trees. He knew she'd like that because she was always weeding her window box, and growing plants in pots from apple pips and cherry stones.

Little Pig went to see Mr Green, the gardener. "I'm sure your mom would love an orchard," said Mr Green, "but your back yard is too small, and trees take years to grow. It was a good idea, Little Pig, but I'm afraid you'll have to think of something else."

On Thursday, Little Pig knew what he had to do. He raided his piggy bank and took his pennies to the shop.

He would buy his mom a silk gown, and a warm coat, and shiny shoes, and furry gloves, and glittering jewels for her to wear around her neck.

But the shopkeeper counted Little Pig's pennies and said, "I'm sorry, Little Pig, but you don't have enough money for any of those things."

"Not even for the gloves?" asked Little Pig.

"Not even for one glove," said the shopkeeper.

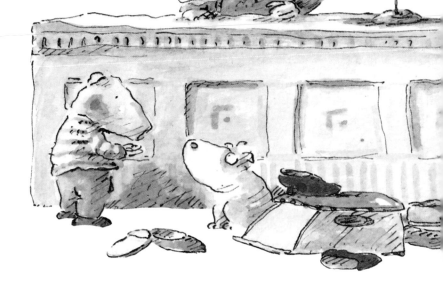

On Friday, Little Pig felt sad. In two days it would be his mom's birthday and Little Pig had nothing to give her. What was he to do?

He asked his dad.

"Why don't you make her something?" suggested Dad.

So Little Pig set to work.

He'd make her a useful box for keeping things in.

He fetched the tools, and found some old pieces of wood in the shed. The wood splintered. The box broke.

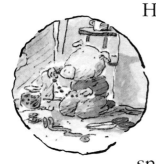

He'd make her a beautiful necklace of beads. He got the beads from the odds and ends drawer, and threaded the beads on cotton. The cotton snapped and the beads spilled all over the floor.

He'd do a painting in rainbow colours.

He got out the paints and a large sheet of white paper. But he knocked over the pot of black paint and spoiled his painting with an ugly blot.

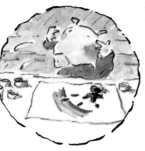

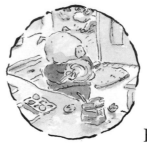

He'd bake some cakes.

He mixed up flour and milk and eggs and sultanas and dates, and greased the baking tray with margarine. But the cakes burnt and came out of the oven as hard as stones.

On Saturday, Little Pig was in despair. He thought and thought until his brain hurt.

And then he had a brain wave.

He gathered together the things he would need.

A piece of paper, a pen and a red ribbon.

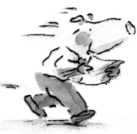

On Sunday, it was Little Pig's mom's birthday. After breakfast Little Pig and Dad sang *Happy Birthday to You*. Then Dad gave Mom a present… and while no one was looking, Little Pig slipped away.

Mom unwrapped her packet. Inside was a watch.

"That's because I want you to have a good time," Dad said. And Mom gave Dad a kiss.

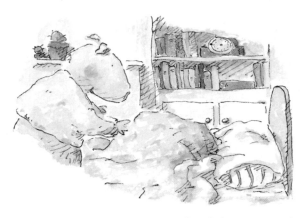

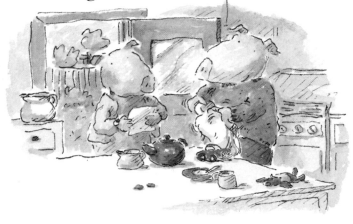

Then, on the table, Mom found a note. It said:

To Mom.

Your present is upstairs in your bed. Happy Birthday! Lots of love from Little Pig.

Mom went up to the bedroom. There was certainly something in the bed. She pulled back the covers and there was…

Little Pig, with a red ribbon tied around him in a bow. "Happy Birthday, Mom!" said Little Pig.

"Oh, Little Pig," said Mom, "this is the best present you could possibly have given me. There's nothing in the world I'd rather have."

Mom hugged Little Pig and gave him a big sloppy kiss. And Little Pig beamed from ear to ear.

Noah's Ark

A long time ago there lived a man called Noah.

Noah was a good man, who trusted in God.

There were also many wicked people in the world.

God wanted to punish the wicked people,

so he said to Noah…

I shall make a flood of water and wash all the wicked people away. Build an ark for your family and all the animals.

Noah worked for years and years and years to build the ark.

At last the ark was finished.

Noah and his family gathered lots of food.

Then the animals came,

two by two,

two by two,

into the ark.

by Lucy Cousins

When the ark was full Noah felt a drop of rain. It rained and rained and rained. It rained for forty days and forty nights. The world was covered with water.

At last the rain stopped and the sun came out. Noah sent a dove to find dry land. The dove came back with a leafy twig.

"Hurrah!" shouted Noah. "The flood has ended."

But many more days passed before the ark came to rest on dry land.

Then Noah and all the animals came safely out of the ark, and life began again on the earth.

DUDLEY
AND THE
STRAWBERRY SHAKE

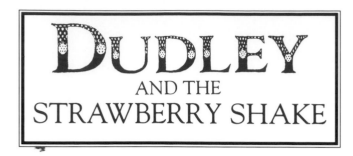

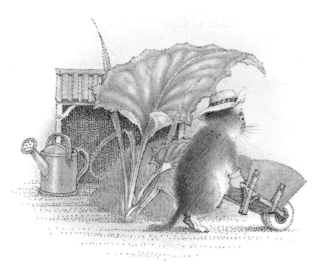

PETER CROSS
Text by JUDY TAYLOR

There was a soft breeze blowing in Shadyhanger and it carried the scent of strawberries through the open window.

Dudley had been awake since early morning searching for his special gloves. Today he was going strawberry picking.

The sun was shining strongly and the ground felt warm.

Dudley set off with his berry-barrow down the lane to the strawberry patch, and long before he got there his mouth was watering.

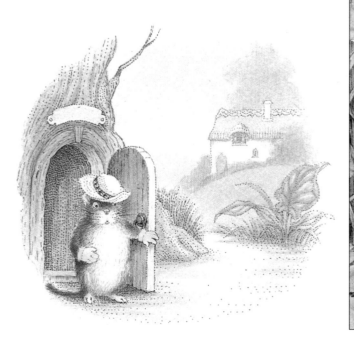

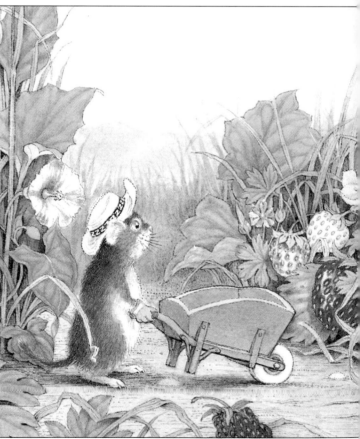

As he turned the corner, there they were before him – row upon row of fat, juicy strawberries.

Dudley picked a big strawberry very carefully with his special gloves.

He took a bite to see if it was ripe. It was.

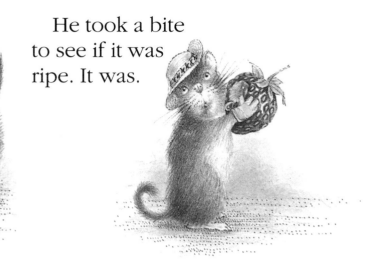

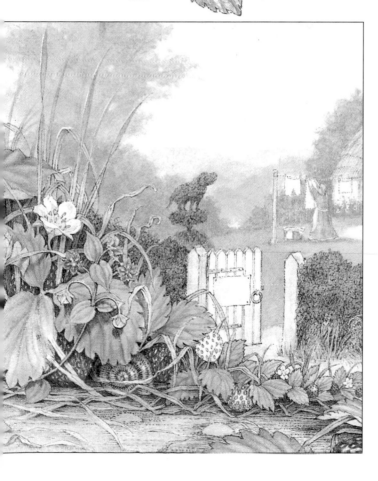

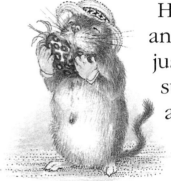

He took another bite just to make sure … and another and another …

until there was nothing left.

Dudley was quite full up.

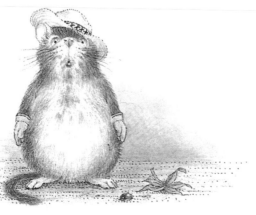

Just then, over by the hedge, Dudley spied an extra large strawberry, the largest he had ever seen.

"That's the one I'll take home for lunch," he said.

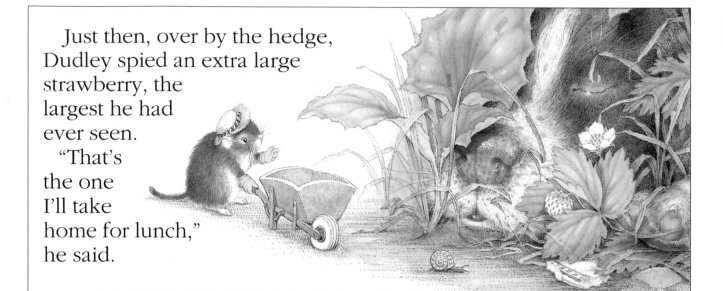

Dudley gripped the strawberry firmly with his gloves but it wouldn't come.

He tried again, pulling and pulling with all his might.

Suddenly the strawberry
began to shake
violently.

Dudley hung
on until he felt
his hands slipping
out of his gloves.
   Then he was sailing
through the air. He landed
on the grass with a BUMP.
   "What an odd
strawberry," thought
Dudley, feeling
rather giddy.

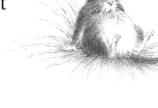

Dudley waited until the world
had stopped going round.
   "It feels like time for a nap," he
said, hurrying home.

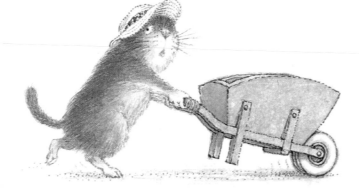

And just as he
was drifting off
to sleep,
Dudley
remembered
he had left
his gloves
bchind.

Oh, Little Jack

by Inga Moore

It was a windy day. Little Jack Rabbit went into the garden. Mommy was in her vegetable patch. She was pulling out onions. "Can I help?" asked Little Jack. Little Jack Rabbit found an onion with a brown curly top. He tugged and he tugged. He tugged as hard as he could. But he couldn't pull it out of the ground.

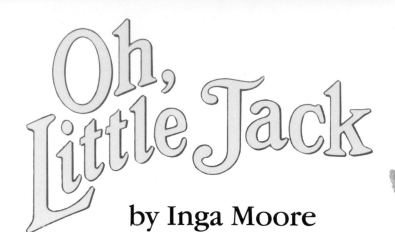

"Oh, Little Jack!" said Mommy. "I think you are too small to pull out onions."

In the garden the wind was blowing down the leaves. "I shall have to sweep up these leaves," said Daddy.

"Can I do it?" asked Little Jack. Little Jack Rabbit ran to fetch the broom. But the broom was very long. He couldn't make it sweep. "Oh, Little Jack!" said Daddy. "I think you are too small to sweep up leaves."

Little Jack Rabbit went to Heathery Heath with his sister Nancy and his big brother Buck. Buck flew his new blue kite.

"Can I fly it?" asked Little Jack.
Little Jack Rabbit held the kite
by its string. He held it as tightly
as he could. But the wind pulled
and pulled. It nearly pulled
the kite away.

"Oh, Little Jack!" said Buck.
"I think you are too small to
fly a kite."
On the way home Nancy rode
her billy-cart down the hill.
"Can I have a turn?" asked Little
Jack.
Little Jack Rabbit sat in the
billy-cart.
He rode
it down
the hill.
But he couldn't
make it stop
at the
bottom.

"Oh, Little
Jack!" said
Nancy.
"I think you
are too small
to ride in a
billy-cart."

115

At home, Little Jack Rabbit went into the kitchen. His sisters Rhona and Rita were helping Mommy to make the tea. She was going to take some to Granpa.

"Can I take it?" asked Little Jack. Little Jack Rabbit picked up the cup. He carried it as carefully as he could. But he spilt the tea into the saucer.

"Oh, Little Jack!" said Rita. "I think you are too small to carry a cup of tea."

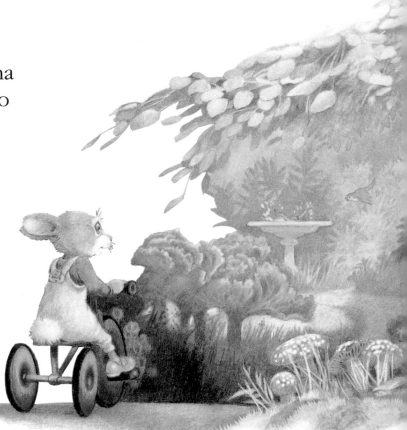

Poor Little Jack Rabbit ran to find his granpa.

"What's the matter, Little Jack?" Granpa asked.

"I am too small," said Little Jack.

"Too small for what?" asked Granpa.

"I am too small for everything," said Little Jack.

Granpa had been busy in his workshop.

He had been fixing something. It was a little red tricycle.

"Who is it for?" asked Little Jack.

"It can't be for me," said Mommy. "I am too big. And it can't be for Daddy. He's much too big."

"Is it for Buck?" asked Little Jack. No, the tricycle was not for Buck. It was not for Nancy or Rhona or Rita. They were all too big to ride it.

"Can I ride it?" asked Little Jack.

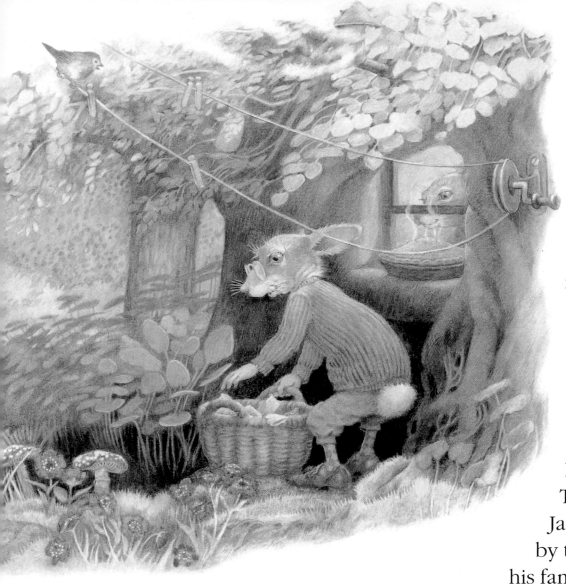

It was better than flying a kite. It was even better than riding in a billy-cart. And it was much better than carrying a cup of tea. "Thank you, Granpa," said Little Jack.

That night Little Jack Rabbit sat by the fire with his family. Now he was glad he was small. And not only because of the little red tricycle. There was something else, something he had forgotten. He was just the right size to sit on Granpa's knee.

Little Jack Rabbit climbed on to the little red tricycle. He was not too big and he was not too small. "Why, Little Jack!" said Granpa. "You are just the right size. The tricycle must be for you."
Little Jack Rabbit rode his little red tricycle round and round the garden. It was better than pulling up onions or sweeping leaves.

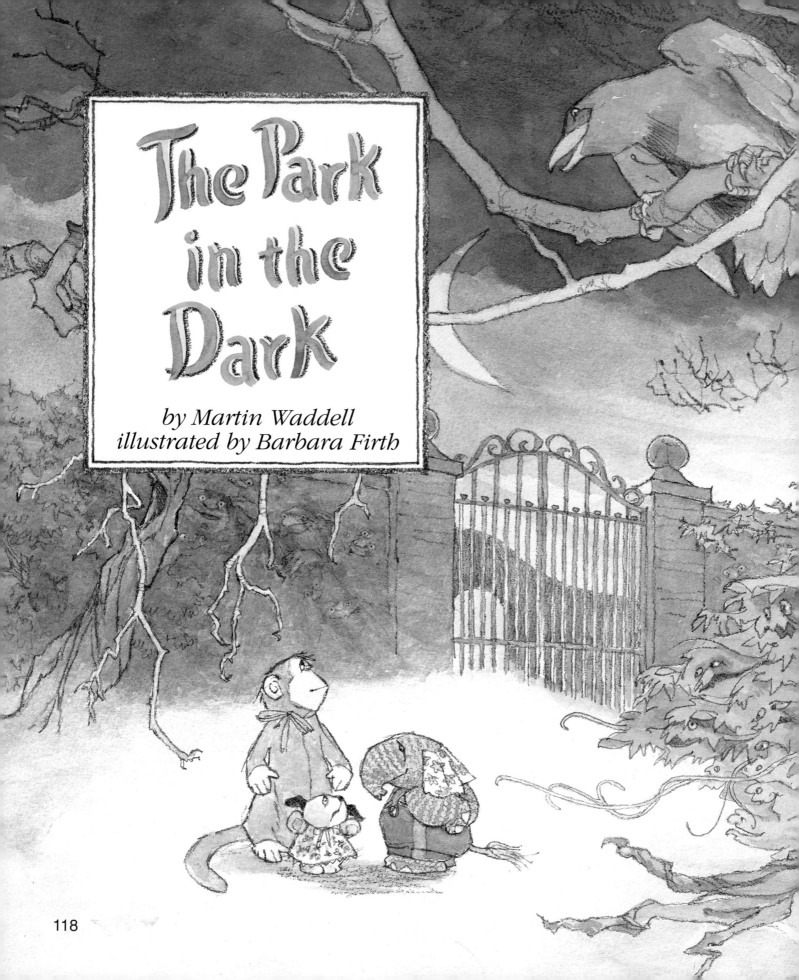

The Park in the Dark

by Martin Waddell
illustrated by Barbara Firth

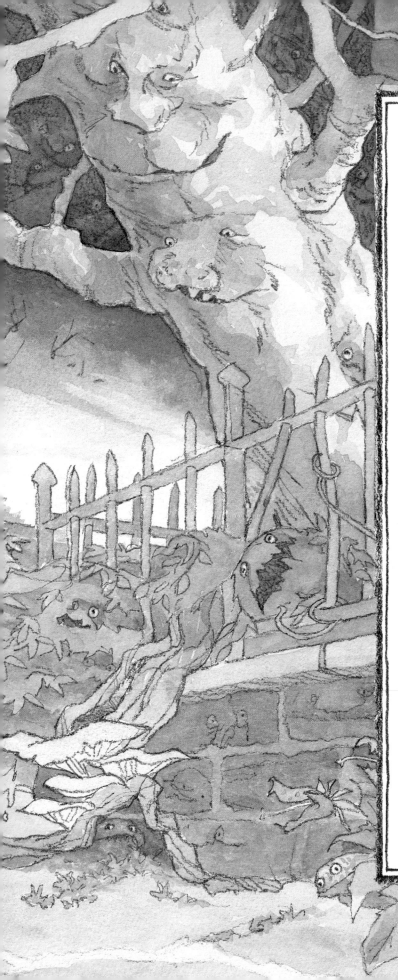

When the sun goes down
and the moon comes up
and the old swing creaks in the dark,
that's when we go to the park,
　me and Loopy and Little Gee,
　　all three.

Softly down the staircase,
through the haunty hall,
trying to look small,
　me and Loopy and Little Gee,
　　we three.

It's shivery out in the dark
on our way to the park,
down dustbin alley,
past the ruined mill, so still,
　just me and Loopy and Little Gee,
　　just three.

And Little Gee doesn't like it.
He's scared of the things he might see
in the park in the dark
with Loopy and me.
　That's me and Loopy and Little Gee,
　　the three.

There might be moon witches
or man-eating trees
or withers that wobble
or old Scrawny Shins
or hairy hobgoblins,
or black boggarts' knees in the trees,
or things we can't see,
　me and Loopy and Little Gee,
　　all three.

But there's not, says Loopy,
and I agree,
and Little Gee gets up on my back
and we pass the Howl Tree,
   me and Loopy and Little Gee.
      We're heroes, we three.

In the park in the dark
by the lake and the bridge,
that's when we see
where we want to be,
   me and Loopy
      and Little Gee.
         WHOOPEE!

And we swing and we slide
and we dance and we jump
and we chase all over the place,
me and Loopy
   and Little Gee,
      the Big Three!

And then the THING comes!
Y A A A A A
A A A I I I
O O O O O E E E E E E !

RUN RUN RUN
shouts Little Gee to Loopy and me
and we flee,
   me and Loopy
      and Little Gee,
         scared three.

Back where we've come
through the park in the dark
and the THING is roaring
and following, see?
  After me and Loopy
    and Little Gee,
      we three.

Up to the
house, to the stair,
to the bed where we ought to be,
me and Loopy and Little Gee,
  safe as can be,
    all three.

FLY BY NIGHT

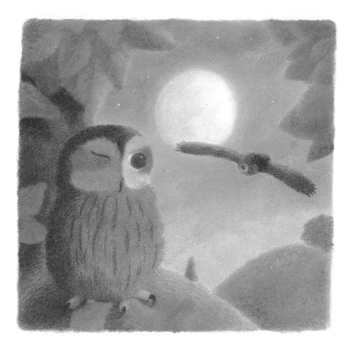

Once, at the edge of a wood, lived two owls, a mother owl and her young one, Blink. Every day, all day long, they slept. Every night, all night long, the mother owl flew and Blink waited.

One day, when the sun was still low in the sky, Blink opened one eye and said, "Now? Is it time?"

"Soon," said his mother. "Soon. Go back to sleep."

Blink tried to sleep. When the sun rose and warmed the earth, he opened the other eye. "*Now* is it time?"

"Not yet," said his mother. "Soon. Go back to sleep."

Blink tried.

Butterflies looped and drifted past him. Beetles scuttled in the undergrowth. Near by, a woodpecker tapped on a tree trunk. Blink couldn't sit still.

"Is it time *yet*?" he said. His mother opened her eyes. "You are old enough and strong enough – " Blink dithered with excitement – "but you must wait." His mother closed her eyes.

The sun was at its highest. A squirrel leapt from tree to tree, quicker than a thought. Along Blink's branch it came, right past him, its tail streaming out behind. Blink wriggled and jiggled. He *couldn't* sit still. All that long afternoon, he watched and waited. He shuffled and fidgeted. Below, in the clearing, a deer and its fawn browsed on leaves and twigs. High above, a kestrel hovered, dipped and soared again into the sky.

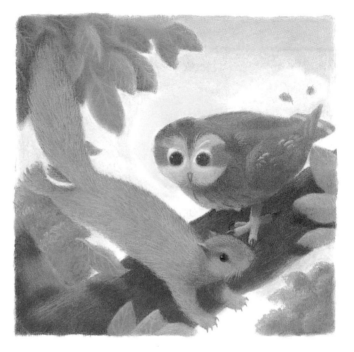

"When will it be *my* time?" said Blink to himself. Towards dusk, a sudden gust of wind, sweeping through the wood, lifting leaves on their branches, seemed to gather Blink from his branch as if it would lift him too. "Time to fly," it seemed to say. Blink fluffed out his feathers. He shifted his wings. But the wind swirled by. It was all puff and nonsense.

Blink sighed.

He closed his eyes.

123

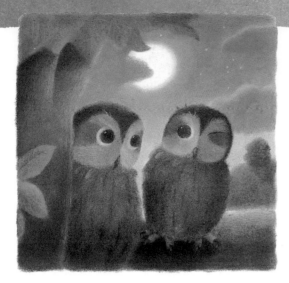

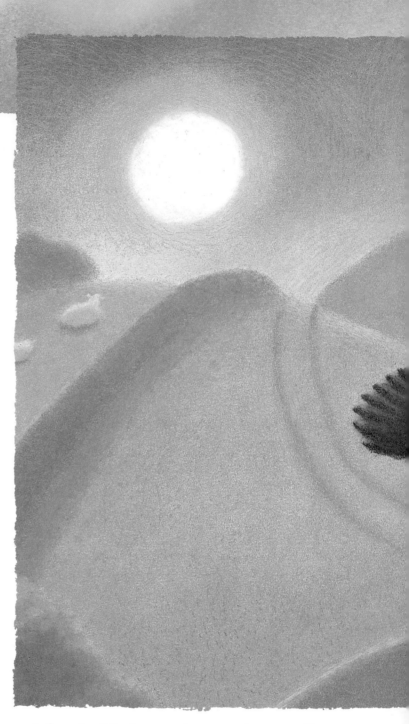

The sun slipped behind the
fields. The moon rose pale and
clear. A night breeze stirred.
"Time to fly."
"Puff and nonsense,"
muttered Blink.
"*Time to fly*," said his
mother beside him.
Blink sat up. "Is it?" he said.
"Is it? *Really*?"
The grey dusk had deepened.
Blink heard soft whisperings.
He saw the stars in the sky
He felt the dampness of the
night air. He knew it was time to fly.
He gathered his strength. He drew
himself up. He stretched out his wings
and – lifted into the air.

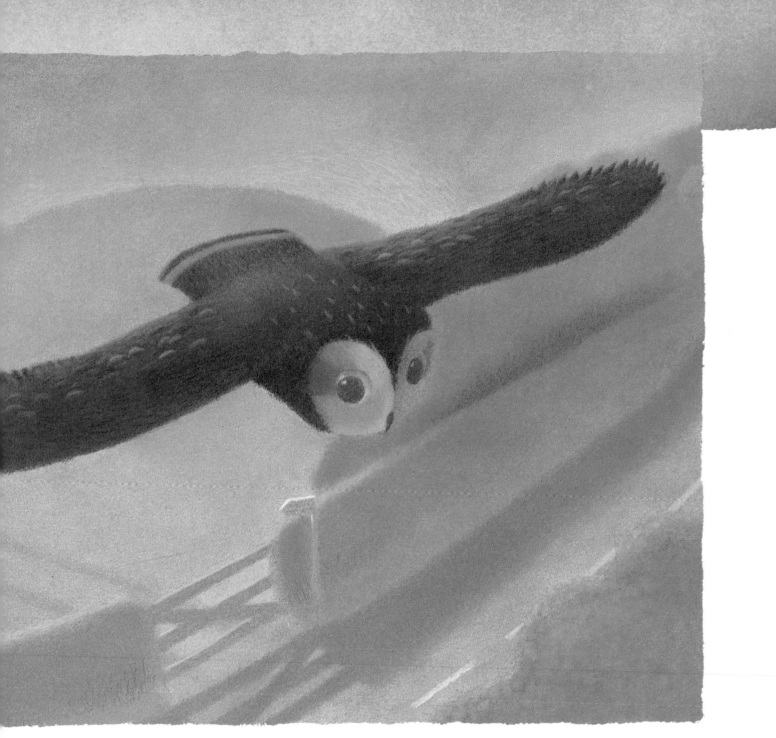

Higher and higher. He flew. Further and further. Over the wood, over the fields, over the road and the sleeping city. High in the sky, his wing-beats strong,

Blink flew on over the sleeping city – and over the fields and the winding river. His first flight; a fly-by-night.

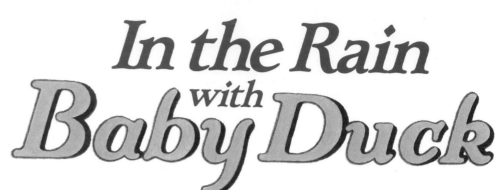

In the Rain with Baby Duck

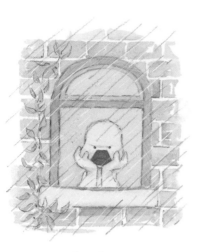

P*it-pat.*
Pit-a-pat.
Pit-a-pit-a-pat.
Oh, the rain came down. It poured and poured. Baby Duck was cross. She did not like walking in the rain. But it was Pancake Sunday, a Duck family tradition, and Baby loved pancakes.

And she loved Grandpa, who was waiting on the other side of town.
Pit-pat. Pit-a-pat. Pit-a-pit-a-pat.
"Follow us! Step lively!" Mr and Mrs Duck left the house arm in arm.
"Wet feet," wailed Baby.
"Don't dally, dear. Don't drag behind," called Mr Duck.

by Amy Hest
illustrated by Jill Barton

"Wet face," pouted Baby. "Water in my eyes."

Mrs Duck pranced along. "See how the rain rolls off your back!"

"Mud," muttered Baby. "Mud, mud, mud."

"Don't dawdle, dear! Don't lag behind!"

Mr and Mrs Duck skipped ahead. They waddled. They shimmied. They hopped in all the puddles. Baby dawdled. She dallied and pouted and dragged behind.

She sang a little song.

I do not like the rain one bit
Splashing down my neck.
Baby feathers soaking wet,
I do not like this mean old day."

"Are you singing?" called Mr and Mrs Duck. "What a fine thing to do in the rain!"

Baby stopped singing.

Grandpa was waiting at the front door. He put his arm round Baby.

"Wet feet?" he asked.

"Yes," Baby said.

"Wet face?" Grandpa asked.

"Yes," Baby said.

"Mud?" Grandpa asked.

"Yes," Baby said. "Mud, mud, mud."

"I'm afraid the rain makes Baby cranky," clucked Mr Duck.

"I've never heard of a duck who doesn't like rain," worried Mrs Duck.

"Oh, really?" Grandpa kissed Baby's cheeks.

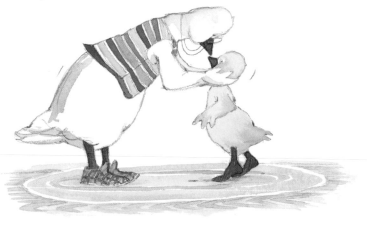

Grandpa took Baby's hand.

"Come with me, Baby."

They went upstairs to the attic.

"We are looking for a tall, green bag," Grandpa said.

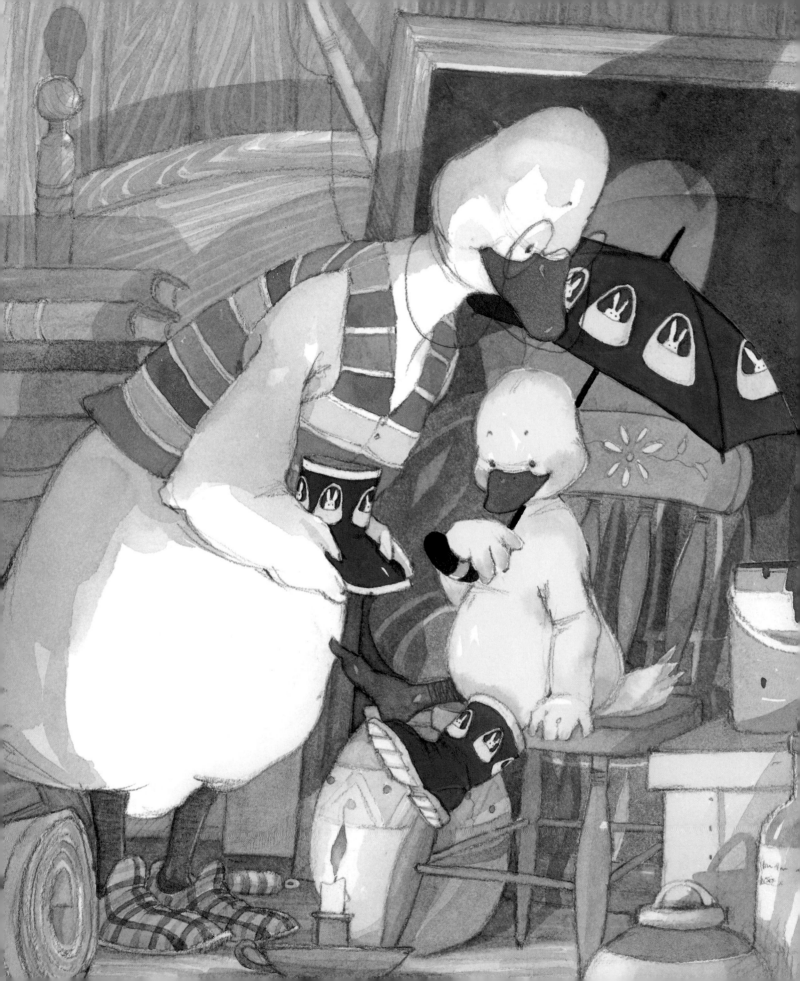

Finally they found it. Inside was a beautiful red umbrella. There were matching boots, too.

"These used to be your mother's," Grandpa whispered. "A long time ago, she was a baby duck who did not like rain."

Baby opened the umbrella. The boots were just the right size.

Baby and Grandpa marched downstairs.

"My boots!" cried Mrs Duck. "And my bunny umbrella!"

"No, mine!" said Baby.

"You look lovely," said Mrs Duck.

Mr Duck put a plate of pancakes on the table. After that, Baby and Grandpa went outside.

Pit-pat. Pit-a-pat. Pit-a-pit-a-pat.

Oh, the rain came down. It poured and poured. Baby Duck and Grandpa walked arm in arm in the rain.

They waddled.

They shimmied.

They hopped in all the puddles.

And Baby Duck sang a new song.

"I really like the rain a lot
Splashing my umbrella.
Big red boots on baby feet,
I really love this rainy day."

We're the noisy dinosaurs, *crash, bang, wallop!*
We're the noisy dinosaurs, *crash, bang, wallop!*
If you're sleeping, we'll wake you up!
We're the noisy dinosaurs, *crash, bang, wallop!*

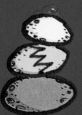

We're the hungry dinosaurs, *um, um, um!*
We're the hungry dinosaurs, *um, um, um!*
We want eggs with jam on top!
We're the hungry dinosaurs, *um, um, um!*

We're the busy dinosaurs, *play, play, play!*
We're the busy dinosaurs, *play, play, play!*
We've got toys to share with you!
We're the busy dinosaurs, *play, play, play!*

We're the happy dinosaurs, *ha, ha, ha!*
We're the happy dinosaurs, *ha, ha, ha!*
We tell jokes and tickle each other!
We're the happy dinosaurs, *ha, ha, ha!*

We're the dancing dinosaurs, *quick, quick, slow!*
We're the dancing dinosaurs,
quick, quick, slow!
Hold our hands but don't step
on our feet!
We're the dancing dinosaurs,
quick, quick, slow!

DINOSAURS!

BY JOHN WATSON

We're the thirsty dinosaurs, *slurp, slurp, glug!*
We're the thirsty dinosaurs, *slurp, slurp, glug!*
We'll drink the sea and your bathwater too!
We're the thirsty dinosaurs, *slurp, slurp, glug!*

CRASH!

We're the angry dinosaurs, *roar, roar, roar!*
We're the angry dinosaurs, *roar, roar, roar!*
Get out of our way or we'll eat you up!
We're the angry dinosaurs, *roar, roar, roar!*

We're the naughty dinosaurs, *bad, bad, bad!*
We're the naughty dinosaurs, *bad, bad, bad!*
We say sorry and promise to be good!
We're the naughty dinosaurs, *bad, bad, bad!*

We're the quiet dinosaurs, *shh, shh, shh!*
We're the quiet dinosaurs, *shh, shh, shh!*
We read books and play hide-and-seek!
We're the quiet dinosaurs, *shh, shh, shh!*

We're the dirty dinosaurs, *scrub, scrub, scrub!*
We're the dirty dinosaurs, *scrub, scrub, scrub!*
We wash our necks and brush our teeth!
We're the dirty dinosaurs, *scrub, scrub, scrub!*

We're the sleepy dinosaurs, *yawn, yawn, yawn!*
We're the sleepy dinosaurs, *yawn, yawn, yawn!*
Send us to bed with a great big kiss!
We're the sleepy dinosaurs,
yawn, yawn, yawn!

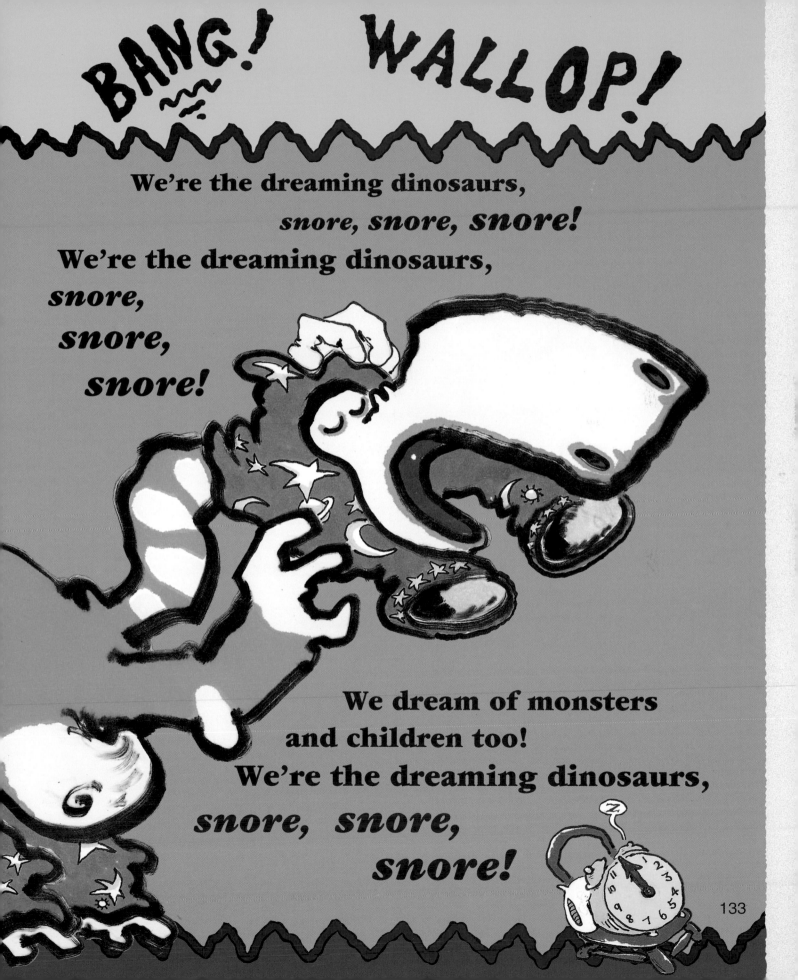

BANG! WALLOP!

We're the dreaming dinosaurs,
snore, snore, snore!
We're the dreaming dinosaurs,
snore,
snore,
snore!

We dream of monsters
and children too!
We're the dreaming dinosaurs,
snore, snore,
snore!

The Three Billy Goats Gruff

illustrated by

Charlotte Voake

Once upon a time three billy-goats lived together in a field on a hillside. Their names were Big Billy-goat Gruff, Middle Billy-goat Gruff, and Little Billy-goat Gruff.

A river ran beside the billy-goats' field, and one day they decided to cross it, to eat the grass on the other side. But first they had to go over the bridge, and under the bridge lived a great ugly Troll.

First Little Billy-goat Gruff stepped on to the bridge.

TRIP TRAP, TRIP TRAP, went his hoofs.

"Who's that tripping over my bridge?" roared the Troll.

"It is only I, Little Billy-goat Gruff, going across the river to make myself fat," said Little Billy-goat Gruff, in such a small voice.

"Now I'm coming to gobble you up," said the Troll.

"Oh please don't eat me, I'm so small," said Little Billy-goat Gruff. "Wait for the next billy-goat, he's much bigger."

"Well, be off with you," said the Troll.

A little while later, Middle Billy-goat Gruff stepped on to the bridge. TRIP TRAP, TRIP TRAP, went his hoofs.

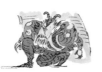

"Who's that tripping over my bridge?" roared the Troll.

"It is only I, Middle Billy-goat Gruff, going across the river to make myself fat," said Middle Billy-goat Gruff, whose voice was not so small.

"Now I'm coming to gobble you up," said the Troll.

"Oh no, don't eat me," said Middle Billy-goat Gruff. "Wait for the next billy-goat, he's the biggest of all."

"Very well, be off with you," said the Troll.

It wasn't long before Big Billy-goat Gruff stepped on to the bridge.

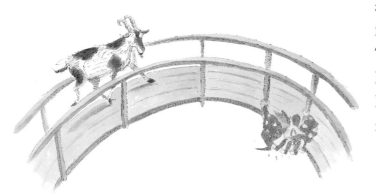

TRIP TRAP, TRIP TRAP, TRIP TRAP, went his hoofs, and the bridge groaned under his weight.

"Who's that tramping over my bridge?" roared the Troll.

"It is I, Big Billy-goat Gruff," said Big Billy-goat Gruff, who had a rough, roaring voice of his own.

"Now I'm coming to gobble you up," said the Troll, and at once he jumped on to the bridge, immensely horrible and hungry.

But Big Billy-goat Gruff was very fierce and strong. He put down his head and

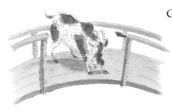

charged the Troll and butted him so hard he flew high into the air and then fell down, down, down, *splash* into the middle of the river. And the great ugly Troll was never seen again.

Then Big Billy-goat Gruff joined Middle Billy-goat Gruff and Little Billy-goat Gruff in the field on the far side of the river. There they got so fat that they could hardly walk home again, and if the fat hasn't fallen off them, they're still fat now.

So *snip, snap, snout,* this tale's told out!

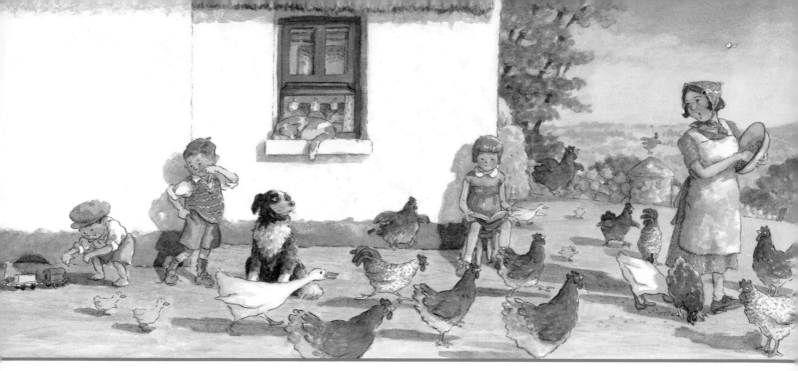

John Joe and the Big Hen

by Martin Waddell   illustrated by Paul Howard

"It's your day for minding John Joe," Mammy told Sammy, so he had to stay with John Joe. Mary read her book and Mammy went on with her work. Splinter the dog sat in the sun and got toasted.

Sammy got bored minding John Joe. Sammy wanted to play with his friend, Willie Brennan. "I'm away down Cow Lane to the Brennans'," Sammy told Mary.

"Take John Joe with you," said Mary, but Sammy took Splinter instead of John Joe.

"I'm left by myself!" John Joe told Mary. "You'd better tell Mammy!"

"Let Mammy get on with her work," Mary said. "I'll settle our Sammy!"

Mary took John Joe by the hand and set off down Cow Lane to find Sammy.

They went to the Brennans', but there was no sign of Sammy! Mary was mad, for it wasn't her day for minding John Joe.

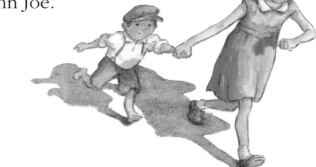

"Do you think they'd be down by the stream?" asked John Joe.

"I'd look, but you are too little to go," Mary said. "And I can't leave you here with no one to mind you."

"I'll mind myself!" said John Joe.

The Brennans' big hen came to look at John Joe. John Joe was used to the hens at his house, but he didn't know the Brennans' big hen.

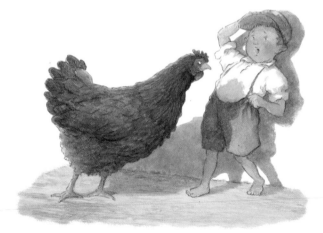

"I'm not scared of you!" John Joe told the hen.

"I'll whack your backside," John Joe told the hen.

"Go away home, hen!" John Joe told the hen … but the big hen didn't go.

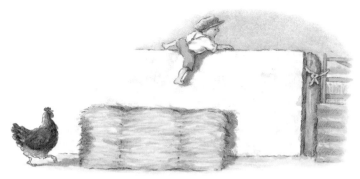

John Joe climbed on the wall, for he thought that the Brennans' big hen might eat him.

"MRS BRENNAN!" shouted John Joe, but Mrs Brennan was out.

"MARY!" yelled John Joe, but Mary had gone after Sammy and she couldn't hear him.

"OH MAMMY!" wailed John Joe, but Mammy was safe back at home.

That left John Joe alone with the Brennans' big hen and so … John Joe ran away from the hen!

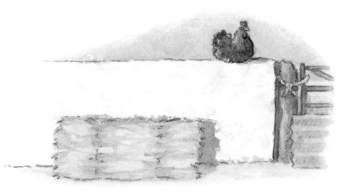

Mary came back to the Brennans' with Sammy and Splinter, but...

"Where's our John Joe?" Sammy said.

"JOHN JOE! JOHN JOE! OUR JOHN JOE!" shouted Sammy.

"JOHN JOE!" shouted Mary.

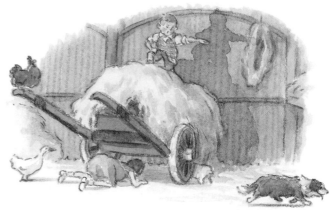

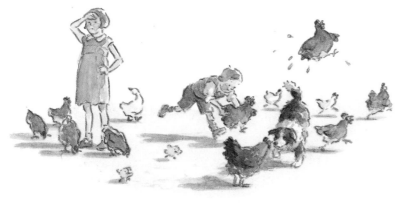

No John Joe with the hens in the yard.
No John Joe with the pigs in the sty.

No John Joe in the ditch.
No John Joe in the barn.

"Go find John Joe, Splinter!" said Sammy.

Splinter walked round and sniffed at the ground ... and the wall ... and the top of the wall.

Then Splinter dived into the corn.

Splinter barked and he barked and he barked...

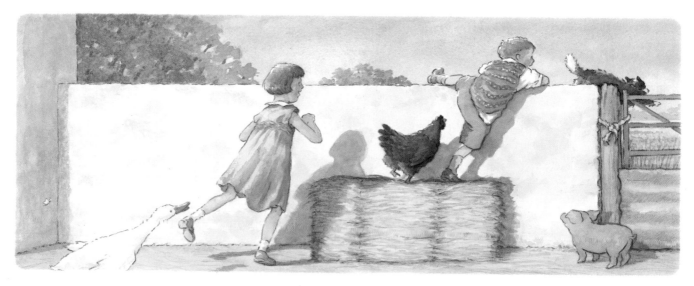

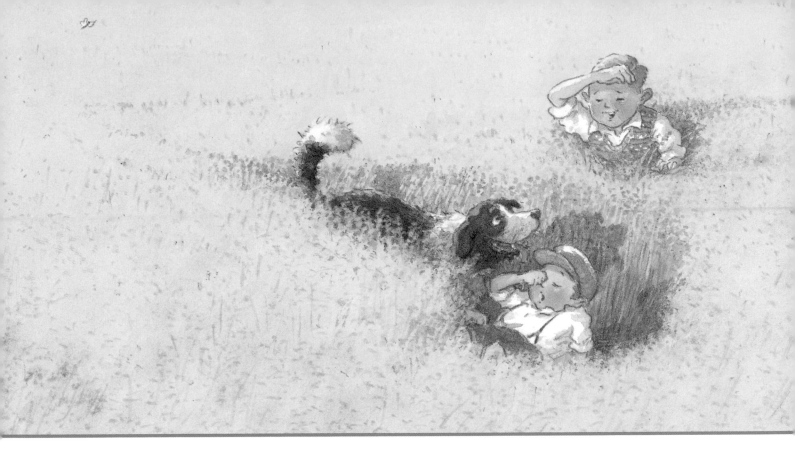

WOOF! WOOF! WOOF!

John Joe was asleep in the corn.

"The big hen chased me!" said John Joe.

"We thought you were lost," said Mary, as she carried John Joe up the lane.

"John Joe was scared by the Brennans' big hen," Mary told Mammy. "He hid away in the corn. We thought that we'd lost our little John Joe."

"There's no way I'm losing my little John Joe!" Mammy said.

"It was your day for minding John Joe," Mary told Sammy.

"Sure, I minded myself," said John Joe.

Contrary Mary by Anita Jeram

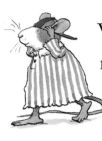

When Mary got up this morning she was feeling contrary. She put her cap on back to front and her shoes on the wrong feet.

"Are you awake, Mary?" her mom called.

"No!" said Contrary Mary.

For breakfast there was hot toast with peanut butter.

"What would you like, Mary?" asked Mom.

"Roast potatoes and gravy, please," said Contrary Mary.

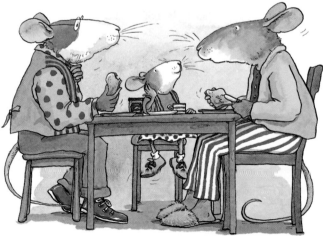

When they went to the shops it was raining.

"Come under the umbrella, Mary," said Mom.

But Contrary Mary didn't. She just danced about, getting wet. All day long, Contrary Mary did contrary things.

She rode her bicycle, backwards. She went for a walk, on her hands. She read a book upside down.

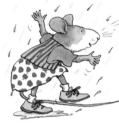

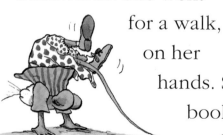

She flew her kite along the ground.

Mary's mom shook her head.

"Mary, Mary, quite contrary," she said.

And then she had an idea.

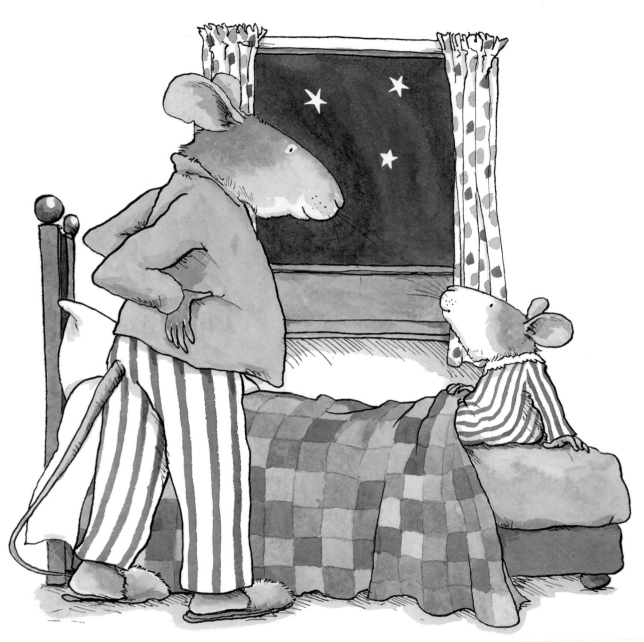

That evening, at bedtime, instead of tucking Mary in the right way round, Mary's mom tucked her in upside down.

Then she opened the curtains, turned on the light, kissed Mary's toes and said, "Good morning!"

Mary laughed and laughed. "Contrary Mom!" she said.

"Do you love me, Contrary Mary?" asked Mary's mom, giving her a cuddle.

"No!" said Contrary Mary. And she gave her mom a great big kiss.

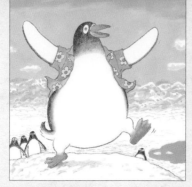

CUDDLY DUDLEY

Dudley loved to play. He loved to play jumping, diving and splashing. But most of all Dudley loved to play ... all by himself.

The trouble was, Dudley was such a lovely cuddly penguin that whenever his brothers and sisters found him on his own they just couldn't resist having a huddle and a waddle and a cuddle with him.

"Go away," Dudley would say. "Leave me alone."

"We can't," came the reply. "You're just too cuddly, Dudley."

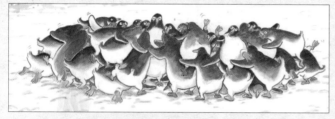

"I'm fed up with all your huddling and waddling and cuddling," said Dudley one day. "I'm going to find a place where I can play all on my own."

And off he went.

He waddled and he toddled for many, many miles until, quite by chance, he found a little wooden house which looked perfect for a penguin.

And it seemed to be empty.

"At last!" said Dudley. "A house of my own — a place where I can jump about all day without being disturbed."

Just then there came a rap-tap-tap at the little wooden door.

"It's us," said two of Dudley's sisters. "We followed your waddleprints. Can we come in?"

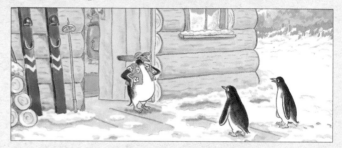

"No, you jolly well can't," said Dudley. "I'm very busy and I don't want to be disturbed, so please go away." And he shut the little wooden door and was alone once more.

"At last!" said Dudley. "A house of my own – a place where I can splash about all day without being..."

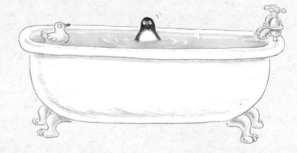

Just then there came a rap-tap-tap at the little wooden door.

"It's us," said his brothers and sisters. "We followed your waddleprints. Can we come in and...?"

"No, you jolly well can't," said Dudley. "I don't want

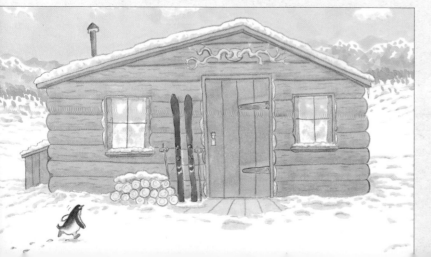

BY JEZ ALBOROUGH

to huddle and waddle and cuddle. So for the very last time . . . STOP FOLLOWING ME AROUND!"

He slammed the little wooden door and was alone once more.

"At last!" sighed Dudley. "A house of my own . . ."

BANG, BANG, BANG went the little wooden door.

"That does it," he said. "When I catch those penguins I'll . . ."

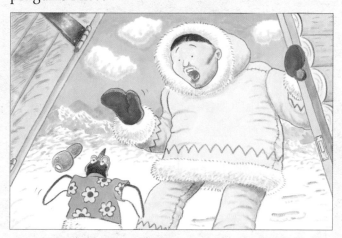

But it wasn't the penguins at the little wooden door. It was a great big man.

"My word!" said the great big man. "What an adorable penguin! *Give us a cuddle!*" he cried, and chased Dudley all round the house and out into the snow.

Dudley ran and ran and escaped from the man. Then he decided to head back home. But which way was home?

Crunch, crunch, crunch went Dudley, looking for some waddleprints to follow. But when night came, he was still alone . . . and completely lost . . . and now, for the first time, he was lonely. He climbed a hill to get a better view, and at the top

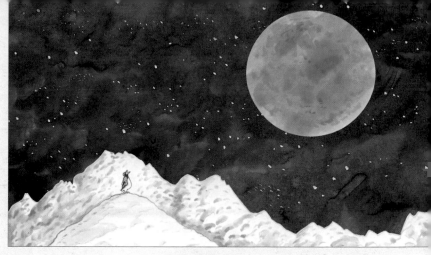

he saw an enormous orange moon with hundreds of tiny sparkling stars huddled all around.

"Excuse me," said a penguin from the foot of the hill. "Have you finished being alone yet? Only we wondered, now that you're back . . . if you wouldn't mind . . . whether we could . . . it's just that you're so . . . *so* . . ."

"CUDDLY!" shouted Dudley. And he bounced down the hill as fast as he could.

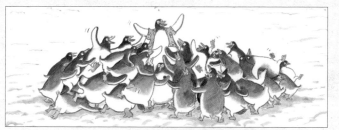

Then Dudley and all his brothers and sisters had the best huddling, waddling, cuddling session that they'd *ever* had. UNTIL . . .

"GIVE US A CUDDLE!"

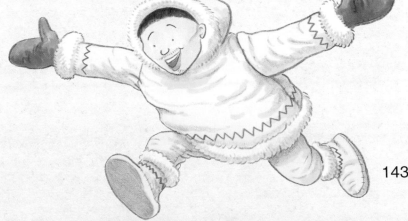

143

Quacky quack-quack!

by **Ian Whybrow**   illustrated by **Russell Ayto**

This little baby had some bread;
His mummy gave it to him
  for the ducks,
But he started eating it instead.

Lots of little ducky things
  came swimming along,
Thinking it was feeding time,
  but they were wrong!

The baby held on to the bag,
  he wouldn't let go;
And the crowd of noisy ducky birds
  started to grow.

They made a lot of ducky noises …
  quacky quack-quack!
Then a whole load of geese swam up
  and went *honk! honk!* at the back.

And when a band went marching by,
  in gold and red and black,
Nobody could hear the tune –
  all they could hear was …
  honk! honk! quacky quack-quack!

honk!
honk!

quacky quack-
quack!

toot! toot!

"Louder, boys," said the bandmaster,
  "give it a bit more puff."
So the band went *toot! toot!*
  ever so loud,
But it still wasn't enough.

Then all over the city,
  including the city zoo,
All the animals heard the noise and
  started making noises too.

All the donkeys went *ee-aw! ee-aw!*
All the dogs went *woof! woof!*
All the snakes went *sss-ssss!*
All the crocodiles went *snap! snap!*
All the mice went *squeaky-squeaky!*
All the lions went …

roar!

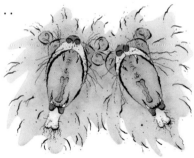

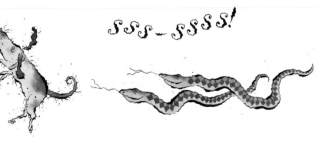

ee-aw! ee-aw!

woof! woof!

sss-ssss!

snap! snap!

squeaky-squeaky!

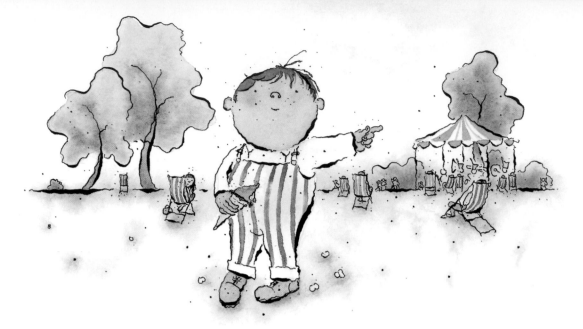

Then one little boy piped up and said,
"I know what this is all about.
That's my baby brother with the
  bag of bread;
I'll soon have this sorted out."

He ran over to where the baby
  was holding his bag of bread
And not giving any to the birdies,
  but eating it instead.

And he said, "What about some
  for the ducky birds?"
But the baby started to …

So his brother said, "If you let me
  hold the bag,
I'll let you hold my ice-cream."

Then the boy said, "Quiet all
  you quack-quacks!
And stop pushing, you're all
  going to get fed."
And he put his hand in the paper bag
  and brought out a handful of bread.

So all the birds went quiet
  and the band stopped playing too…
And all the animals stopped
  making a noise,
Including the animals in the zoo.

And suddenly the baby realized
  they were all waiting for a crumb!
So he gave the ice-cream back
  and he took a great big handful
    of bread and …
Threw all the ducky birds some.

scream!

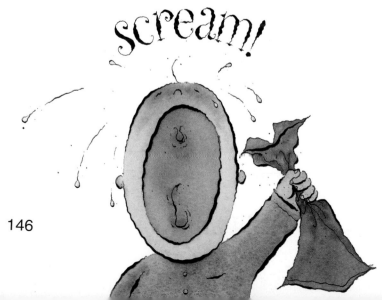

146

Then all the hungry ducky birds
were ever so glad they'd come,
And instead of going …
honk! honk! quacky quack-quack!
All the birdies said …

YUM! YUM!

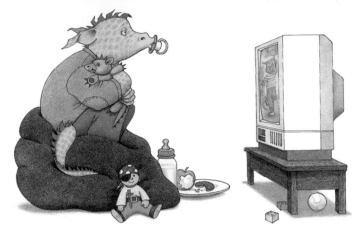

Marlon sat on the floor watching TV. Marlon's granny sat in the armchair, watching Marlon.

"He's getting too old for that dummy," she said sternly to Marlon's mom.

"It's a noo-noo," said Marlon.

"He calls it a noo-noo," explained Marlon's mom.

"Well, what*ever* he calls it," said Marlon's granny, "he looks like an idiot with that stupid great *thing* stuck in his mouth all the time."

"He doesn't have it *all* the time," soothed Marlon's mom. "Only at night or if he's a bit tired. He's a bit tired now – aren't you, pet?"

"Mmmmm," said Marlon.

"His teeth will start sticking out," warned Marlon's granny.

"Monsters' teeth stick out anyway," observed Marlon.

"Don't answer back," said Marlon's granny. "You should just throw them *all* away," she continued. "At this rate he'll be starting *school* with a dummy. At this rate he'll be starting *work* with a dummy. You'll just have to be firm with him."

"Well," said Marlon's mom, "I am *thinking* about it. We'll start next week, won't we Marlon? Now you're a big boy, we'll just get rid of all those silly noo-noos, won't we?"

"No," said Marlon.

"You see!" said Marlon's granny. "One word from you and he does as he likes."

There was no doubt about it. Marlon was a hopeless case.

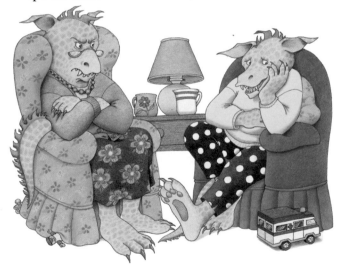

Marlon's mom decided to take drastic action. She gathered up every single noo-noo she could find and dumped them all in the dustbin five minutes before the rubbish truck arrived. But Marlon had made plans just in case the worst should happen. He had secret noo-noo supplies all over the house.

NOO-NOO
by Jill Murphy

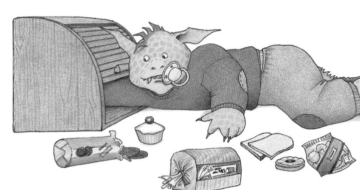

"Who's his mommy's little darling?" cooed Boomps-a-daisy.

Marlon always ignored their taunts.

"You're just jealous," he replied.

"You all wish you'd got one too."

There was a yellow one down the side of the armchair, a blue one at the back of the breadbin, various different types in his toy ambulance and his favourite pink one was lurking in the toe of his wellington boot.

His mother and granny were astonished. They could not think where he kept finding them.

"You'll be teased when you go out to play," warned his granny. "A great big monster like you with a baby's dummy."

Marlon knew about this already. The other monsters had been teasing him for ages, but he loved his noo-noos so much that he didn't care.

The other monsters often lay in wait and jumped out on Marlon as he passed by with his noo-noo twirling.

"Who's a big baby, then?" jeered Basher.

"Does the little baby need his dummy, then?" sneered Alligatina.

Gradually, the secret supply of noo-noos dwindled. Marlon's mom refused to buy any more and they all began to be lost, or thrown away by Marlon's mom. Finally, there was only one left, the pink one. Marlon kept it with him all the time. Either in his mouth or under his pillow or in the toe of his wellington boot, where no one thought to look.

To his delight, Marlon found one extra noo-noo that his mom had missed. It was a blue one, which had fallen down the side of his bed and been covered up by a sock. He knew his best pink noo-noo wouldn't last for ever, so he crept out and planted the blue one in the garden.

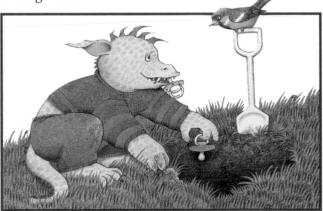

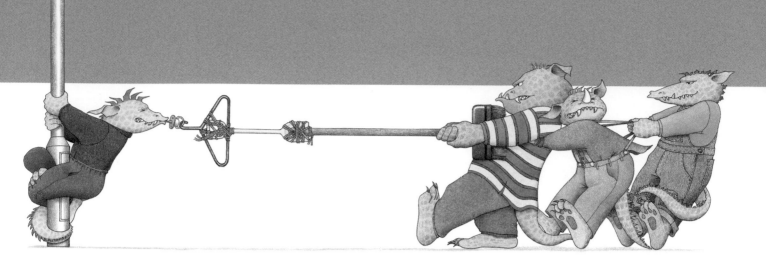

All the other monsters decided to gang up on Marlon. They collected lots of different bits of junk and fixed them all together until they had made just what they wanted. It was a noo-noo snatcher.

Then they waited behind a bush until Marlon came past with his pink noo-noo twirling.

"Here he comes," said Alligatina.

"Grab it!" yelled Boomps-a-daisy.

"Now!" said Basher.

With one quick hooking movement, they caught the ring of the noo-noo with the noo-noo snatcher and pulled!

But Marlon clenched his teeth and held on. Monsters have the most powerful jaws in the world. Once they have decided to hang on, that's *it*. Marlon hung on, the monsters hung on to the noo-noo snatcher and there they stayed, both sides pulling with all their monster might.

And there they would *still* be, if Marlon had not decided, just at that very moment, that perhaps he was too old to have a noo-noo any more.

So, he let go. And all the other monsters went whizzing off down the road, across the park and into the pond with a mighty splash.

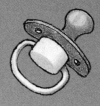

Marlon went home. "I've given up my noo-noo," he said. "I sort of threw it into the pond."

"Good gracious me!" exclaimed Marlon's mom, sitting down suddenly with the shock.

"I told you," said Marlon's granny. "You just have to be firm."

"Actually," said Marlon, "I've planted one, so I'll have a noo-noo tree — just in case I change my mind."

"That's nice, dear," said Marlon's mom.

"Nonsense!" said Marlon's granny. "Dummies don't grow on trees. A noo-noo tree! How ridiculous!"

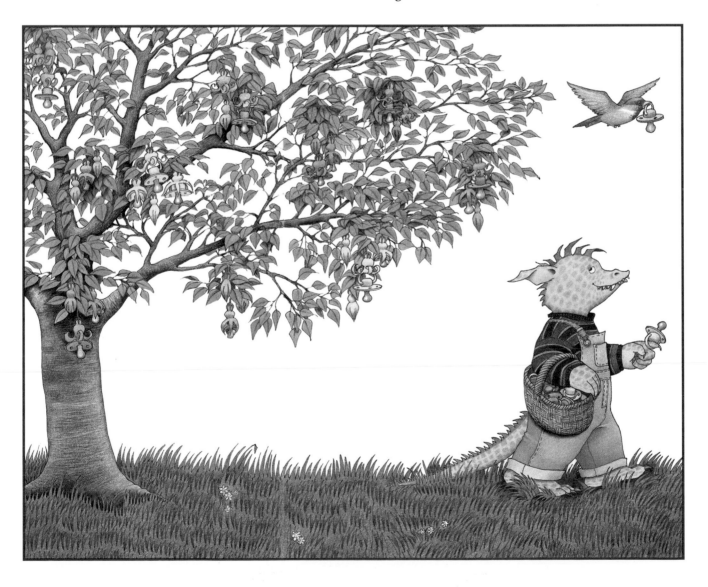

Two Shoes, New Shoes

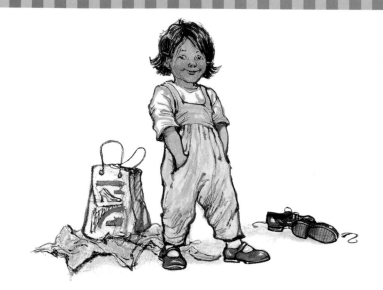

Two shoes, new shoes,
  Bright shiny blue shoes.

High-heeled ladies' shoes
  For standing tall,
Button-up baby's shoes,
  Soft and small.

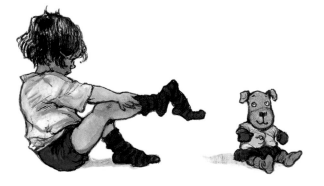

Slippers, warm by the fire,
  Lace-ups in the street.
Gloves are for hands
  And socks are for feet.

A crown made of paper,
  A hat with a feather,
Sun hats, fun hats,
  Hats for bad weather.

by Shirley Hughes

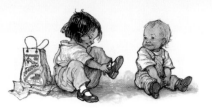

A clean white T-shirt
  Laid on the bed,
Two holes for arms
  And one for the head.

Zip up a zipper,
  Button a coat,
A shoe for a bed,
  A hat for a boat.

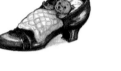

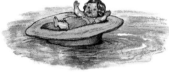

Wearing it short
  And wearing it long,
Getting it right
  And getting it wrong.

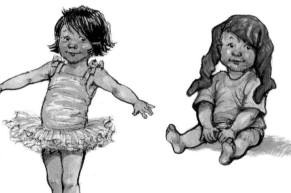

Trailing finery,
  Dressed for a ball
And into the bath
  Wearing nothing at all!

THIS IS THE BEAR
— AND THE —
BAD LITTLE GIRL

by Sarah Hayes   *illustrated by* Helen Craig

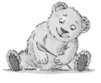 This is the bear who went out to eat.
This is the dog who stayed in the street.

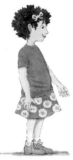 This is the girl with the curly hair
who said she really liked the bear.

This is the dog who put out a paw
and tripped the woman who came in the door …

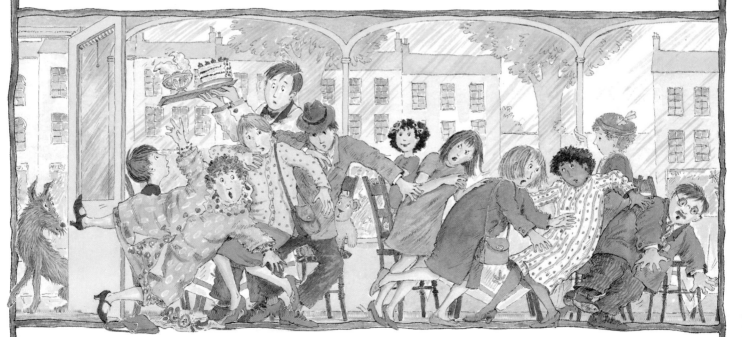

which pushed the people waiting to pay
and made the waiter drop the tray.

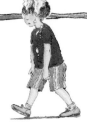

This is the boy all covered in cream
who went to the kitchen to wash his face clean.

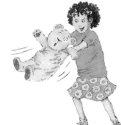

This is the girl with the curly hair
who said, "You're coming with me, bear."

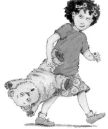

This is the girl who walked down the street
holding the bear by one of his feet.

This is the dog who thought it was fun
when the bad little girl began to run.

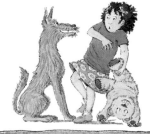

This is the girl who ran faster and faster
but this is the dog who ran right past her.

This is the girl
who gave the bear back
and said he was
only a baggy old sack.
This is the boy
who said, "I don't care
if he's saggy or baggy,
he's still *my* bear."

My Mom and Dad Make Me Laugh

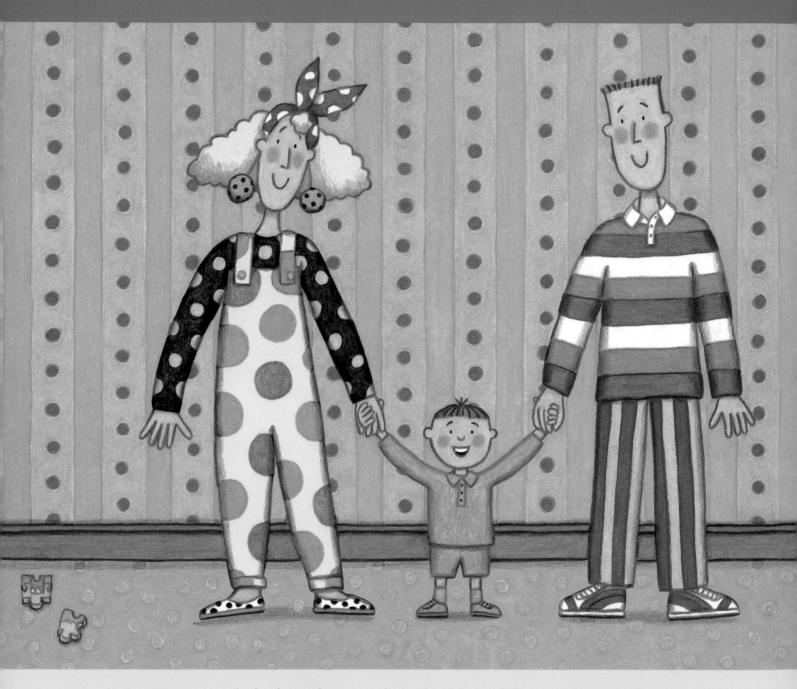

My mom and dad make me laugh. One likes spots and the other likes stripes.

My mom likes spots in winter and spots in summer. My dad likes stripes on weekdays and stripes at weekends.

by Nick Sharratt

Last weekend we went to the
safari park. My mom put on her
spottiest dress and earrings,
and my dad put on his stripiest
suit and tie.
I put on my gray top and
trousers.
"You do like funny clothes!"
said my mom and dad.

We set off in the car and on the way we stopped for something to eat.
My mom had a spotty pizza and my dad had a stripy ice-cream.
I had a bun.
"You do like funny food!" said my mom and dad.

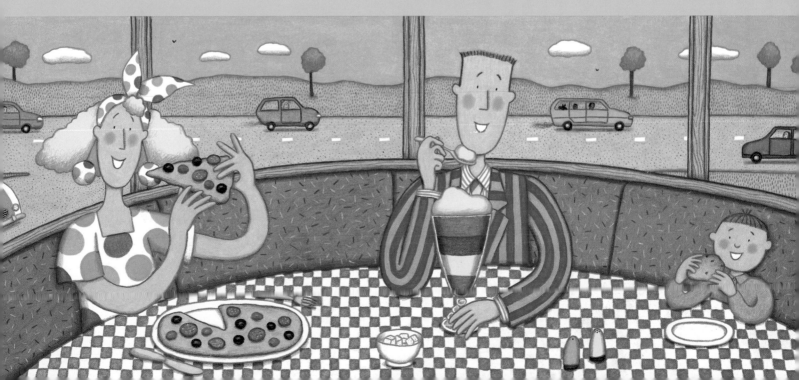

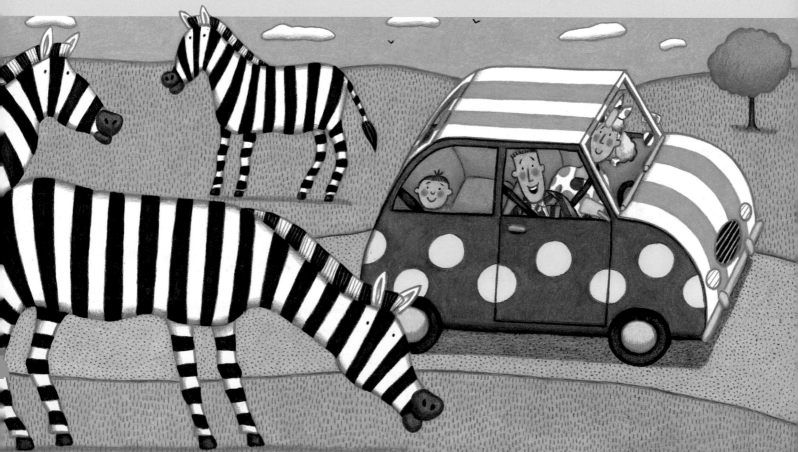

When we got to the safari park it was very exciting.
My mom liked the big cats best.
"Those are splendid spots," she said. "And I should know!"
My dad liked the zebras best.
"Those are super stripes," he said. "And I should know!"

STAY IN
YOUR CAR!

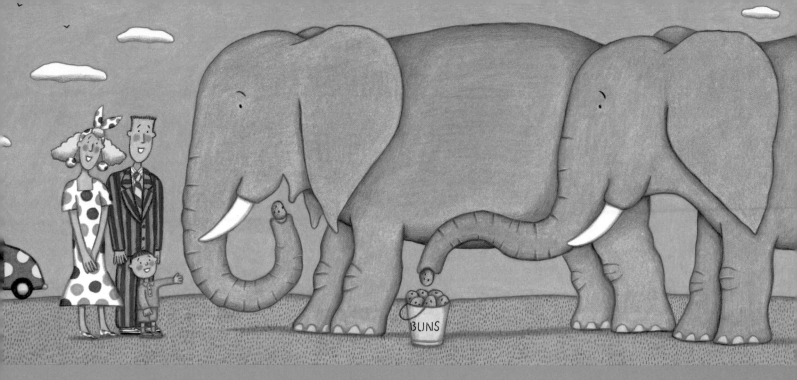

But the animals I liked best didn't have spots and didn't have stripes.
They were big and gray and eating their tea.
"Those are really good elephants," I said.

"And I should know!"

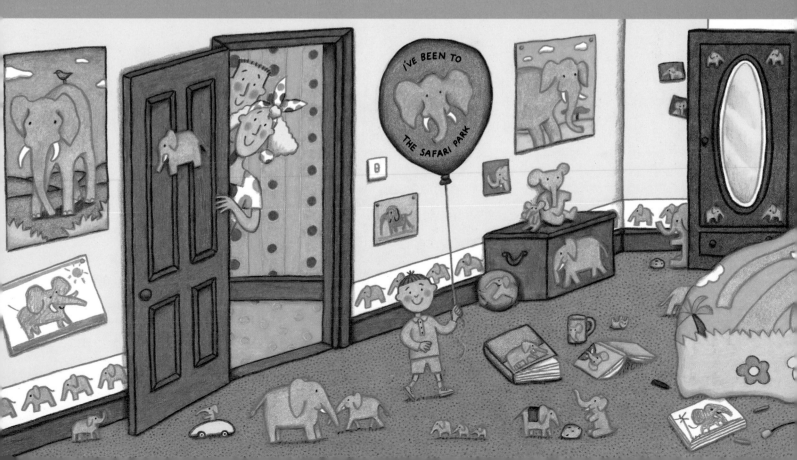

WHERE'S MY MOM?

by Leon Rosselson
illustrated by Priscilla Lamont

Where's my mom?
She's not in the drawer,
Or under the bed,
Or behind the door.

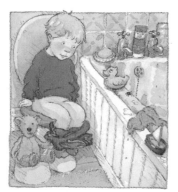

She's not in the bath,
Unless she's got
Turned into
a spider.
I hope she's not!

I'll look in the mirror;
Who can that be
With the scowly face?
It must be me!

She's not in the fridge
With the strawberry jelly,
The chicken, the milk and
The something smelly.

She's not in the cupboard.
What's that noise?
No, she's not
in the box
With all my
toys.

She's not
in the piano
Or under the chair,
Or behind the curtains
Or anywhere.

I'll try the garden.
Where can she be?
She's not in the sky
Or the apple tree.

Look at those ants
racing to
and fro!
Have you seen
my mom?
I think that
means no.

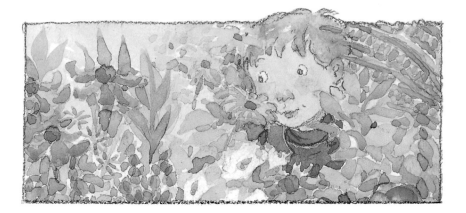

Paint me a picture.
Play games
  with me.
Mom! I'm hungry.
I want my tea.

I can't see a mom
In the garden shed,
And she isn't a flower
In the flowerbed!

Mom! I can hop!
I can jump on the bed!
I can curl in a ball,
I can stand on my head.

Can I drink my milk in
My dinosaur mug?
Get up, Mom …
And I'll give you a hug!

Perhaps she's in *her* bed.
I'll go and explore.
Back into the house;
Push open her door.

There's a lumpy shape—
I'll take a peep …
There's my mom,
And she's fast asleep!

Mom! Mom!
You should be awake.
Tell me a story!
Bake me a cake!

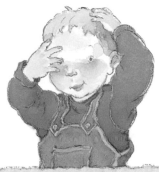

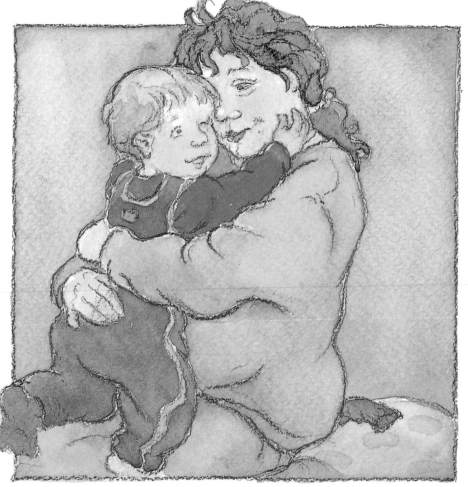

The Fat King

Once upon a time there was a fat king.

He lived in a fat house with his fat wife

and fat children. He had a fat dog

and a fat cat. And fat birds sat in fat trees

under a fat sun. Everything in the garden was fat.

One day the king came downstairs and said hello to his kingdom. "Hello, dog and cat," he said.

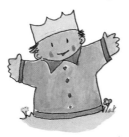

"Hello, cabbages. Hello, potatoes. Hello, trees. Hello, world."

But when he came to the green oak tree he stopped and stared.

"Come and see this," he called to his wife and children. For there, under the tree, sitting in its shade, was a THIN bird.

"Shoo!" said the king and clapped his hands. "Shoo, little thin bird!" he said very loudly indeed.

But the little thin bird did not move. So the king gave him a dish of breadcrumbs and went off to consult the gardener.

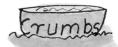

"You could try chasing him," said William.

But the king said, "That will only frighten him. I will go and ask Fido instead."

And on the way to Fido he passed the green oak tree, and put down another dish of crumbs for the little thin bird.

"Hello, Fido," said the king. "I have called about the little thin bird."

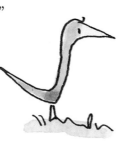

by *Graham Jeffery*

Fido said, "I will come and bark at him." But the king said, "No, I do not want to startle him, I will go and see Tibby instead."

And as he passed the green oak tree he left a dish of milk for the little thin bird.

Tibby said, "I could jump over him and scratch him."

But the king said, "No, that will not do at all. I will go and ask the family. They will think of something kinder."

But his family did not know what to do. And the fisherman didn't know. And the vicar didn't know. And the postman didn't know.

And every time the king passed the green oak tree, he left a bowl of crumbs for the little thin bird.

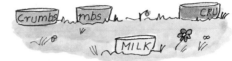

The fat king said to his friends, "It is no good. It is no good at all. Nobody knows what to do about the little thin bird."

But then Fido looked under the green oak tree, and Tibby looked, and the king looked, and everybody looked.

And there under the green oak tree was … the fattest, plumpest bird you ever saw. And he hopped up into the green oak tree and went to sleep under the fat sun.

MOUSE PARTY

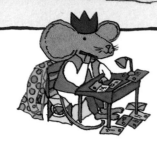

Mouse found a deserted house and decided to make his home there.

But it was a very big house for such a small mouse and he felt a little lonely.

"I know," he thought, "I'll have a party." So he sent invitations to all his friends.

The first to arrive were…

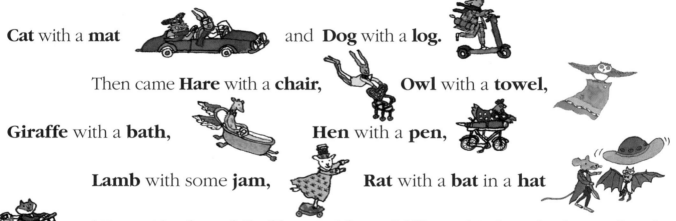

Cat with a **mat**   and **Dog** with a **log.**

Then came **Hare** with a **chair,**   **Owl** with a **towel,**

Giraffe with a **bath,**   **Hen** with a **pen,**

Lamb with some **jam,**   **Rat** with a **bat** in a **hat**

and **Fox** with a **box** full of **lots** and **lots** of different kinds and colours of **socks.**

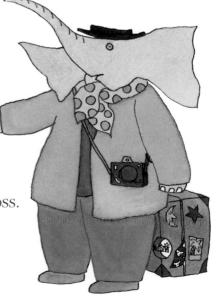

"Let's party!" said Mouse. But…

Rat-a-tat-tat!

It was an elephant with two trunks. He was

blowing through one and carrying the other.

"Hello," said Mouse. "Welcome to my house."

"*Your* house?" said the elephant and he looked rather cross.

"I've just been away on a long holiday.

This house, I must tell you, is mine!"

164

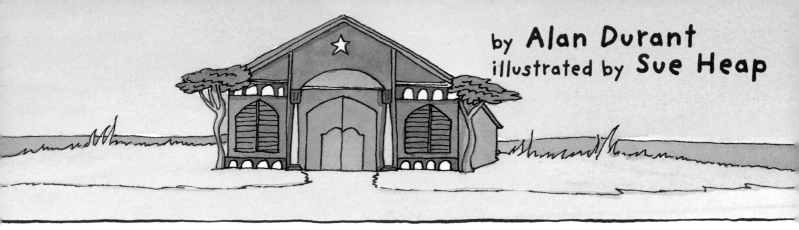

by Alan Durant
illustrated by Sue Heap

"Oh," said Mouse, Lamb, Hare, Rat and Bat.

"Oh," said Hen, Dog, Owl, Fox and Giraffe.

But, "Come in, come in!" said Cat. "You're just in time for the party."

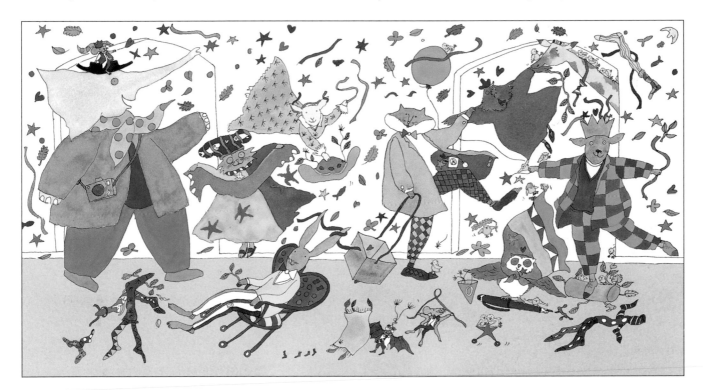

"A party … for me?" said Elephant. "Oh my! Yippee!"

So they drank and they ate and they danced until late and had the most
marvellous party. And later, when the guests had all gone home,
leaving Elephant and Mouse alone,
Elephant said, "I think, little Mouse, perhaps it's true,
there's room for us both in this house, don't you?"

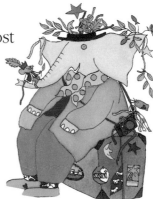

165

The Red Woolen Blanket

by Bob Graham

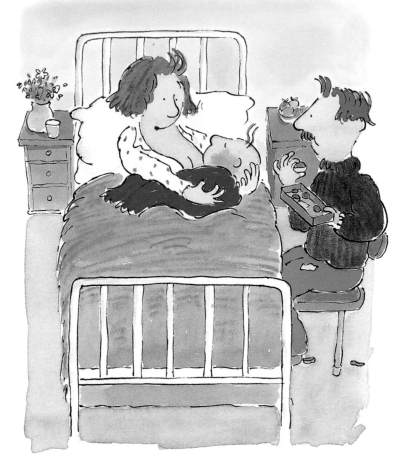

Julia had her own blanket right from the start. Julia was born in the winter. She slept in her special cot wrapped tight as a parcel. She had a band of plastic on her wrist with her name on it.

"She's as bald as an egg," said her father, helping himself to another chocolate.

Julia came home from the hospital with her new red blanket, a bear, a gray woolen dog and a plastic duck.

Waiting at home for her were a large pair of pants with pink flowers and a beautiful blue jacket specially knitted by her grandmother.

"Isn't blue for boys?" said Dad.

"No, it doesn't really matter," said Mom.

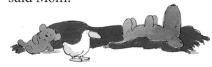

Wrapped up in the red woolen blanket, Julia slept in her own basket or in the front garden in the watery winter sunshine. Her hair sprouted from the holes in her tea-cosy hat. She smiled— nothing worried Julia.

Julia grew. She slept in a cot and sucked and chewed the corners of the not-so-new blanket. She rubbed the red woolen blanket gently against her nose.

Julia's mom carried her to the shops in a pack on her back. The pack was meant to carry the shopping. Julia liked it so much up there that the pushchair was used for the shopping and the pack was used for Julia.

Then Julia was crawling and her blanket went with her. Some of it was left behind ...

Then Julia took her first step.

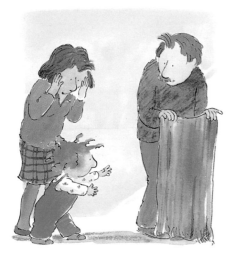

Julia made her own small room from the blanket. It was pink twilight under there. From outside, the "creature" had a mind of its own. It heaved and throbbed.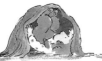

Wherever Julia went her blanket went too. In the spring, the summer, the autumn, and the winter.

Julia was getting bigger. Her blanket was getting smaller.

A sizeable piece was lost under the lawnmower.

"If Julia ran off deep into a forest," said her father, "she could find her way back by the blanket threads left behind."

The day that Julia started school, she had a handy little blanket not much bigger than a postage stamp —because it would never do to take a whole blanket to school … unless you were Billy, who used his blanket as a "Lone Avenger's" cape.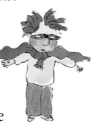

Sometime during Julia's first day at school, she lost the last threads of her blanket.

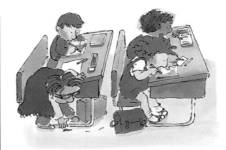

It may have been while playing in the school yard, or having her lunch under the trees. It could have been anywhere at all …

and she hardly missed it.

HANDA'S SURPRISE

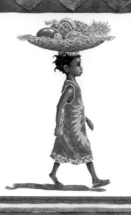

Handa put seven delicious fruits in a basket
for her friend, Akeyo.
She will be surprised, thought Handa
as she set off for Akeyo's village.
I wonder which fruit she'll like best?

Will she like
the soft yellow banana …

or the sweet-
smelling guava?

Will she like the
round juicy orange …

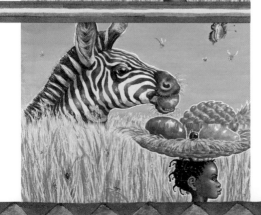

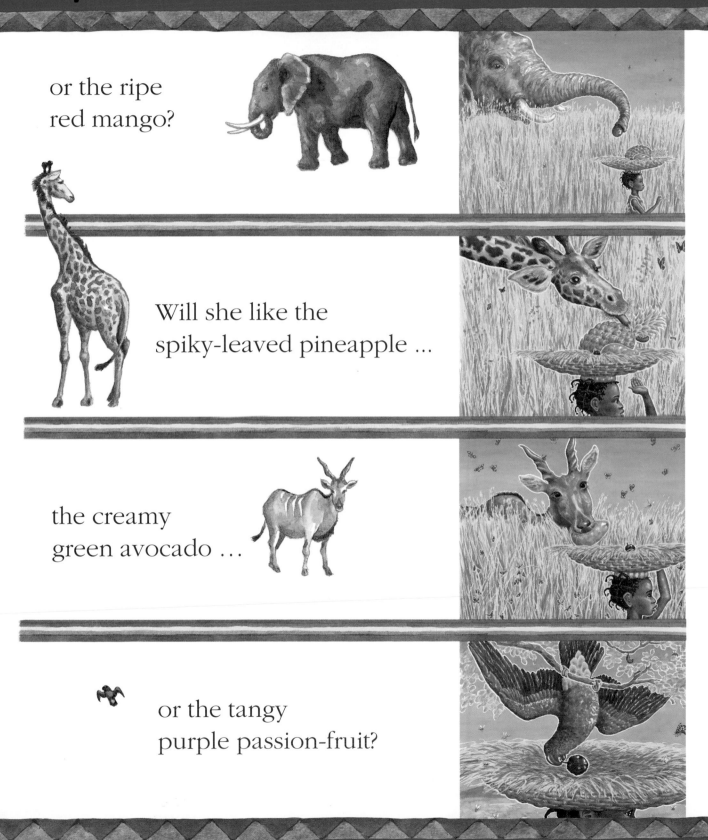

by Eileen Browne

or the ripe
red mango?

Will she like the
spiky-leaved pineapple ...

the creamy
green avocado ...

or the tangy
purple passion-fruit?

169

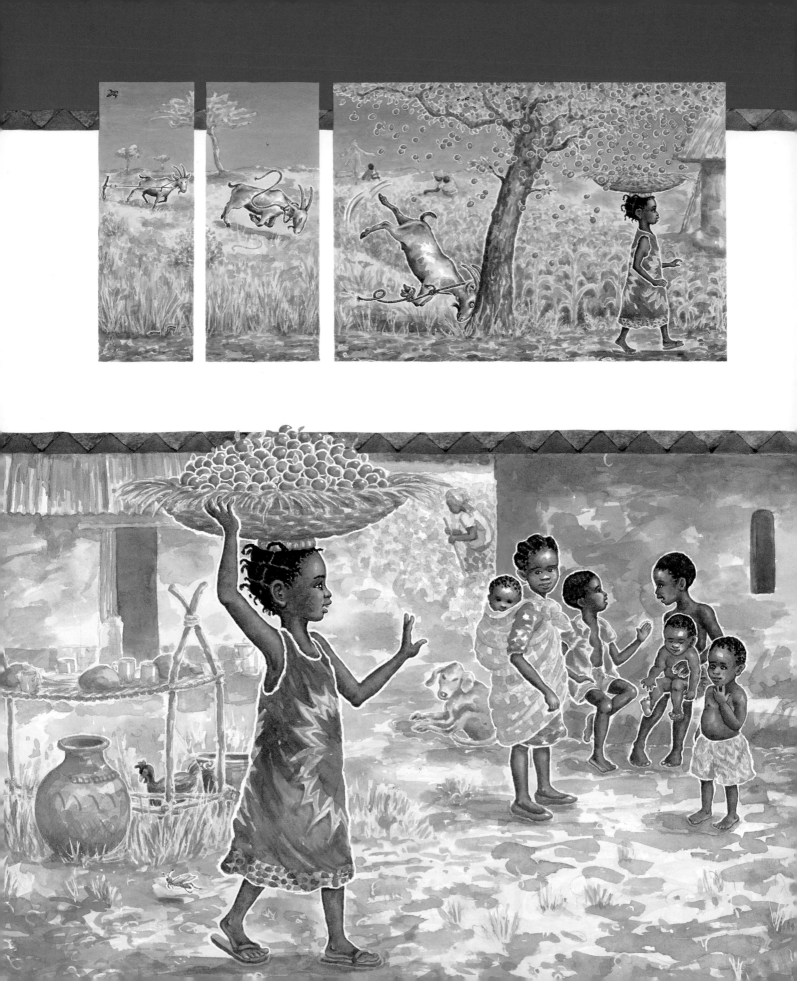

Which fruit will Akeyo like best?

"Hello, Akeyo," said Handa. "I've brought you a surprise."
"Tangerines!" said Akeyo. "My favourite fruit."

"TANGERINES?" said Handa. "That *is* a surprise!"

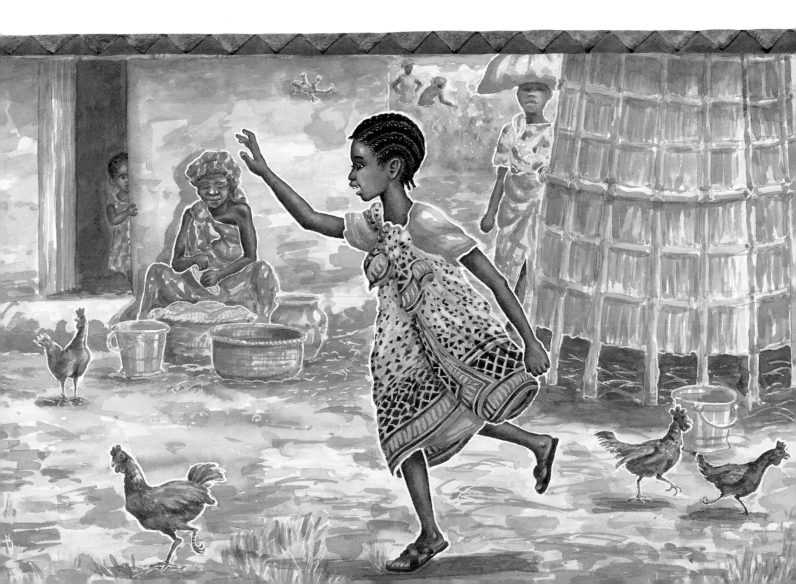

SEBASTIAN'S TRUMPET

by Miko Imai

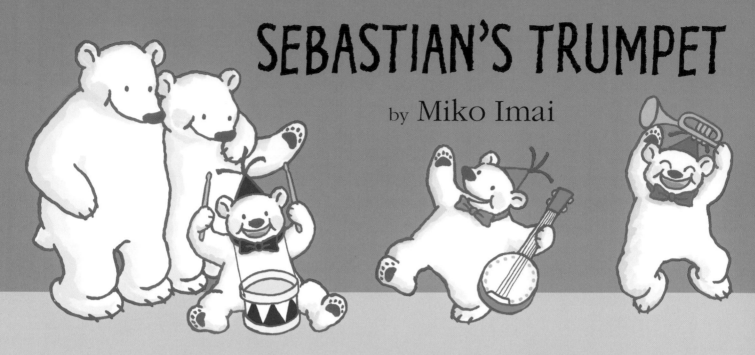

It was the three little bears' birthday. Daddy and Mommy Bear had some special presents for them. Theodore got a drum. Oswald got a banjo. And Sebastian got a trumpet.

"Let's play 'Happy Birthday!'" they shouted.
Theodore banged on his drum. Rat-a-tat-tat.
Oswald strummed his banjo. Twang Twang.
And Sebastian blew into his trumpet.
But the only sound it made was Pfffft.

Pfffft

"What's happened to your trumpet?" asked Theodore. "Let *me* try it … Pfffftt."
"Let *me* try!" said Oswald. "I bet I can do it … Pfffffftt."

Theodore and Oswald played "Happy Birthday" for Daddy and Mommy Bear.

I wish I could play my trumpet,
thought Sebastian.

"Pffftt … I HATE this trumpet!"
Sebastian sobbed.

Rat-a-tat-tat

Twang

Twang

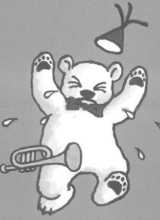

172

"Why did you give me a trumpet, Mommy?
It doesn't even work!"
"Maybe you're trying too hard," said Mommy
Bear. "Why don't you rest now and try
again later?"

When Sebastian woke up, he couldn't
wait to try his trumpet again.
He tiptoed towards it.

Pffooott

He picked it up and started to play.

Troooft

TA-TA-TA-
ROOOOOOOON!
TA-TA-TA-
ROOOOOOON!

"You did it, Sebastian!" his brothers shouted.
And the three little bears all played
"Happy Birthday" together.

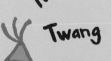

Rat-a-tat-tat

Twang
Twang

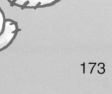

Toot
Toot

MONKEY TRICKS

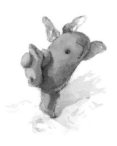 Horatio was practising hopping. HOP HOP HOP
WHOOPS! He fell over a notice board. I'll ask
James what this says, he thought.

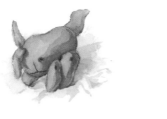 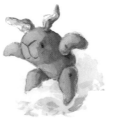

James was looking in his Useful Box. Someone had untidied it.
"What does this say?" asked Horatio.

"Johnny Conqueror Coming Today," said
James. He looked worried.
"That naughty monkey!"
Horatio looked all
around for Johnny
Conqueror.

by Camilla Ashforth

"Jimmies and Jacks! Mind your backs!"
a voice called, and there was Johnny
Conqueror, pulling a wagon.

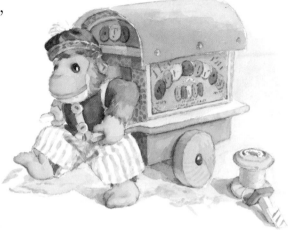

"I'm very good at juggling,"

he boasted.

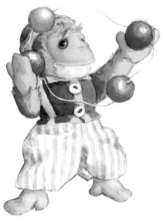

He threw a string
of beads into the
air and held out his hands to catch them. But
he missed and the beads scattered everywhere.
Horatio clapped his hands.

My beads look like this, thought
James, picking one up.

"For my next trick," shouted Johnny Conqueror, "I take a long piece of rope and knot it here and twist it a bit here…"

That rope looks useful, thought James.

He looked in his Useful Box again.

Johnny Conqueror got into a tangle. He needed James to untie him. Horatio thought it was very funny.

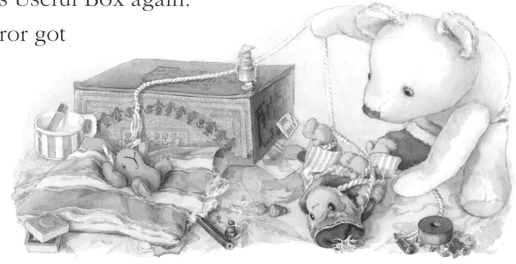

"I'll show you how clever I am at balancing," said Johnny Conqueror, jumping onto a cotton reel! He stood on one leg and spun a dish above him. The cotton reel wobbled.

James looked worried. If that was my dish … he thought.

CRASH! The cotton reel spun away. Johnny Conqueror fell over. The dish broke. Oh dear, thought James.

"Hooray!" shouted Horatio.

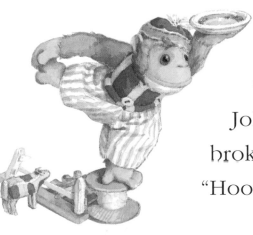

"To end the show," announced Johnny Conqueror, "I do my best trick. I disappear! All close your eyes and count to five."

"One … two …" Horatio began.

"I know who untidied my Useful Box," whispered James.

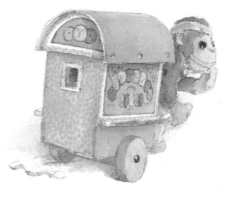

"Three … four …" added Horatio.

"And I'm going to catch him," James said.

"Five!" shouted Horatio and they opened their eyes. Johnny Conqueror had disappeared.

"Bother," said James. "He got away."

James began to tidy up.

"Now I can show you my trick," said Horatio, and he hopped for James. James clapped his hands.

"That really is clever," he said, and gave Horatio a big hug.

The Little Boat

by Kathy Henderson

illustrated by Patrick Benson

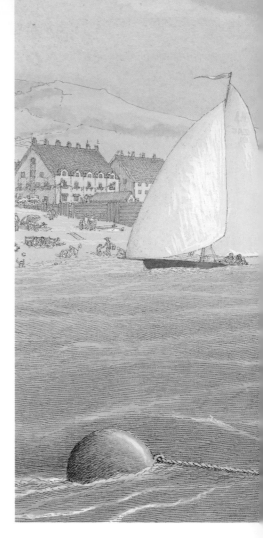

Down by the shore
where the sea meets the land,
licking at the pebbles
sucking at the sand,
and the wind flaps
the sunshades
and the ice-cream man
out-shouts the seagulls
and the people come
with buckets and spades
and suntan lotion
to play on the shore
by the edge of the ocean,

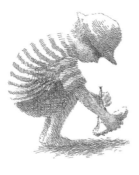

a little boy
made himself a boat
from an old piece of
polystyrene plastic,
with a stick for a mast
and a string tail sail
and he splashed
and he played
with the boat he'd made
digging it a harbour
scooping it a creek,
all day long by the edge
of the sea,
singing
*'We are unsinkable
my boat and me!'*

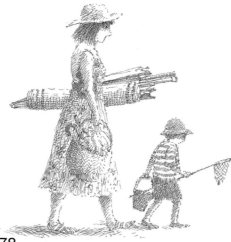

Until he turned his back
and a small wind blew
and the little boat drifted
away from the shore,
out of his reach
across the waves,
past the swimmers
and air beds,
away from the beach.

And the boat
sailed out
in the skim of the wind
past the fishermen
sitting on the end of the pier,

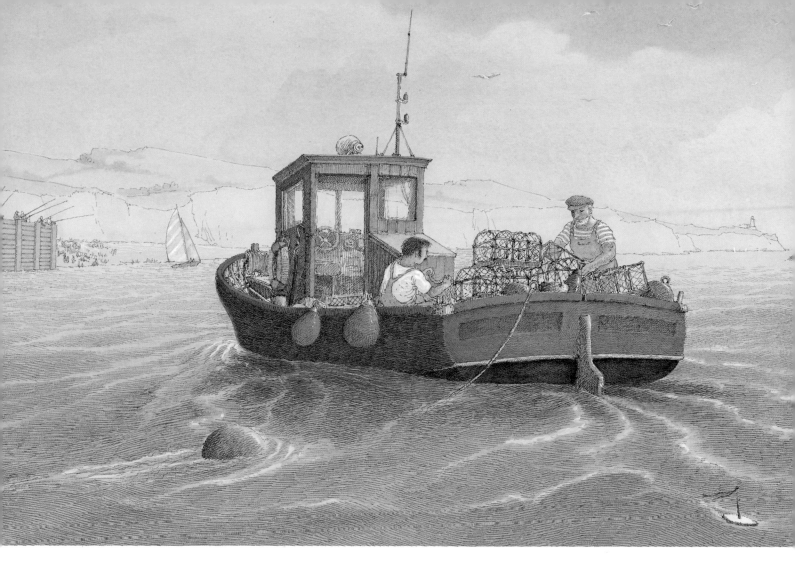

out and out
past a crab boat trailing
a row of floats
and a dinghy sailing
a zig-zag track
across the wind,

out where the lighthouse
beam beats by
where the sea birds wheel
in the sky and dive
for the silvery fish
just beneath the waves,
out sailed the little boat
out and away.

And it bobbed by
a tugboat chugging home
from leading a liner
out to sea
and it churned in the wake,
still further out,
of a giant tanker
as high as a house
and as long as a road,
on sailed the little boat
all alone.

And the further it sailed
the bigger grew
the ocean

until all around
was sea
and not a sign of land,
not a leaf,
not a bird,
not a sound,
just the wind
and heaving sliding
gliding breathing water
under endless sky.

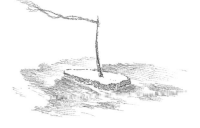

And hours went by
and days went by
and still the little boat
sailed on,
with once a glimpse
of the lights from an oil rig
standing in the distance
on giant's legs
and sometimes
the shape of a ship
like a toy,
hanging in the air
at the rim of the world,

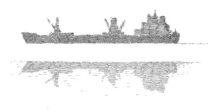

or a bit of driftwood
or rubbish passing,
otherwise nothing,
on and on.

And then came a day
when the sky went dark
and the seas grew uneasy
and tossed about
and the wind
that had whispered
began to roar
and the waves grew bigger
and lashed and tore
and hurled great manes
of spray
in the air
like flames in a fire

and all night long
as the seas grew rougher
the little boat danced
with the wind
and the weather

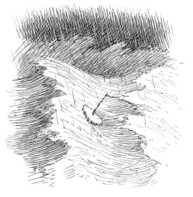

till the morning came
and the storm was over
and all was calm and still
and quiet again.

And then suddenly
up from underneath
with a thrust and a leap
and a mouth full of teeth
came a great fish snapping
for something to eat,
and it grabbed the boat
and dived

deep

deep

deep

down
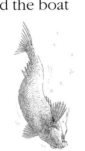
to where the light grows dim
in the depths of the sea,
a world of fins and claws
and slippery things
and rocks and wrecks
of ancient ships
and ocean creatures
no one's seen

where,
finding that plastic
wasn't food,
the fish spat out
the boat again
and up it flew,
up up up up
like the flight of an arrow
towards the light,
burst through the silver skin
of the sea
and floated on
in the calm sunshine.

Then a small breeze came
and the small breeze grew,
steadily pushing
the boat along,
and now sea birds called
in the sky again
and a boat sailed near
and another
and then,
in the beat of the sun
and the silent air,
a sound could be heard,
waves breaking somewhere
and the sea swell curled
and the white surf rolled
the little boat on
and on
towards land.

And there at the shore
where the sea greets the land,
licking at the pebbles
sucking at the sand,
a child was standing,
she stretched out her hand
and picked up the boat
from the waves at her feet
and all day long
she splashed and she played
with the boat she'd found
at the edge of the sea,
singing
*'We are unsinkable
my boat and me!'*

"Not me," said the monkey

"Who keeps dropping
banana skins round here?"
growled the lion.
"Not me," said the monkey.

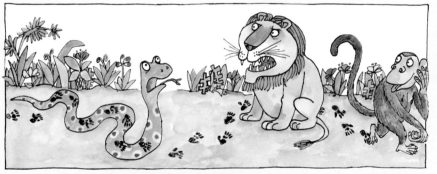

"Who keeps walking
all over me?"
hissed the snake.
"Not me," growled the lion.
"And not me," said the monkey.

"Who keeps throwing coconuts
about?" snorted the rhino.
"Not me," hissed the snake.
"Not me," growled the lion.
"And not me," said
the monkey.

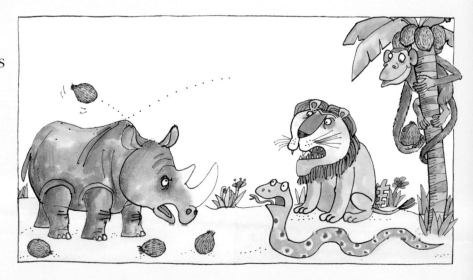

182

by Colin West

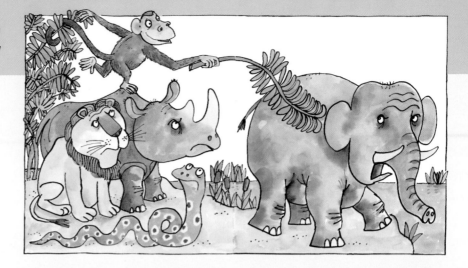

"WHO KEEPS TICKLING ME?"
 roared the elephant.
"Not me," snorted the rhino.
"Not me," hissed the snake.
"Not me," growled the lion.
"And not ME!" said the monkey.

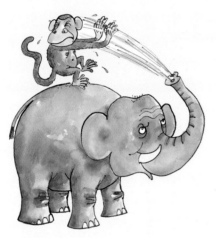

Slurp! Slurp! Slurp! went the elephant.

WHOOOOSH!

"Now who's going to stop all this monkey business?"
laughed the lion, and the snake,
and the rhino,
and the elephant.

"Well…
NOT ME!" said You-Know-Who.

183

THE ELEPHANT TREE
by Penny Dale

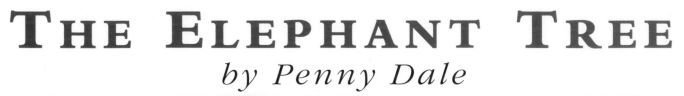

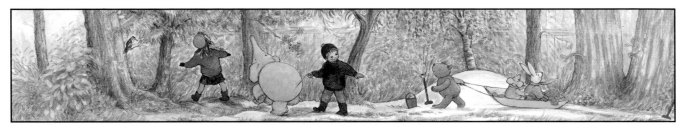

Elephant wanted to climb a tree. So we went to find the elephant tree.

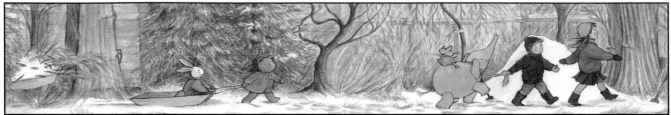

We walked and we walked. We looked and we looked.

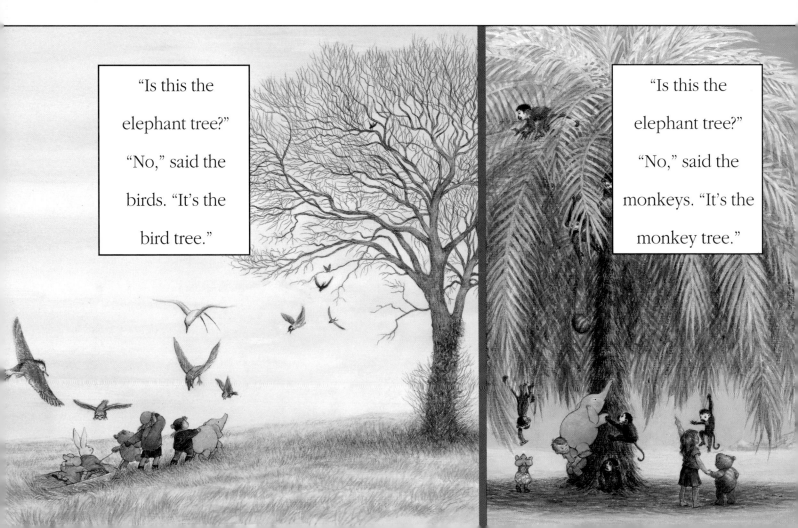

"Is this the elephant tree?" "No," said the birds. "It's the bird tree."

"Is this the elephant tree?" "No," said the monkeys. "It's the monkey tree."

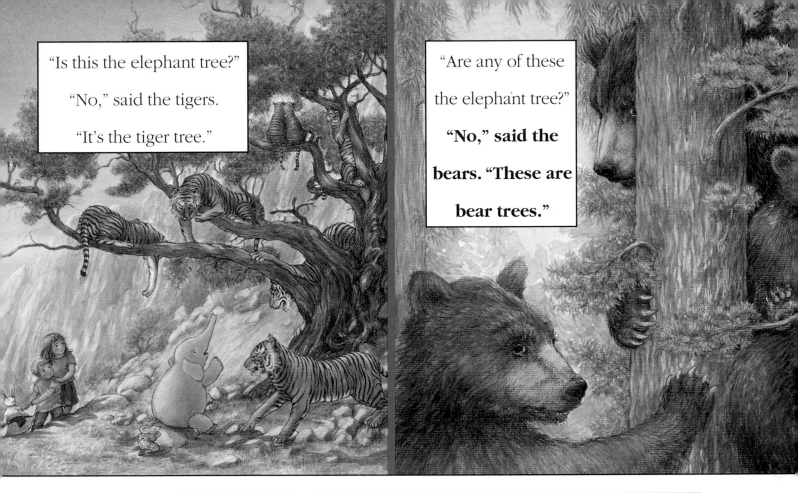

"Is this the elephant tree?"

"No," said the tigers.

"It's the tiger tree."

"Are any of these the elephant tree?"

"No," said the bears. "These are bear trees."

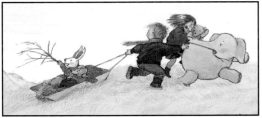

We ran and we ran.

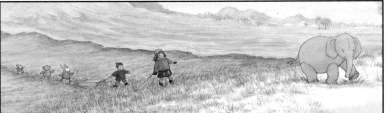

We walked and we walked.

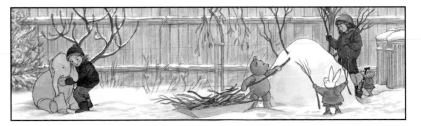

We looked and we looked.

But we still couldn't find the elephant tree.

Never mind, Elephant. Wait and see.

Here it is. Look. The elephant tree.

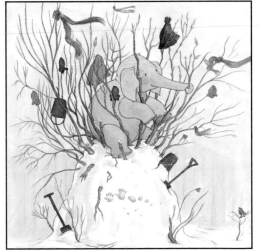

185

MY FRIEND HARRY

The day James bought Harry, Harry's life changed. James talked all the way home. Harry didn't say a thing. He just sat in the car, looking clean and new and neat.

"What are you thinking?" James asked. But Harry never said.

At the beginning of every day, when James woke up, he tossed and rumpled the blankets until Harry fell out of bed.

"Good morning, my friend Harry!" James said. "What shall we do today?" But Harry never said.

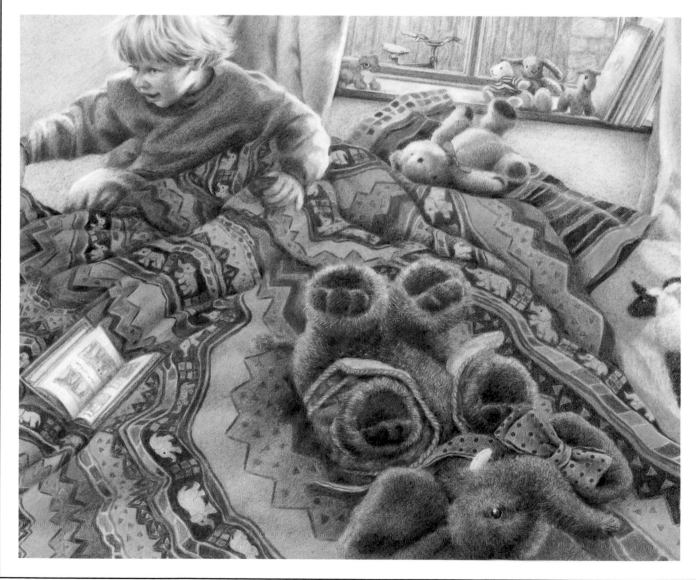

BY KIM LEWIS

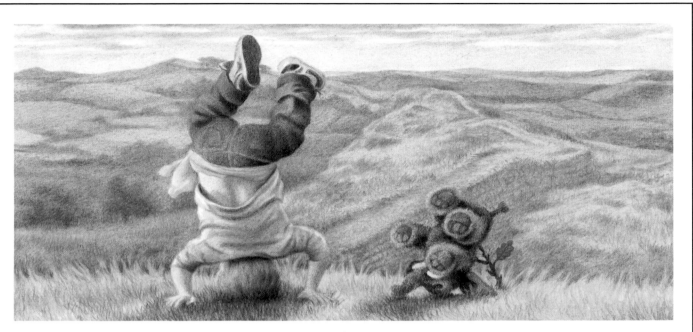

So in the mornings, James and Harry went everywhere. They climbed to the top of the hill and back again, and travelled from one end of the farm to the other.

In the sun and the wind and the rain, Harry's skin soon began to wrinkle. Once he fell off James' bicycle and James had to mend his head.

In the afternoons James and Harry helped his father and mother – gathering sheep, feeding cattle, fixing tractors and bringing in the hay.

Both James and Harry got very dirty. After many bathtimes Harry's jacket shrank and his skin began to fade.

"What are you thinking?" James asked Harry.

But Harry never said, so James hugged him tight until Harry's ears began to flop and his trunk began to sag.

Sometimes James made Harry stand on his head. Harry never complained.

"My friend Harry!" James always said.

At the end of every day James tucked Harry into bed beside him. He read story after story and talked and talked.

"Are you listening?" he yawned.

But Harry lay close to James and never said, until James' dad came in to kiss them.

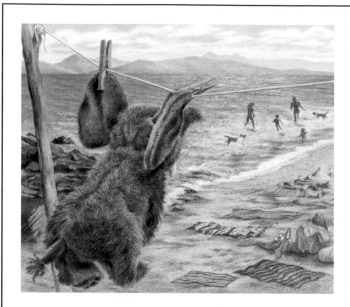

James even took Harry on holiday, squeezing him into the dark in a bag with the apple juice. But the juice spilled and made Harry very sticky. James scrubbed Harry and hung him out to dry. Harry swung in the sea breeze, while James and his mom and dad ran in and out of the waves.

Then one day Harry could no longer sit up straight. James propped him up in a chair.

"I'm going to school today!" James said. "What do you think?"

Harry was quiet. James got dressed in brand new clothes, and went a little quiet too.

Harry stayed cuddled up in James' mother's arms while the children played all around in the school yard. When James went into school, his mother waved, then drove home, very quietly, with Harry.

James' mother tucked Harry into James' bed and softly closed the door. Harry lay very still. Cows mooed faintly in the distance. James' father drove the tractor out of the yard. Birds pecked and peeped in the bushes by the house. The sun rose up and went round, warming Harry where he lay, until it was afternoon.

Harry lay still, waiting all by himself, without James.

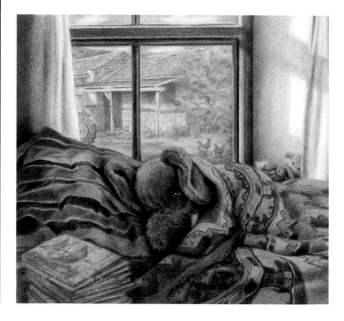

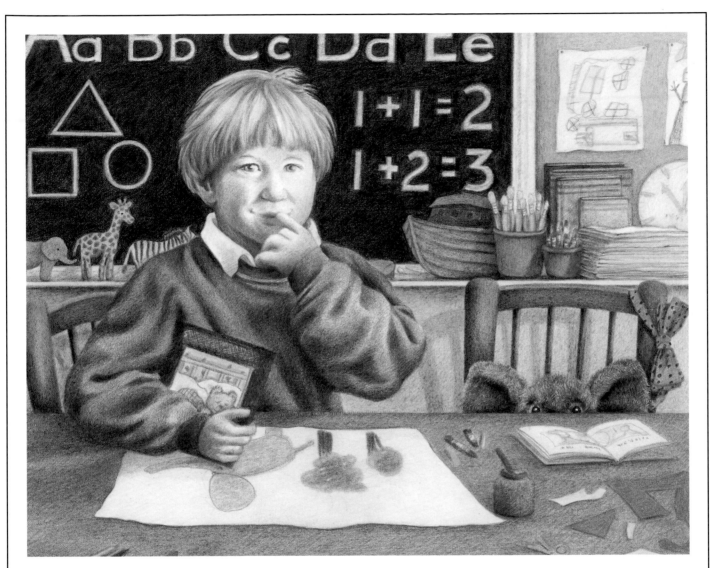

That night, James told Harry about his day. "I expect I'll go to school again tomorrow," he said.

Harry was very quiet.

James stared into the dark for a long time. "Did you miss me, my friend Harry?" he asked.

The next day, James took Harry to school. "Just this once," he said. "Until you get used to being on your own."

Harry sat very close to James and never said a word.

"My friend Harry," said James.

PROWLPUSS

by **Gina Wilson**

illustrated by **David Parkins**

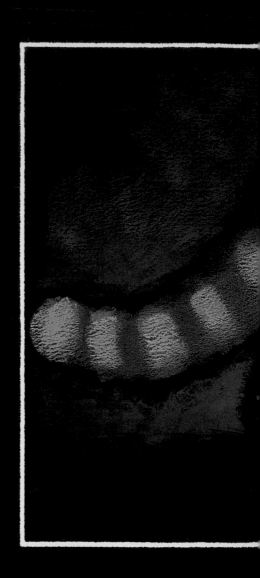

Prowlpuss is cunning
and wily and sly,
A kingsize cat with
one ear and one eye.
He's not a
sit-by-the-fire-
and-purr cat,
A look-at-my-
exquisite-fur cat,
No, he's not!

He's rough and gruff
and very very tough.
Where ya goin',
Prowlpuss?
AHA!

Down in the alley
something stirs!
Is it a burglar?
Is it a witch?

Is it a ghoul with
a bag of bones?
No, it's not!
It's Prowlpuss!

He's not a lap cat,
a cuddle-up-
for-a-chat cat,
No, he's not!

He's not a sit-in-
the-window-
and-stare cat.
He's an I-WAS-
THERE! cat.

Watch out!
Prowlpuss about!

He's not a stay-
at-home cat,
No, he's not!

He's not a sit-on-
the-mat-and-lick-
yourself-down cat.
He's an out-on-
the-town cat,
A racer, a chaser,
A "You're a disgrace"-er!
A "Don't show
your face"-er!

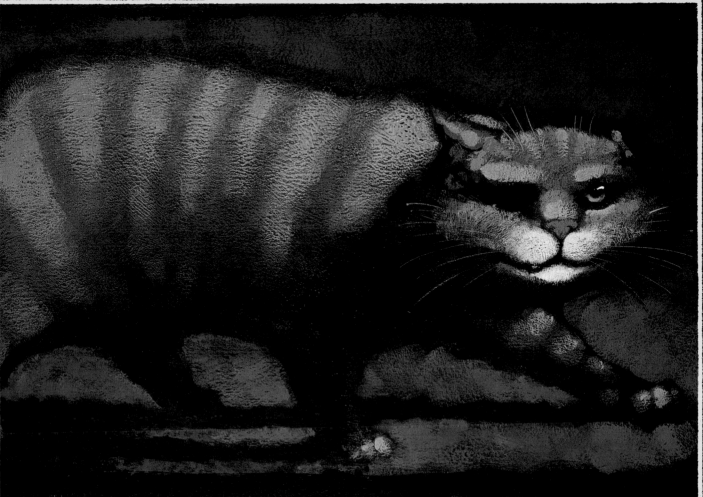

He's not a throat-
   soft-as-silk cat,
A saucer-of-
   milk cat,
No, he's not!
He's a fat cat,
A rat cat,
A "What on earth
   was that?" cat.

So what's it all for –
All the razzle and dazzle,
The crash, bang, wallop,
The yowling,
   the howling,
The "Give us a break!"
"Don't keep us awake!"
"Hoppit!" "Clear off!"
   "Get lost!" "Scram!"

"Good riddance!"
   "Go to the devil!"?

Who is
   he wooing
With his
   hullabalooing
Night after night?

AHA!

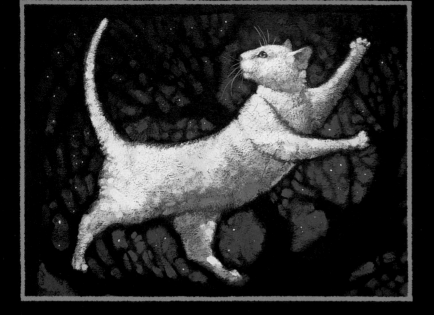

Back through
   the alley
   slinks Prowlpuss
   at dawn,
Love-lost and lorn.

And old
   Nellie Smith
   in her deep
   feather bed
Lifts her head.

"That's Prowly
   come home!
That's my
   jowly Prowly!
My sweet
   Prowly-wowly!
My sleep-all-
   the-day cat,
My let-the-mice-
   play cat,
My what-did-
   you-say? cat,
My soft and dozy,
Oh-so-cosy,
Tickle-my-toes-y,
Stroke-my-nose-y

PROWLPUSS."

High in a tree
   at the alley's end,
Right at the top
   so no one
   can get her
Or fret her
   or pet her,
Lives one little cat –
A tiny-white-star cat,
A twinkle-afar cat.

In the moonlight
   she dances,
Like snowflakes
   on branches,
She spins
   and she whirls.

But not for long!
In a flash
   she's gone!

Now Prowlpuss
   will sing for her –
What he would
   bring for her!
Oh, how he
   longs for her!
Love of his life!

If she'd *only*
   come down…

But she won't!
   No, she won't!

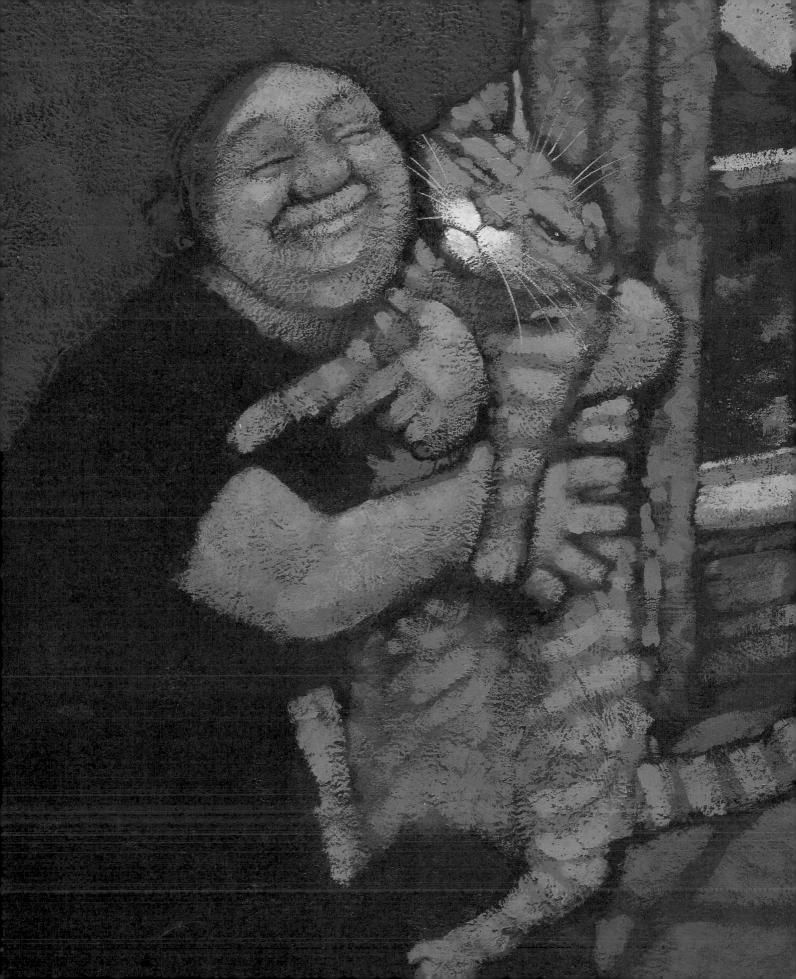

SQUEAK-A-LOT

In an old old house lived a small small mouse
  who had no one to play with.
So the small small mouse went out of the house
  to find a friend to play with.

And he found **a bee**.
"Can I play with you?"
the mouse asked the bee.
"Of course," said the bee.
"What will we play?" asked the mouse.
"We'll play Buzz-a-lot," said the bee.

Buzz buzz buzz buzz!

But the mouse didn't like it a lot.
So he went to find a better friend to play with.

And he found **a dog**.
"Can I play with you?" the mouse asked the dog.
"Of course," said the dog.
"What will we play?" asked the mouse.
"We'll play Woof-a-lot," said the dog.

Woof woof woof woof!

But the mouse didn't like it a lot.
So he went to find a better friend to play with.

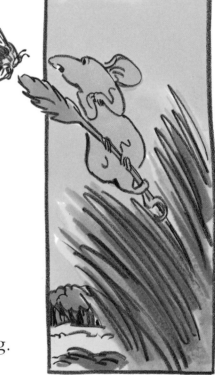

by **Martin Waddell**
illustrated by **Virginia Miller**

And he found **a chicken**.

"Can I play with you?" the mouse asked the chicken.
"Of course," said the chicken.
"What will we play?" asked the mouse.
"We'll play Cluck-a-lot," said the chicken.

Cluck cluck cluck cluck!

But the mouse didn't like it a lot.
So he went to find a better friend to play with.

And he found **a cat**.
"Can I play with you?"
the mouse asked
the cat. And …

WHAM!

BAM!

SCRAM!

The mouse didn't like
it a lot. So he ran away
through the long long grass
playing Squeak-a-lot all by himself.

Squeak squeak squeak squeak!

195

Squeak! Some mice found the mouse.
"Can we play with you?" the mice asked the mouse.
"Of course," said the mouse.
"What will we play?" asked the mice.

"Buzz-a-lot!" said the mouse.

Buzz buzz buzz buzz!

And all of them liked it a lot.

"Woof-a-lot!" said the mouse.

Woof woof woof woof!

And all of them liked it a lot.

"Cluck-a-lot!" said the mouse.

Cluck cluck cluck cluck!

And all of them liked it a lot.

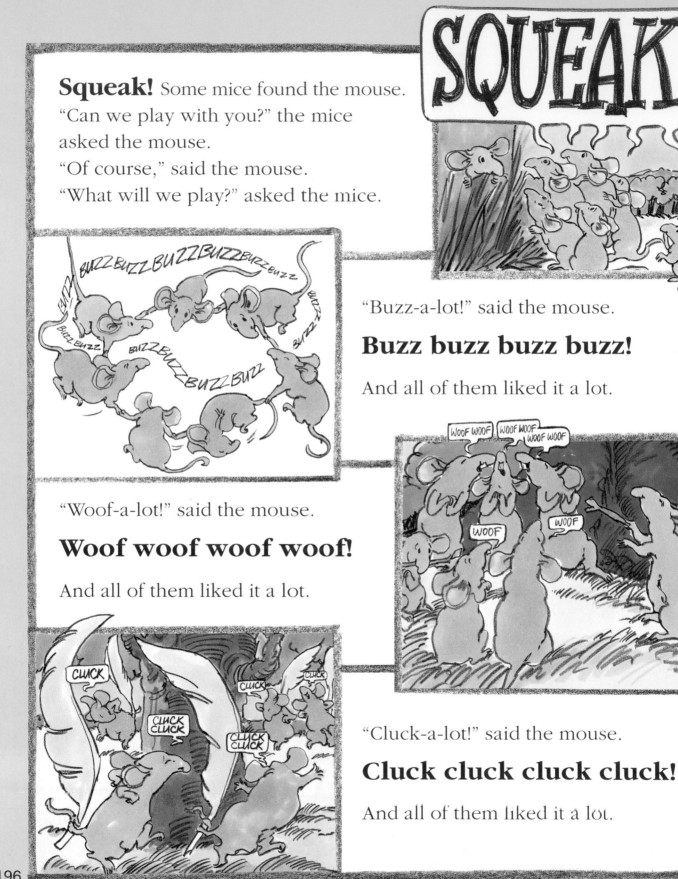

196

"WHAM! BAM! SCRAM!" said the mouse.

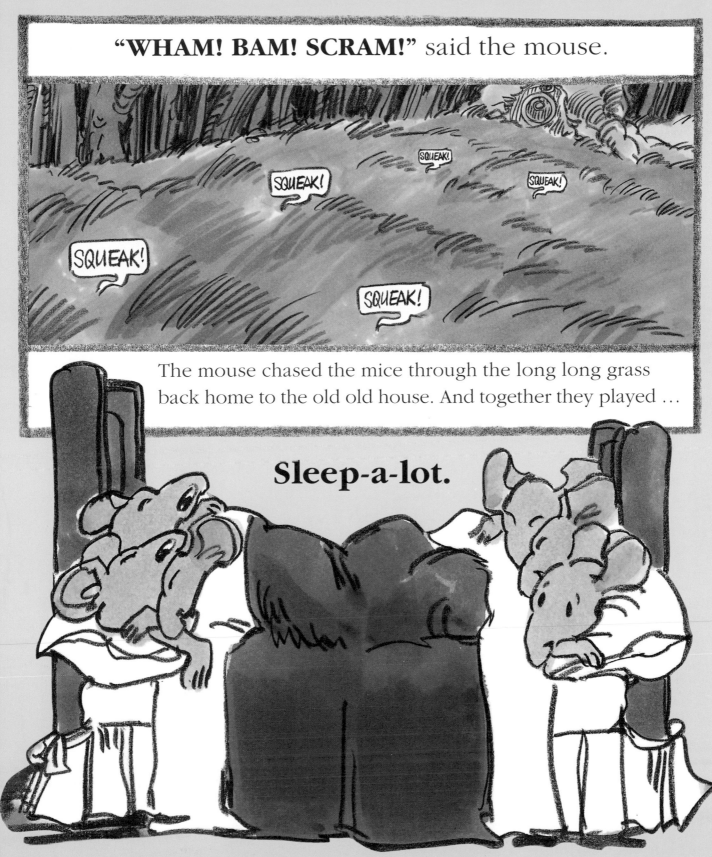

The mouse chased the mice through the long long grass back home to the old old house. And together they played ...

Sleep-a-lot.

The Big Big Sea

by Martin Waddell

illustrated by Jennifer Eachus

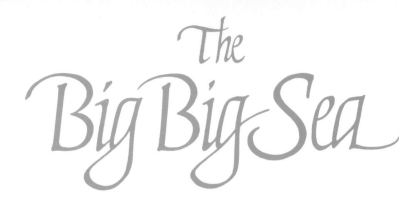

Mom said, "Let's go!"
So we went
   out of the house
      and into the dark
         and I saw…
THE MOON.

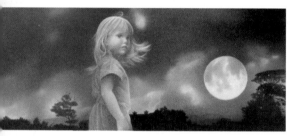

We went over the field
and under the fence
and I saw
the sea in the moonlight,
waiting for me.
Mom said,
"Take off your shoes
and socks!"
And I did.

And I ran
and Mom ran.
We ran and we ran
straight through
the puddles
and out to the sea!

I went right in
to the shiny bit.
There was only me
in the big big sea.

I splashed
and I laughed
and Mom came after me
and we paddled
out deep in the water.

We got all wet.

Then we walked
a bit more
by the edge of the sea
and our feet
made big holes
in the sand.

Far far away
right round the bay
were the town
and the lights
and the mountains.
We felt very small,
Mom and me.

We didn't go to the town.
We just stayed for a while
by the sea.

And Mom said to me,
"Remember this time.
It's the way life should be."

I got cold
and Mom carried me
all the way back.

We sat by the fire,
Mom and me,
and ate hot buttered toast
and I went to sleep
on her knee.

I'll always remember
just Mom and me
and the night
   that we walked
      by the big big sea.

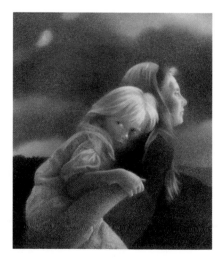

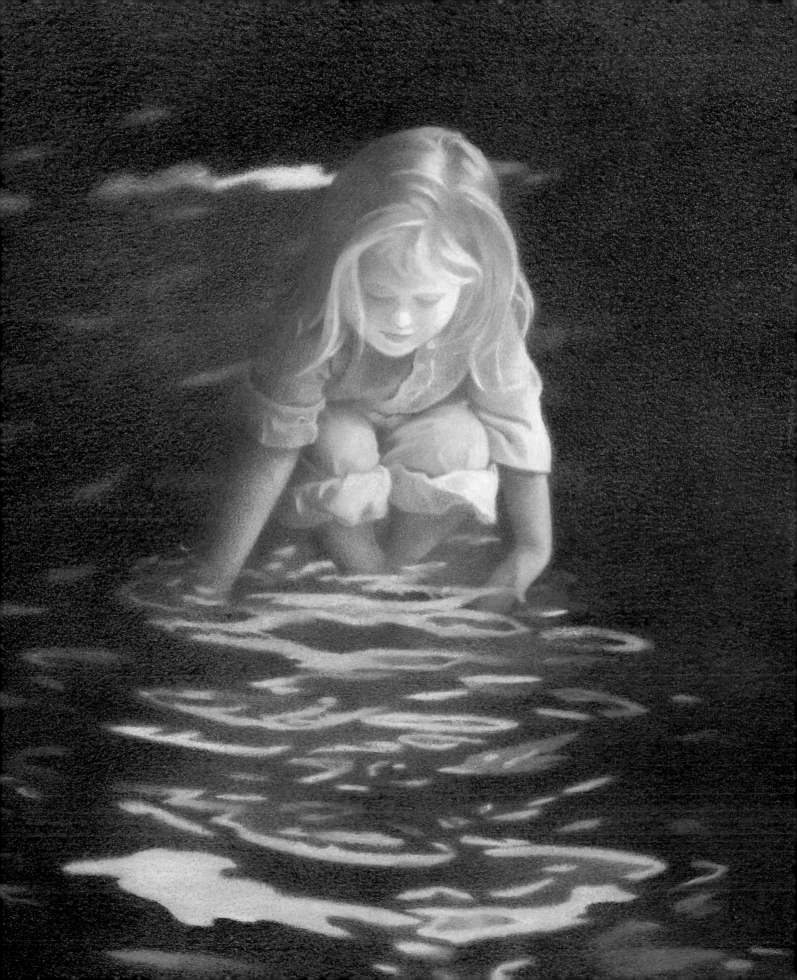

GINGER

by Charlotte Voake

Ginger was a lucky cat. He lived with a little girl who made him delicious meals and gave him a beautiful basket, where he would curl up … and close his eyes.

Here he is, fast asleep.

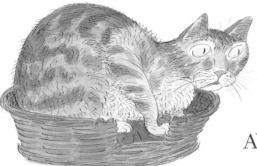

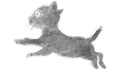

But here he is again, WIDE AWAKE. What's this? A kitten!

"He'll be a nice new friend for you, Ginger," said the little girl. But Ginger didn't want a new friend, especially one like this. Ginger hoped the kitten would go away, but he didn't.

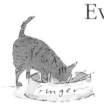

Everywhere Ginger went, the kitten followed, springing out from behind doors, leaping on to Ginger's back, even eating Ginger's food! What a naughty kitten!

But what upset Ginger more than anything was that whenever he got into his beautiful basket, the kitten always climbed in too, and the little girl didn't do anything about it.

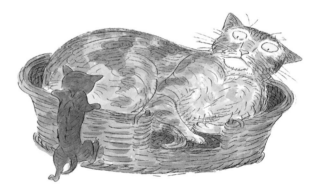

So Ginger decided to leave home.

He went out through the cat flap and he didn't come back.

The kitten waited for a bit, then he got into Ginger's basket.

It wasn't the same without Ginger.

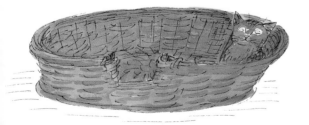

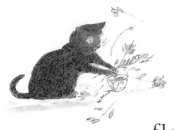

The kitten played with some flowers, then he found somewhere to sharpen his claws. The little girl found him on the table drinking some milk. "You naughty kitten!" she said. "I thought you were with Ginger. Where is he anyway?" She looked in Ginger's basket, but of course he wasn't there. "Perhaps he's eating his food," she said. But Ginger wasn't there either. "I hope he's not upset," she said. "I hope he hasn't run away."

She put on her wellingtons and went out into the garden, and that is where she found him; a very wet, sad, cold Ginger, hiding under a bush.

The little girl carried Ginger and the kitten inside. "It's a pity you can't be friends," she said.

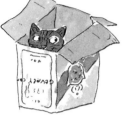

She gave Ginger a special meal. She gave the kitten a little plate of his own. Then she tucked Ginger into his own warm basket.

All she could find for the kitten to sleep in was a little tiny cardboard box. But the kitten didn't mind, because cats love cardboard boxes (however small they are).

So when the little girl went in to see the two cats again, THIS is how she found them.

And now Ginger and the naughty kitten get along very well …

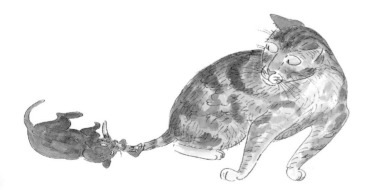

most of the time!

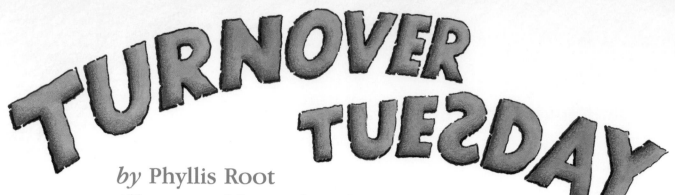

TURNOVER TUESDAY

by **Phyllis Root**
illustrated by **Helen Craig**

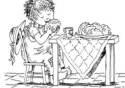

One Tuesday Bonnie Bumble baked six plum turnovers for breakfast. "Delicious," she said, and she ate up five, every bite. There wasn't even a crumb left over for her little dog, Spot.

But when Bonnie Bumble got up from her chair, she turned over upside down.

And nothing could turn her back over again.

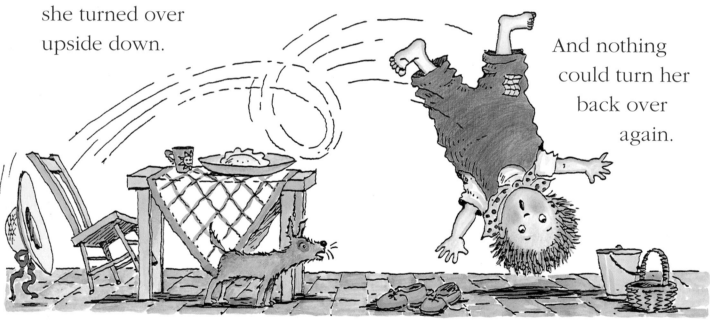

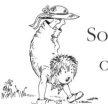

So Bonnie Bumble put her hat on her feet and her shoes on her hands. Then she went to do her chores.

Upside down she milked the cow.
But the milk SPLASHED out of the bucket.

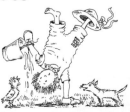

204

Upside down she gathered the eggs. But the eggs SMASHED out of the basket.

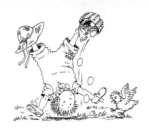

On the way back to the house, the sheep nibbled her hair. And the pig's tail tickled her ear.

"This will never do!" said Bonnie Bumble.

Back into the kitchen she went to find the last plum turnover. Upside down she ate it, almost every bite.

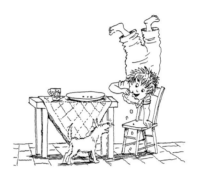

When she got up from the table, she turned back over, right side up! "Thank goodness everything's back to normal," said Bonnie Bumble. And it was …

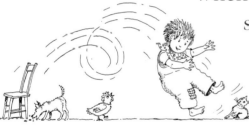

except for Spot, who had eaten up all the crumbs.

Baby Duck
and the
New Eyeglasses

by Amy Hest

illustrated by

Jill Barton

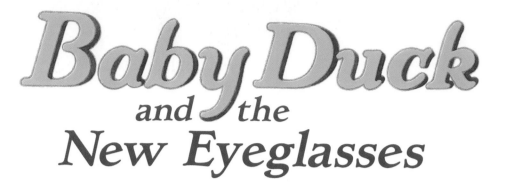

Baby Duck was looking in the mirror. She was trying on her new eyeglasses. They were too big on her baby face. They pushed against her baby cheeks. And she did not look like Baby.

Baby came slowly down the stairs.

"Park time!" said Mr Duck. "Grandpa will be waiting in his boat at the lake!"

"How sweet you look in your new eyeglasses!" cooed Mrs Duck. "Don't you love them?"

"No," Baby said.

"How well you must see in your new eyeglasses!" clucked Mr Duck. "Don't you like them just a little?"

"No," Baby said.

The Duck family went out of the front door. Mr and Mrs Duck hopped along. "Hop down the lane, Baby!"

Baby did not hop. Her glasses might fall off.

Mr and Mrs Duck danced along.

"Dance down the lane, Baby!"

Baby did not dance.

Her glasses might fall off.

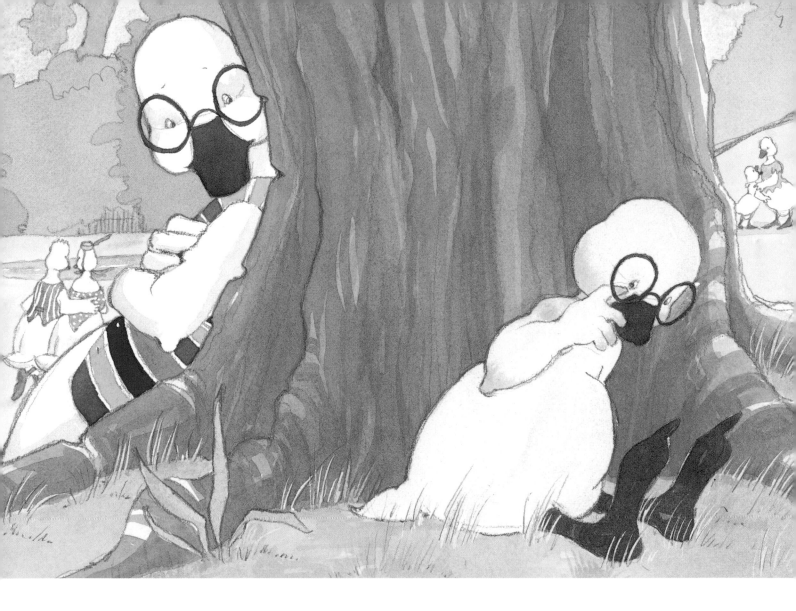

When they got to the park, Baby sat in the grass behind a tree. She sang a little song.

"*Poor, poor Baby, she looks ugly*
In her bad eyeglasses.
Everyone can play but me,
Poor, poor, poor, poor Baby."

Grandpa came up the hill. "Where's that Baby?" he called.

"I'm afraid she is hiding," Mrs Duck sighed.

"She does not like her new eyeglasses," worried Mr Duck.

Grandpa sat in the grass behind the tree. "I like your hiding place," he whispered.

"Thank you," Baby said.

Grandpa peered round the side of the tree. "I see new eyeglasses," he

207

whispered. "Are they blue?"

"No," Baby said.

"Green?" Grandpa whispered.

"No," Baby said.

"Cocoa brown?" Grandpa whispered.

Baby came out from behind the tree.

Grandpa folded his arms. "Well," he said, "I think those eyeglasses are *very* fine."

"Why?" Baby asked.

"Because they are red like mine!" Grandpa said.

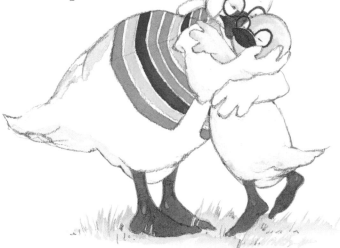

Grandpa kissed Baby's cheek. "Can you still run to the lake and splash about?"

Baby ran and splashed. Then she splashed harder. Her glasses did not fall off.

"Can you still twirl three times without falling down?"

Baby twirled. One, two, three. She did not fall down. And her glasses did not fall off.

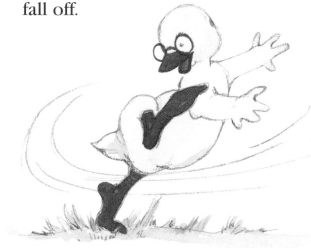

"Come with me, Baby. I have a surprise," Grandpa said.

They walked down to the pier. Grandpa's boat was bobbing on the water. There was another boat, too.

"Can you read what it says?" Grandpa asked.

Baby read, "B-a-b-y."

The letters were very clear. Then Grandpa and Mr and Mrs Duck sat in Grandpa's boat.

But Baby sat in *her* boat and
sang a new song.

"*I have nice new eyeglasses!*
I look like my grandpa.
My rowing-boat is lots of fun,
And I can read my name on it."

CALAMITY

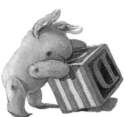

James and Horatio were building a tower.

"One, two, three," said James as he balanced the blocks.

"Seven, four," added Horatio.

"HEE-HAW!" BUMP! Something crashed into the Useful Box and sent everything flying.

"What was that?" asked Horatio.

"It's a calamity," said James, looking at the mess.

"What were you doing, Calamity?" asked Horatio.

"Racing," Calamity said. "And I won."

"Can I race?" asked Horatio.

"Find yourself a jockey," Calamity said. "Here's mine." She turned round.

But that's a bobbin, thought James. He started to tidy up.

by Camilla Ashforth

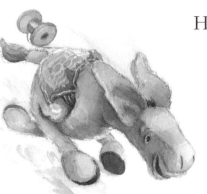

Horatio looked for a jockey. I like this one, he thought. It was James's clock.

"Are you ready?" asked Calamity.

They waited a moment.

"One, two, three, go!" Calamity called. She hurtled round the Useful Box. Twice.

Horatio tried to move his jockey.

He pushed it and pulled it. Then he rolled it over. His jockey would not budge.

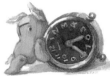

Calamity screeched to a halt. "Hee-haw! I won!" she bellowed. "Let's race again."

James turned round. He picked up Horatio's jockey.

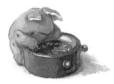

"That's my clock," said James and he put it in his Useful Box. Horatio looked for another jockey.

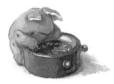

"One, two, three, go!" Calamity called. She galloped very fast.
Backwards and forwards.

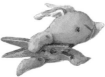

Horatio looked around. I'll go this way, he thought, and he set off with his new jockey.

"Hee-haw! Won again!" cried Calamity, stopping suddenly.

Horatio looked puzzled.

"One more race," Calamity said. "I'm good at this."

"James," whispered Horatio, "can you help me win this time?"

"What you need is a race track," said James. "I'll make you one. This block is the start," he said. "And this string is the finishing line. Ready, steady, go!"

Calamity thundered off. She was going the wrong way.

Horatio headed for the finishing line as fast as he could.

Calamity turned in a circle and headed back towards James.

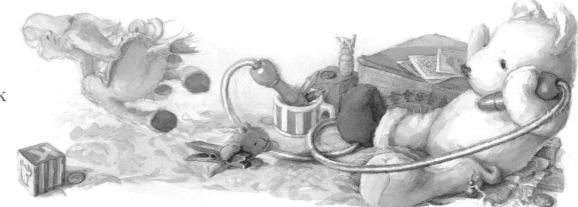

"Stop!"
James cried.

As Horatio crossed the line,
Calamity collided with the Useful Box. CRASH!

"That was a good race. Who won?" asked Calamity.

"I think you both did," James said, and squeezed Horatio tight.

Bathwater's Hot

by Shirley Hughes

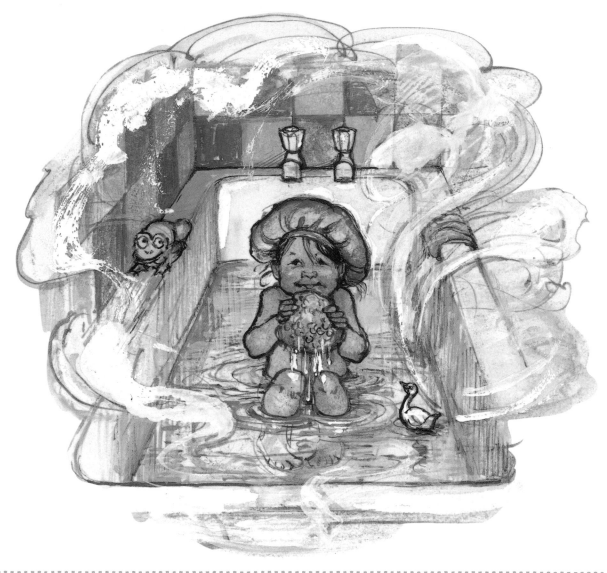

Bathwater's hot,
  Seawater's cold,
Ginger's kittens are *very* young
  But Buster's getting old.

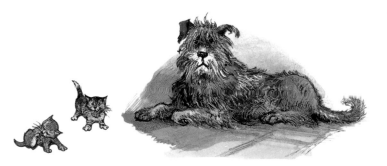

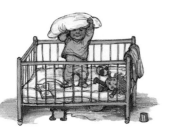

Some things you can throw away,
Some are nice to keep.
Here's someone who is wide awake,
Shhh, he's fast asleep!

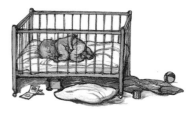

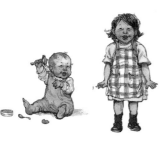

Some things are hard as stone,
Some are soft as cloud.
Whisper very quietly…
SHOUT OUT LOUD!

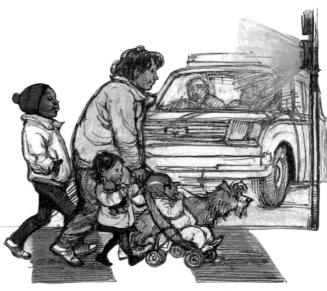

It's fun to run very fast
Or to be slow.
The red light says 'stop'
And the green light says 'go'.

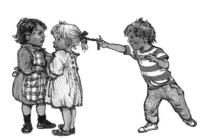

It's kind to be helpful,
Unkind to tease,
Rather rude to push and grab,
Polite to say 'please'.

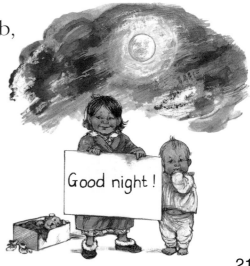

Good night!

Night time is dark,
Day time is light.
The sun says 'good morning'
And the moon says 'good night'.

Grandad's Magic

by Bob Graham

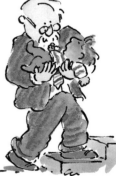

Three dogs lived in Alison's house. Two sat high on the shelf. They were very precious to Alison's mom. They were very breakable. Alison was not to touch them even if she could reach. She didn't like them anyway.

Alison much preferred Rupert. He lived on the armchair. Rupert only left the chair to have his dinner or go to the toilet. He wouldn't leave the chair for Alison's mom *or* her dad, and certainly not for Max, who often tried to pull his tail.

Rupert wouldn't even get out of his chair when Grandma and Grandad came to lunch on Sunday. Alison held Max for Grandma to kiss. He curled his fists and kicked his legs.

"Give him to me," said Grandad. "I know how to handle this young chap. Now for my magic…"

Grandad reached into Max's shirt and slowly pulled out a chocolate bear.

"Have you been keeping that in your shirt all this time?" he said. Max's face lit up with pleasure. Then Grandad lost the bear … and found it again under Rupert's collar!

"It's magic," said Alison.

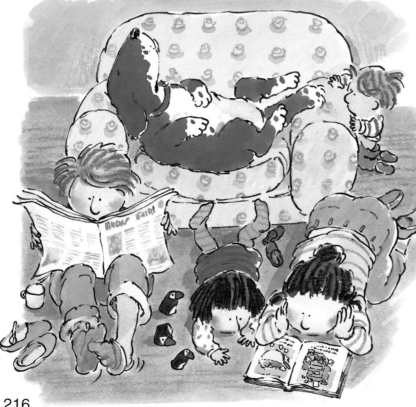

216

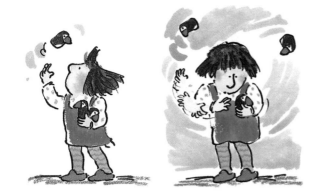

"Watch me, Grandad," said Alison. She had a trick of her own. She was learning to juggle with three puffins filled with sand that Grandad had given her. This *sounded* easy, but she

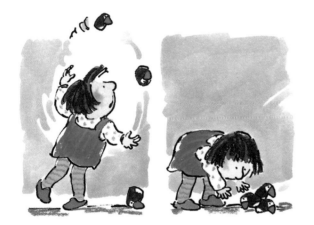

had to keep them going from hand to hand. The idea was to have three puffins in the air all at once.

"Try one at a time, Alison," said Grandad. "Backwards and forwards, and when you

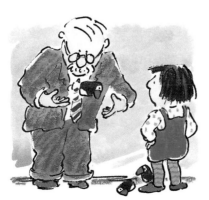

learn that, try two, and when you learn that, try three."

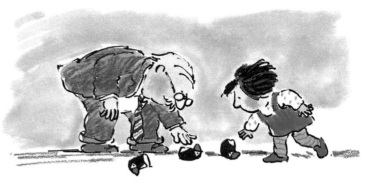

"I'm not as good as I used to be," said Grandad.

Sunday was the only day the china dogs came down from the shelf. Alison's mom used them as a table decoration. They guarded the fruit. Every Sunday Grandad picked his table napkin out of the air like an apple off a tree. And he talked of his best trick of all …

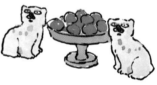

"I used to be able to take this tablecloth, give it a pull in a certain kind of way, and it would whip out from under all this stuff and leave everything standing there. But that was a long time ago."

Then one Sunday, Grandad noticed how well Alison juggled, and …

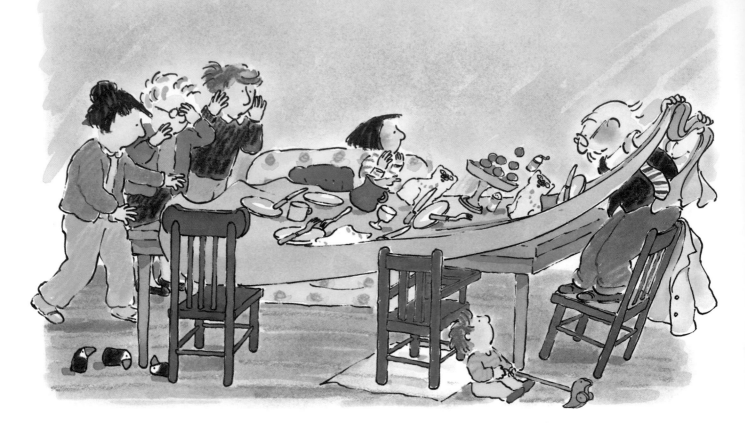

without warning, he removed his coat and climbed on to the chair.

"One good trick deserves another," he said. And he gave the tablecloth a short, snapping tug.

There was a moment of silence. Mom looked pale.

"You did it!" said Alison.
Grandad did a triumphant dance round the room. And *that's* when it happened.

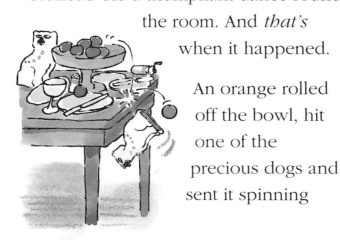

An orange rolled off the bowl, hit one of the precious dogs and sent it spinning

into mid-air … just as Rupert happened to be making a trip to the toilet. It settled on his very broad back …

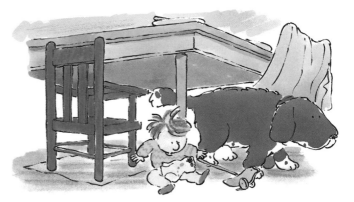

then landed safely in Max's lap. Alison held her breath. Would Grandad get into trouble? But Mom smiled thinly as she put the dogs back on the shelf.

"Don't *you* try that trick, Ally," said Grandad.

218

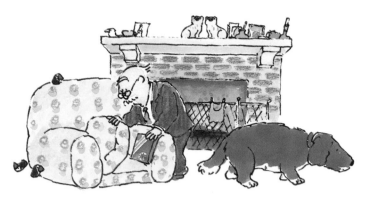

The following Sunday there were a number of changes in Alison's house. When Grandma and Grandad came to lunch, the dogs stayed on the shelf. And the table was set with unbreakable plastic plates and place mats.

Just before lunch, Rupert found a box of chocolates hidden under his cushion.

Later, Grandad made the chocolates appear just like magic. They were for Mom, who had such a shock last week.

Alison was dismayed. "That's not magic, it's a trick! You put them there, Grandad. The price is still on them!"

"We performers can't get it right all the time, Alison," Grandad said, "but the chocolates have certainly vanished.

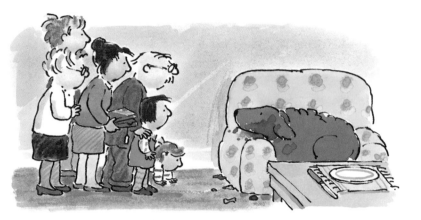

Now let's see how long *you* can spin this plastic plate on the end of your finger!"

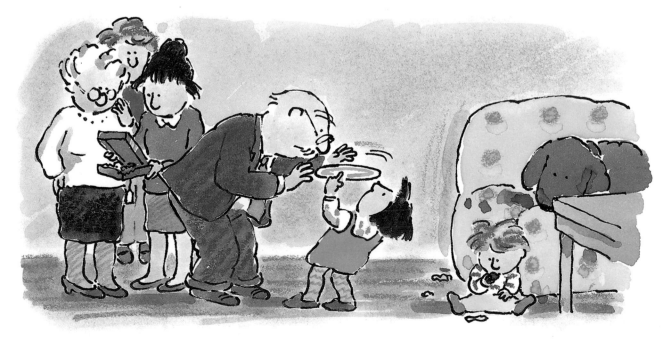

YOU AND ME, LITTLE BEAR

by
Martin Waddell

illustrated by
Barbara Firth

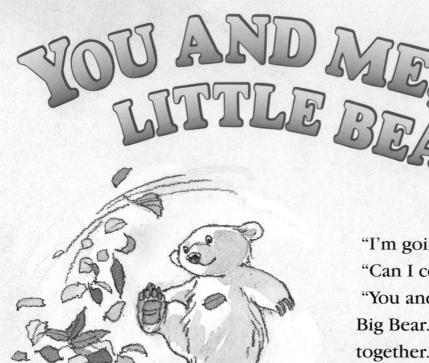

Once there were two bears, Big Bear and Little Bear. Big Bear is the big bear and Little Bear is the little bear.

Little Bear wanted to play, but Big Bear had things to do.
 "I want to play!" Little Bear said.
 "I've got to get wood for the fire," said Big Bear.
 "I'll get some too," Little Bear said.
 "You and me, Little Bear," said Big Bear. "We'll fetch the wood in together!"

"What shall we do now?" Little Bear asked.

"I'm going for water," said Big Bear.
"Can I come too?" Little Bear asked.
"You and me, Little Bear," said Big Bear. "We'll go for the water together."

"Now we can play," Little Bear said.
 "I've still got to tidy our cave," said Big Bear.
 "Well … I'll tidy too!" Little Bear said.
 "You and me," said Big Bear. "You tidy your things, Little Bear. I'll look after the rest."

"I've tidied my things, Big Bear!" Little Bear said.
 "That's good, Little Bear," said Big Bear. "But I'm not finished yet."
 "I want you to play!" Little Bear said.
 "You'll have to play by yourself, Little Bear," said Big Bear. "I've still got plenty to do!"

Little Bear went to play by himself, while Big Bear got on with the work.

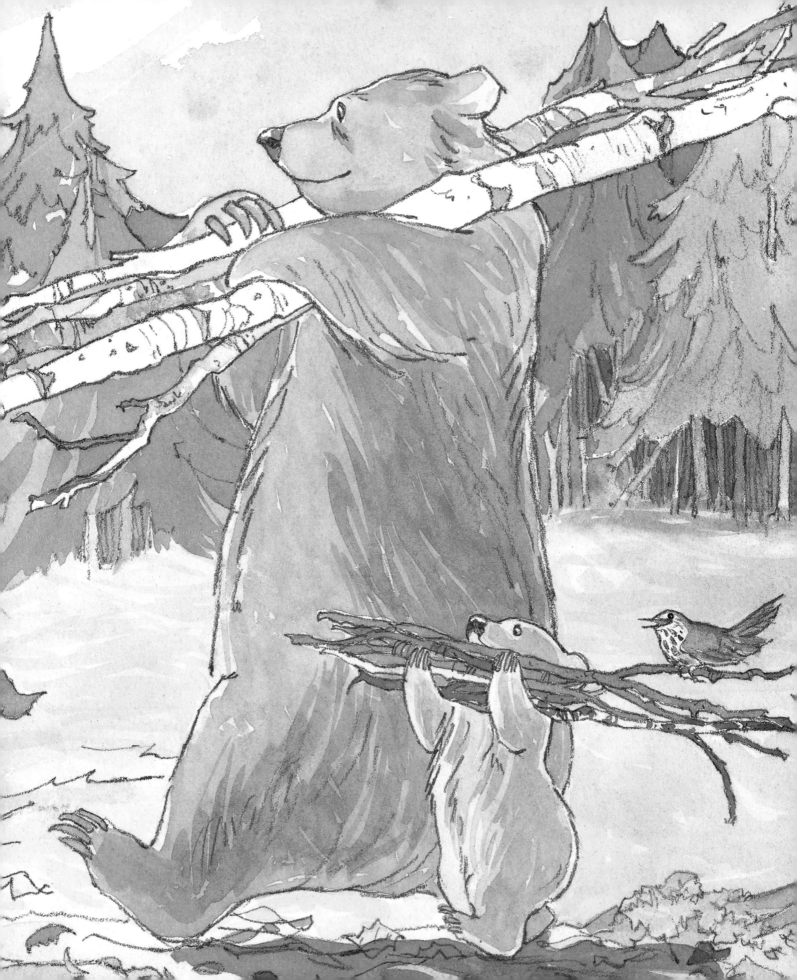

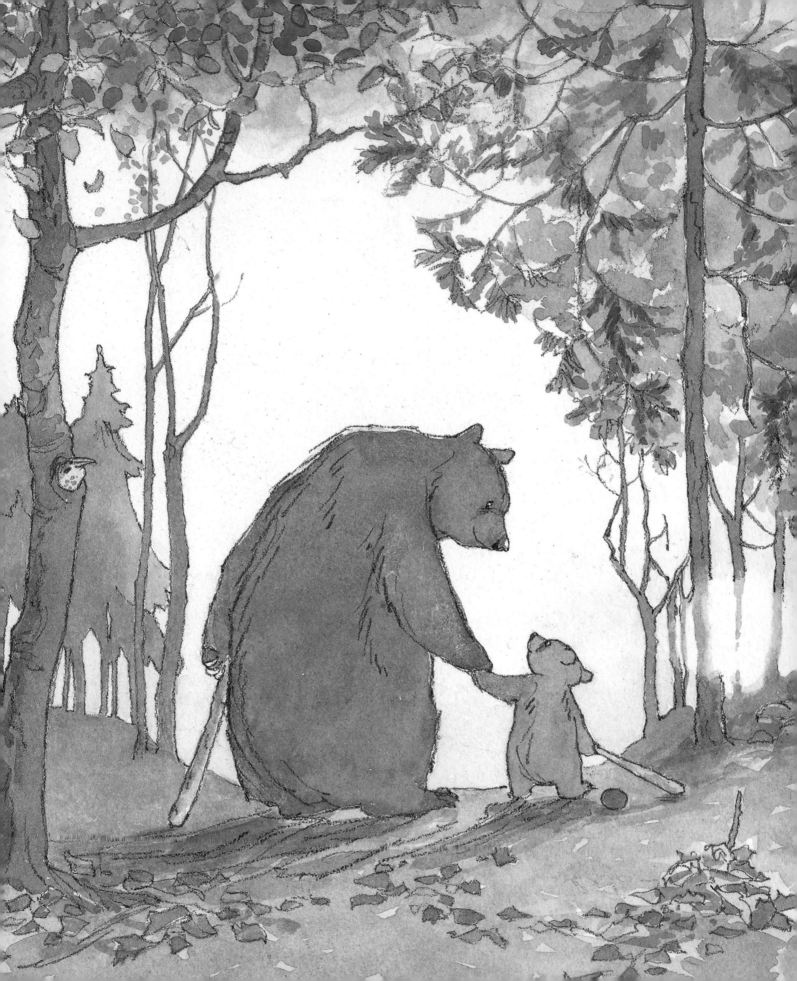

Little Bear
played bear-jump.
Little Bear played bear-slide. Little
Bear played bear-swing. Little Bear
played bear-tricks-with-bear-sticks.
Little Bear played bear-stand-on-his-
head and Big Bear came out to sit on
his rock. Little Bear played bear-run-
about-by-himself and Big Bear closed
his eyes for a think.

Little Bear went to speak to Big Bear,
but Big Bear was … asleep!
 "Wake up, Big Bear!" Little Bear said.
Big Bear opened his eyes. "I've played
all my games by myself," Little
Bear said.

Big Bear thought for a bit, then he
said, "Let's play hide-and-seek,
Little Bear."
 "I'll hide and you seek," Little Bear
said, and he ran off to hide.
 "I'm coming now!" Big Bear called,
and he looked till he found Little
Bear. Then Big Bear hid, and
Little Bear looked.

"I found you, Big Bear!" Little Bear
said. "Now I'll hide again."

They played lots of bear-games. When
the sun slipped away through the
trees, they were still playing. Then
Little Bear said, "Let's go home now,
Big Bear."

Big Bear and Little Bear went home
to their cave.
 "We've been busy today, Little Bear!"
said Big Bear.
 "It was lovely, Big Bear," Little Bear
said. "Just you and me playing …

together."

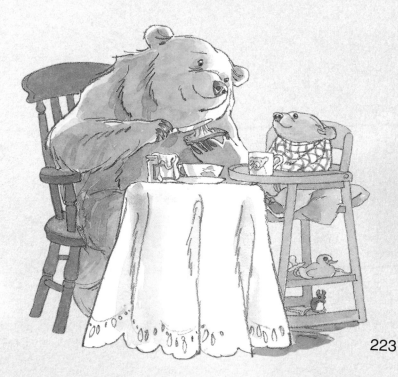

223

The Teeny Tiny WOMAN

A Traditional Tale
illustrated by **Arthur Robins**

Once upon a time a teeny tiny woman who lived in a teeny tiny house put on her teeny tiny hat and went out for a teeny tiny walk.

When the teeny tiny woman had gone a teeny tiny way, she went through a teeny tiny gate into a teeny tiny churchyard.

In the teeny tiny churchyard the teeny tiny woman found a teeny tiny bone on a teeny tiny grave. Then the teeny tiny woman said to her teeny tiny self, "This teeny tiny bone will make some teeny tiny soup for my teeny tiny supper."

So the teeny tiny woman took the teeny tiny bone back to her teeny tiny house. When she got home she felt a teeny tiny tired, so she put the teeny tiny bone in her teeny tiny cupboard and got into her teeny tiny bed for a teeny tiny sleep.

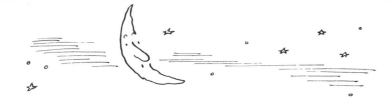

After a teeny tiny while the teeny tiny woman was woken by a teeny tiny voice that said, "Give me my bone!"

The teeny tiny woman was a teeny tiny frightened, so she hid her teeny tiny head under her teeny tiny sheet.

The teeny tiny voice said a teeny tiny closer and a teeny tiny louder, **"Give me my bone!"**

This made the teeny tiny woman a teeny tiny more frightened, so she hid her teeny tiny head a teeny tiny further under her teeny tiny sheet.

Then the teeny tiny voice said a teeny tiny closer and a teeny tiny louder, **"Give me my bone!"**

The teeny tiny woman was a teeny tiny more frightened, but she put her teeny tiny head out from under her teeny tiny sheet and said in her **loudest** teeny tiny voice …

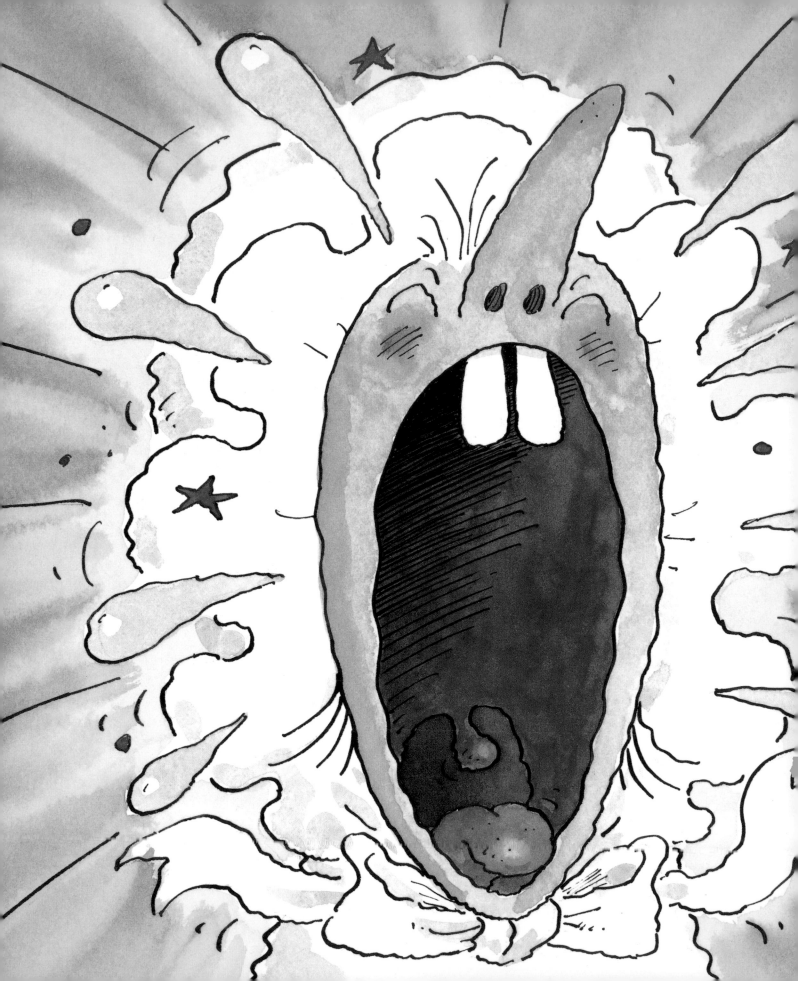

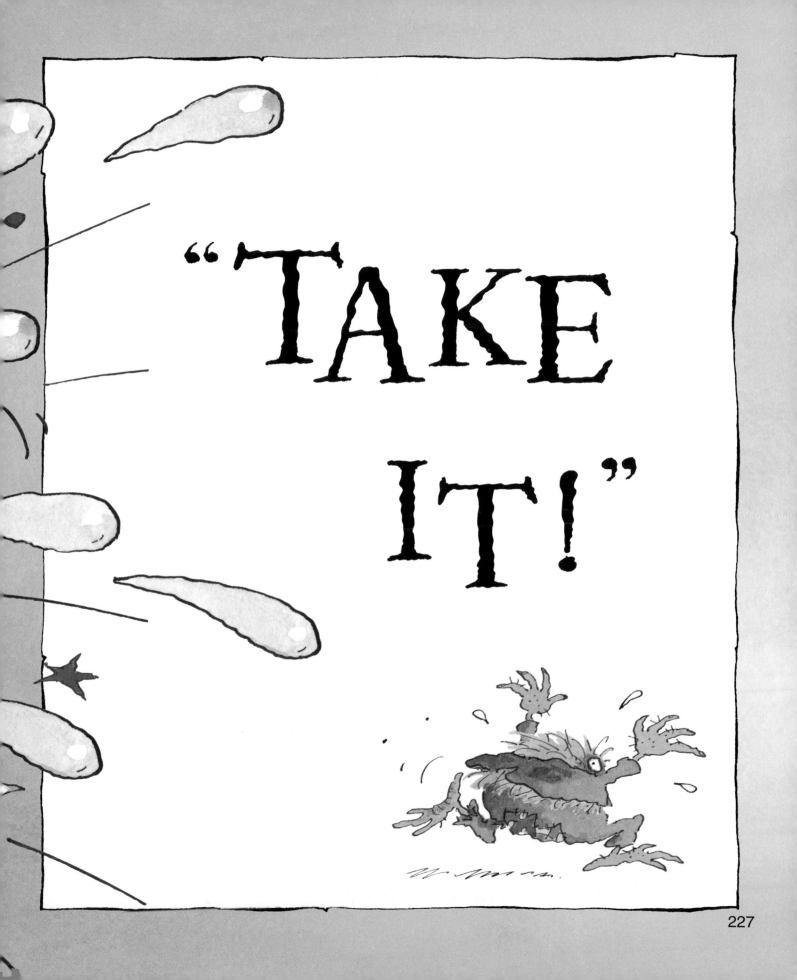

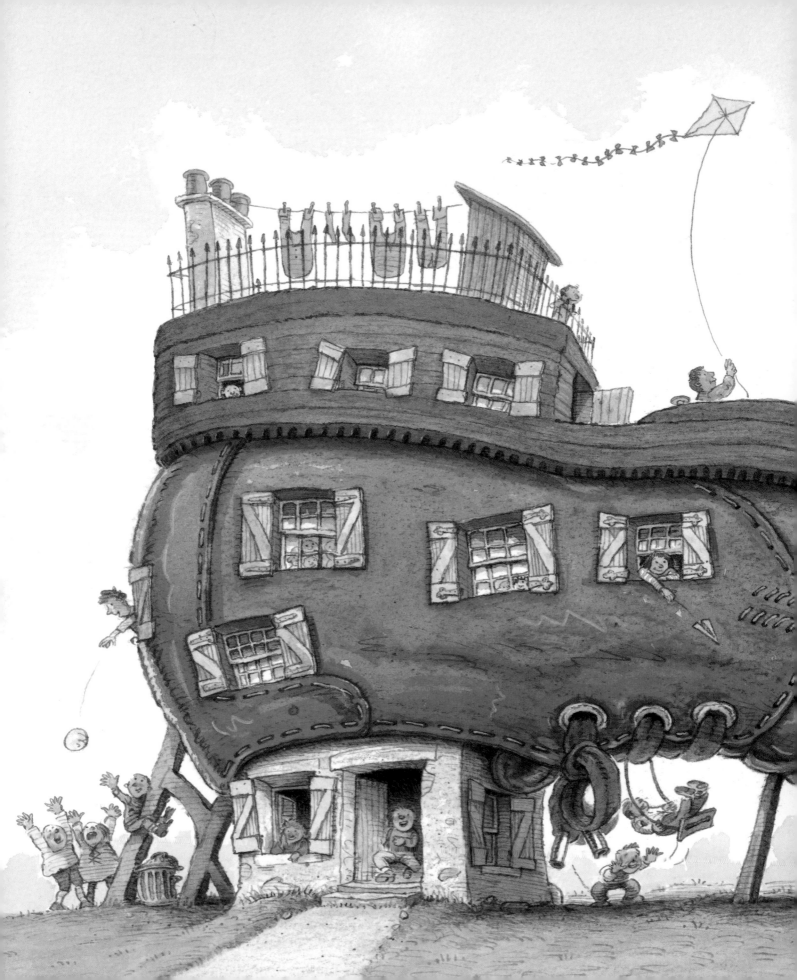

That's the Way to Do It!

by Colin McNaughton

There was an old woman
   Who lived in a shoe,
She had so many children
   She didn't know what to do;
So she sought the advice
   Of her friend Mr Punch,
Who said fry them with onions
   And eat them for lunch!

Friends

by Kim Lewis

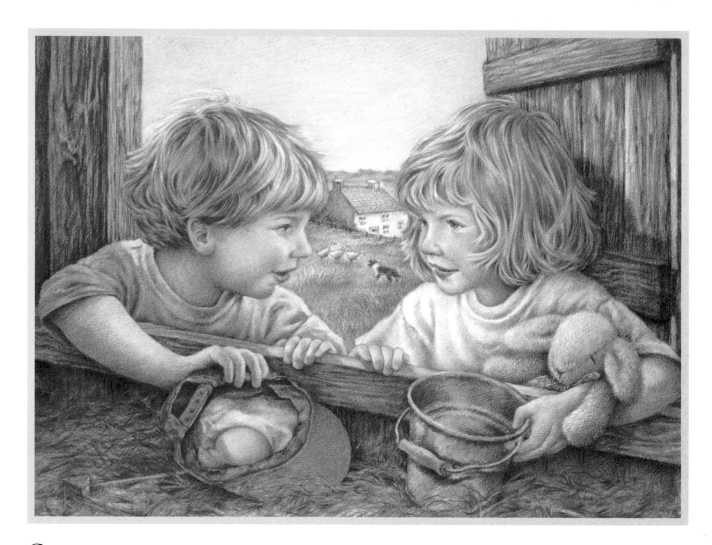

Sam's friend Alice came to play on the farm. They were in the garden when they heard loud clucking coming from the hen house.

"Listen!" said Sam. "That means a hen has laid an egg."

"An egg!" said Alice. "Let's go and find it."

Sam and Alice ran to the hen house.

"Look," said Alice. "There's the egg!"

"I can put it in my hat," said Sam.

"I can put your hat in my bucket,"

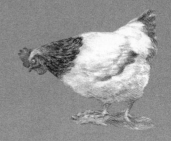

said Alice, "and put the bucket in the wheelbarrow."

"Then we can take it home," said Sam.

The geese stood across the path.

"I'm afraid of geese," said Alice.

"Come on," said Sam. "We can go the long way round."

Alice pushed the wheelbarrow through the trees.

"It's my turn now," said Sam, and he pulled it through the long grass and thistles.

Together, they lifted it over a ditch.

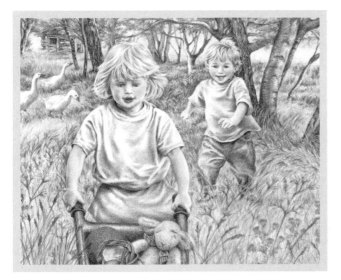

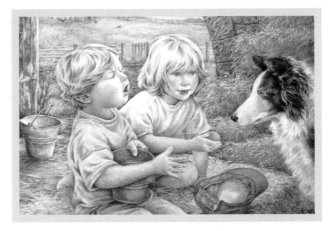

Sam and Alice went into the barn. They were followed by Glen, the old farm dog.

"Is the egg all right?" asked Alice.

Sam and Alice looked in the hat. The egg was safe and smooth, without a crack.

"Look what we've found!" said Alice, holding out the egg to Glen.

"No!" cried Sam. "He'll eat it!"

Sam reached out to take the egg.

Alice held it tight.

"It's mine!" said Sam.

"It's not!" said Alice. "I found it!"

"They're my hens!" said Sam, pushing Alice.

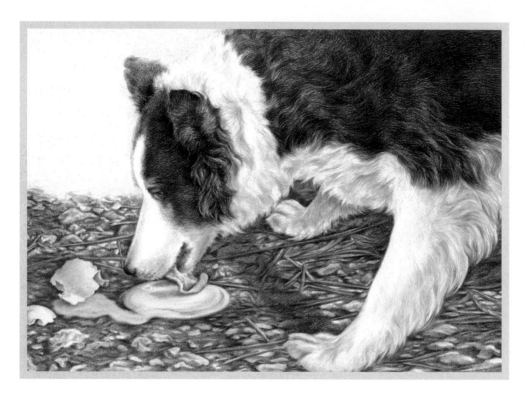

Just then loud clucking came from the hen house. Sam ran out of the barn.

"Another egg!" he cried.

Sam and Alice looked at each other.

"We can go and find it," said Sam.

"Yes, let's!" said Alice, and smiled.

SMASH went the egg as it fell on the ground. Glen started to eat it.

"I don't like you any more," said Alice. She picked up her bucket and went out of the barn.

Sam put on his empty hat. He did like Alice and he didn't like Alice and he felt he was going to cry.

Sam put the egg in his hat. He gave the hat to Alice who put it in her bucket. They tiptoed past the geese and Glen and walked back to the house.

"What have you two been doing?" asked Mom.

"Finding eggs," said Sam.

"Together!" said Alice.

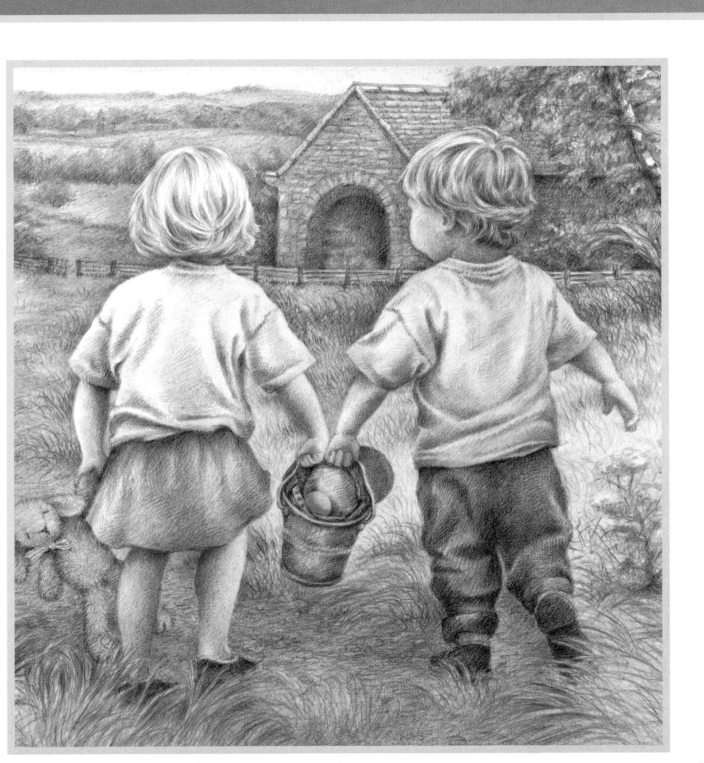

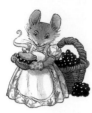

Mimi and the Blackberry Pies

by Martin Waddell   illustrated by Leo Hartas

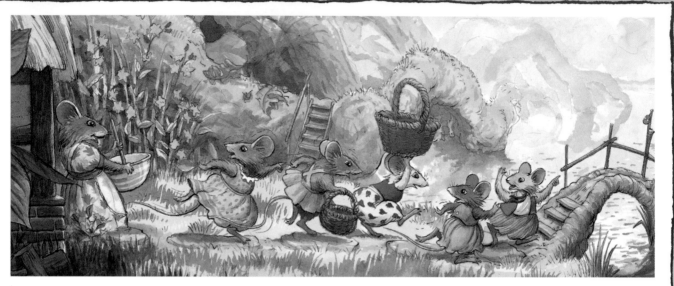

Mimi lived with her mouse sisters and brothers beneath the big tree. It was blackberry time in the hedge.

"I'm going to make blackberry pies," Mimi told her mouse sisters.

"We'll help you, Mimi!" her mouse sisters said. "We'll pick the best berries to go in the pies!" They all loved Mimi's blackberry pies.

Mimi's mouse sisters took their baskets out to the hedge, and they started to pick the juicy blackberries, but the berries were nice and they ate a lot more than they picked.

They ate and they ate and they ate and they ate

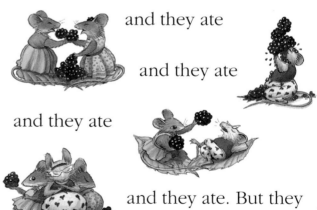

and they ate. But they didn't pick many berries for Mimi.

"This isn't much help!" Mimi said, when she'd counted the berries they'd picked.

"We'll help you, Mimi," her mouse brothers cried. "We'll pick trillions of berries!" They all loved Mimi's blackberry pies.

Mimi's mouse brothers climbed up into the hedge and got busy. But soon some-brother-mouse splatted some-other-brother-mouse with a berry! Mouse-brother-splatting looked fun. They forgot all about picking berries for Mimi, and started mouse-splatting each other instead.

They splatted

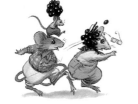

and they splatted

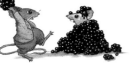

and they splatted

and they splatted

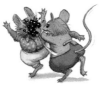

and they splatted.

But they didn't pick many berries for Mimi.

"This isn't much help!" Mimi sighed. And she went out to the hedge and picked all the berries she needed herself.

Mimi made blackberry pies. A sweet berry smell drifted over Mimi's sisters and brothers.

Their noses twitched

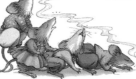

and they twitched

and they twitched

and they twitched

and they twitched.

The rich berry smell was so good that Mimi's sisters and brothers ran to her house. Mimi came out with the pies that she'd made on a tray. Mimi's blackberry pies were bursting with berries and juice.

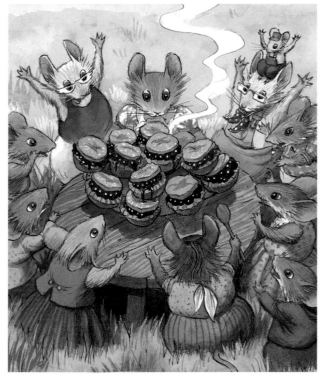

"This time I'm sure that you'll help!" Mimi said. And her mouse sisters and brothers helped Mimi eat all her blackberry pies!

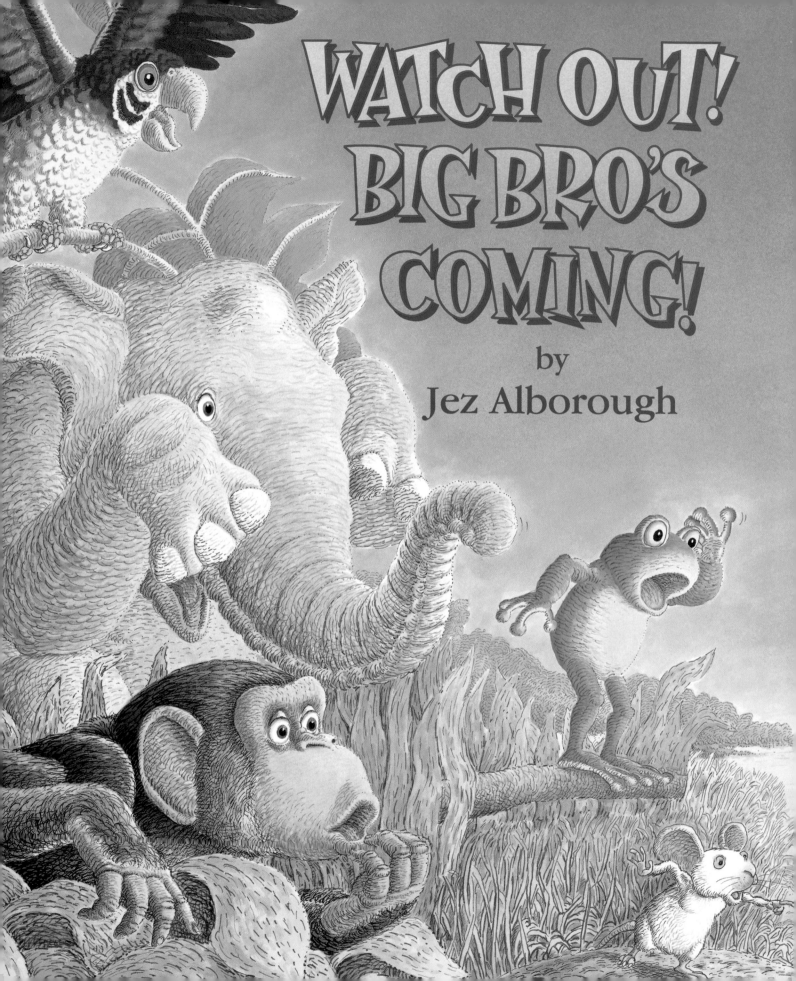

WATCH OUT! BIG BRO'S COMING!

by

Jez Alborough

"Help!" squeaked a mouse. "He's coming!"

"Who's coming?" asked a frog.

"Big Bro," said the mouse. "He's rough, he's tough, and he's big."

"Big?" said the frog. "How big?"

The mouse stretched out his arms as wide as they could go. "This big," he cried, and he scampered off to hide.

"Look out!" croaked the frog. "Big Bro's coming!"

"Big who?" asked the parrot.

"Big Bro," said the frog. "He's rough, he's tough, and he's really big."

"Really big?" said the parrot. "How big?"

The frog stretched out his arms as wide as they could go. "This big," he cried, and he hopped off to hide.

"Watch out!" squawked the parrot. "Big Bro's coming!"

"Who's he?" asked the chimpanzee.

"Don't you know Big Bro?" asked the parrot. "He's rough, he's tough, and he's ever so big."

"Ever so big?" said the chimpanzee. "How big?"

The parrot stretched out his wings as wide as they could go. "This big," he cried, and he flapped off to hide.

"Ooh-ooh! Look out!" whooped the chimpanzee. "Big Bro's coming!"

"Big Joe?" said the elephant.

"No," said the chimpanzee. "Big Bro. He's rough, he's tough, and everybody knows how big Big Bro is."

The elephant shook his head. "I don't," he said.

The chimpanzee stretched out his arms as wide as they could go. "This big," he cried.

"That big?" gulped the elephant. "Let's hide!"

So there they all were, hiding and waiting, waiting and hiding.

"Where is he?" asked the elephant.

"Shhh," said the chimpanzee. "I don't know."

"Why don't you creep out and have a look around?" whispered the elephant.

"Not me," said the chimpanzee.

"Not me," said the parrot.

"Not me," said the frog.

"All right," said the mouse. "As you're all so frightened, I'll go."

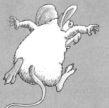

The mouse tiptoed ever so slowly out from his hiding place. He looked this way and that way to see if he could see Big Bro.

And then … "He's coming!" shrieked the mouse.

"H … h … h … hide!"

Big Bro came closer and closer and closer. Everyone covered their eyes.

"Oh no," whispered the frog.

"Help," gasped the parrot.

"I can hear something coming," whined the chimpanzee.

"It's him," whimpered the elephant. *"It's… it's…"*

"BIG BRO!" shrieked the mouse.

"Is that Big Bro?" asked the frog.

"He's tiny," said the parrot.

"Teeny weeny," said the chimpanzee.

"He's a mouse," said the elephant.

Big Bro looked up at them all, took a deep breath, and said …

"BOO!"

"Come on,
Little Bro," said
Big Bro. "Mom wants you back
home *now!*"
　"Wow," said the elephant.
　"Phew," said the chimpanzee.
　"He is rough," said the parrot.
　"And tough," said the frog.
　"Rough and tough," said
Little Bro, looking
back over his
shoulder.

"And I *told* you he was big!"

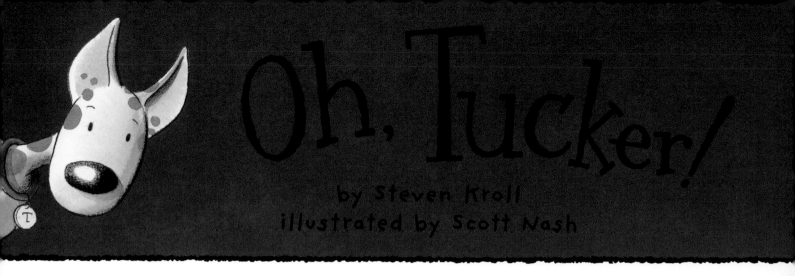

Oh, Tucker!

by Steven Kroll
illustrated by Scott Nash

"**TUCKER!** Time for breakfast!"
Tina called.

Tucker came running.
WHAM! He
knocked over
a dustbin.

He jumped
up and licked
Tina's chin.
"Oh, Tucker!" Tina giggled.

Tucker pushed open the front door
and raced into the house.
WHAM! He
knocked over a
vase of flowers.
WHAM! He
knocked a china
plate on to the floor.
"Oh, Tucker!" Tina groaned.

Tucker ran for the stairs.
"Tucker, no!" Tina cried.
"It's breakfast-time!"
But Tucker didn't listen. He had

to say good morning to Tina's parents.
He bounded up the stairs.

Mom and Dad were fast
asleep. Tucker didn't mind.
WHAM! He landed on
the bed.

"OOF!" said Mom.
"OOF!" said Dad.

Tucker licked their faces and wagged
his tail. **WHAM!** He knocked over the
bedside lamp. **WHAM!** He knocked
over the clock and the radio and a
glass of water.
"Oh, Tucker!" said Tina.

Tucker barked. He ran back to the
stairs – and
slipped!

Tucker flew
through
the air.

240

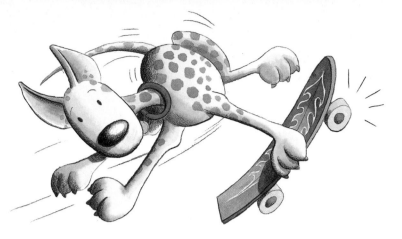

WHAM! He hit the wall and a picture fell. He scrambled to his feet. **WHAM!** He knocked over a table and a lamp. The lampshade plopped on his head.

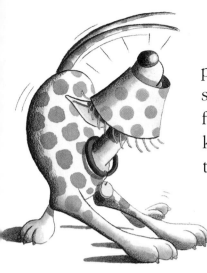

Tucker couldn't see but that didn't stop him. He zigzagged through the living room.

"Oh, Tucker, WAIT!" Tina cried. But Tucker didn't listen.

WHAM! He knocked over a chair. **WHAM!** He knocked over a vase. **WHAM!** He knocked over a plant and a bowl and a china cat.

WHAM! WHAM! WHAM!

Tucker stepped on Tina's skateboard and zoomed down the hall! Tina hid her eyes. "Oh, Tucker!"

WHAM! He crashed against the kitchen sink. The lampshade flew off his head. Tina hurried in. Mom and Dad hurried in, too.

"Here, Tucker, look," Tina said. She set his dish down in front of him. They all held their breath. Tucker dug in. "Finally," said Tina.

Mom and Dad sighed with relief. Tina smiled. Such a nice dog. Such a friendly dog. Who could possibly scold him?

WHAM! WHAM! WHAM!
WHAM! WHAM! WHAM! WHAM!

"Oh, Tucker!"

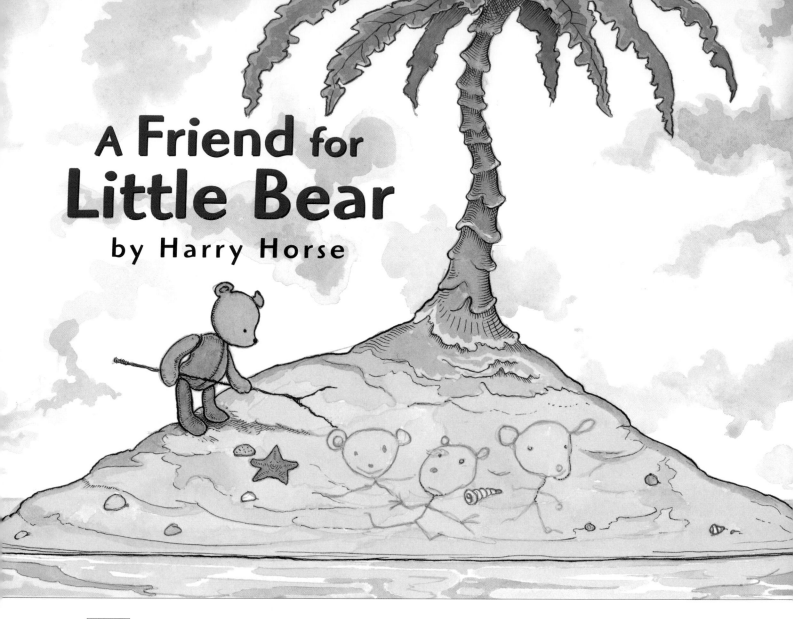

A Friend for Little Bear
by Harry Horse

Little Bear lived all alone on a desert island. "I wish I had something to play with," he said.

A stick came floating by. Little Bear picked it out of the sea. He drew a picture in the sand. Then he drew some more. "I need something else to play with," he said. He was tired of drawing pictures.

A bottle came floating by. Little Bear picked it out of the sea. He filled it up with water, then poured out the water on the sand.

"I need a cup," said Little Bear, "to pour the water into."

242

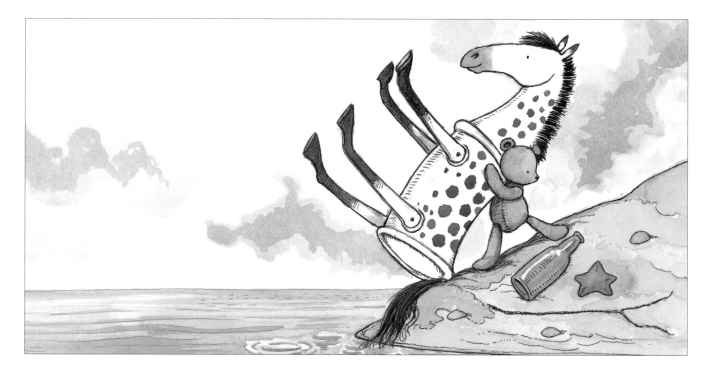

Then something spotted came floating by. Little Bear wondered what it was. "It isn't a cup," he said, but he pulled it out of the sea anyway. It was a wooden horse.

The wooden horse ran round the island. Little Bear ran after him. The wooden horse hid. Little Bear looked for him. They had a lovely time. They drew pictures in the sand and filled the bottle again and again. They played all day long and then went to sleep under the tall palm tree.

Little Bear woke up. He rubbed his eyes. "Look!" he cried. "Lots of things floating in the water!" He stretched with his stick and pulled out as many as he could. "I don't know what these things are," he said, "but I need them, all the same." He piled them into a heap. Then he sighed. "I still do wish I had a cup."

243

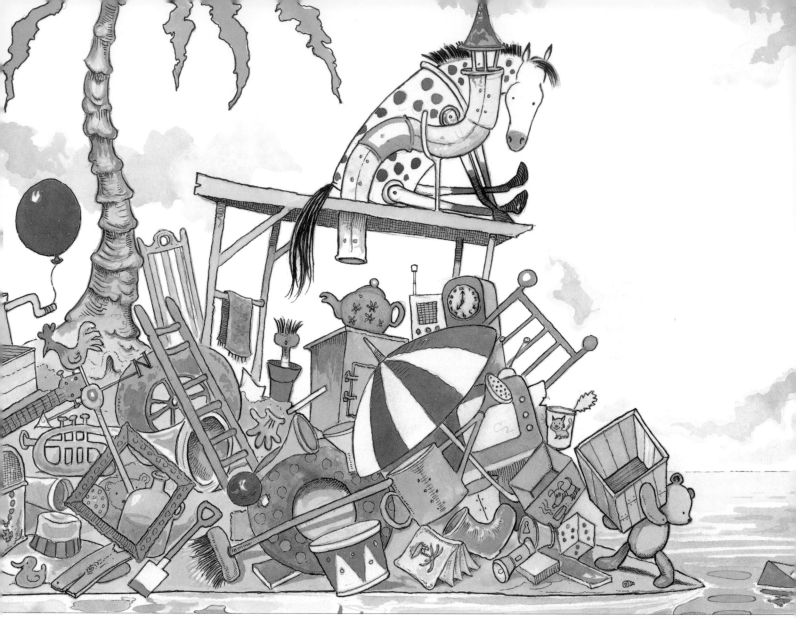

There wasn't much room on the island now. Little Bear
had filled it up. He told the wooden horse to get
out of the way. "Climb on to that," said Little
Bear. "I need more room for these boxes."

"Look!" cried Little Bear. "A cup!"

SNAP!

The roof broke. The wooden
horse fell into the sea and floated away.

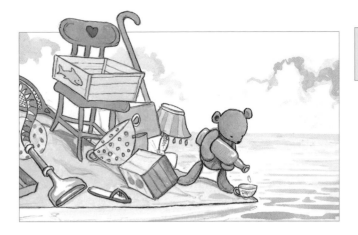

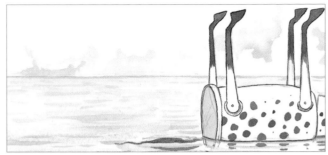

He ran and pulled it out of the sea.

Little Bear was filling his bottle with water and pouring the water into his cup. "Watch me!" he cried. He filled up the bottle again. "Watch me!" But no one was there. He looked up. He put the bottle down. He walked all round the island. "Where are you?" he called. "I need you!" but no one answered.

"I only need you, Wooden Horse," he said, and the two of them danced for joy on the sand.

"I need my *friend*," said Little Bear. "I don't need that cup!" He threw all his things back into the sea and they floated away.

He sat underneath the tall palm tree and began to cry.

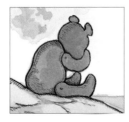

245

Pog had

by Peter Haswell

Pog had a banana. "I wonder what a banana does," said Pog.

He put it on his head. 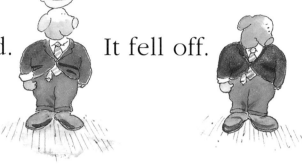 It fell off.

He dropped it on the floor.

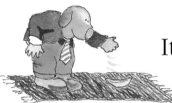 It didn't bounce.

He put it in a vase.

It didn't grow.

Pog peeled the banana.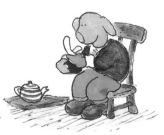

He threw away the skin.

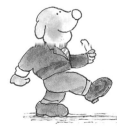 Pog walked…

246

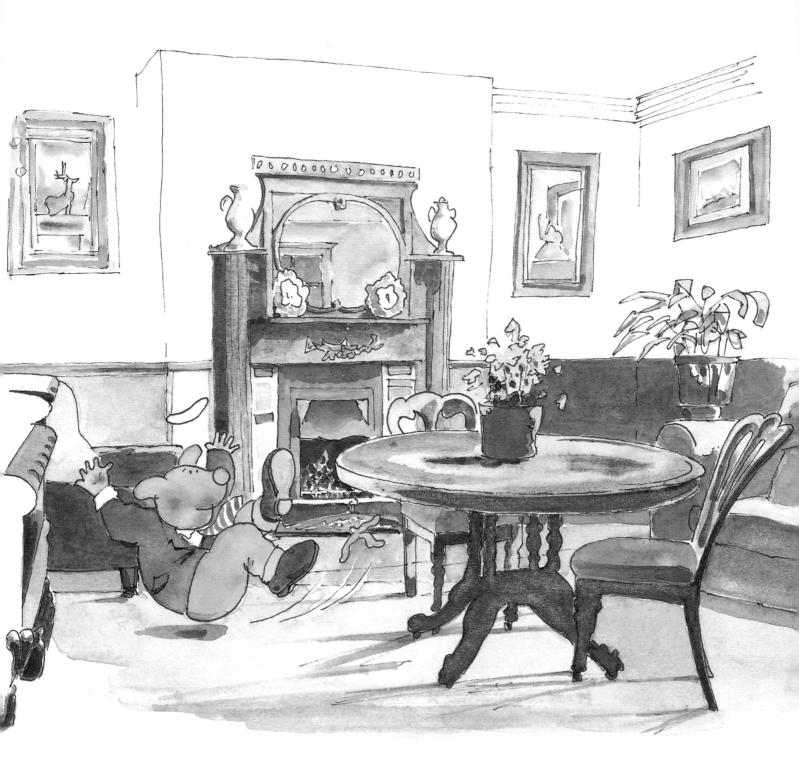

"Now I know what a banana does," said Pog.

"It makes you fall down!"

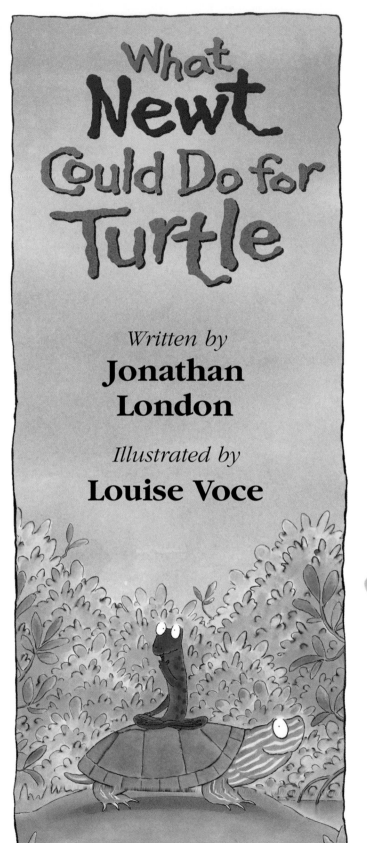

What Newt Could Do for Turtle

Written by
Jonathan London

Illustrated by
Louise Voce

Spring had come to the swamp.

A red-spotted newt crawled out from his winter bed in the mud.

"Help!" cried Newt. "I'm stuck!"

A painted turtle yawned, greeting the spring.

"Coming, dear Newt!" cried Turtle.

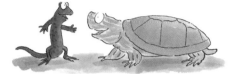

Pock! went the mud as Turtle pulled Newt free.

"Thanks, Turtle! You're the best!"

"That's what friends are for!" said Turtle.

"Yep," said Newt. His spots turned a deeper red, and he wondered, *What can I do for Turtle?*

That spring the swamp buzzed with life. There were catfish and dragonflies, cat's-tails and dogwoods, polecats and tadpoles. Turtle took good care of Newt, and Newt and Turtle were happy just to be together. But sometimes, when Newt sat alone on his thinking rock, he wondered, *What can I do for Turtle?*

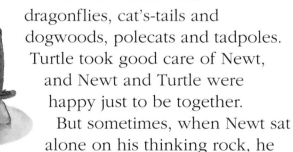

In the summer Newt and Turtle played in their favourite swimming holes.

They swooshed down muddy banks and crashed into the water together – *splash!*

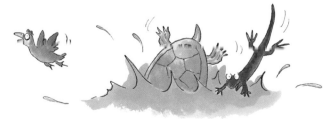

Playing hide-and-seek, Newt climbed on to Turtle's back.
"*Yoo-hoo!* Turtle! Where are you?"

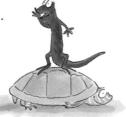

He thought he was on a rock.
"*Boo!*" said Turtle, poking his head out.
Newt jumped high into the air.

One day, a cottonmouth snake slithered off a branch and whispered through the water. Snake swam straight towards Newt.
He was about to strike when Newt heard Turtle's voice,
"*Newt! A snake!*"

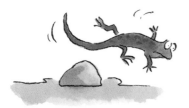

Newt plunged into the water and hid at the bottom of the swamp.
Once again, Newt wondered, *What can I do for Turtle?*

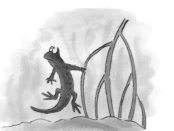

Autumn came and the leaves of the swamp trees sailed down like little umbrellas.
One day, Newt was paddling a leaf when an alligator glided up to him.
Turtle was watching but he was so scared he hit the water with a great *smack!* and went under.
Alligator turned her head to look, and at that moment Newt dived away.

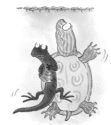

Newt and Turtle hid together beneath the duckweed. Newt sighed, happy to be alive, and his spots turned redder. Now, more than ever, he wondered, *What can I do for Turtle?*

Then, one day, a curious bobcat slunk through the reeds, twitched his whiskers and *pounced* – right on to Turtle's back.
"*Yikes!*" yelled Turtle, pulling his head inside his shell.
Bobcat batted with his paws and flipped Turtle over. Then he grew bored and trotted back into the forest.

249

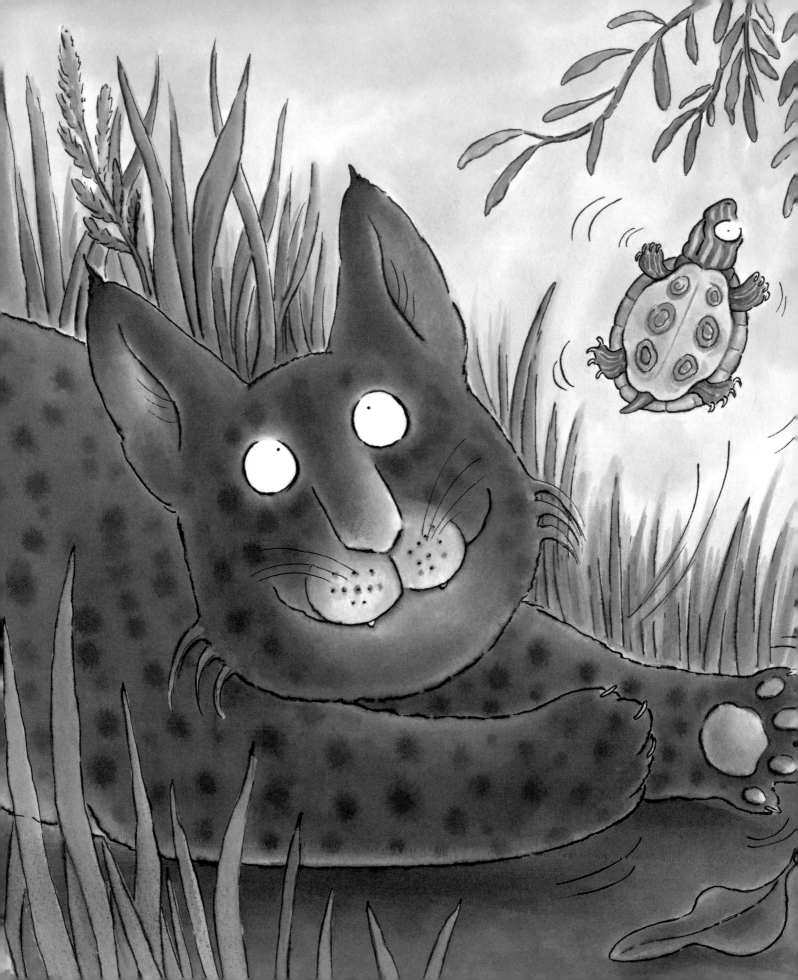

Poor Turtle wriggled back and forth. If he could not roll over, he would dry up and die!

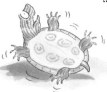

"Newt, oh Newt!" he cried. "Where are you?"

Now, across the swamp, Newt was dreaming that Turtle was in trouble. "*What can I do for Turtle?*" he said.

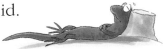

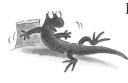

His own words woke him up! His heart bumped and stumbled, just like his feet. He scurried to and fro, searching for his friend.

At last, beneath a weeping willow, Newt found him.

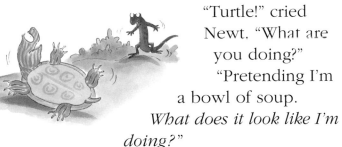

"Turtle!" cried Newt. "What are you doing?"

"Pretending I'm a bowl of soup. *What does it look like I'm doing?*"

"Don't worry," said Newt. "I'll help you." This was his big chance! Newt went to his thinking rock, and thought and thought.

"*Aha!*" he said at last. He hauled a big stick over to Turtle and stuck it under his shell.

He pushed a rock beneath the stick then he sprang up, grabbed hold, and swung.

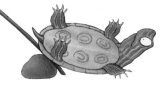

"*Rock 'n' roll!*" cried Newt. Turtle wobbled, teetered on edge …

and toppled over.

"Hooray!" shouted Turtle. "You *did* it!"

"That's what friends are for!" sang Newt. Turtle stretched out his neck and gently nuzzled Newt. Newt's spots turned so dark they were almost purple.

The days were getting shorter. Ducks splashed off, chattering news of winter.

Newt licked a toe and held it up, testing the breeze. "Yep," he said. "Winter has finally come."

Turtle nodded with a drowsy smile.

"Well," said Newt, "it's nice knowing what we can do for each other."

"Yes," said Turtle wisely, "these things are worth remembering."

"Goodnight, Turtle," said Newt. "See you next spring!"

"Goodnight, Newt!" said Turtle.

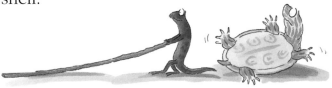

And they slipped deep into the swamp mud, where it was snug and cosy and warm.

"Sleep tight!" murmured Turtle.

And that is what they did.

All winter.

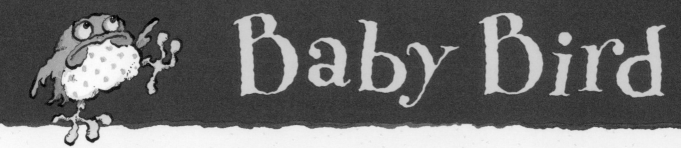

Baby Bird

This is the bird that climbed out of the nest and …

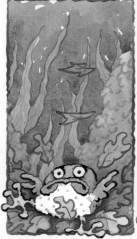 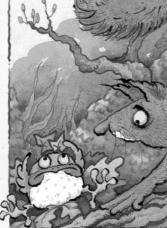 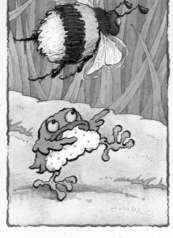 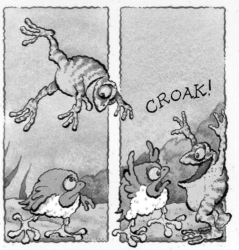

flop
flop
flop …
he fell!

This is the
squirrel that
sniffed at the
bird that fell.

This is the bee
that buzzed
round the
bird that fell.

This is the frog
that hopped
over the bird
that fell.

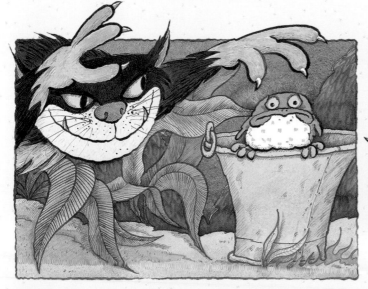 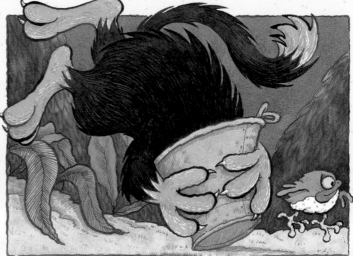

This is the cat that stalked
the bird …

and fell himself
(which was just as well).

252

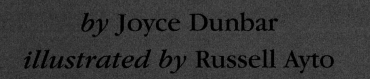

by Joyce Dunbar
illustrated by Russell Ayto

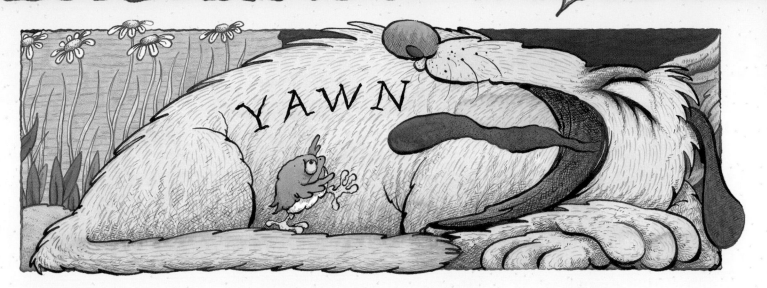

This is the dog that opened wide and a bird that nearly walked inside.

A baby bird that wanted to fly up, up above, up above in the sky …
and thought he would have just one more try …

flap   flap   flap   flap …

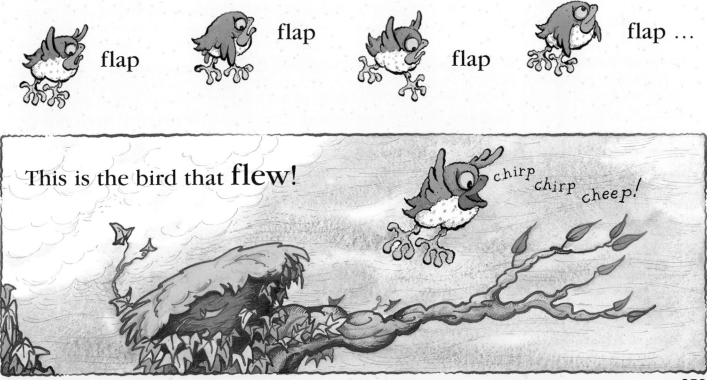

This is the bird that **flew!**

chirp chirp cheep!

COWBOY BABY

SUE HEAP

It was getting late and Sheriff Pa said, "Cowboy Baby, time for bed."

But Cowboy Baby wouldn't go to bed, not without Texas Ted and Denver Dog and Hank the Horse.

"Off you go and find them," said Sheriff Pa. "Bring them safely home."

Cowboy Baby put on his hat and his boots,

and he set off on the trail of Texas Ted, Denver Dog and Hank the Horse. He went down the dusty path and through the barnyard gate.

Over by the hen-house he found ... **Texas Ted.** "Howdy, Texas Ted," said Cowboy Baby.

Cowboy Baby and Texas Ted crossed the rickety bridge.

Down by the old wagon wheel they found ... **Denver Dog.** "Howdy, Denver Dog," said Cowboy Baby.

Cowboy Baby, Texas Ted and Denver Dog crawled through the long grass and out into the big, wide desert.

There by the little rock they found ...

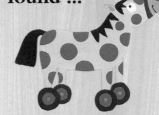

Hank the Horse. "Howdy, Hank the Horse," said Cowboy Baby.

"I'VE FOUND THEM," Cowboy Baby shouted to Sheriff Pa. "That's dandy," Sheriff Pa called back. "Bring them home now, safe and sound."

Cowboy Baby and his gang sat down on the little rock. None of them wanted to go home. "Let's hide!" said Cowboy Baby. "Hey, Sheriff Pa," he shouted. "I bet you can't find us, NO SIRREE!"

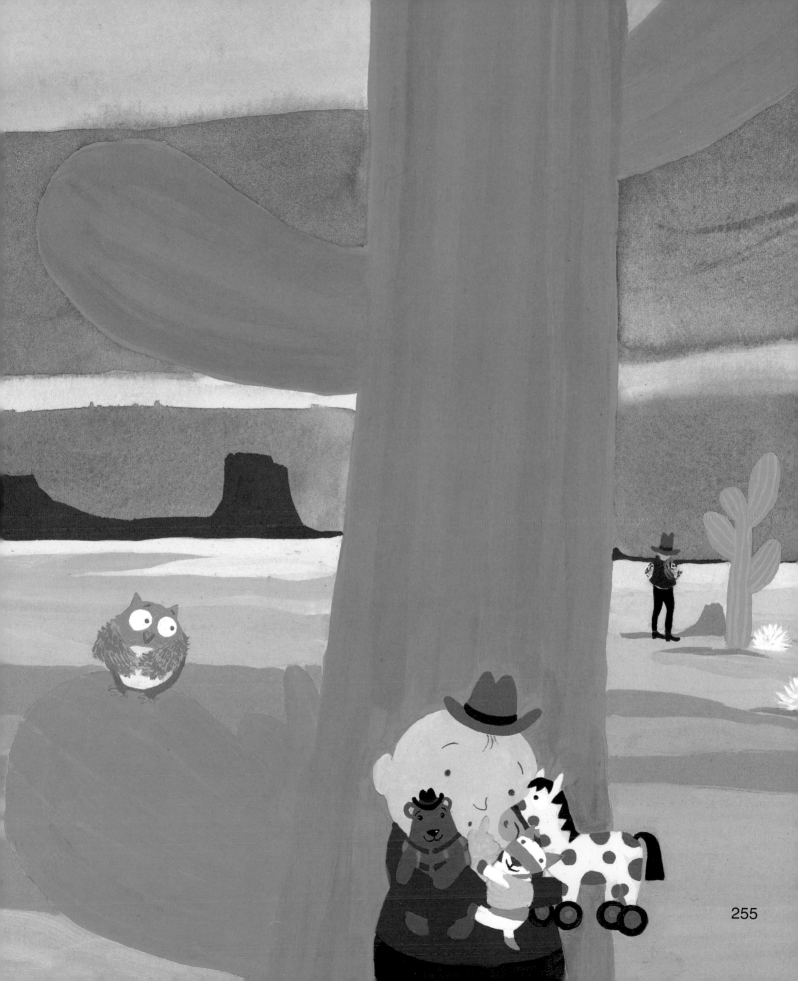

255

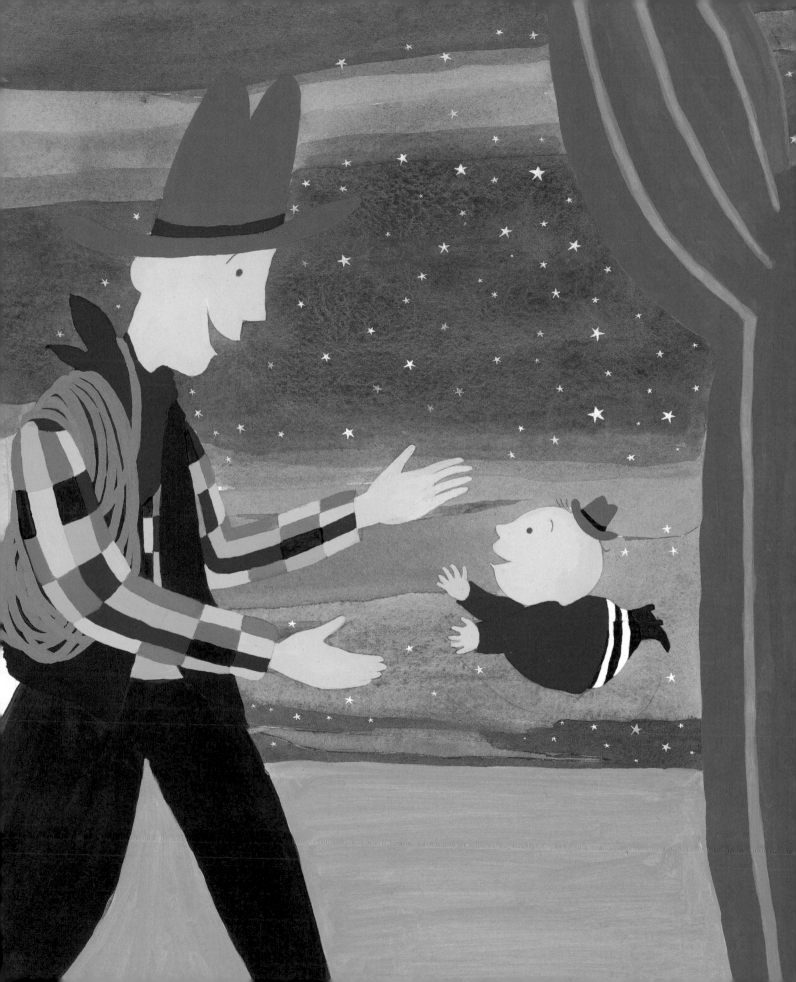

Sheriff Pa came to the big, wide desert.
 "Shh!" said Cowboy Baby to his gang.
 Sheriff Pa looked. He looked ... and he looked ... and he looked. But he couldn't find Cowboy Baby. No sirree!

"You got me beat, Cowboy Baby," called Sheriff Pa. "But if you come out, there'll be a big surprise, just for you!"
 Out jumped Cowboy Baby. "Howdy, Sheriff Pa!"

The sheriff threw his lasso. It twisted and turned in the starlit sky and it caught ... a twinkling star.

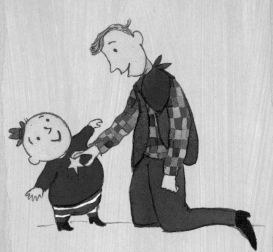

"Look!" said Sheriff Pa, and he gave the star to Cowboy Baby.
 "Now you're my deputy," he said.

Then Cowboy Baby picked up Texas Ted and Denver Dog and Hank the Horse, and Sheriff Pa picked up Cowboy Baby.

And all together they went home to bed.

"Nighty night, Cowboy Baby," said Sheriff Pa. But Cowboy Baby was already fast asleep.

YES SIRREE!

SOMETHING'S COMING!

by Richard Edwards ● *illustrated by* Dana Kubick

"Something's coming!" said Elephant, sitting up.

"Nothing's coming," said Frog sleepily.

"Something's coming," said Elephant.

"Nothing's coming," said Little Rabbit.

"Something's coming," said Elephant.

"Nothing's coming," said Frog and

Little Rabbit together.

"I'm sure something's coming,"

said Elephant.

Little Rabbit pushed back the blanket and

looked out of the box.

"If Elephant thinks something's coming, we'll never get any sleep until

we've found out what it is. Come on, let's have a look round."

And with the others following close behind,

Little Rabbit climbed out of the box and

dropped silently to the floor.

It was very quiet in the moonlit room.

They crept to the door and listened, but

there was no sound of anything coming. They

climbed on to the window-sill and peered out,

but there was no sight of anything coming.

They looked up the chimney. They looked in

the cupboards. They looked under the sofa.

They looked everywhere.

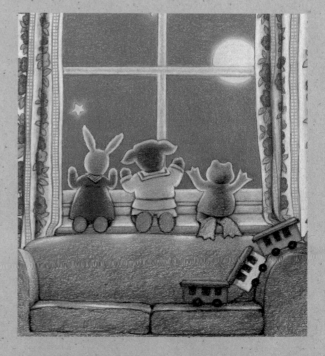

"See," said Little Rabbit. "Nothing's coming. Not a single thing."

Elephant raised his trunk. "Something's coming," he insisted. " I can feel it."

"Then what is it?" asked Frog.

"It's a … It's a …

It's a … a … a …

T C H O O !"

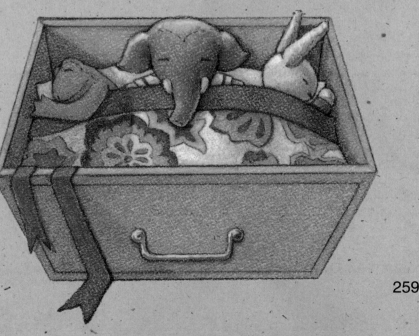

And Elephant sneezed so hard that Frog and Little Rabbit went flying across the room and landed in a tangled heap in the corner.

"Is that what was coming?" asked Little Rabbit, picking herself up.

"Yes," said Elephant. "A … a … a … a … TCHOO!" And he sneezed again, even harder than before.

"I knew something was coming," said Elephant, breathing deeply through his nice clear trunk. "Let's go back to bed now."

Soon they were fast asleep.

259

Nasty Kids, Nice Kids

What are nasty kids like?

They pull your hair,
    they call you names,

They tell you lies,
    they spoil your games,

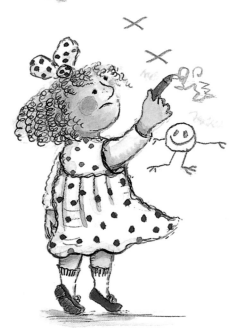

They draw on walls,
    scream on the floor.

Nasty kids want **more, more, more.**

by Catherine and Laurence Anholt

What are nice kids like?

They make you laugh,
they hold your hand,

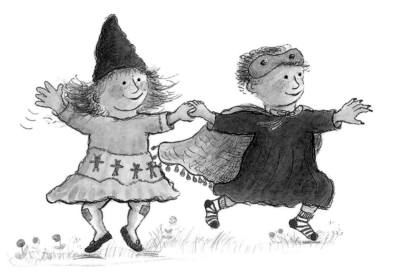

Nice kids always
understand.

They share their toys,
they let you play,

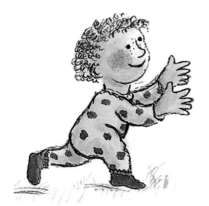

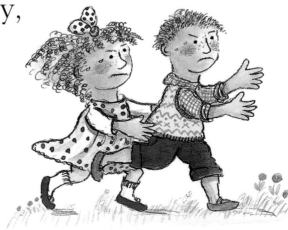

They chase the nasty kids away.

Let the LYNX Come In

Jonathan London
∞
illustrated by
Patrick Benson

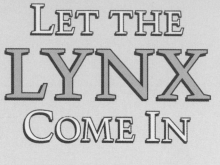

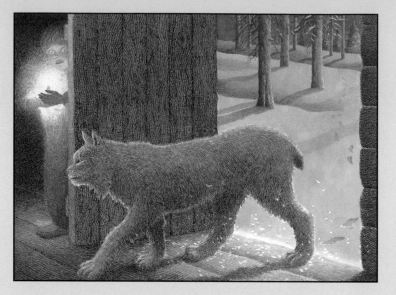

As the fire snaps
and roars
in the pot-belly stove,
my father snores,
but I can't sleep.
It was his idea
to come
to the north woods
where I've never
been before.

There are wolves
and bears out there.
And a lynx.

I hear a scratching
coming from
outside.

I get up,
creep to the door,
open it a crack,
then jump back ...

A WILDCAT!

The lynx steps in,
shakes first
one paw
then the other;
stands still
as a stone,
quiet as an owl,
in the middle
of the room.
Firelight glows
in its yellow eyes.

I shiver
in the warm room
as the lynx grows
and grows
and grows,
till its whiskers
touch the walls!

Great Lynx
commands
with his silence.

I grab fistfuls of fur
and climb up and up
on to the back
of the enormous cat.
And the next thing
I know ...

we're outside in
the snow!

Bunched like a fist
I clench fur as
Great Lynx creeps
on big cat's feet.
If I cry, my tears
will turn to ice.
In the trees
the moon trembles
on a bare
black branch,
then rolls
along with us
through the hard
northern night.

Great Lynx leaps
across
a frozen river,
steps across
glittering snow,
stalking some
invisible thing.
We climb a ridge
of ice and
there it is!

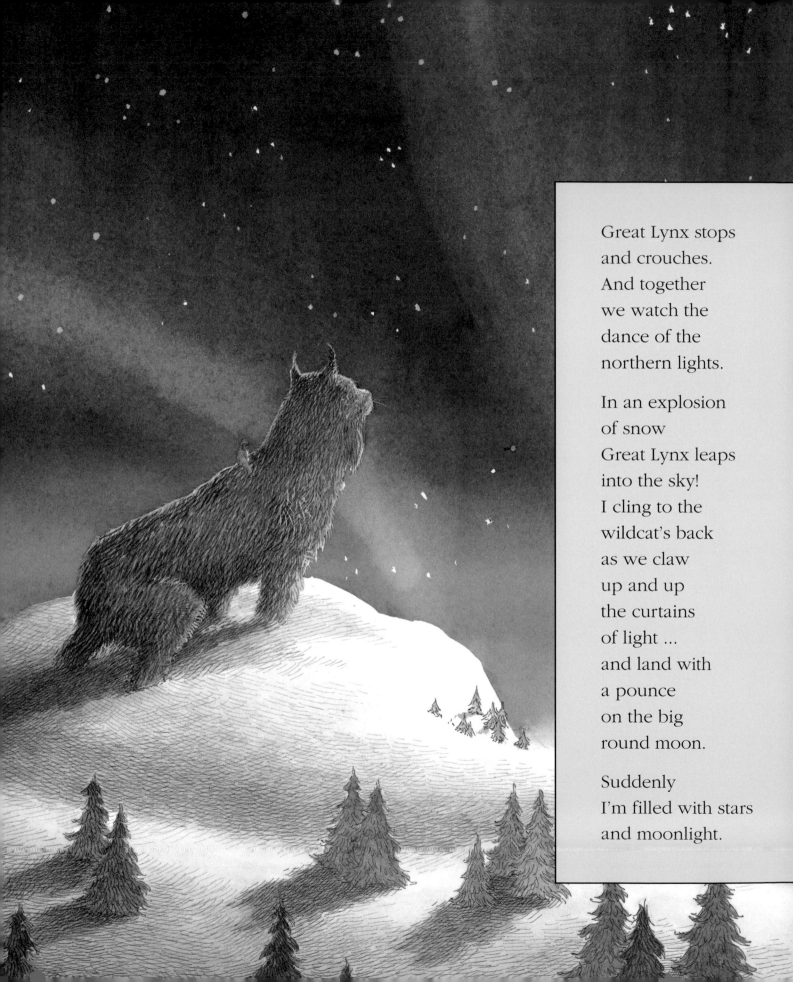

Great Lynx stops
and crouches.
And together
we watch the
dance of the
northern lights.

In an explosion
of snow
Great Lynx leaps
into the sky!
I cling to the
wildcat's back
as we claw
up and up
the curtains
of light ...
and land with
a pounce
on the big
round moon.

Suddenly
I'm filled with stars
and moonlight.

Great Lynx purrs
and if I could
I would purr too.

I yawn and
drowsily say,
"Lynx, let's go home!"

Down and down
we ripple
through the night,
down the curtains
of light ...
till we flop
like a pile of snow
before my cabin.

I climb off,
turn at the door.
Before my eyes
Great Lynx shrinks
down and down.

He crouches and
I feel his gaze
inside me

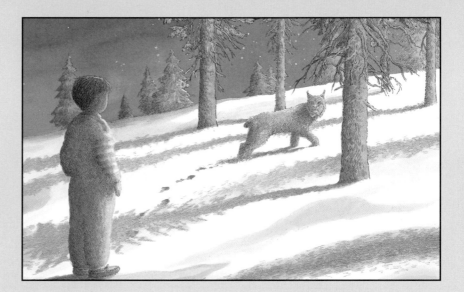

like fire
from
the northern lights.

He shakes a paw
and slowly
bounds away
through
the silent night.

The pot-belly's
still chugging.
My dad's
still snoring.

I curl up and
gaze at the fire.
As I close my eyes
and sink
into sleep,
I say ...

"Let the lynx
come in."

And the lynx
sleeps curled
in my dream
like the moon.

NOISY

Noisy noises!

Pan lids clashing,

Dog barking,

Plate smashing,

Telephone ringing,

Baby bawling,

Midnight cats

Cat-a-wauling,

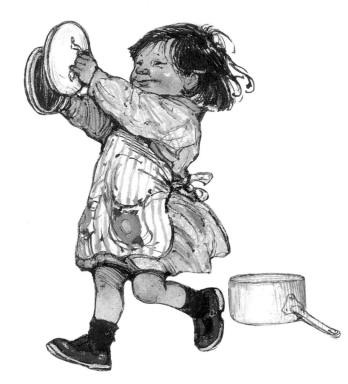

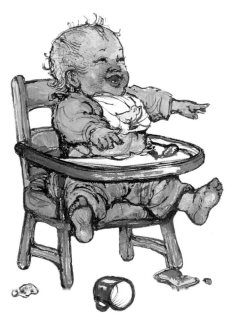

Door slamming,

Aeroplane zooming,

Vacuum cleaner

Vroom-vroom-vrooming,

And if I dance and sing a tune,

Baby joins in with a saucepan and spoon.

by Shirley Hughes

Gentle noises...
Dry leaves swishing,
Falling rain
Splashing, splishing,
Rustling trees
Hardly stirring,
Lazy cat
Softly purring.

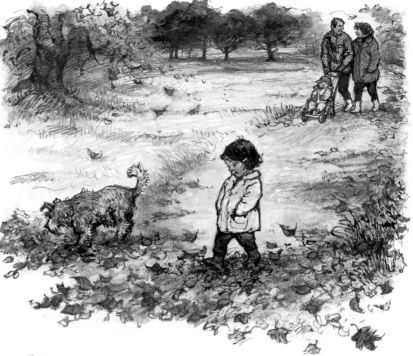

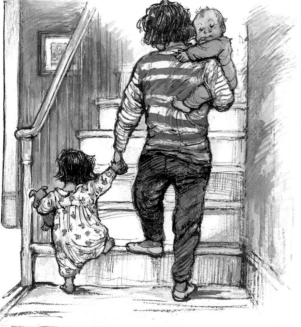

Story's over,
Bedtime's come,
Crooning baby
Sucks his thumb.
All quiet, not a peep,
Everyone is fast asleep.

"ONLY JOKING!"
LAUGHED THE LOBSTER
BY COLIN WEST

"Look out, Fish, there's a
shark following you!
... only joking!"
laughed the lobster.

"Look out, Eel,
there's a great big
shark following you!
... only joking!" laughed the lobster.

"Look out, Crab, there's a great
big ugly shark following you!
... only joking!" laughed the lobster.

"Look out, Turtle, there's a great big
ugly wild-looking shark following you!
... only joking!" laughed the lobster.

"Look out, Octopus, there's a
great big ugly wild-looking
mean old shark following you!
... only joking!" laughed the lobster.

"Look out, Shark, there's a
great big ugly wild looking
mean old hungry shark ..."

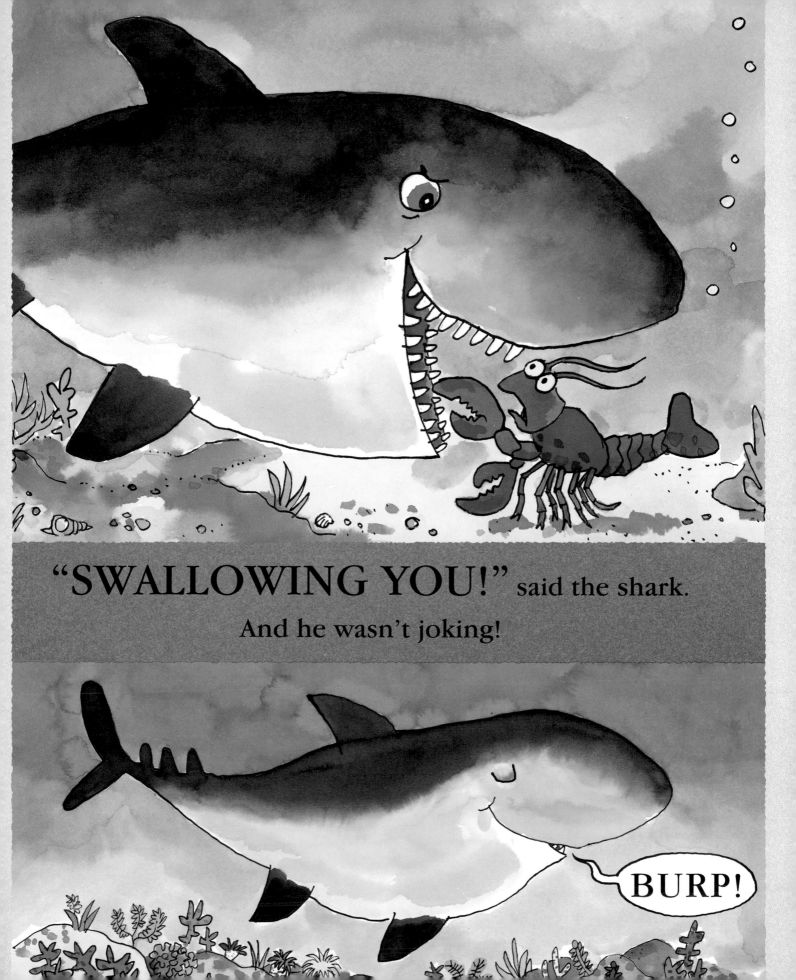

"SWALLOWING YOU!" said the shark.
And he wasn't joking!

BURP!

One Summer Day

BY KIM LEWIS

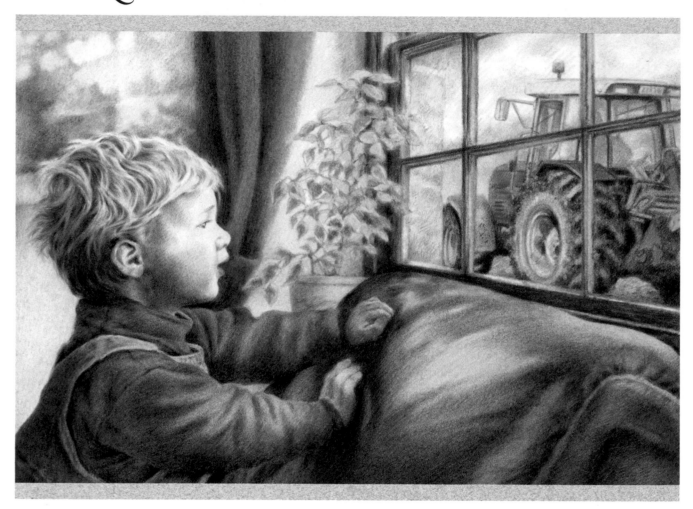

One day Max saw a huge red tractor with a plough roar by.

"Go out," said Max, racing to find his shoes and coat and hat. He hurried back to the window and looked out.

Two boys walked along with fishing-rods. Max's friend Sara cycled past in the sun. Max pressed his nose to the window, but the tractor was gone.

As Max looked out, suddenly Sara looked in.

"Peekaboo!" she said.

Then Max heard a knock at the door. "Can Max come out?"

"It's a summer day," laughed Sara, helping Max take off his coat. The sun was hot and the grass smelled sweet. Max and Sara walked down the farm road.

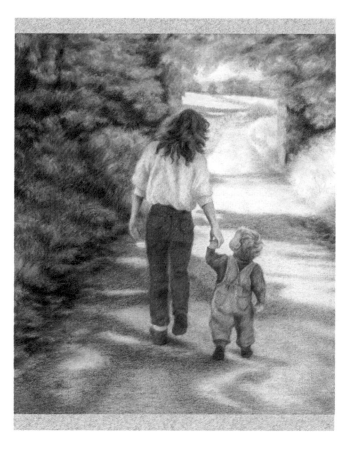

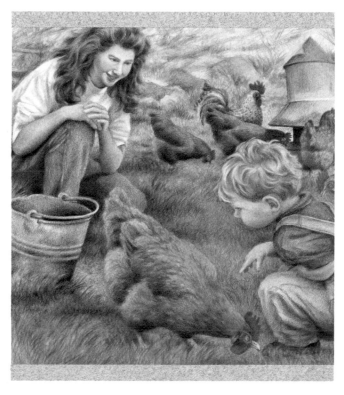

Max and Sara stopped to watch the hens feeding. One hen pecked at Max's foot.

"Shoo!" cried Max and sent the hens flapping.

Max and Sara ran through a field where the grass was very high. A cow with her calf mooed loudly. Max made a small "Moo!" back.

271

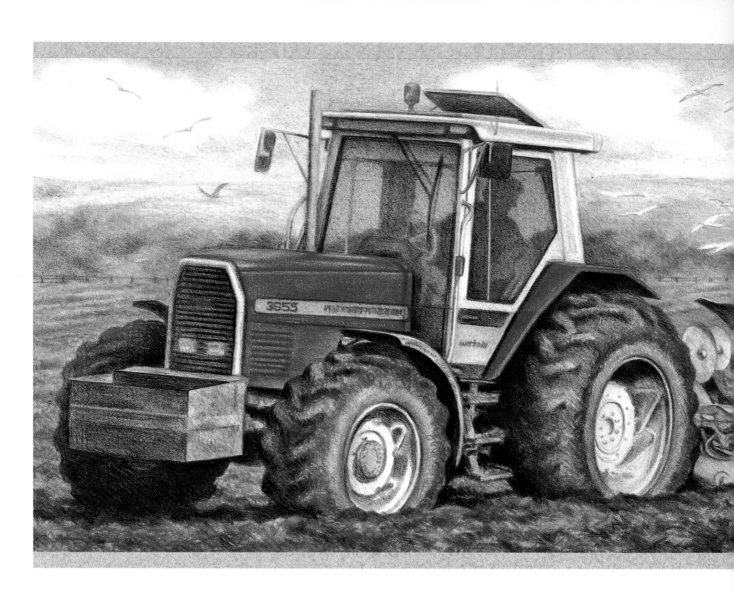

Max and Sara came to the river.

"Look, the boys are fishing." said Sara.

Sara caught Max and took off his shoes before he ran in to paddle.

Then Max and Sara reached a gate. Sara sat Max on top. They heard a roar in the field coming nearer and louder.

"Tractor!" shouted Sara and Max.

Max clung to the gate as the tractor loomed past. It pulled a huge plough which

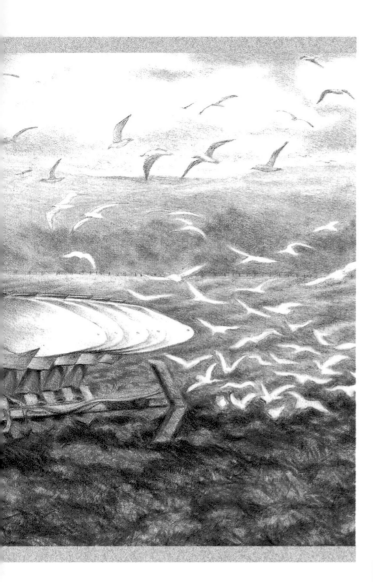

Sara carried Max back up the road.

"Tractor," sighed Max and closed his eyes.

Max woke up when they reached his house.

"Goodbye, Max," said Sara. "See you soon."

Max raced inside to the window. Sara looked in as Max looked out.

"Peepo!" said Max, and pressed his nose to the glass.

flashed in the sun. The field was full of gulls.

"Let's go home," said Sara to Max.

They walked beside the freshly ploughed field, along by the river and through the grass.

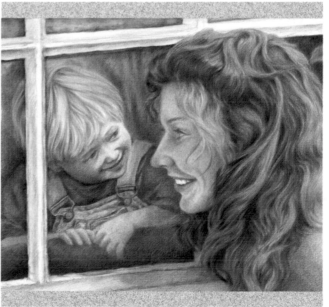

Danny's Duck

A duck flew over the land, looking for a
good woody place. Down she flew to a
pile of brushwood at the edge of a school
playground. No one saw her come.
        Except Danny.

    At playtime he looked for her.
    He had to look hard. Her colours
    were so like the colours of the
twigs and branches.
    But Danny saw her.
And she saw him.

by *June Crebbin* • *illustrated by Clara Vulliamy*

In school Danny drew the duck sitting.

"How lovely," said his teacher. "A duck on her nest."

When Danny visited the pile of brushwood again, the duck was still there, sitting very still. Again she saw him. Then she stood up and stretched.

Danny saw her eggs. He looked and counted.

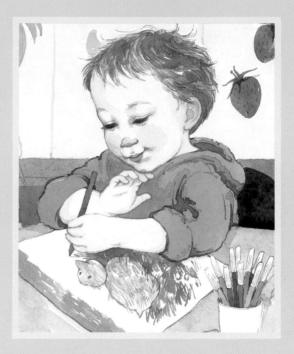

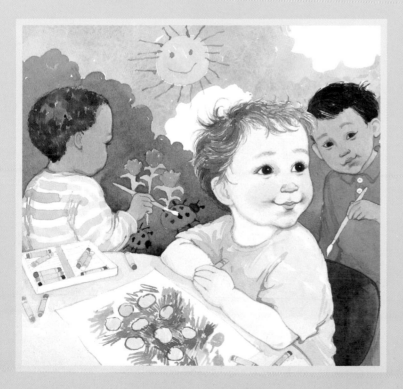

In school he drew a picture of the nest with nine pale green eggs in it.

"How lovely," said his teacher. "They'll have ducklings inside, growing."

Danny visited the duck every day. Children played in the playground. Parents passed close by on the footpath. But no one saw.

275

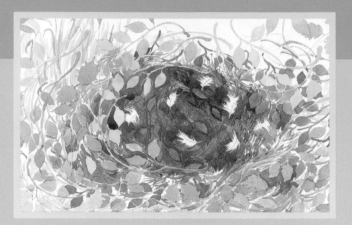

One sunny morning, just as he always did, Danny ran into the playground and over to the pile of brushwood.

But the duck wasn't there. Nor were her eggs. The nest was empty. Danny cried. He cried and cried.

In school he drew a picture of the empty nest. But when his teacher saw the picture – she smiled!

"The mother duck eats the egg-shells," she said, "after the eggs have hatched."

At lunch-time, Danny took his teacher across the playground to the pile of brushwood.
There was the nest.

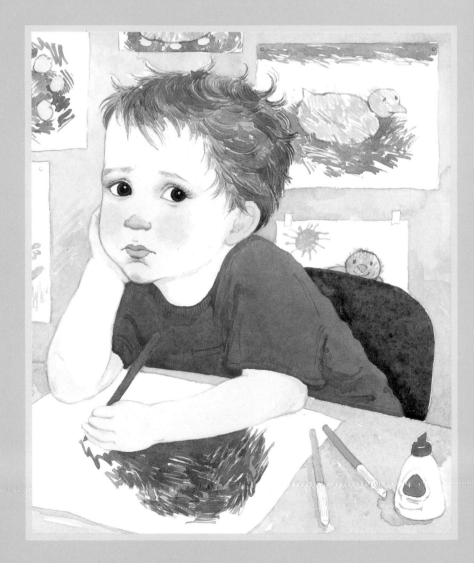

276

Then his teacher took Danny
across the school field, to the pond.
Danny looked.
"There's my duck!" he shouted.
"And – one, two, three, four, five,
six, seven, eight, *nine ducklings!*"
And everyone came to see.

Rosie's Babies

by **Martin Waddell**

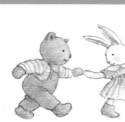

illustrated by **Penny Dale**

Mom was putting the baby to bed and Rosie said,
"I've got two babies and you've only got one."
"Two, including you," said Mom.
"I'm not a baby, I'm four years old," said Rosie.
"Tell me about your babies," Mom said.

And Rosie said,
"My babies live in a bird's nest and they are nearly as big as me. They go out in the garden all by themselves and sometimes they make me cross!"
"Do they?" said Mom.
"Yes, when they do silly things!" said Rosie.
"What silly things do they do?" asked Mom.

And Rosie said,
"My babies climbed a big mountain. That was silly, because they couldn't get down. They jumped, and they bumped on their bottoms!"
"Silly babies," said Mom. "Did they hurt themselves?"

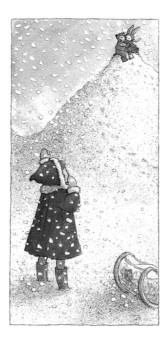

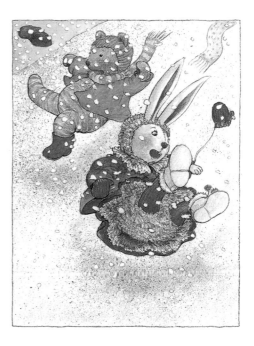

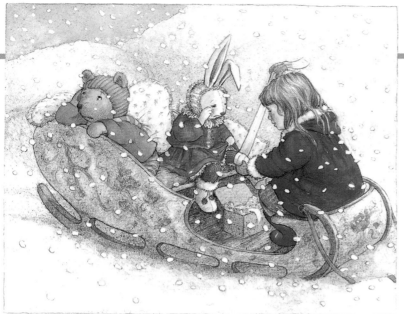

rockers and dinosaurs. They go to the park when it's dark and there are no moms and dads who can see, only me!"
"Gracious!" said Mom.
"Aren't they scared?"

And Rosie said,
"One of my babies hurt her knee. I bandaged it up and she cried and I said 'Never mind' because I am kind."
"I'm sure you are," said Mom.
"What else do your babies do?"

And Rosie said,
"My babies drive cars that are real ones and lorries and dumpers and boats. My babies are very good drivers."
"What do your babies like doing best?" asked Mom.

And Rosie said,
"My babies like swings and

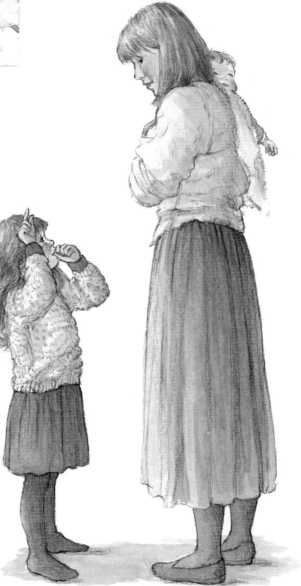

279

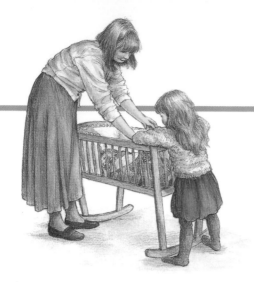

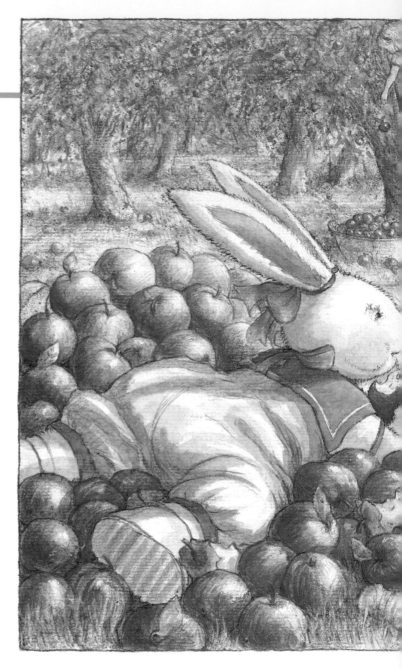

And Rosie said,
"My babies are scared of the
big dog, but I'm not.
I know the big dog. I go
'Blackie, sit,' and he does."
"They are not very scared
then?" said Mom.
"My babies know I will
look after them," said Rosie.
"I'm their mom."
"How do you look after
them?" Mom asked.

And Rosie said,
"I make their teas and I tell
them stories and I take them for
walks and I talk to them and I tell
them that I love them."
"That's a good way to look after
babies!" said Mom. "Do you
make them nice things to eat,
like pies?"

And Rosie said,
"My babies make their own
pies, but they never eat them."
"What do they eat?" asked Mom.

And Rosie said,
"My babies eat apples and

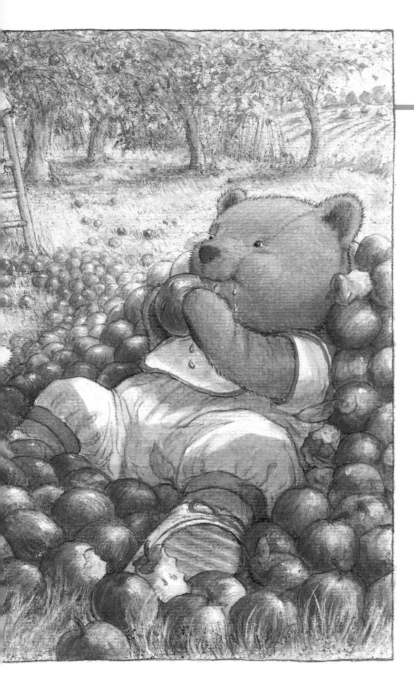

And Rosie thought and thought and thought and then Rosie said,
"My babies have gone to bed."
"Just like this one," said Mom.
"I don't want to talk about my babies any more because they are asleep," said Rosie. "I don't want them to wake up, or they'll cry."
"We could talk very softly," said Mom.
"Yes," said Rosie.
"What will we talk about?" asked Mom.

And Rosie said
"ME!"

apples and apples all the time. And grapes and pears but they don't like the pips."
"Most babies don't," said Mom.
"Are you going to tell me more about your babies?"

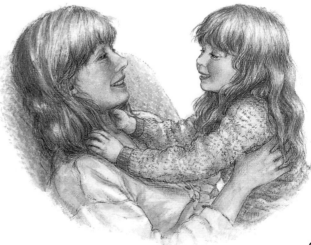

281

Can't You Sleep, Little Bear?

by Martin Waddell ● *illustrated by Barbara Firth*

Once there were two bears. Big Bear and Little Bear. Big Bear is the big bear, and Little Bear is the little bear.

They played all day in the bright sunlight. When night came, and the sun went down, Big Bear took Little Bear home to the Bear Cave.

Big Bear put Little Bear to bed in the dark part of the cave.

"Go to sleep, Little Bear," he said.

And Little Bear tried.

Big Bear settled in the Bear Chair and read his Bear Book, by the light of the fire. But Little Bear couldn't get to sleep.

"Can't you sleep, Little Bear?" asked Big Bear, putting down his Bear Book (which was just getting to the interesting part) and padding over to the bed.

"I'm scared," said Little Bear.

"Why are you scared, Little Bear?" asked Big Bear.

"I don't like the dark," said Little Bear.

"What dark?" said Big Bear.

"The dark all around us," said Little Bear.

Big Bear looked, and he saw that the dark part of the cave was very dark, so he went to the Lantern Cupboard and took out the tiniest lantern that was there. Big Bear lit the tiniest lantern, and put it near to Little Bear's bed.

"There's a tiny light to stop you being scared, Little Bear," said Big Bear.

"Thank you, Big Bear," said Little Bear, cuddling up in the glow.

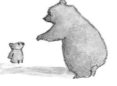

"Now go to sleep, Little Bear," said Big Bear, and he padded back to the Bear Chair and settled down to read the Bear Book, by the light of the fire.

Little Bear tried to go to sleep, but he couldn't.

"Can't you sleep, Little Bear?" yawned Big Bear, putting down his Bear Book (with just four pages to go to the interesting bit) and padding over to the bed.

"I'm scared," said Little Bear.

"Why are you scared, Little Bear?" asked Big Bear.

"I don't like the dark," said Little Bear.

"What dark?" asked Big Bear.

"The dark all around us," said Little Bear.

"But I brought you a lantern!" said Big Bear.

"Only a tiny-weeny one," said Little Bear. "And there's lots of dark!"

Big Bear looked, and he saw that Little Bear was quite right, there was still lots of dark. So Big Bear went to the Lantern Cupboard and took out a bigger lantern. Big Bear lit the lantern, and put it beside the other one.

"Now go to sleep, Little Bear," said Big Bear and he padded back to the Bear Chair and settled down to read the Bear Book, by the light of the fire.

Little Bear tried and tried to go to sleep, but he couldn't.

"Can't you sleep, Little Bear?" grunted Big Bear, putting down his Bear Book (with just three pages to go) and padding over to the bed.

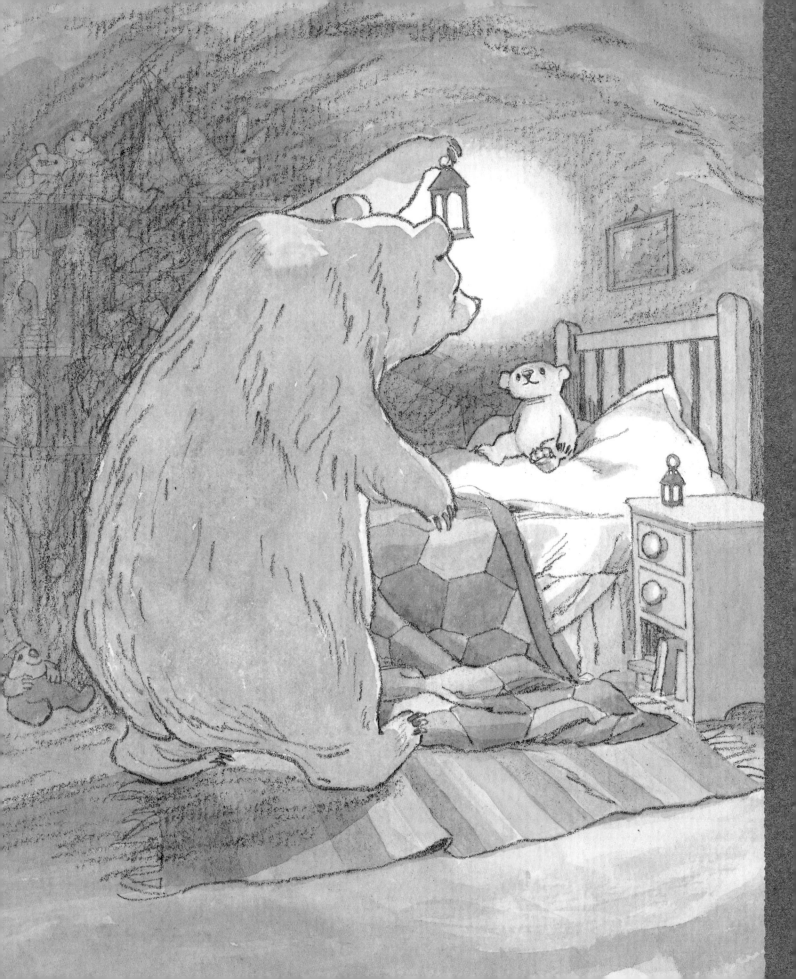

"I'm scared," said Little Bear.

"Why are you scared, Little Bear?" asked Big Bear.

"I don't like the dark," said Little Bear.

"What dark?" asked Big Bear.

"The dark all around us," said Little Bear.

"But I brought you two lanterns!" said Big Bear. "A tiny one and a bigger one!"

"Not much bigger," said Little Bear. "And there's still lots of dark."

Big Bear thought about it, and then he went to the Lantern Cupboard and took out the Biggest Lantern of Them All, with two handles and a bit of chain. He hooked the lantern up above Little Bear's bed.

"I've brought you the Biggest Lantern of Them All!" he told Little Bear. "That's to stop you being scared!"

"Thank you, Big Bear," said Little Bear, curling up in the glow and watching the shadows dance.

"Now go to sleep, Little Bear," said Big Bear and he padded back to the Bear Chair and settled down to read the Bear Book, by the light of the fire.

Little Bear tried and tried and tried to go to sleep, but he couldn't.

"Can't you sleep, Little Bear?" groaned Big Bear, putting down his Bear Book (with just two pages to go) and padding over to the bed.

"I'm scared," said Little Bear.

"Why are you scared, Little Bear?" asked Big Bear.

"I don't like the dark," said Little Bear.

"What dark?" asked Big Bear.

"The dark all around us," said Little Bear.

"But I brought you the Biggest Lantern of Them All, and there isn't any dark left," said Big Bear.

"Yes, there is!" said Little Bear. "There is, out there!" And he pointed out of the Bear Cave, at the night.

Big Bear saw that Little Bear was right. Big Bear was very puzzled. All the lanterns in the world couldn't light up the dark outside.

Big Bear thought about it for a long time, and then he said, "Come on, Little Bear."

"Where are we going?" asked Little Bear.

"Out!" said Big Bear.

"Out into the darkness?" said Little Bear.

"Yes!" said Big Bear.

"But I'm scared of the dark!" said Little Bear.

"No need to be!" said Big Bear, and he took Little Bear by the paw and led him out from the cave into the night and it was … DARK!

"Ooooh! I'm scared," said Little Bear, cuddling up to Big Bear. Big Bear lifted Little Bear, and cuddled him, and said, "Look at the dark, Little Bear." And Little Bear looked.

"I've brought you the moon, Little Bear," said Big Bear. "The bright yellow moon, and all the twinkly stars."

But Little Bear didn't say anything, for he had gone to sleep, warm and safe in Big Bear's arms.

Big Bear carried Little Bear back into the Bear Cave, fast asleep and he settled down with Little Bear on one arm and the Bear Book on the other, cosy in the Bear Chair by the fire.

And Big Bear read the Bear Book right to …

THE END

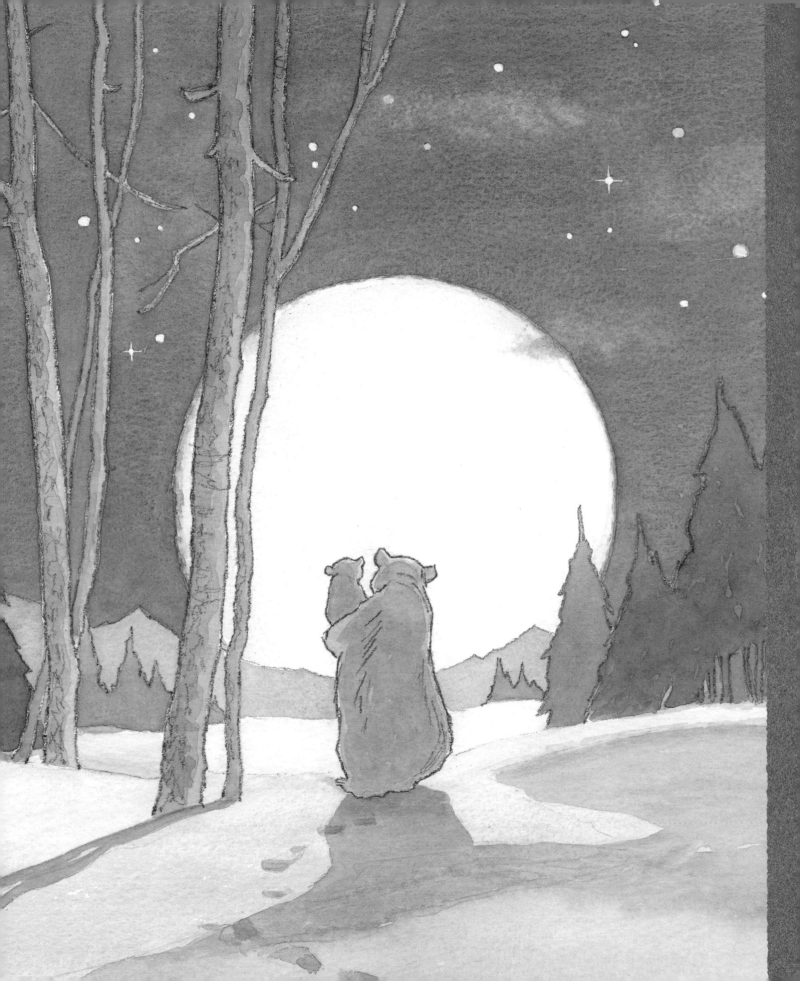

Index

Acknowledgments

Baby Bird Text copyright © 1998 Joyce Dunbar; Illustrations copyright © 1998 Russell Ayto · *Baby Duck and the New Eyeglasses* Text copyright © 1996 Amy Hest; Illustrations copyright © 1996 Jill Barton · *Bathwater's Hot* Copyright © 1985 Shirley Hughes · *Beaky* Copyright © 1990 Jez Alborough · *Bears in the Forest* Text copyright © 1994 Karen Wallace; Illustrations copyright © 1994 Barbara Firth · *The Big Big Sea* Text copyright © 1994 Martin Waddell; Illustrations copyright © 1994 Jennifer Eachus · *Calamity* Copyright © 1993 Camilla Ashforth · *Can't You Sleep, Little Bear?* Text copyright © 1988 Martin Waddell; Illustrations copyright © 1988 Barbara Firth · *Chi-li the Panda* Text copyright © 1984 and 1988 Derek Hall; Illustrations copyright © 1984 John Butler · *Contrary Mary* Copyright © 1995 Anita Jeram · *Cowboy Baby* Copyright © 1998 Sue Heap · *Cuddly Dudley* Copyright © 1993 Jez Alborough · *Daisy Dare* Copyright © 1995 Anita Jeram · *Daley B* Text copyright © 1992 Jon Blake; Illustrations copyright © 1992 Axel Scheffler · *Danny's Duck* Text copyright © 1995 June Crebbin; Illustrations copyright © 1995 Clara Vulliamy · *Duck* Text copyright © 1984 and 1988 David Lloyd; Illustrations copyright © 1984 and 1988 Charlotte Voake · *Dudley and the Strawberry Shake* Text copyright © 1986 Judy Taylor; Illustrations copyright © 1986 Peter Cross · *The Elephant Tree* Copyright © 1991 Penny Dale · *Farmer Duck* Text copyright © 1991 Martin Waddell; Illustrations copyright © 1991 Helen Oxenbury · *The Fat King* Copyright © 1990 Graham Jeffrey · *The Fibbs* Copyright © 1987 Chris Riddell · *Floss* Copyright © 1992 Kim Lewis · *Fly by Night* Text copyright © 1993 June Crebbin; Illustrations copyright © 1993 Stephen Lambert · *A Friend for Little Bear* Copyright © 1996 Harry Horse · *Friends* Copyright © 1997 Kim Lewis · *Ginger* Copyright © 1997 Charlotte Voake · *Giving* Copyright © 1993 Shirley Hughes · *Grandad's Magic* Copyright © 1989 Blackbird Design Pty. Ltd. · *Handa's Surprise* Text copyright © 1994 Eileen Browne · *The Happy Hedgehog Band* Text copyright © 1991 Martin Waddell; Illustrations copyright © 1991 Jill Barton · *Horatio's Bed* Copyright © 1992 Camilla Ashforth · *In the Middle of the Night* Text copyright © 1992 Kathy Henderson; Illustrations copyright © 1992 Jennifer Eachus · *In the Rain with Baby Duck* Text copyright © 1995 Amy Hest; Illustrations copyright © 1995 Jill Barton · *John Joe and the Big Hen* Text copyright © 1995 Martin Waddell; Illustrations copyright © 1995 Paul Howard · *The Last Noo-noo* Copyright © 1995 Jill Murphy · *Let the Lynx Come In* Text copyright © 1996 Jonathan London; Illustrations copyright © 1996 Patrick Benson · *Let's Go Home, Little Bear* Text copyright © 1991 Martin Waddell; Illustrations copyright © 1991 Barbara Firth · *The Little Boat* Text copyright © 1995 Kathy Henderson; Illustrations copyright © 1995 Patrick Benson · 'A Little Boy Came Down to Breakfast' from *Hard-Boiled Legs: The Breakfast Book* Text copyright © 1987 Michael Rosen; Illustrations copyright © 1987 Quentin Blake · *Little Pig's Tale* Text copyright © 1990 Nigel Gray; Illustrations copyright © 1990 Mary Rees · *Mimi and the Blackberry Pie* Text copyright © 1996 Martin Waddell; Illustrations copyright © 1996 Leo Hartas · *Monkey Tricks* Copyright © 1992 Camilla Ashforth · *The Most Obedient Dog in the World* Copyright © 1993 Anita Jeram · *Mouse Party* Text copyright © 1995 Alan Durant; Illustrations copyright © 1995 Sue Heap · *Mrs. Goose's Baby* Copyright © 1989 Charlotte Voake · *My Friend Harry* Copyright © 1995 Kim Lewis · *My Mom and Dad Make Me Laugh* Copyright © 1994 Nick Sharratt · *My Old Teddy* Copyright © 1991 Dom Mansell · 'Nasty Kids, Nice Kids' from *Kids* Copyright © 1992 Catherine and Laurence Anholt · *Noah's Ark* Copyright © 1993 Lucy Cousins · *Noisy* Copyright © 1985 Shirley Hughes · *Nonsense Rhymes* Copyright © 1985 and 1987 Nicola Bayley · 'Not me,' said the Monkey Copyright © 1987 Colin West · *Oh, Little Jack* Copyright © 1992 Inga Moore · *Oh, Tucker!* Text copyright © 1998 Steven Kroll; Illustrations copyright © 1998 Scott Nash · *One Summer Day* Copyright © 1996 Kim Lewis · 'Only Joking!' Laughed the Lobster Copyright © 1995 Colin West · *Over the Moon* Copyright © 1985 Charlotte Voake · *Owl Babies* Text copyright © 1992 Martin Waddell; Illustrations copyright © 1992 Patrick Benson · *The Owl and the Pussy Cat* Illustrations copyright © 1991 Louise Voce · *The Park in the Dark* Text copyright © 1989 Martin Waddell; Illustrations copyright © 1989 Barbara Firth · *Parrot Cat* Copyright © 1984 Nicola Bayley · *A Piece of Cake* Copyright © 1989 Jill Murphy · 'Pog Had' from *Pog* Copyright © 1989 Peter Haswell · *Prowlpuss* Text copyright © 1994 Gina Wilson; Illustrations copyright © 1994 David Parkins · *Quacky Quackquack!* Text copyright © 1991 Ian Whybrow; Illustrations copyright © 1991 Russell Ayto · *The Red Woolen Blanket* Copyright © 1987 Blackbird Design Pty. Ltd. · *Robert the Great* Copyright © 1985 Philippe Dupasquier · *Rosie's Babies* Text copyright © 1990 Martin Waddell; Illustrations copyright © 1990 Penny Dale · *Sally and the Limpet* Copyright © 1991 Simon James · *Sebastian's Trumpet* Copyright © 1995 Miko Imai · *Something's Coming!* Text copyright © 1995 Richard Edwards; Illustrations copyright © 1995 Dana Kubick · *Squeak-a-lot* Text copyright © 1991 Martin Waddell; Illustrations copyright © 1991 Virginia Miller · *The Teeny Tiny Woman* Copyright © 1998 Arthur Robins · *Tell Us a Story* Text copyright © 1986 Allan Ahlberg; Illustrations copyright © 1986 Colin McNaughton · *Ten in the Bed* Copyright © 1988 Penny Dale · *Terrible, Terrible Tiger* Copyright © 1987 Colin and Jacqui Hawkins · 'That's the Way to Do It!' from *Who's Been Sleeping in My Porridge?* Copyright © 1990 Colin McNaughton · *This Is the Bear* Text copyright © 1986 Sarah Hayes; Illustrations copyright © 1986 Helen Craig · *This Is the Bear and the Bad Little Girl* Text copyright © 1995 Sarah Hayes; Illustrations copyright © 1995 Helen Craig · 'The Three Billy Goats Gruff' from *The Three Little Pigs and Other Favourite Nursery Stories* Copyright © 1992 Charlotte Voake · *Turnover Tuesday* Text copyright © 1998 Phyllis Root; Illustrations copyright © 1998 Helen Craig · *Two Shoes, New Shoes* Copyright © 1986 Shirley Hughes · *Under the Bed* Text copyright © 1986 Michael Rosen; Illustrations copyright © 1986 Quentin Blake · *Watch Out! Big Bro's Coming!* Copyright © 1997 Jez Alborough · *We Love Them* Text copyright © 1990 Martin Waddell; Illustrations copyright © 1990 Barbara Firth · *We're the Noisy Dinosaurs!* Copyright © 1992 John Watson · *What Newt Could Do for Turtle* Text copyright © 1996 Jonathan London; Illustrations copyright © 1996 Louise Voce · *Where's My Mom?* Text copyright © 1994 Leon Rosselson; Illustrations copyright © 1994 Priscilla Lamont · *Who's Been Sleeping in My Porridge?* Copyright © 1990 Colin McNaughton · *You and Me, Little Bear* Text copyright © 1996 Martin Waddell; Illustrations copyright © 1996 Barbara Firth · *A Zoo in Our House* Text copyright © 1988 Heather Eyles; Illustrations copyright © 1988 Andy Cooke

The stories and poems in this collection were previously published individually by Candlewick Press or its sister company, Walker Books Ltd., London.

Candlewick Press
2067 Massachusetts Avenue
Cambridge, MA 02140

visit us at www.candlewick.com